The latest **evolution** in learning

Evolve provides online access to free learning resources and activities designed specifically for the textbook you are using in your class. The resources will provide you with information that enhances the material covered in the book and much more.

Visit the Web address listed below to start your learning evolution today!

LOGIN: http://evolve.elsevier.com/Waugh/anatomy

Ross and Wilson Anatomy and Physiology in Health and Illness, 9th Edition

Evolve Learning Resources for Students:

■ **WebLinks**

An exciting resource that lets you link to websites carefully chosen to supplement the content of the textbook.

Ross and Wilson Anatomy and Physiology in Health and Illness, 9th Edition

Evolve Learning Resources for Lecturers:

■ **Image bank**

The complete collection of images from the book in JPEG and PDF format as well as PowerPoint slides.

Think outside the book...**evolve.**

Ninth Edition

Ross and Wilson

Anatomy
and
Physiology
in Health and Illness

For Churchill Livingstone:

Senior Commissioning Editor: Sarena Wolfaard
Designer: Sarah Russell
Project Development Editor: Mairi McCubbin
Page Layout: Alan Palfreyman

Ninth Edition

Ross and Wilson

Anatomy
and
Physiology
in Health and Illness

Anne Waugh BSc(Hons) MSc CertEd SRN RNT ILTM
Senior Lecturer, School of Acute and Continuing Care Nursing,
Napier University, Edinburgh, UK

Allison Grant BSc PhD RGN
Lecturer, School of Biological and Biomedical Sciences,
Glasgow Caledonian University, Glasgow, UK

Illustrations by Graeme Chambers

ELSEVIER
CHURCHILL
LIVINGSTONE

EDINBURGH LONDON NEW YORK OXFORD PHILADELPHIA ST LOUIS SYDNEY TORONTO 2001

CHURCHILL LIVINGSTONE
An imprint of Elsevier Limited

First edition 1963
Second edition 1966
Third edition 1968
Fourth edition 1973
Fifth edition 1981
Sixth edition 1987
Seventh edition 1990
Eighth edition 1996
Ninth edition 2001
Reprinted 2001, 2002, 2003, 2004, 2005

International Student Edition
First published 1991
Eighth edition 1996
Ninth edition 2001
Reprinted 2001, 2002, 2003 (twice), 2004, 2005

ISBN 0 443 06469 5

ISBN 0 443 06468 7

British Library Cataloguing in Publication Data
A catalogue record for this book is available from the British Library

Library of Congress Cataloging in Publication Data
A catalog record for this book is available from the Library of Congress

Note
Medical knowledge is constantly changing. As new information becomes available, changes in treatment, procedures, equipment and the use of drugs become necessary. The authors and the publishers have taken care to ensure that the information given in this text is accurate and up to date. However, readers are strongly advised to confirm that the information, especially with regard to drug usage, complies with the latest legislation and standards of practice.

ELSEVIER your source for books,
journals and multimedia
in the health sciences
www.elsevierhealth.com

Working together to grow
libraries in developing countries
www.elsevier.com | www.bookaid.org | www.sabre.org

ELSEVIER   BOOK AID International   Sabre Foundation

The publisher's policy is to use **paper manufactured from sustainable forests**

Printed in China

Contents

Preface

Ross and Wilson has been a core text for students of anatomy and physiology for almost 40 years. This latest edition is aimed at health care professionals including nurses, nursing students, students of the professions allied to medicine, paramedics, ambulance technicians and complementary therapists. It retains the straightforward approach to the description of body systems and how they work, and the normal anatomy and physiology is followed by a section that covers common disorders and diseases: the pathology.

The human body is described system by system. The reader must, however, remember that physiology is an integrated subject and that, although the systems are considered in separate chapters, they must all function together for the human body to operate as a healthy unit. The first three chapters provide an overview of the body and describe its main constituents. A new section on introductory biochemistry is included, forming the basis of a deeper understanding of body function.

The later chapters are gathered together into three further sections, reflecting three areas essential for normal body function: communication; intake of raw materials and elimination of waste; and protection and survival. Much of the material for this edition has been extensively revised and rewritten. There is a new chapter on immunology, reflecting the growing importance of this subject in physiology.

The artwork has been completely redrawn using full colour, and many new diagrams have been included.

A new list of common prefixes, suffixes and roots has been prepared for this edition, giving meanings and providing examples of common terminology used in the study of anatomy and physiology. Some biological values have been extracted from the text and presented as an Appendix for easy reference. In some cases, slightly different 'normals' may be found in other texts and used by different medical practitioners.

Edinburgh 2001

Anne Waugh
Allison Grant

Acknowledgements

The ninth edition of this textbook would not have been possible without the efforts of many people. In preparing this edition, we have built on the foundations established by Kathleen Wilson and we would like to acknowledge her immense contribution to the success of this title.

We are grateful to Graeme Chambers for the preparation of the new artwork for the ninth edition.

We are grateful to readers of the eighth edition for their constructive comments, many of which have influenced the content of the ninth.

We are also grateful to the staff of Churchill Livingstone, particularly Mairi McCubbin and Kirsty Guest, for their support and hospitality.

Thanks are also due to our families, Andy, Michael, Seona and Struan, for their patience and acceptance of lost evenings and weekends.

Common prefixes, suffixes and roots

The terminology used in the book is easier to learn and use when it is understood. To facilitate this, the common parts of such terms: prefixes (beginnings), roots (middle parts) and suffixes (endings), are listed here, in alphabetical order. Meanings are also given, along with some examples of their uses.

Prefix/suffix/root	To do with	Examples in the text
a-/an-	lack of	anuria, agranulocyte, asystole, anaemia
-aemia	of the blood	anaemia, hypoxaemia, uraemia, hypovolaemia
angio-	vessel	angiotensin, haemangioma
anti-	against	antidiuretic, anticoagulant, antigen, antimicrobial
-blast	germ, bud	reticuloblast, osteoblast
brady-	slow	bradycardia
broncho-	bronchus	bronchiole, bronchitis, bronchus
card-	heart	cardiac, myocardium, tachycardia
chole-	bile	cholecystokinin, cholecystitis, cholangitis
cyto-/-cyte	cell	erythrocyte, cytosol, cytoplasm, cytotoxic
derm-	skin	dermatitis, dermatome, dermis
dys-	difficult	dysuria, dyspnoea, dysmenorrhoea, dysplasia
-ema	swelling	oedema, emphysema, lymphoedema
endo-	inner	endocrine, endocytosis, endothelium
erythro-	red	erythrocyte, erythropoietin, erythropoiesis
exo-	outside	exocytosis, exophthalmos
extra-	outside	extracellular, extrapyramidal
-fferent	carry	afferent, efferent
gast-	stomach	gastric, gastrin, gastritis, gastrointestinal
-gen-	origin/production	gene, genome, genetic, antigen, pathogen, allergen
-globin	protein	myoglobin, haemoglobin
haem-	blood	haemostasis, haemorrhage, haemolytic
-hydr-	water	dehydration, hydrostatic, hydrocephalus
hepat-	liver	hepatic, hepatitis, hepatomegaly, hepatocyte
hyper-	excess/above	hypertension, hypertrophy, hypercapnia
hypo-	below/under	hypoglycaemia, hypotension, hypovolaemia
intra-	within	intracellular, intracranial, intraocular
-ism	condition	hyperthyroidism, dwarfism, rheumatism
-itis	inflammation	appendicitis, hepatitis, cystitis, gastritis
lact-	milk	lactation, lactic, lacteal
lymph-	lymph tissue	lymphocyte, lymphatic, lymphoedema
lyso-/-lysis	breaking down	lysosome, glycolysis, lysozyme
-mega-	large	megaloblast, acromegaly, splenomegaly, hepatomegaly
micro-	small	microbe, microtubules, microvilli
myo-	muscle	myocardium, myoglobin, myopathy, myosin
neo-	new	neoplasm, gluconeogenesis, neonate
nephro-	kidney	nephron, nephrotic, nephroblastoma, nephrosis
neuro-	nerve	neurone, neuralgia, neuropathy
-oid	resembling	myeloid, sesamoid, sigmoid
-oma	tumour	carcinoma, melanoma, fibroma
-ophth-	eye	xerophthalmia, ophthalmic, exophthalmos
-ory	referring to	secretory, sensory, auditory, gustatory
osteo-	bone	osteocyte, osteoarthritis, osteoporosis
-path-	disease	pathogenesis, neuropathy, nephropathy
-plasm	substance	cytoplasm, neoplasm
pneumo-	lung/air	pneumothorax, pneumonia, pneumotoxic
poly-	many	polypeptide, polyuria, polycythaemia
-rrhagia	excessive flow	menorrhagia
-rrhoea	discharge	dysmenorrhoea, diarrhoea, rhinorrhoea
sub-	under	subphrenic, subarachnoid, sublingual
tachy-	excessively fast	tachycardia
thrombo-	clot	thrombocyte, thrombosis, thrombin, thrombus
-tox-	poison	toxin, cytotoxic, hepatotoxic
-uria	urine	anuria, polyuria, haematuria, nocturia
vas, vaso-	vessel	vasoconstriction, vas deferens, vascular

The body and its constituents

1

1
Introduction to the human body

The human body is complex, like a highly technical and sophisticated machine. It operates as a single entity, but is made up of a number of operational parts that work interdependently. Each part is associated with a specific, and sometimes related, function that is essential for the well-being of the individual. The component parts do not operate independently, but rather in conjunction with all the others. Should one part fail, the consequences are likely to extend to other parts, and may reduce the ability of the body to function normally. Integrated working of the body parts ensures the ability of the individual to survive. The human body is therefore complex in both its structure and function, and the aim of this book is to explain the fundamental structures and processes involved.

Anatomy is the study of the structure of the body and the physical relationships involved between body parts. *Physiology* is the study of how the parts of the body work, and the ways in which they cooperate together to maintain life and health of the individual. *Pathology* is the study of abnormalities and how they affect body functions, often causing illness. Building on the normal anatomy and physiology, relevant illnesses are considered at the end of the later chapters.

LEVELS OF STRUCTURAL COMPLEXITY

Learning outcome

After studying this section you should be able to:

■ state the levels of structural complexity within the body.

Within the body there are different levels of structural organisation and complexity (Fig. 1.1). The lowest level is chemical. *Atoms* combine to form *molecules*, of which there is a vast range in the body. The structures, properties and functions of important biological molecules are considered in Chapter 2. *Cells* are the smallest independent units of living matter and there are millions in the body. They are too small to be seen with the naked eye, but when magnified using a microscope different types can be distinguished by their size, shape and the dyes they absorb when stained in the laboratory. Each cell type has become *specialised*, and carries out a particular function that contributes to body needs. In complex organisms such as the human body, cells with similar structures and functions are found together, forming *tissues*. The structure and functions of cells and tissues are explored in Chapter 3.

Organs are made up of a number of different types of tissue and carry out a specific function. *Systems* consist of a number of organs and tissues that together contribute to one or more survival needs of the body. The human body has several systems, which work interdependently carrying out specific functions. All are required for health. The body systems are considered in later chapters.

THE INTERNAL ENVIRONMENT AND HOMEOSTASIS

Learning outcomes

After studying this section you should be able to:

■ define the terms internal environment and homeostasis

■ compare and contrast negative and positive feedback control mechanisms

■ outline the potential consequences of homeostatic imbalance.

The *external environment* surrounds the body and provides the oxygen and nutrients required by all the cells of the body. Waste products of cellular activity are eventually excreted into the external environment. The skin provides a barrier between the dry external environment and the watery environment of most body cells.

The *internal environment* is the water-based medium in which body cells exist. Cells are bathed in fluid called *interstitial* or *tissue fluid*. Oxygen and other substances they require must pass from the internal transport systems through the interstitial fluid to reach them. Similarly, cell waste products must move through the interstitial fluid to the transport systems to be excreted.

Cells are surrounded by the *cell membrane*, which provides a potential barrier to substances entering or leaving. The structure of membranes (p. 30) confers certain properties, in particular *selective permeability* or *semipermeability*. This prevents large molecules moving between the cell and the interstitial fluid (Fig. 1.2). Smaller particles can usually pass through the membrane, some more readily than others, and therefore the chemical composition of the fluid inside is different from that outside the cell.

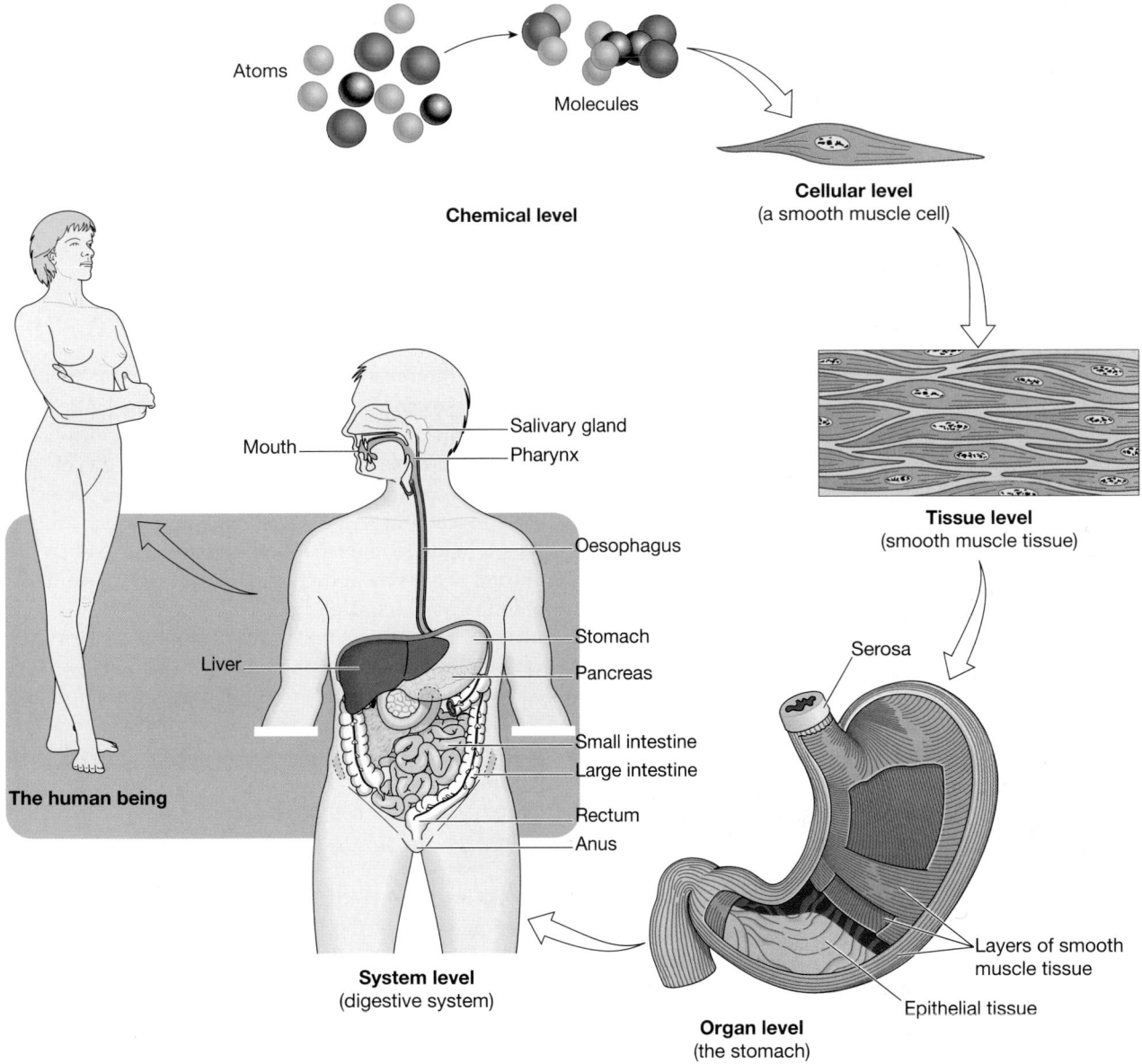

Figure 1.1 The levels of structural complexity.

Homeostasis

The composition of the internal environment is maintained within narrow limits, and this fairly constant state is called *homeostasis*. Literally, this term means 'unchanging', but in practice it describes a dynamic, ever-changing situation kept within narrow limits. When this balance is threatened or lost, there is a serious risk to the well-being of the individual. There are many factors in the internal environment which must be maintained within narrow limits and some of these are listed in Box 1.1.

Homeostasis is maintained by control systems which detect and respond to changes in the internal environment. A control system (Fig. 1.3) has three basic components: detector, control centre and effector. The *control centre* determines the limits within which the variable factor should be maintained. It receives an input from the *detector* or *sensor*, and integrates the incoming information. When the incoming signal indicates that an adjustment is needed the *control centre* responds and its output to the *effector* is changed. This is a dynamic process that maintains homeostasis.

Small particles able to pass through pores in the cell membrane

Large particles outside – cannot pass into the cell

Large particles inside – cannot pass out of the cell

Large particles inside and outside – cannot pass through cell membrane

Figure 1.2 Diagram of a cell with a semipermeable membrane.

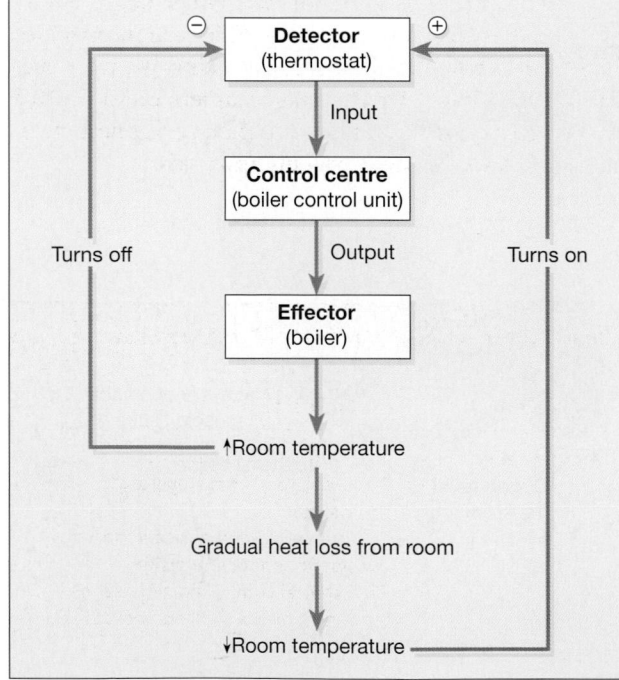

Figure 1.3 Example of a negative feedback mechanism: control of room temperature by a domestic boiler.

Negative feedback mechanisms

In systems controlled by negative feedback the effector response decreases or negates the effect of the original stimulus, restoring homeostasis (thus the term negative feedback). Control of body temperature is similar to the non-physiological example of a domestic central heating

system. The thermostat (temperature detector) is sensitive to changes in room temperature (variable factor). The thermostat is connected to the boiler control unit (control centre), which controls the boiler (effector). The thermostat constantly compares the information from the detector with the preset temperature and, when necessary, adjustments are made to alter the room temperature. When the thermostat detects the room temperature is low it sends an input to the boiler control unit, switching it on. The result is output of heat by the boiler, warming the room. When the preset temperature is reached, the system is reversed. The thermostat detects the higher room temperature and sends an input to the boiler control unit, turning it off. The output of heat from the boiler stops and the room slowly cools as heat is lost. This series of events is a negative feedback mechanism and it enables continuous self-regulation or control of a variable factor within a narrow range.

Body temperature is a physiological variable controlled by negative feedback (Fig. 1.4). When body temperature falls below the preset level, this is detected by specialised temperature sensitive nerve endings. They transmit this information as an input to groups of cells in the hypothalamus of the brain which form the control centre. The output from the control centre activates mechanisms that raise body temperature (effectors). These include:

- stimulation of skeletal muscles causing shivering
- narrowing of the blood vessels in the skin reducing the blood flow to, and heat loss from, the peripheries
- behavioural changes, e.g. we put on more clothes or curl up.

When body temperature rises to within the normal range, the temperature sensitive nerve endings no longer stimulate the cells of the control centre and therefore the output of this centre to the effectors ceases.

Most of the homeostatic controls in the body use negative feedback mechanisms to prevent sudden and serious changes in the internal environment. Many more of these are explained in the following chapters.

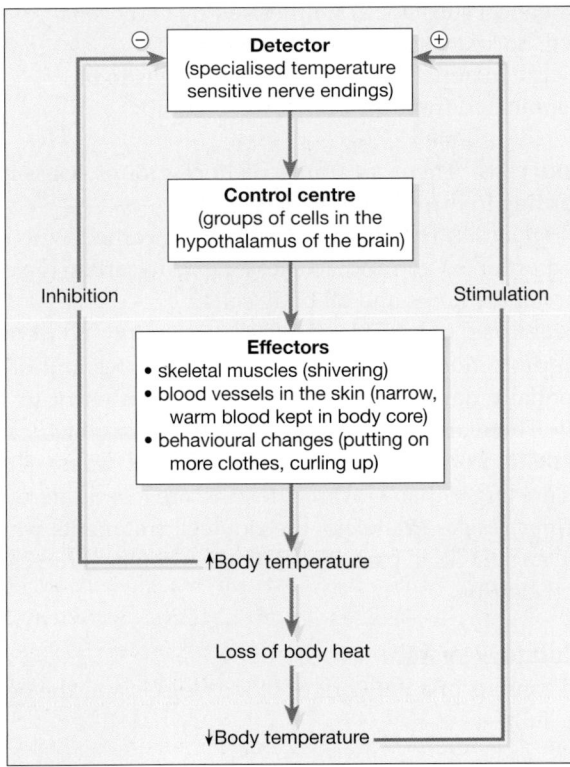

Figure 1.4 Example of a physiological negative feedback mechanism: control of body temperature.

Positive feedback mechanisms

There are only a few of these *amplifier* or *cascade systems* in the body. In positive feedback mechanisms, the stimulus progressively increases the response, so that as long as the stimulus is continued the response is progressively being amplified. Examples include blood clotting and uterine contractions during labour.

During labour, contractions of the uterus are stimulated by the hormone oxytocin. These force the baby's head into the cervix of the uterus stimulating stretch receptors there. In response to this, more of the hormone oxytocin is released, further strengthening the contractions and maintaining labour. After the baby is born the stimulus (stretching of the cervix) is no longer present and the release of oxytocin stops (see Fig. 9.5, p. 219).

Homeostatic imbalance

This arises when the fine control of a factor in the internal environment is inadequate and the level of the factor falls outside the normal range. If control cannot achieve homeostasis, an abnormal state develops that may threaten health, or even life. Many of these situations are explained in later chapters.

SURVIVAL NEEDS OF THE BODY

Learning outcomes

After studying this section you should be able to:

- describe the role of the body transport systems

- outline the roles of the nervous and endocrine systems in internal communication

- outline how raw materials are absorbed by the body

- state the waste materials eliminated from the body

- outline activities undertaken by an individual for protection and survival.

By convention, the body systems are described separately in the study of anatomy and physiology, but in reality they are all interdependent. This section provides an introduction to body activities linking them to survival needs (Table 1.1). The later chapters build on this framework, exploring human structure and functions in health and illness using a systems approach.

Table 1.1 Survival needs and related body activities	
Survival need	**Body activities**
Communication	Transport systems: blood, circulatory system, lymphatic system Internal communication: nervous system, endocrine system External communication: special senses, verbal and non-verbal communication
Intake of raw materials and elimination of waste	Intake of oxygen Dietary intake Elimination of waste: carbon dioxide, urine, faeces
Protection and survival	Protection against the external environment: skin Resistance and immunity: non-specific and specific defence mechanisms Body movement Reproduction

Communication

In this section, transport and communication are considered. Transport systems ensure that all cells have access to the internal and external environments; the blood, the circulatory system and lymphatic system are involved. All communication systems involve receiving, collating and responding to appropriate information.

There are different systems for communicating with the internal and external environments. Internal communication involves mainly the nervous and endocrine systems; these are important in the maintenance of homeostasis and regulation of vital body functions. Communication with the external environment involves the special senses, and verbal and non-verbal activities, and all of these also depend on the nervous system.

Transport systems

Blood

The blood transports substances around the body through a large network of blood vessels. In adults the body contains 5 to 6 l of blood (Ch. 4). It consists of two parts—a sticky fluid called plasma and cells which are suspended in the plasma.

Plasma. This is mainly water with a wide range of substances dissolved or suspended in it. These include:

- nutrients absorbed from the alimentary canal
- oxygen absorbed from the lungs
- chemical substances synthesised by body cells, e.g. hormones
- waste materials produced by body cells to be eliminated from the body by excretion.

Blood cells. There are three distinct groups, classified according to their functions (Fig. 1.5).

Erythrocytes (red blood cells) are concerned with the transport of oxygen and, to a lesser extent, carbon dioxide between the lungs and all body cells.

Leukocytes (white blood cells) are mainly concerned with protection of the body against microbes and other potentially damaging substances that gain entry to the body. There are several types of leukocytes which carry out their protective functions in different ways. These cells are larger than erythrocytes and are less numerous.

Thrombocytes (platelets) are tiny cell fragments which play an essential part in the very complex process of blood clotting.

Circulatory system (Ch. 5)

This consists of a network of blood vessels and the heart (Fig. 1.6).

Blood vessels. There are three types:

- *arteries*, which carry blood away from the heart
- *veins*, which return blood to the heart
- *capillaries*, which link the arteries and veins.

Capillaries are tiny blood vessels with very thin walls consisting of only one layer of cells. They are the site of

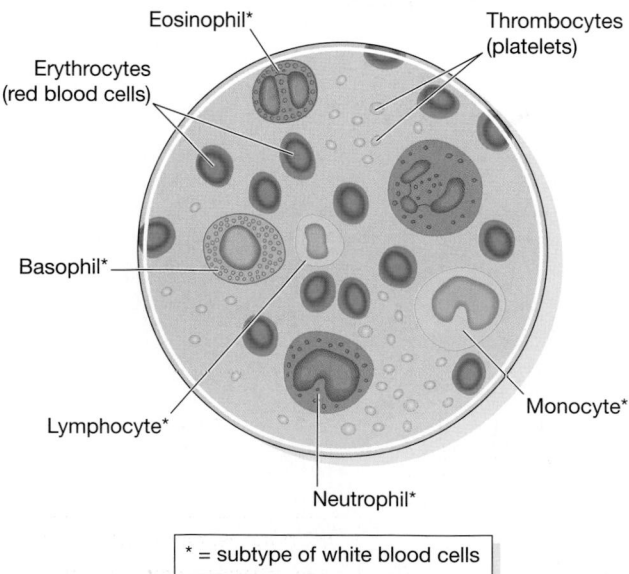

Eosinophil*
Thrombocytes (platelets)
Erythrocytes (red blood cells)
Basophil*
Lymphocyte*
Neutrophil*
Monocyte*

* = subtype of white blood cells

Figure 1.5 Blood cells after staining in the laboratory viewed through a microscope.

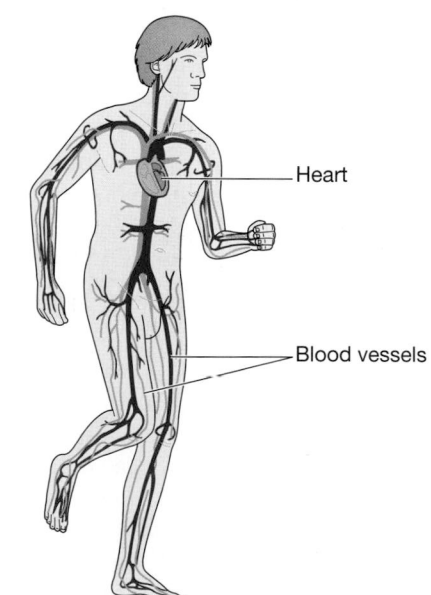

Heart
Blood vessels

Figure 1.6 The circulatory system.

exchange of substances between the blood and body tissues, e.g. nutrients, oxygen and cellular waste products. Blood vessels form a network that transports blood to:

- the lungs (*pulmonary circulation*) where oxygen is absorbed from the air in the lungs and at the same time carbon dioxide is excreted from the blood into the air
- cells in all parts of the body (*general* or *systemic circulation*).

Heart. The heart is a muscular sac. It pumps the blood round the body and maintains the blood pressure in the lungs and general circulation. This is essential for life.

The heart muscle is not under conscious (voluntary) control. At rest, the heart contracts between 65 and 75 times per minute. The rate may be greatly increased during physical exercise, when the oxygen and nutritional needs of the muscles moving the limbs are increased, and in some emotional states.

The rate at which the heart beats can be counted by taking the *pulse*. The pulse can be felt most easily where an artery lies close to the surface of the body and can be pressed gently against a bone. The wrist is the site most commonly used for this purpose.

Lymphatic system
The lymphatic system (Ch. 6) consists of a series of *lymph vessels*, which begin as blind-ended tubes in the spaces between the blood capillaries and tissue cells (Fig. 1.7). Structurally they are similar to veins and blood capillaries but the pores in the walls of the lymph capillaries are larger than those of the blood capillaries. *Lymph* is tissue fluid containing large molecules, e.g. proteins, fragments of damaged tissue cells and microbes. It is transported along lymph vessels and is returned to the bloodstream.

There are collections of *lymph nodes* situated at various points along the length of the lymph vessels. Lymph is filtered as it passes through the lymph nodes, and microbes, noxious substances and some waste materials are removed.

The lymphatic system provides the sites for formation and maturation of *lymphocytes*, the white blood cells involved in immunity.

Internal communication

Communication and the nervous system
The nervous system is a rapid communication system (Ch. 7). The main components are shown in Figure 1.8.

The central nervous system consists of:

- the *brain*, situated inside the skull
- the *spinal cord*, which extends from the base of the skull to the lumbar region and is protected from injury by the bones of the spinal column.

The peripheral nervous system is a network of nerve fibres, which are:

- *sensory* or *afferent*, providing the brain with 'input' from organs and tissues, or
- *motor* or *efferent*, which convey nerve impulses carrying 'output' from the brain to effector organs: the muscles and glands.

Figure 1.7 The lymphatic system: lymph nodes and vessels.

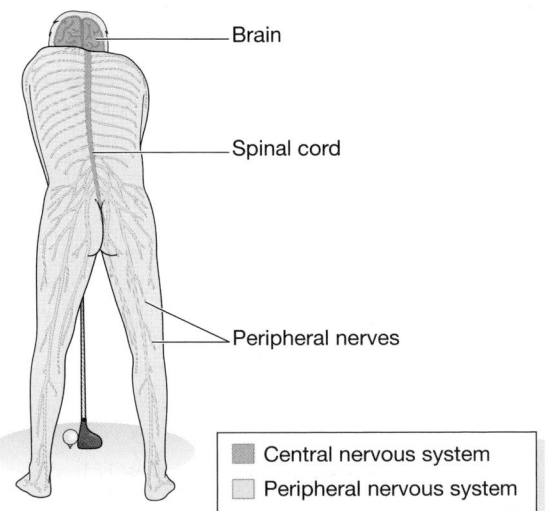

Brain

Spinal cord

Peripheral nerves

| | Central nervous system |
| | Peripheral nervous system |

Figure 1.8 The nervous system.

The somatic (common) senses are pain, touch, heat and cold, and they arise following stimulation of specialised sensory receptors at nerve endings found throughout the skin. There are different receptors in muscles and joints that respond to changes in the position and orientation of the body, maintaining posture and balance. Yet other receptors are activated by stimuli in internal organs and maintain control of vital body functions, e.g. heart rate, respiratory rate and blood pressure. Stimulation of any of these receptors sets up impulses that are conducted to the brain in sensory (afferent) nerves. Communication along nerve fibres (cells) is by electrical impulses that are generated when nerve endings are stimulated.

Communication between nerve cells is also required, since more than one nerve is involved in the chain of events occurring between the initial stimulus and the physiological reaction to it. Nerves communicate with each other by releasing a chemical (the *neurotransmitter*) into tiny gaps between them. The neurotransmitter quickly travels across the gap and either stimulates or inhibits the next nerve cell, thus ensuring the message is transmitted.

Sensory nerves and chemical substances circulating in the blood provide information to appropriate parts of the brain, which collates it and then responds via motor nerves to effector organs, often through a negative feedback mechanism (Fig. 1.3). Some of these activities are understood and perceived, e.g. pain, whereas others take place subconsciously, e.g. changes in blood pressure. Nerve impulses travel at great speed along nerve fibres leading to rapid responses; adjustments to many body functions occur within a few seconds.

Communication and the endocrine system

The endocrine system consists of a number of *endocrine glands* situated in different parts of the body. They synthesise and secrete chemical messengers called *hormones* that circulate round the body in the blood. Hormones stimulate *target glands* or *tissues*, influencing metabolic and other cellular activities and regulating body growth and maturation. Endocrine glands detect and respond to levels of particular substances in the blood, including specific hormones. Changes in blood hormone levels are controlled by negative feedback mechanisms (Fig. 1.3). The endocrine system provides slower and more precise control of body functions than the nervous system.

Communication with the external environment

Special senses

These senses arise following stimulation of specialised sensory receptor cells located in sensory organs or tissues in the head. The senses and the special organs involved are shown in Box 1.2.

Although these senses are usually considered separate and different from each other, one sense is rarely used alone (Fig. 1.9). For example, when the smell of smoke is perceived then other senses such as sight and sound are used to try and locate the source of a fire. Similarly, taste and smell are closely associated in the enjoyment, or otherwise, of food. The brain collates incoming information with information from the memory and initiates a response by setting up electrical impulses in motor (efferent) nerves to effector organs, muscles and glands. Such responses enable the individual to escape from the fire, or to prepare the digestive system for eating.

Verbal communication

Sound is a means of communication and is produced in the larynx as a result of blowing air through the space between the *vocal cords* during expiration. Speech is the manipulation of sound by contraction of the muscles of the throat and cheeks, and movements of the tongue and lower jaw.

Non-verbal communication

Posture and movements are associated with non-verbal communication, e.g. nodding the head and shrugging the

> **Box 1.2** The senses and related sense organs
>
> Sight – eyes
>
> Hearing – ears
>
> Balance – ears
>
> Smell – nose
>
> Taste – tongue

Figure 1.9 Combined use of the special senses: vision, hearing, smell and taste.

shoulders. The skeletal system provides the bony framework of the body (Ch. 16), and movement takes place at joints between bones. Skeletal muscles which move the bones lie between them and the skin. They are stimulated by the part of the nervous system under conscious (voluntary) control. Some non-verbal communication, e.g. changes in facial expression, may not involve the movement of bones.

Intake of raw materials and elimination of waste

This section considers the substances that must be taken into and excreted from the body. Oxygen, water and food are the substances the body needs to take in, and carbon dioxide, urine and faeces are those excreted.

Intake of oxygen

Oxygen is a gas that makes up about 21% of atmospheric air. A continuous supply is essential for human life because most chemical activities that take place in the body cells can occur only in its presence. Oxygen is needed in the series of chemical reactions that result in the release of energy from nutrients.

The respiratory system carries air between the nose and the lungs during breathing (Ch. 10). Air passes through a system of passages consisting of the pharynx (also part of the alimentary canal), the larynx (voice box), the trachea, two bronchi (one bronchus to each lung) and a large number of bronchial passages (Fig. 1.10). These

end in alveoli, millions of tiny air sacs in each lung. They are surrounded by a network of tiny capillaries and are the sites where the vital process of gas exchange between the lungs and the blood takes place (Fig. 1.11).

Nitrogen, which makes up about 80% of atmospheric air, is breathed in and out but, in this gaseous form, it cannot be used by the body. The nitrogen needed by the body is present in protein-containing foods, mainly meat and fish.

Dietary intake

Nutrition is considered in Chapter 11. A balanced diet is important for health and provides *nutrients*, substances that are absorbed, often following digestion, and promote body function. Nutrients include water, carbohydrates, proteins, fats, vitamins and mineral salts. They are required for:

- maintaining water balance within the body
- energy production, mainly carbohydrates and fats
- synthesis of large and complex molecules, using mineral salts, proteins, fats, carbohydrates and vitamins
- cell building, growth and repair, especially proteins.

Digestion

The digestive system has developed because the food eaten is chemically complex and seldom in a form the body cells can use. Its function is to break down or *digest* food so that it can be absorbed into the circulation and then used by body cells. The digestive system consists of the alimentary tract and accessory glands (Fig. 1.12).

Alimentary canal. This is a tube that begins at the mouth and continues through the pharynx, oesophagus, stomach, small and large intestines, rectum and anus.

Glands. The accessory organs situated outside the alimentary canal with ducts leading into it are the *salivary*

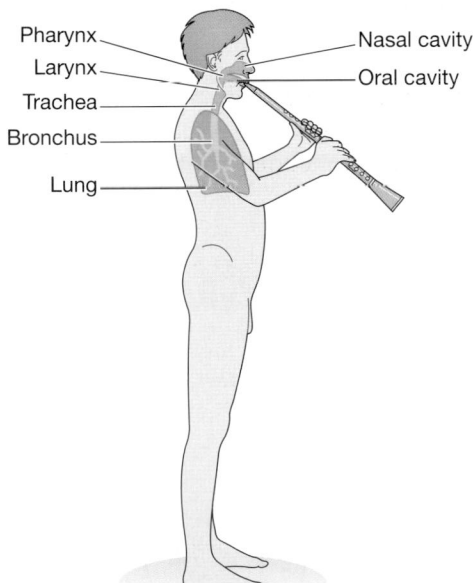

Pharynx
Larynx
Trachea
Bronchus
Lung
Nasal cavity
Oral cavity

Figure 1.10 The respiratory system.

Arteriole
Respiratory bronchiole
Venule
Alveoli
Alveolar duct
Capillaries

Figure 1.11 Alveoli: the site of gas exchange.

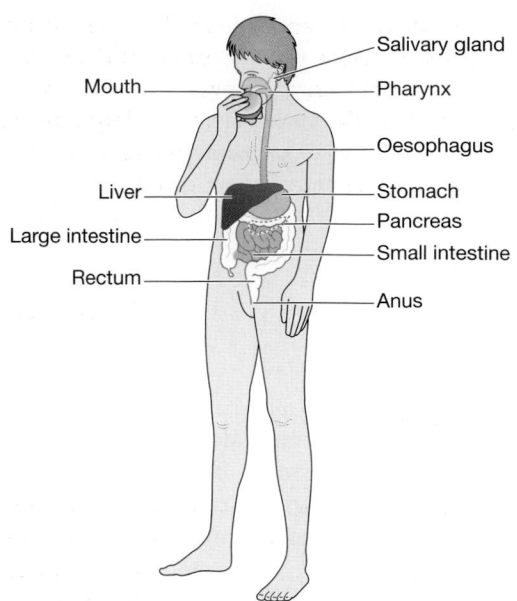

Figure 1.12 The digestive system.

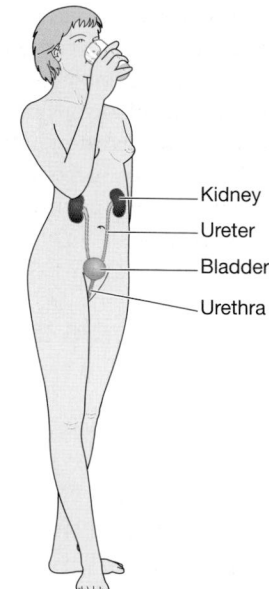

Figure 1.13 The urinary system.

glands, the *pancreas* and the *liver*. There are also many small glands situated in the walls of the alimentary canal. Most of these glands synthesise *digestive enzymes* that are involved in the chemical breakdown of food.

Metabolism

This is the sum total of the chemical activity in the body. It consists of two groups of processes:

- *anabolism*, building or synthesising large and complex substances
- *catabolism*, breaking down substances to provide energy and raw materials for anabolism, and substances for excretion as waste.

The sources of energy are mainly the carbohydrates and fats provided by the diet. If these are in short supply, proteins are used.

Elimination of waste

Carbon dioxide

This is continually excreted by the respiratory system, as described above. Carbon dioxide is a waste product of cellular metabolism. It dissolves in water to form an acid that must be excreted in appropriate amounts to maintain the pH (acidity or alkalinity) of the blood in its normal range.

Urine

This is formed by the kidneys, which are part of the urinary system (Ch. 13). The organs of the urinary system are shown in Figure 1.13. Urine consists of water and waste products mainly of protein breakdown, e.g. urea. Under the influence of hormones from the endocrine system the kidneys regulate water balance within the body. They also play a role in maintaining blood pH within the normal range. The bladder stores urine until it is excreted during *micturition*. The process of micturition (passing urine) also involves the nervous system.

Faeces

The waste materials from the digestive system are excreted as faeces containing:

- indigestible food residue that remains in the alimentary canal because it cannot be absorbed
- bile from the liver, which contains the waste products from the breakdown of red blood cells
- large numbers of microbes.

Elimination of faeces (*defecation*) also involves the nervous system.

Protection and survival

In this section relevant activities will be outlined under the following headings: protection against the external environment, resistance and immunity, movement and reproduction.

Protection against the external environment

On the body surface, the skin (Ch. 14) mainly provides this. It consists of two layers: the epidermis and the dermis.

The epidermis lies superficially and is composed of several layers of cells that grow towards the surface from its deepest layer. The surface layer consists of dead cells that are constantly being rubbed off and replaced from below. The epidermis constitutes the barrier between the moist environment of the living cells of the body and the dry atmosphere of the external environment.

The dermis contains tiny *sweat glands* that have little canals or ducts, leading to the surface. Hairs grow from follicles in the dermis. The layers of the skin form a barrier against:

- invasion by microbes
- chemicals
- dehydration.

Sensory nerve endings present in the dermis are stimulated by pain, temperature and touch. If the finger touches a very hot plate, it is removed immediately. This cycle of events is called a *reflex action* and is a very rapid motor response (contraction of muscles) to a sensory stimulus (stimulation of sensory nerve endings in the skin). This type of reflex action is an important protective mechanism that is mediated by the nervous system.

The skin also plays an important role in the regulation of body temperature.

Resistance and immunity

The body has many means of self-protection from invaders (Ch. 15). They are divided into two categories: specific and nonspecific defence mechanisms.

Nonspecific defence mechanisms

These are effective against any invaders. The protection provided by the skin is outlined above. In addition there are other protective features at body surfaces, e.g. mucus secreted by mucous membranes traps microbes and other foreign materials on its sticky surface. Some body fluids contain antimicrobial substances, e.g. gastric juice contains hydrochloric acid, which kills most ingested microbes. Following successful invasion other nonspecific processes may occur including the inflammatory response, which is also involved in tissue healing.

Specific defence mechanisms

The body generates a specific (immune) response against any substance it identifies as foreign. Such substances are called *antigens* and include:

- bacteria and other microbes
- cancer cells or transplanted tissue cells
- pollen from flowers and plants.

Following exposure to an antigen, lifelong immunity against further invasion by the same antigen usually develops. Over a lifetime, an individual gradually builds up immunity to millions of antigens. Allergic reactions are abnormally powerful immune responses to an antigen that usually poses no threat to the body.

Movement

Movement of the whole body or parts of it are essential for:

- obtaining food
- avoiding injury
- reproduction.

Most body movement is under conscious (voluntary) control. The exceptions include protective movements which are carried out before the individual is aware of them, e.g. the reflex action of removing the finger from a very hot surface.

The skeleton provides the bony framework of the body and movement takes place at joints between two or more bones. *Skeletal muscles* (Fig. 1.14) move the *joints* and they are stimulated to contract by the nervous system. A brief description of the skeleton is given in Chapter 3, and a more detailed account of bones, muscles and joints is presented in Chapters 16, 17 and 18.

Skeletal muscles

Tendon

Figure 1.14 The skeletal muscles.

Reproduction (Ch. 19)

Successful reproduction is essential in order to ensure the continuation of a species from one generation to the next. *Bisexual reproduction* results from the fertilisation of a female egg cell or *ovum* by a male sperm cell or *spermatozoon*. Ova are produced by two *ovaries* situated in the female pelvis (Fig. 1.15). Usually only one ovum is released at a time and it travels towards the *uterus* in the *uterine tube*. The spermatozoa are produced in large numbers by the two *testes*, situated in the *scrotum*. From each testis spermatozoa pass through a duct called the *deferent duct (vas deferens)* to the *urethra*. During sexual intercourse (coitus) the spermatozoa are deposited in the female *vagina*.

They then pass upwards through the uterus and fertilise the ovum in the uterine tube. The fertilised ovum (*zygote*) then passes into the uterus, embeds itself in the uterine wall and grows to maturity during pregnancy or gestation, in about 40 weeks. The newborn baby is entirely dependent on others for food and protection that was provided by the mother's body before birth.

One ovum is produced about every 28 days during the child-bearing years between *puberty* and the *menopause*.

Deferent duct
Prostate gland
Penis
Testis
Uterine tube
Ovary
Uterus
Vagina

Figure 1.15 The reproductive systems: male and female.

When the ovum is not fertilised it passes out of the uterus accompanied by bleeding, called *menstruation*. The cycle in the female, called the *menstrual cycle*, has phases associated with changes in the concentration of hormones involving the endocrine system. There is no similar cycle in the male but hormones similar to those of the female are involved in the production and maturation of the spermatozoa.

INTRODUCTION TO THE STUDY OF ILLNESS

Learning outcomes

After studying this section you should be able to:

- list factors that commonly cause disease
- define the following terms: aetiology, pathogenesis and prognosis
- name some common disease processes that can affect many of the body systems.

In order to understand the specific diseases described in later chapters, a knowledge of the relevant anatomy and physiology is necessary, as well as familiarity with the pathological processes outlined below.

Many different illnesses, disorders and diseases are known, and these vary from minor, but often very troublesome conditions, to the very serious. The study of abnormalities can be made much easier when a systematic approach is adopted. In order to achieve this in later chapters where specific diseases are explained, the headings shown in Box 1.3 will be used as a guide. Causes (*aetiology*) are outlined first when there are clear links between them and the effects of the abnormality (*pathogenesis*).

Box 1.3 Suggested framework for understanding diseases

Aetiology: cause of the disease

Pathogenesis: the nature of the disease process and its effect on normal body functioning

Complications: other consequences which might arise if the disease progresses

Prognosis: the likely outcome

Aetiology

Disease is usually caused by one or more of a limited number of factors including:

- genetic abnormalities, either inherited or acquired
- infection by microbes or parasites, e.g. viruses, bacteria or worms
- chemicals
- ionising radiation
- physical trauma
- degeneration, e.g. excessive use or ageing.

In some diseases more than one of the aetiological factors listed above is involved, while in others, no specific cause has been identified and these may be described as *essential, idiopathic* or *spontaneous*. For some diseases of which the precise cause is unknown, links may have been established with *predisposing factors*, or *risk factors*. *Iatrogenic* conditions are those that result from harm caused by members of the caring professions.

Pathogenesis

The main processes causing illness or disease are as follows.

- *Inflammation* (p. 375) — this is a tissue response to damage by, e.g. trauma, invasion of microbes*. Inflammatory conditions are recognised by the suffix -itis, e.g. appendicitis.
- *Tumours* (p. 53) — these arise when the rate of cell production exceeds that of normal cell destruction causing a mass to develop. Tumours are recognised by the suffix -oma, e.g. carcinoma.

---

*The term **microbe**, used throughout the text, includes all types of organisms that can only be seen by using a microscope. Specific microbes are named where appropriate.

- *Abnormal immune mechanisms* (p. 383) — these are a response of the normally protective immune system that causes undesirable effects.
- *Thrombosis, embolism* and *infarction* (p. 117) — these are the effects and consequences of abnormal changes in the blood and/or blood vessel walls.
- *Degeneration* — this is often associated with normal ageing but also arises prematurely when structures deteriorate causing impaired function.
- *Metabolic abnormalities* — cause undesirable effects (e.g. phenylketonuria (p. 185)).
- *Genetic abnormalities* — may be either inherited or caused by environmental factors such as exposure to ionising radiation.

Box 1.4 is a glossary of disease-associated terminology.

Box 1.4 Glossary of terminology associated with disease

Acute: a disease with sudden onset often requiring urgent treatment (compare with chronic).

Acquired: a disorder which develops any time after birth (compare with congenital).

Chronic: a long-standing disorder which cannot usually be cured (compare with acute).

Congenital: a disorder which one is born with (compare with acquired).

Sign: an abnormality seen or measured by people other than the patient.

Symptom: an abnormality described by the patient.

Syndrome: a collection of signs and symptoms which tend to occur together.

15

2

Introduction to the chemistry of life

In all the following chapters, the cells, tissues and organs of the body will be studied in more depth. However, on a smaller scale even than the cell, all living matter is made up of chemical building blocks. The basis of anatomy and physiology is therefore a chemical one, and before launching into the study of the subject it is necessary to consider briefly some aspects of chemistry and biochemistry.

ATOMS, MOLECULES AND COMPOUNDS

Learning outcomes

After studying this section, you should be able to:

- define the following terms: atomic number, atomic weight, isotope, molecular weight, ion, electrolyte, pH, acid and alkali
- describe the structure of an atom
- discuss the types of bonds that hold molecules together
- outline the concept of molar concentration
- discuss the importance of buffers in the maintenance of body pH.

The *atom* is the smallest particle of an element which can exist as a stable entity. An *element* is a chemical substance whose atoms are all of the same type; e.g. iron contains only iron atoms. *Compounds* contain more than one type of atom; for instance, water is a compound containing both hydrogen and oxygen atoms.

There are 92 naturally occurring elements. The body structures are made up of a great variety of combinations of four elements: carbon, hydrogen, oxygen and nitrogen. In addition small amounts of others are present, collectively described as *mineral salts* (p. 276).

Atomic structure

Atoms are made up of three main types of particles.

- *Protons* are particles present in the nucleus or central part of the atom. Each proton has *one unit of positive electrical charge* and *one atomic mass unit*.
- *Neutrons* are also found in the nucleus of the atom. They have *no electrical charge* and *one atomic mass unit*.
- *Electrons* are particles which revolve in orbit around the nucleus of the atom at a distance from it (Fig. 2.1), as the planets revolve round the sun. Each electron

Table 2.1 **Characteristics of subatomic particles**		
Particle	Mass	Electric charge
Proton	1 unit	1 positive
Neutron	1 unit	neutral
Electron	negligible	1 negative

carries *one unit of negative electrical charge* and its mass is so small that it can be disregarded when compared with the mass of the other particles.

Table 2.1 summarises the characteristics of these subatomic particles.

In all atoms the number of positively charged protons in the nucleus is *equal to* the number of negatively charged electrons in orbit around the nucleus and therefore an atom is electrically neutral.

Atomic number and atomic weight

What makes one element different from another is the number of protons in the nuclei of its atoms. For instance, hydrogen has only one proton per nucleus, oxygen has eight and sodium has 11. The number of protons in the nucleus of an atom is called the atomic number; the atomic numbers of hydrogen, oxygen and sodium are therefore 1, 8 and 11 respectively. It therefore follows that each element has its own atomic number (Fig. 2.2). The atomic weight of an element is the sum of the protons and neutrons in the atomic nucleus (Fig. 2.2).

The electrons are shown in Figure 2.1 to be in concentric rings round the nucleus. These shells diagrammatically represent the different energy levels of the electrons

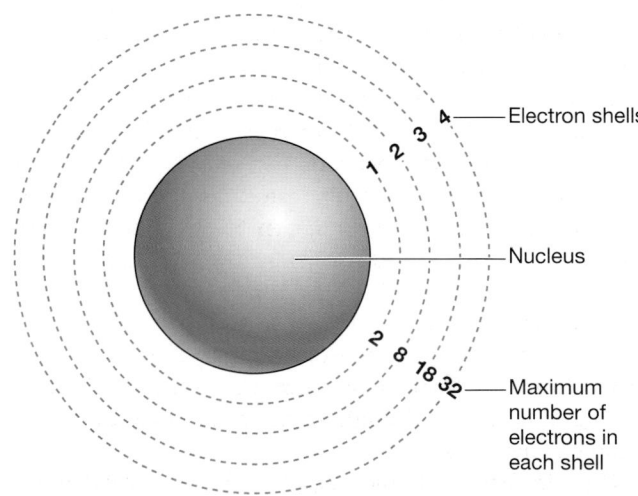

Figure 2.1 The atom showing the nucleus and four electron shells.

18

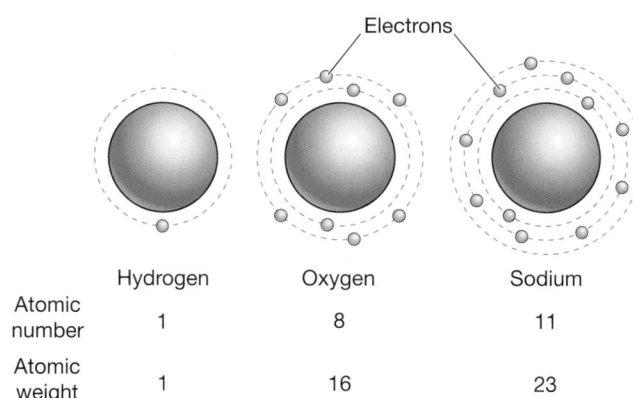

Figure 2.2 The atomic structures of the elements hydrogen, oxygen and sodium.

	Hydrogen	Oxygen	Sodium
Atomic number	1	8	11
Atomic weight	1	16	23

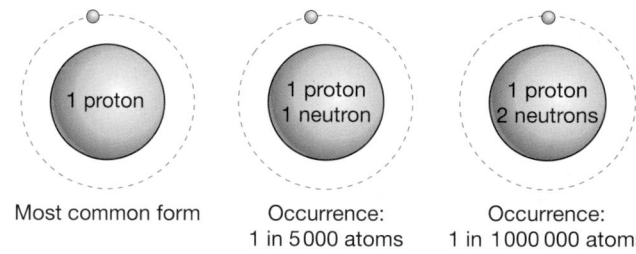

Figure 2.3 The isotopes of hydrogen.

in relation to the nucleus, not their physical positions. The first energy level can hold only two electrons and is filled first. The second energy level can hold only eight electrons and is filled next. The third and subsequent energy levels hold increased numbers of electrons, each containing more than the preceding level.

The *electron configuration* denotes the distribution of the electrons in each element, e.g. sodium is 2 8 1 (Fig. 2.2).

An atom is most stable when its outermost electron shell is full. Once electrons have filled the first two shells, the atom can reach a level of stability by having either the full complement of 18, or exactly eight, electrons in its third shell. When the outermost shell does not have a stable number of electrons, the atom is reactive and will combine with other reactive atoms, forming the wide range of the complex molecules of life. This will be described more fully in the section discussing molecules and compounds.

Isotopes. These are atoms of an element in which there is a *different number of neutrons in the nucleus*. This does not affect the electrical activity of these atoms because neutrons carry no electrical charge, but it does affect their atomic weight. For example, there are three forms of the hydrogen atom. The most common form has one proton in the nucleus and one orbiting electron. Another form has one proton and *one neutron* in the nucleus. A third form has one proton and *two neutrons* in the nucleus and one orbiting electron. These three forms of hydrogen are called *isotopes* (Fig. 2.3).

Taking into account the isotopes of hydrogen and the proportions in which they occur, the atomic weight of hydrogen is 1.008, although for many practical purposes it can be taken as 1.

Chlorine has an atomic weight of 35.5, because it exists in two forms; one isotope has an atomic weight of 35 (with 18 neutrons in the nucleus) and the other 37 (with 20 neutrons in the nucleus). Because the proportion of these two forms is not equal, the *average atomic weight* is 35.5.

Molecules and compounds

It was mentioned earlier that the atoms of each element have a specific number of electrons around the nucleus. When the number of electrons in the outer shell of an element is the optimum number (Fig. 2.1), the element is described as inert or chemically unreactive, i.e. it will not easily combine with other elements to form compounds. These elements are the inert or noble gases—helium, neon, argon, krypton, xenon and radon.

Molecules consist of two or more atoms which are chemically combined. The atoms may be of the same element, e.g. a molecule of atmospheric oxygen (O_2) consists of two oxygen atoms. Most molecules, however, contain two or more different elements; e.g. a water molecule (H_2O) contains two hydrogen atoms and an oxygen atom. As mentioned earlier, when two or more elements combine, the resulting molecule can also be referred to as a compound.

Compounds which contain the element carbon are classified as *organic*, and all others as *inorganic*. The body contains both.

Covalent and ionic bonds. The vast array of chemical processes on which body functioning is based is completely dependent upon the way atoms come together, bind and break apart. For example, the simple water molecule is a crucial foundation of all life on Earth. If water was a less stable compound, and the atoms came apart easily, human biology could never have evolved. On the other hand, the body is dependent upon the breaking down of various molecules (e.g. sugars, fats) to release energy for cellular activities. When atoms are joined together, they form a chemical bond which is generally one of two types: *covalent* or *ionic*.

Covalent bonds are formed when atoms share their electrons with each other. Most atoms use this type of bond when they come together; it forms a strong and stable link between them, because atoms are most stable

19

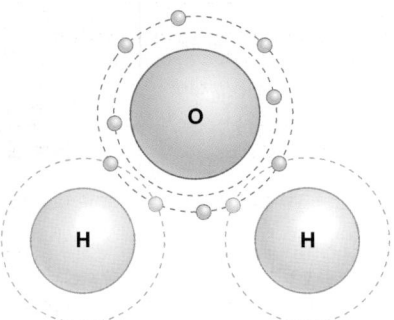

Figure 2.4 A water molecule, showing the covalent bonds between hydrogen (yellow) and oxygen (green).

when their outer electron shells are filled. A water molecule is built using covalent bonds. Hydrogen has one electron in its outer shell, but the optimum number for this shell is two. Oxygen has six electrons in its outer shell, but the optimum number for this shell is eight. Therefore, if one oxygen atom and two hydrogen atoms combine, each hydrogen atom will share its electron with the oxygen atom, giving the oxygen atom a total of eight outer electrons and thereby conferring stability. The oxygen atom shares one of its electrons with each of the two hydrogen atoms, so that each hydrogen atom has two electrons in its outer shell and they too are stable (Fig. 2.4).

Ionic bonds are weaker than covalent bonds and are formed when electrons are transferred from one atom to another. For example, when sodium (Na) combines with chlorine (Cl) to form sodium chloride (NaCl) there is a transfer of the only electron in the outer shell of the sodium atom to the outer shell of the chlorine atom. (Fig. 2.5).

This leaves the sodium atom of the compound with eight electrons in its outer (second) shell, and therefore stable. The chlorine atom also has eight electrons in its outer shell, which, although not filling the shell, is a stable number.

The number of electrons is the only change which occurs in the atoms in this type of reaction. There is no change in the number of protons or neutrons in the nuclei of the atoms. The chloride atom now has *18 electrons*, each with one negative electrical charge, and *17 protons*, each with one positive charge. The sodium atom has lost one electron, leaving *10 electrons* orbiting round the nucleus with *11 protons*. When sodium chloride is dissolved in water the two atoms separate, i.e. they *ionise*, and the imbalance of protons and electrons leads to the formation of two *charged particles* called *ions*. Sodium, with the positive charge, is a *cation*, written Na+, and chloride is an *anion*, written Cl-. By convention the number of electrical charges carried by an ion is indicated by the superscript plus or minus signs.

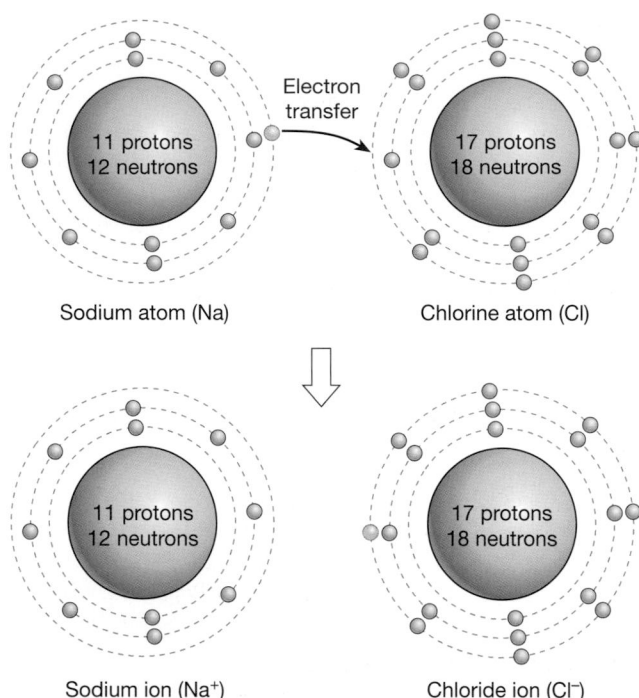

Figure 2.5 Formation of the ionic compound, sodium chloride.

Electrolytes

An ionic compound, e.g. sodium chloride, in solution in water is called an *electrolyte* because it can conduct electricity. Electrolytes are important body constituents because:

- some conduct electricity, essential for muscle and nerve function
- some exert osmotic pressure, keeping body fluids in their own compartments
- some function in acid–base balance, as buffers to resist pH changes in body fluids.

In this discussion, sodium chloride has been used as an example of the formation of an ionic compound and to illustrate electrolyte activity. There are, however, many other electrolytes within the human body which, though in relatively small quantities, are equally important. Although these substances may enter the body in the form of compounds, such as sodium bicarbonate, they are usually discussed in the ionic form, that is, as sodium ions (Na^+) and bicarbonate ions (HCO_3^-).

The bicarbonate part of sodium bicarbonate is derived from carbonic acid (H_2CO_3). All inorganic acids contain hydrogen combined with another element, or with a group of elements called a *radical* which acts like a single element. Hydrogen combines with chlorine to form hydrochloric acid (HCl) and with the *phosphate radical* to form phosphoric acid (H_3PO_4). When these two acids ionise they do so thus:

$$HCl \rightarrow H^+ \, Cl^-$$
$$H_3PO_4 \rightarrow 3H^+ \, PO_4^{3-}$$

In the second example, three atoms of hydrogen have each lost one electron, all of which have been taken up by one unit, the phosphate radical, making a phosphate ion with three negative charges.

A large number of compounds present in the body are not ionic and therefore have no electrical properties when dissolved in water, e.g. carbohydrates.

Molecular weight

The molecular weight of a molecule is the sum of the atomic weights of the elements which form its molecules, e.g.:

Water (H.OH)

2 hydrogen atoms	(atomic weight 1)	2
1 oxygen atom	(atomic weight 16)	16
	Molecular weight	= 18

Sodium bicarbonate (NaHCO$_3$)

1 sodium atom	(atomic weight 23)	23
1 hydrogen atom	(atomic weight 1)	1
1 carbon atom	(atomic weight 12)	12
3 oxygen atoms	(atomic weight 16)	48
	Molecular weight	= 84

Molecular weight, like atomic weight, is expressed simply as a figure until a scale of measurement of weight is applied.

Molar concentration

This is the term recommended in the *Système Internationale* for expressing the concentration of substances present in the body fluids (SI units).

The mole (mol) is the molecular weight in grams of a substance (formerly called 1 gram molecule). One mole of any substance contains 6.023×10^{23} molecules or atoms. For example, 1 mole of sodium bicarbonate (the example above) is 84 grams.

A molar solution is a solution in which 1 mole of a substance is dissolved in 1 litre of solvent. In the human body the solvent is water or fat. A molar solution of sodium bicarbonate is therefore prepared using 84 g of sodium bicarbonate dissolved in 1 litre of solvent.

Molar concentration may be used to measure quantities of electrolytes, non-electrolytes, ions and atoms, e.g. molar solutions of the following substances mean:

1 mole of sodium chloride molecules (NaCl)	= 58.5 g per litre
1 mole of sodium ions (Na$^+$)	= 23 g per litre
1 mole of carbon atoms (C)	= 12 g per litre
1 mole of atmospheric oxygen (O$_2$)	= 32 g per litre

Table 2.2 Examples of normal plasma levels

Substance	Amount in SI units	Amount in other units
Chloride	97–106 mmol/l	97–106 mEq/l
Sodium	135–143 mmol/l	135–143 mEq/l
Glucose	3.5–5.5 mmol/l	60–100 mg/100 ml
Iron	14–35 µmol/l	90–196 µg/100 ml

In physiology this system has the advantage of being a measure of the number of particles (molecules, atoms, ions) of substances present because molar solutions of different substances contain the same number of particles. It has the advantage over the measure milliequivalents per litre* because it can be used for non-electrolytes, in fact for any substance of known molecular weight.

Many of the chemical substances present in the body are in very low concentrations so it is more convenient to use smaller metric measures, e.g. *millimoles per litre* (mmol/l) or micromoles per litre (µmol/l) as a biological measure (Table 2.2).

For substances of unknown molecular weight, e.g. insulin, concentration may be expressed in International Units per millilitre (IU/ml).

Acids, alkalis and pH

The number of hydrogen ions present in a solution is a measure of the acidity of the solution. The maintenance of the normal hydrogen ion concentration ([H$^+$]) within the body is an important factor in maintaining a stable environment, i.e. homeostasis.

The pH scale

A standard scale for the measurement of the hydrogen ion concentration in solution has been developed: the pH scale. Not all acids ionise completely when dissolved in water. The hydrogen ion concentration is a measure, therefore, of the amount of *dissociated acid* (ionised acid) rather than of the total amount of acid present. Strong acids dissociate more freely than weak acids, e.g. hydrochloric acid

*Milliequivalents per litre (mEq/l)

$$\text{Equivalent weight} = \frac{\text{atomic weight}}{\text{number of electrical charges}}$$

Concentration is expressed:

$$\text{mEq/l} = \frac{\text{mg/l}}{\text{atomic weight}} \times \text{number of electrical charges}$$

Figure 2.6 The pH scale.

Table 2.3 **pH values of body fluids**	
Body fluid	**pH**
Blood	7.35 to 7.45
Saliva	5.4 to 7.5
Gastric juice	1.5 to 3.5
Bile	6 to 8.5
Urine	4.5 to 8.0

dissociates freely into H^+ and Cl^-, while carbonic acid dissociates much less freely into H^+ and HCO_3^-. The number of *free hydrogen ions* in a solution is a *measure of its acidity* rather than an indication of the type of molecule from which the hydrogen ions originated.

The alkalinity of a solution depends on the number of hydroxyl ions (OH^-). Water is a neutral solution because every molecule contains one hydrogen ion and one hydroxyl radical. For every molecule of water (H.OH) which dissociates, one hydrogen ion (H^+) and one hydroxyl ion (OH^-) are formed, neutralising each other.

The scale for measurement of pH was developed taking water as the standard.

In a neutral solution such as water, where the number of hydrogen ions is balanced by the same number of hydroxyl ions, the pH = 7. The range of this scale is from 0 to 14.

A pH reading *below* 7 indicates an *acid solution*, while readings *above* 7 indicate *alkalinity* (Fig. 2.6). A change of one whole number on the pH scale indicates a tenfold change in [H^+]. Therefore, a solution of pH 5 contains ten times as many hydrogen ions as a solution of pH 6.

Ordinary litmus paper indicates whether a solution is acid or alkaline by colouring blue for alkaline and red for acid. Other specially treated absorbent papers give an approximate measure of pH by a colour change. When accurate measurements of pH are required, sensitive pH meters are used.

pH values of the body fluids

Body fluids have pH values that must be maintained within relatively narrow limits for normal cell activity. The pH values are not the same in all parts of the body; e.g. the normal range of pH values of certain body fluids are shown in Table 2.3.

The pH value in an organ is produced by its secretion of acids or alkalis which establishes the optimum level. The highly acid pH of the gastric juice is maintained by hydrochloric acid secreted by the parietal cells in the walls of the gastric glands. The low pH value in the stomach provides the environment best suited to the functioning of the enzyme pepsin that begins the digestion of dietary protein. Saliva has a pH of between 5.4 and 7.5 which is the optimum value for the action of salivary

amylase, the enzyme present in saliva which initiates the digestion of carbohydrates. The action of salivary amylase is inhibited when food containing it reaches the stomach and is mixed with acid gastric juice.

Blood has a pH value between 7.35 and 7.45. The pH range of blood compatible with life is 7.0 to 7.8. The metabolic activity of the body cells produces certain acids and alkalis which alter the pH of the tissue fluid and blood. To maintain the pH within the normal range, there are substances present in blood that act as *buffers*.

Buffers

The optimum pH level is maintained by the balance between acids and bases produced by cells. Bases are substances that accept (or bind) hydrogen ions and when dissolved in water they produce an alkaline solution. Buffers are substances such as phosphates, bicarbonates and some proteins that maintain the [H^+] within normal, but narrow, limits. Some buffers 'bind' hydrogen ions and others 'bind' hydroxyl ions, reducing their circulating levels and preventing damaging changes. For example, if there is sodium hydroxide (NaOH) and carbonic acid (H_2CO_3) present, both will ionise to some extent, but they will also react together to form sodium bicarbonate ($NaHCO_3$) and water (H.OH). One of the hydrogen ions from the acid has been 'bound' in the formation of the bicarbonate radical and the other by combining with the hydroxyl radical to form water.

NaOH	+ H_2CO_3	→ $NaHCO_3$	+ H.OH
sodium hydroxide	carbonic acid	sodium bicarbonate	water

Acidosis and alkalosis

The substances in the complex buffer system that 'bind' hydrogen ions are called the *alkali reserve* of the blood. When the pH is below 7.35, and all the reserves of alkaline buffer are used up, the condition of *acidosis* exists. When the reverse situation pertains and the pH is above 7.45, and the increased alkali uses up all the *acid reserve*, the state of *alkalosis* exists.

The buffer systems maintain *homeostasis* by preventing dramatic changes in the pH values in the blood, but can only function effectively if there is some means by which excess acid or alkali can be excreted from the body. The organs most active in this way are the *lungs* and the *kidneys*. The lungs are important regulators of blood pH because they excrete carbon dioxide (CO_2). CO_2 increases [H^+] in body fluids because it combines with water to form carbonic acid, which then dissociates into a bicarbonate ion and a hydrogen ion.

$$CO_2 + H_2O \rightarrow H_2CO_3 \rightarrow H^+ + HCO_3^-$$

| carbon dioxide | water | carbonic acid | hydrogen ion | bicarbonate ion |

In acidosis, the brain detects the rising [H^+] in the blood and stimulates breathing, causing increased CO_2 loss and a fall in [H^+]. Conversely, in alkalosis, the brain can reduce the respiration rate to increase CO_2 levels and increase [H^+], restoring pH towards normal.

The kidneys have the ability to form ammonia, an alkali, which combines with the acid products of protein metabolism which are then excreted in the urine.

The buffer and excretory systems of the body together maintain the *acid–base balance* so that the pH range of the blood remains within normal, but narrow, limits.

IMPORTANT BIOLOGICAL MOLECULES

Learning outcomes

After studying this section, you should be able to:

- describe in simple terms the chemical nature of sugars, protein, lipids, nucleotides and enzymes
- discuss the biological importance of each of these important groups of molecules.

Carbohydrates

The carbohydrates are the sugars. Carbohydrates are composed of carbon, oxygen and hydrogen and the carbon atoms are normally arranged in a ring, with the oxygen and hydrogen atoms linked to them. The structures of glucose, fructose and sucrose are shown in Figure 2.7. When two sugars link up, the reaction occurring expels a molecule of water and the resulting bond is called a *glycosidic linkage*.

Simple sugars, like glucose, can exist as single units, and are referred to as *monosaccharides*. Glucose is the main form in which sugar is used by cells, and blood levels are tightly controlled. Frequently, the monosaccharides are linked together, the resultant molecule ranging from two sugars or *disaccharides*, e.g. sucrose (table sugar), to long chains containing many thousands of sugars. Such complex carbohydrates are called *polysaccharides*, e.g. starch.

Glucose can be broken down (metabolised) in either the presence (*aerobically*) or the absence (*anaerobically*) of oxygen, but the process is much more efficient when O_2 is used. During this process, energy, water and carbon dioxide are released (p. 315) This family of molecules:

- serves as a ready source of energy to fuel cellular activities (p. 272)
- provides a form of energy storage, e.g. glycogen (p. 315)
- forms an integral part of the structure of DNA and RNA (p. 25)
- can act as receptors on the cell surface, allowing the cell to recognise other molecules and cells.

Amino acids and proteins

Amino acids always contain carbon, hydrogen, oxygen and nitrogen, and many in addition carry sulphur. In human biochemistry, 20 amino acids are used as the principal building blocks of protein, although there are

Figure 2.7 The combination of glucose and fructose to make sucrose.

Figure 2.8 Amino acid structures: A. Common structure, R = variable side chain. B. Glycine, the simplest amino acid. C. Alanine. D. Phenylalanine.

others; for instance, there are some amino acids used only in certain proteins, and some seen only in microbial products. Of the amino acids used in human protein synthesis, there is a basic common structure, including an amino group (NH_2), a carboxy group (COOH) and a hydrogen atom. What makes one amino acid different from the next is a variable side chain. The basic structure and three common amino acids are shown in Figure 2.8. As in formation of glycosidic linkages, when two amino acids join up the reaction expels a molecule of water and the resulting bond is called a *peptide bond*.

Proteins are made from amino acids joined together, and are the main family of molecules from which the human body is built. Protein molecules vary enormously in size, shape, chemical constituents and function. Many important groups of biologically active substances are proteins, e.g.:

- carrier molecules, e.g. haemoglobin (p. 63)
- enzymes (p. 26)
- many hormones, e.g. insulin (p. 225)
- antibodies (p. 380).

Proteins can also be used as an alternative energy source, usually in dietary inadequacy, although the process is much less efficient than when carbohydrates or fats are broken down.

Lipids

Lipids are made up of carbon, hydrogen and oxygen atoms. One group of lipids, the *phospholipids*, form an integral part of the cell membrane. One notable feature of lipid molecules is that they are strongly hydrophobic

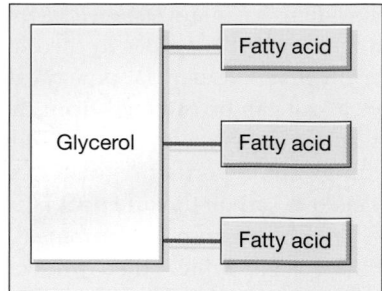

Figure 2.9 Core structure of the fats.

(water hating) and therefore lipids do not mix with water. This is important in their function in the cell membrane (p. 30).

Other types of lipids include certain vitamins (e.g. E and K), an important group of hormones called *steroids*, and the *fats*. A molecule of fat consists of three fatty acids, each linked to a molecule of glycerol (Fig. 2.9). Fats are a source of energy, and provide a convenient form in which to store excess calorific intake. When fats are broken down, they release energy, but the process is less efficient than when carbohydrates are used, since it requires more energy for the breakdown reaction to take place. They are used in the body for:

- insulation
- protection of body parts
- energy storage.

Nucleotides

Nucleic acids

These are the largest molecules in the body and are built from components called nucleotides, which consist of three subunits:

- a sugar unit
- a base
- one or more phosphate groups linked together.

Deoxyribonucleic acid (DNA)

This is a double strand of nucleotides arranged in a spiral (helix) which resembles a twisted ladder (Fig. 2.10). *Chromosomes* are clusters of DNA molecules consisting of functional subunits called *genes*. The nucleotides contain the sugar deoxyribose, phosphate groups and one of four bases: adenine [A], thymine [T], guanine [G] and cytosine [C]. A in one chain is paired with T in the other, and G with C. In this way, nucleotides are arranged in a precisely ordered manner in which one chain is complementary to the other. DNA acts as the template for protein synthesis and is stored safely in the nucleus.

Figure 2.10 Deoxyribonucleic acid (DNA).

Ribonucleic acid (RNA)

This is a single-stranded chain of nucleotides which contains the sugar ribose instead of the deoxyribose found in DNA. It contains no thymine, but uses uracil [U] instead. It is synthesised in the nucleus from the DNA template, and carries the message instructing synthesis of a new protein from the DNA (which cannot leave the nucleus) to the protein-synthesising apparatus in the cell cytoplasm.

Protein synthesis. When cells require new protein, a single strand of RNA is made using DNA as the template; the RNA leaves the nucleus. RNA acts as the messenger which carries the instructions for the assembly of the new protein to tiny structures in the cytoplasm called ribosomes (p. 32). Ribosomes read the message and, following the instructions, assemble the new protein from amino acids in the cell cytoplasm (Fig. 2.11). New chains of protein are often large molecules which coil up in a particular way to maintain stability of the molecule.

Adenosine triphosphate (ATP)

ATP is a nucleotide which contains ribose (the sugar unit), adenine (the base) and three phosphate groups attached to the ribose (Fig. 2.12A). It is sometimes known as the energy currency of the body, which implies that the body has to 'earn' (synthesise) it before it can 'spend' it. Many of the body's huge number of reactions release energy, e.g. the breakdown of sugars in the presence of O_2. The body captures the energy released by these reactions, using it to make ATP from adenosine diphosphate (ADP). When the body needs chemical energy to fuel cellular activities, ATP releases its stored energy, water and a phosphate group through the splitting of a high-energy phosphate bond, and reverts to ADP (Fig. 2.12B).

The body needs chemical energy to:

- drive synthetic reactions (i.e. building biological molecules)
- fuel movement
- transport substances across membranes.

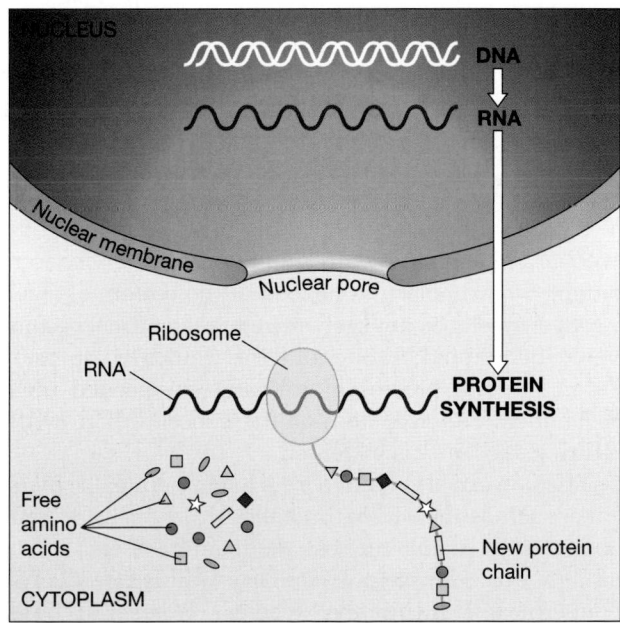

Figure 2.11 The relationship between DNA, RNA and protein synthesis.

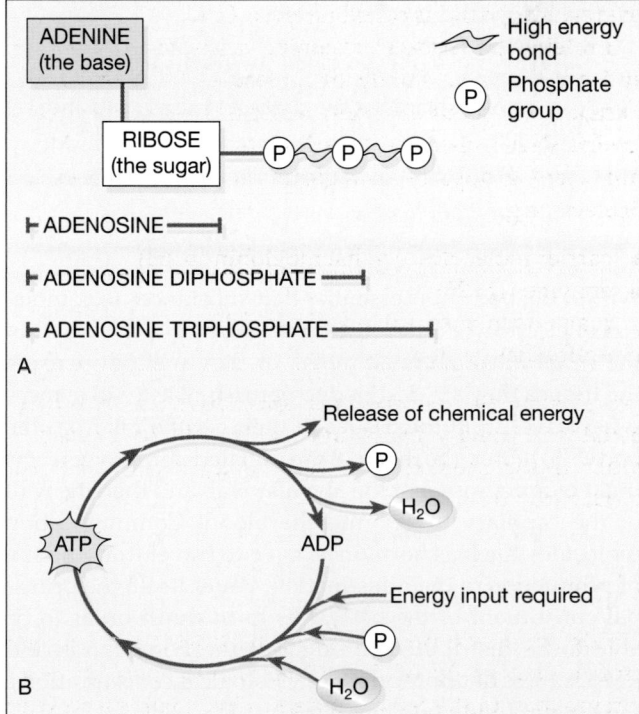

Figure 2.12 ATP and ADP: A. Structures. B. Conversion cycle.

Enzymes

Many of the body's chemical reactions can be reproduced in a test-tube. Surprisingly, the rate at which the reactions then occur usually plummets to the extent that, for all practical purposes, chemical activity ceases. The cells of the body have developed a solution to this apparent problem—they are equipped with a huge array of enzymes. Enzymes are proteins which act as *catalysts* for biochemical reactions—that is, they speed the reaction up but are not themselves changed by it, and therefore can be used over and over again. Enzymes are very selective and will usually catalyse only one specific reaction. The molecule(s) entering the reaction is called the *substrate* and it binds to a very specific site on the enzyme, called the *active site*. Whilst the substrate(s) is bound to the active site the reaction proceeds, and once it is complete the product(s) of the reaction breaks away from the enzyme and the active site is ready for use again (Fig. 2.13).

Enzymes can catalyse both synthesis and breakdown reactions, and their names (almost always!) end in ~ase.

MOVEMENT OF SUBSTANCES WITHIN THE BODY

Learning outcomes

After studying this section, you should be able to:

■ compare and contrast the processes of osmosis and diffusion

■ using these concepts, describe how molecules move within and between body compartments.

Within the body, it is essential that substances (e.g. molecules, electrolytes) move around. Nutrients absorbed in the small intestine must move, or they will never reach the tissues they are destined to nourish. Waste substances must travel from the tissues to their exit points from the body. To enter the body from inhaled air, oxygen gas must move across first the alveolar wall and then the wall of the capillary to get into the blood. Communication molecules, such as hormones, have to travel from the site of production to their destination. Water itself, the principal constituent of the body, has to move in order to be able to be distributed throughout the body fluids and keep solutes at appropriate physiological concentrations, thus maintaining homeostasis.

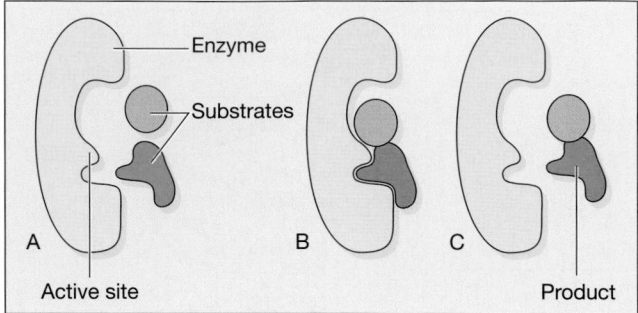

Figure 2.13 Action of an enzyme: A. Enzyme and substrates. B. Enzyme–substrate complex. C. Enzyme and product.

From a physical point of view, substances will always travel from an area of high concentration to one of low concentration, assuming that there is no barrier in the way. Between two such areas, there exists a *concentration gradient* and movement of substances occurs *down* the concentration gradient, or downhill. No energy is required for such movement; this process is therefore described as *passive*.

$$\text{high concentration} \xrightarrow{\text{Net movement of substance}} \text{low concentration}$$

There are many examples in the body of substances moving *uphill*, i.e. against the concentration gradient; in this case, chemical energy is required, usually in the form of ATP. These processes are described as *active*. Movement of substances across cell membranes by active transport is described on page 34.

Passive movement of substances in the body proceeds usually in one of two main ways—*diffusion* or *osmosis*.

Diffusion

Diffusion refers to the movement of a chemical substance from an area of high concentration to an area of low concentration, and occurs mainly in gases, liquids and solutions. This process enables the transfer of oxygen from the alveoli of the lungs (high concentration) through the alveolar and capillary walls into the blood (low concentration). Sugar molecules heaped at the bottom of a cup of coffee which has not been stirred will, in time, become evenly distributed throughout the liquid by diffusion (Fig. 2.14). The process of diffusion is speeded up if the temperature rises and/or the concentration of the diffusing substance is increased.

Diffusion can also occur across a semipermeable membrane, such as the plasma membrane; in this case, only those molecules able to cross the membrane can diffuse through. For example, the capillary wall is effectively a semipermeable membrane; whereas water can travel freely in either direction across it, large proteins in the

A Before diffusion   B After diffusion

Figure 2.14 The process of diffusion: a spoonful of sugar in a cup of coffee.

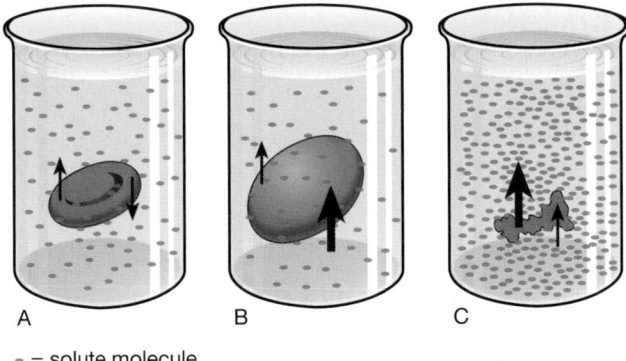

• = solute molecule

Figure 2.15 The process of osmosis. Net water movement when a red blood cell is suspended in solutions of varying concentrations (tonicity): A. Isotonic solution. B. Hypotonic solution. C. Hypertonic solution.

plasma and red blood cells are too large to cross and therefore remain in the blood.

Osmosis

Osmosis is the movement of water down its concentration gradient across a semipermeable membrane when equilibrium cannot be achieved by diffusion of solute molecules. This is usually because the solute molecules are too large to pass through the pores in the membrane. The force with which this occurs is called the *osmotic pressure*. Water crosses the membrane down its concentration gradient from the side with the lower solute concentration to the side with the greater solute concentration. This dilutes the more concentrated solution, and concentrates the more dilute solution. Osmosis proceeds until equilibrium is reached, at which point the solutions on each side of the membrane are of the same concentration and are said to be *isotonic*. Osmosis can be illustrated using the semipermeable membrane of the red blood cell as an example.

The concentration of water and solutes in the plasma is maintained within a very narrow range because if the plasma water concentration rises, i.e. the plasma becomes more dilute than the intracellular fluid within the red blood cells, then water will move down its concentration gradient across the membranes and into the red blood cells. This may cause the red blood cells to swell and burst. In this situation, the plasma is said to be *hypotonic*. Conversely, if the plasma water concentration falls so that the plasma becomes more concentrated than the intracellular fluid within the red blood cells (the plasma becomes *hypertonic*), water passively moves by osmosis from the blood cells into the plasma and shrinkage of the blood cells occurs (Fig. 2.15).

BODY FLUIDS

Learning outcomes

After studying this section, you should be able to:

■ define the terms intra- and extracellular fluid

■ using examples, explain why homeostatic control of the composition of these fluids is vital to body function.

The total body water in adults of average build is about 60% of body weight. This proportion is higher in young people and in adults below average weight. It is lower in the elderly and in obesity in all age groups. About 22% of body weight is extracellular water and about 38% is intracellular water (Fig. 2.16).

Extracellular fluid

The extracellular fluid (ECF) consists of blood, plasma, lymph, cerebrospinal fluid and fluid in the interstitial spaces of the body. Interstitial or intercellular fluid (tissue fluid) bathes all the cells of the body except the outer layers of skin. It is the medium through which substances pass from blood to the body cells, and from the cells to blood. Every body cell in contact with the ECF is directly dependent upon the composition of that fluid for its well-being. Even slight changes can cause permanent damage, and any change is therefore resisted by the body, through one or more of its many control mechanisms; this is homeostasis. For example, a fall in plasma calcium levels

Figure 2.16 Distribution of body water in a 70 kg person.

causes *tetany* (abnormal spasmodic muscle contractions) and convulsions (fits), because of increased excitability of muscle and nervous tissue. Rising blood calcium depresses muscle and nerve function, and can even cause the heart to stop beating. Calcium levels in the ECF are only one of the many parameters under constant, careful adjustment by the homeostatic mechanisms of the body.

Intracellular fluid

The composition of intracellular fluid (ICF) is largely controlled by the cell itself, because there are selective uptake and discharge mechanisms present in the cell membrane. The composition of ICF can therefore be very different from ECF. Thus, sodium levels are nearly ten times higher in the ECF than in the ICF. This concentration difference occurs because although sodium diffuses into the cell down its concentration gradient there is a pump in the membrane which selectively pumps it back out again. This concentration gradient is essential for the function of excitable cells (mainly nerve and muscle). Conversely, many substances are found inside the cell in significantly higher amounts than outside, e.g. ATP, protein and potassium.

3

The cells, tissues and organisation of the body

Cells are the smallest functional units of the body. They are grouped together to form *tissues*, each of which has a specialised function, e.g. blood, muscle, bone. Different tissues are grouped together to form *organs*, e.g. heart, stomach, brain. Organs are grouped together to form *systems*, each of which performs a particular function that maintains homeostasis and contributes to the health of the individual (p. 5). For example, the digestive system is responsible for taking in, digesting and absorbing food and involves a number of organs, including the stomach and intestines.

THE CELL: STRUCTURE AND FUNCTIONS

Learning outcomes

After studying this section you should be able to:

- describe the structure of the plasma membrane

- explain the functions of the following organelles: nucleus, mitochondria, ribosomes, endoplasmic reticulum, Golgi apparatus, lysosomes, microtubules and microfilaments

- outline the two types of cell division

- define the term 'mutation'

- compare and contrast active, passive and bulk transport of substances across cell membranes.

The human body develops from a single cell called the *zygote*, which results from the fusion of the ovum (female egg cell) and the spermatozoon (male germ cell). Cell multiplication follows and, as the fetus grows, cells with different structural and functional specialisations develop, all with the same genetic make-up as the zygote. Individual cells are too small to be seen with the naked eye. However, they can be seen when thin slices of tissue are stained in the laboratory and magnified by a microscope.

A cell consists of a *plasma membrane* inside which there are a number of *organelles* floating in a watery fluid called *cytosol* (Fig. 3.1). Organelles are small structures with highly specialised functions, many of which are contained within a membrane. They include: the *nucleus, mitochondria, ribosomes, endoplasmic reticulum, Golgi apparatus, lysosomes, microfilaments* and *microtubules*.

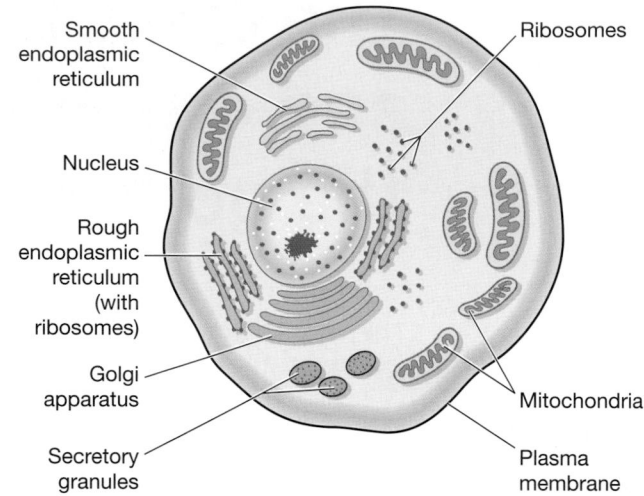

Figure 3.1 The simple cell.

Figure 3.2 The plasma membrane.

Plasma membrane

The plasma membrane (Fig. 3.2) consists of two layers of phospholipids (fatty substances (p. 24)) with some protein molecules embedded in them. Those that extend all the way through the membrane may provide channels that allow the passage of, for example, electrolytes and non-lipid-soluble substances.

The phospholipid molecules have a head which is electrically charged and *hydrophilic* (meaning 'water loving') and a tail which has no charge and is *hydrophobic* (meaning 'water hating'). The phospholipid bilayer is arranged like a sandwich with the hydrophilic heads aligned on the outer surfaces of the membrane and the hydrophobic tails forming a central water-repelling layer. These differences influence the transfer of substances across the membrane.

The membrane proteins perform several functions:

- branched carbohydrate molecules attached to the outside of some membrane protein molecules give the cell its immunological identity
- they can act as specific receptors for hormones and other chemical messengers
- some are enzymes
- some are involved in transport across the membrane.

Organelles

Nucleus

Every cell in the body has a nucleus, with the exception of mature erythrocytes (red blood cells). Skeletal muscle and some other cells contain several nuclei. The nucleus is the largest organelle and is contained within a membrane similar to the plasma membrane but it has tiny pores through which some substances can pass between it and the *cytoplasm*, i.e. the cell contents excluding the nucleus.

The nucleus contains the body's genetic material, which directs the activities of the cell. This is built from DNA (p. 24) and proteins called *histones* coiled together forming a fine network of threads called *chromatin*. Chromatin resembles tiny strings of beads. During cell division the chromatin replicates and becomes more tightly coiled forming *chromosomes* (Fig. 3.3).

The functional subunits of chromosomes are called *genes*. Each cell contains the total complement of genes required to synthesise all the proteins in the body but most cells synthesise only the defined range of proteins that are appropriate to their own specialised functions. This means that only part of the *genome* or genetic code is used by each cell. Metabolic processes occur in a series of steps, each of which is catalysed by a specific enzyme (p. 26) and each enzyme can be produced only if the controlling gene is present. This is the 'one gene, one enzyme' concept. Therefore, when a gene is missing the associated enzyme is also missing and the chemical change it should catalyse does not occur (Fig. 3.4). This means that the intermediate metabolite upon which the enzyme should act accumulates. In physiological quantities such metabolites are harmless but when they accumulate they may become toxic. There are a number of diseases caused by such inborn errors of metabolism, e.g. phenylketonuria, abnormal haemoglobin and some immune deficiencies (see later chapters).

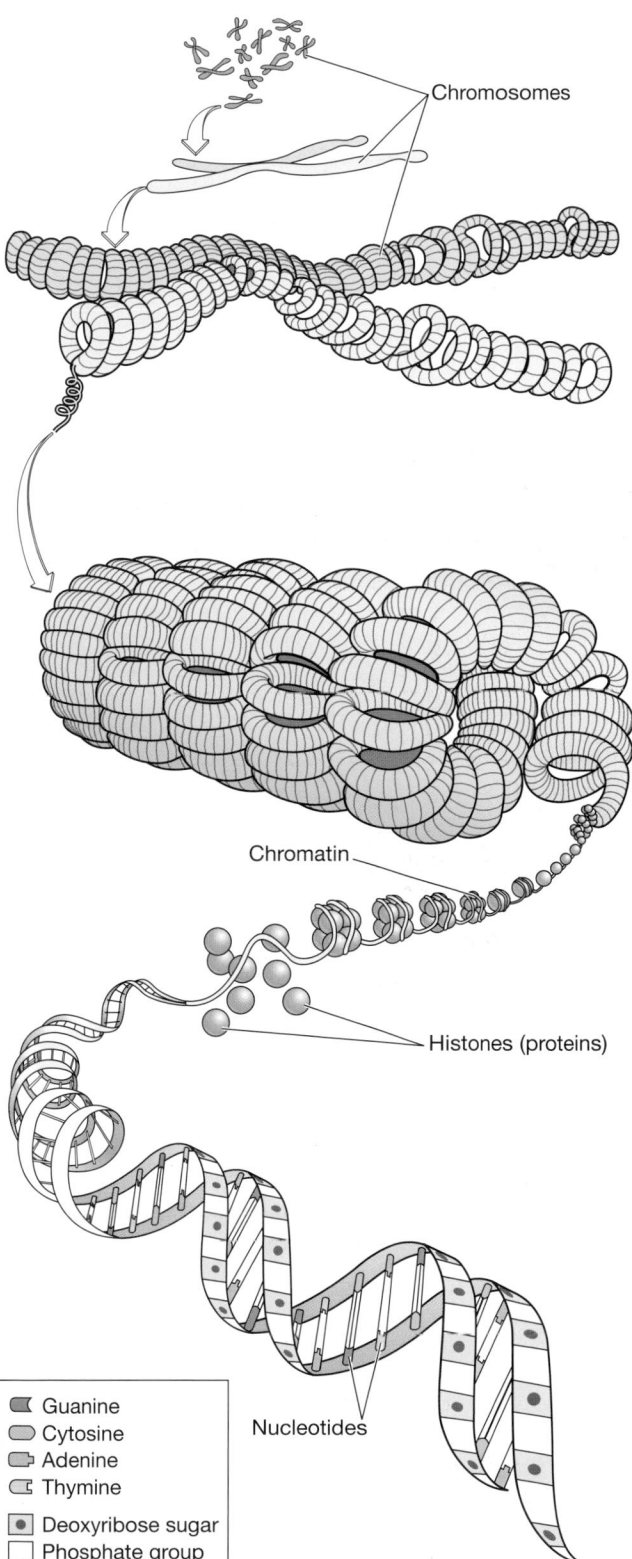

Chromosomes

Chromatin

Histones (proteins)

	Guanine
	Cytosine
	Adenine
	Thymine
	Deoxyribose sugar
	Phosphate group

Nucleotides

Figure 3.3 The structural relationship between DNA, chromatin and chromosomes.

31

Figure 3.4 The relationship between genes, enzymes and protein synthesis: A. Enzyme synthesised. B. Effect when enzyme not synthesised.

Mitochondria

Mitochondria are sausage-shaped structures in the cytoplasm, sometimes described as the 'power house' of the cell. They are involved in aerobic respiration, the processes by which chemical energy is made available in the cell. This is in the form of ATP, which releases energy when the cell breaks it down (see Fig. 2.12, p. 25). Synthesis of ATP is most efficient in the final stages of aerobic respiration, a process requiring oxygen (p. 315).

Ribosomes

These are tiny granules composed of RNA and protein. They synthesise proteins from amino acids, using RNA as the template (see Fig. 2.11, p. 25). When present in free units or in small clusters in the cytoplasm, the ribosomes make proteins for use within the cell. Ribosomes are also found on the outer surface of rough endoplasmic reticulum (see below).

Endoplasmic reticulum (ER)

Endoplasmic reticulum is a series of interconnecting membranous canals in the cytoplasm. There are two types: smooth and rough. Smooth ER synthesises lipids and steroid hormones, and is also associated with the detoxification of some drugs. Rough ER is studded with ribosomes. These are the site of synthesis of proteins that are 'exported' (extruded) from cells, i.e. enzymes and hormones that pass out of their parent cell to be used by other cells in the body.

Golgi apparatus

The Golgi apparatus consists of stacks of closely folded flattened membranous sacs. It is present in all cells but is larger in those that synthesise and export proteins. The proteins move from the endoplasmic reticulum to the Golgi apparatus where they are 'packaged' into membrane-bound vesicles called *secretory granules*. The vesicles are stored and, when needed, move to the plasma membrane, through which the proteins are exported.

Lysosomes

Lysosomes are one type of secretory vesicle formed by the Golgi apparatus. They contain a variety of enzymes involved in breaking down fragments of organelles and large molecules (e.g. RNA, DNA, carbohydrates, proteins) inside the cell into smaller particles that are either recycled, or extruded from the cell as waste material.

Lysosomes in white blood cells contain enzymes that digest foreign material such as microbes.

Microfilaments and microtubules

Microfilaments. These are tiny strands of protein that provide structural support and maintain the characteristic shape of the cell.

Microtubules. These are contractile protein structures in the cytoplasm involved in the movement of the cell and of organelles within the cell, the movement of cilia (small projections from the free border of some cells) and possibly the organisation of proteins in the plasma membrane.

Cell division (Fig. 3.5)

There are two types of cell division: *mitosis* and *meiosis*.

Mitosis

Beginning with the fertilised egg, or zygote, cell division is an ongoing process. As the fetus develops in the mother's uterus, its cells multiply and grow into all the specialities that provide the sum total of the body's physiological functions. The life span of most individual cells is limited. Many become worn out and die, and are replaced by identical cells by the process of mitosis.

Mitosis occurs in two stages: replication of DNA, in the form of 23 pairs of chromosomes, then division of the cytoplasm. DNA is the only type of molecule capable of independently forming a duplicate of itself. When the two identical sets of chromosomes have moved to the opposite poles of the parent cell, a 'waist' forms in the cytoplasm, and the cell divides. There is then a complete

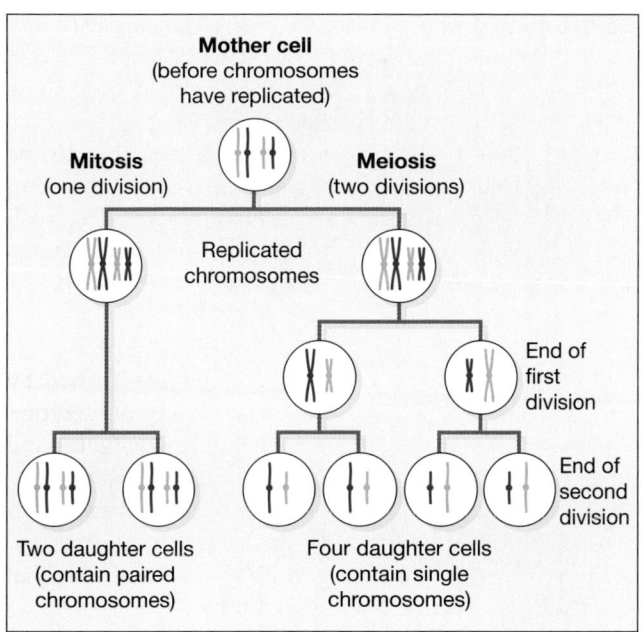

Figure 3.5 Cell division. Simplified diagram of mitosis and meiosis.

set of chromosomes in each daughter cell. The organelles in the cytoplasm of the daughter cells are incomplete at cell division but they develop as the cell grows to maturity.

The frequency with which cell division occurs varies with different types of cell (p. 42).

Meiosis

This is the process of cell division that occurs in the formation of reproductive cells (*gametes* — the ova and spermatozoa). The ova grow to maturity in the ovaries of the female and the spermatozoa in the testes of the male. In meiosis four daughter cells are formed after two divisions. During meiosis the pairs of chromosomes separate and one from each pair moves to opposite poles of the 'parent' cell. When it divides, each of the 'daughter' cells has only 23 chromosomes, called the *haploid number*. This means that when the ovum is fertilised the resultant zygote has the full complement of 46 chromosomes (the *diploid number*), half from the father and half from the mother. Thus the child has some characteristics inherited from the mother and some from the father, such as colour of hair and eyes, height, facial features, and some diseases.

Determination of sex depends upon one particular pair of chromosomes: the *sex chromosomes*. In the female both sex chromosomes are the same size and shape and are called X chromosomes. In the male there is one X chromosome and a slightly smaller Y chromosome. When the ovum is fertilised by an X-bearing spermatozoon the child is female and when it is fertilised by a Y-bearing spermatozoon the child is male.

Sperm X + ovum X → child XX = female
Sperm Y + ovum X → child XY = male

Mutation

Cells are said to mutate when their genetic make-up is altered in any way. Mutation may cause:

- no significant change in cell function
- modification of cell function that may cause physiological abnormality but does not prevent cell growth and multiplication, e.g. inborn errors of metabolism, defective blood clotting
- the death of the cell.

Some mutations occur by chance, which may be accounted for by the countless millions of cell divisions and DNA replications that occur in the body throughout life. Others may be caused by extraneous factors, such as X-rays, ultraviolet rays or some chemicals.

The most important mutations are those that occur in the ova and spermatozoa. Genetic changes in these cells are passed on to subsequent generations although they do not affect the parent.

Transport of substances across cell membranes

Passive transport

This occurs when substances can cross plasma and organelle (semipermeable) membranes and move down the concentration gradient (downhill) without using energy.

Diffusion

This was described on page 26. Small substances diffuse down the concentration gradient crossing membranes by:

- dissolving in the lipid part of the membrane, e.g. lipid-soluble substances: oxygen, carbon dioxide, fatty acids, steroids
- passing through water-filled channels, or pores in the membrane, e.g. small water-soluble substances: sodium, potassium, calcium.

Facilitated diffusion

This passive process is utilised by some substances that are unable to diffuse through the semipermeable membrane unaided, e.g. glucose, amino acids. Specialised protein carrier molecules in the membrane have specific sites that attract and bind substances to be transferred,

33

like a lock and key mechanism. The carrier then changes its shape and deposits the substance on the other side of the membrane (Fig. 3.6). The carrier sites are specific and can be used by only one substance. As there are a finite number of carriers, there is a limit to the amount of a substance which can be transported at any time. This is known as the *transport maximum*.

Osmosis

Osmosis is passive movement of water *down its concentration gradient* towards equilibrium across a semipermeable membrane and is explained on page 27.

Active transport

This is the transport of substances *up their concentration gradient* (uphill), i.e. from a lower to a higher concentration. Chemical energy in the form of ATP (p. 25) drives specialised protein carrier molecules that transport substances across the membrane in either direction (see Fig. 3.6). The carrier sites are specific and can be used by only one substance; therefore the rate at which a substance is transferred depends on the number of sites available.

The sodium pump

This active transport mechanism maintains homeostasis of the electrolytes sodium (Na^+) and potassium (K^+). It may utilise up to 30% of the ATP required for cellular metabolism.

The principal cations are: K^+ intracellularly and Na^+ extracellularly. There is a tendency for these ions to diffuse down their concentration gradients, K^+ outwards and Na^+ into the cell. Homeostasis is maintained as excess Na^+ is pumped out across the cell membrane in exchange for K^+.

Bulk transport (Fig. 3.7)

Transfer of particles too large to cross cell membranes occurs by *pinocytosis* or *phagocytosis*. These particles are

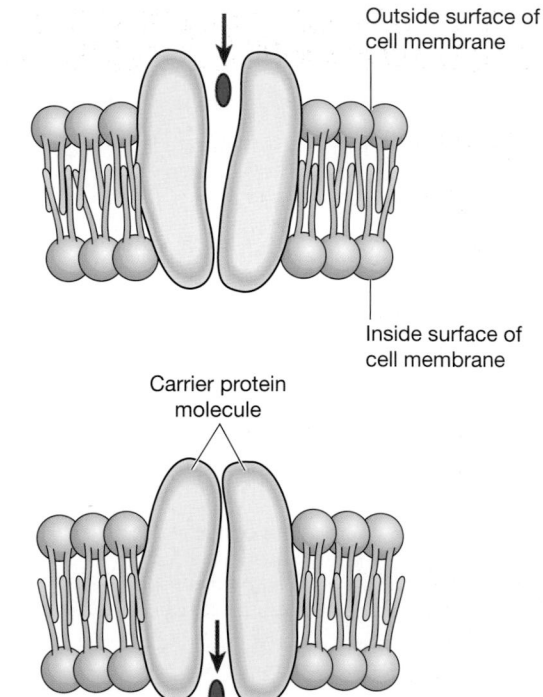

Figure 3.6 Specialised protein carrier molecules involved in facilitated diffusion and active transport.

engulfed by extensions of the cytoplasm which enclose them, forming a membrane-bound vacuole. When the vacuole is small, pinocytosis occurs. In phagocytosis larger particles, e.g. cell fragments, foreign materials, microbes, are taken into the cell. Lysosomes then adhere to the vacuole membrane, releasing enzymes which digest the contents.

Extrusion of waste material by the reverse process through the plasma membrane is called *exocytosis*. Secretory granules formed by the Golgi apparatus usually leave the cell in this way, as do any indigestible residues of phagocytosis.

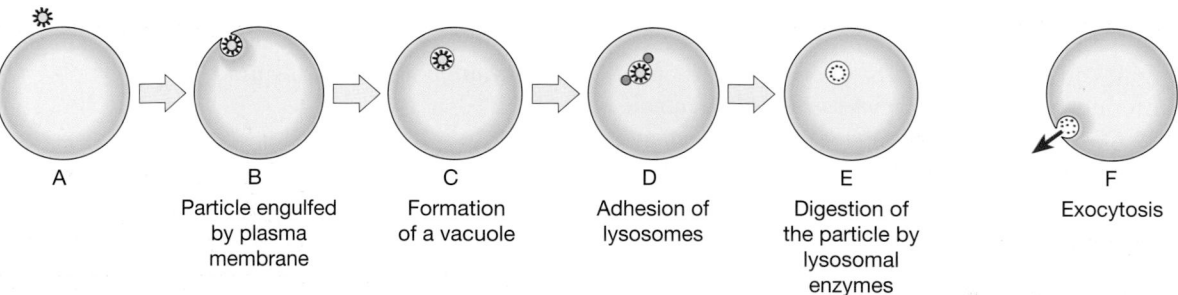

A	B	C	D	E	F
	Particle engulfed by plasma membrane	Formation of a vacuole	Adhesion of lysosomes	Digestion of the particle by lysosomal enzymes	Exocytosis

Figure 3.7 Bulk transport across plasma membranes: A–E. Phagocytosis. F. Exocytosis.

TISSUES

The tissues of the body consist of large numbers of cells and they are classified according to the size, shape and functions of these cells. There are four main types of tissue, each of which has subdivisions.

They are:

- epithelial tissue or epithelium
- connective tissue
- muscle tissue
- nervous tissue.

Epithelial tissue

This group of tissues is found covering the body and lining cavities and tubes. It is also found in glands. The structure of epithelium is closely related to its functions which include:

- protection of underlying structures from, for example, dehydration, chemical and mechanical damage
- secretion
- absorption.

The cells are very closely packed and the intercellular substance, called the *matrix*, is minimal. The cells usually lie on a *basement membrane*, which is an inert connective tissue.

Epithelial tissue may be:

- *simple*: a single layer of cells
- *stratified*: several layers of cells.

Simple epithelium

Simple epithelium consists of a single layer of identical cells and is divided into four types. It is usually found on

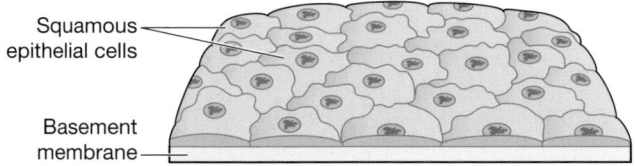

Figure 3.8 Squamous epithelium.

absorptive or secretory surfaces, where the single layer enhances these processes, and not usually on surfaces subject to stress. The types are named according to the shape of the cells, which differs according to their functions. The more active the tissue, the taller are the cells.

Squamous (pavement) epithelium

This is composed of a single layer of flattened cells (Fig. 3.8). The cells fit closely together like flat stones, forming a thin and very smooth membrane.

Diffusion takes place freely through this thin, smooth, inactive lining of the following structures:

- heart ⎫ where it is
- blood vessels ⎬ also known as
- lymph vessels ⎭ endothelium
- alveoli of the lungs.

Cuboidal (cubical) epithelium

This consists of cube-shaped cells fitting closely together lying on a basement membrane (Fig. 3.9). It forms the tubules of the kidneys and is found in some glands. Cuboidal epithelium is actively involved in secretion, absorption and excretion.

Columnar epithelium

This is formed by a single layer of cells, rectangular in shape, on a basement membrane (Fig. 3.10). It is found

Figure 3.9 Cuboidal epithelium.

Figure 3.10 Columnar epithelium.

Figure 3.11 Ciliated columnar epithelium.

lining the organs of the alimentary tract and consists of a mixture of cells; some absorb the products of digestion and others secrete *mucus*. Mucus is a thick sticky substance secreted by modified columnar cells called *goblet cells*.

Ciliated epithelium (Fig. 3.11)

This is formed by columnar cells each of which has many fine, hair-like processes, called *cilia*. The cilia consist of microtubules inside the plasma membrane that extends from the free border (luminal border) of the columnar cells. The wave-like movement of many cilia propels the contents of the tubes, which they line in one direction only.

Ciliated epithelium is found lining the uterine tubes and most of the respiratory passages. In the uterine tubes the cilia propel ova towards the uterus (Ch. 19) and in the respiratory passages they propel mucus towards the throat (Ch. 10).

Stratified epithelia

Stratified epithelia consist of several layers of cells of various shapes. The superficial layers grow up from below. Basement membranes are usually absent. The main function of stratified epithelium is to protect underlying structures from mechanical wear and tear. There are two main types: stratified squamous and transitional.

Stratified squamous epithelium (Fig. 3.12)

This is composed of a number of layers of cells of different shapes representing newly formed and mature cells. In the deepest layers the cells are mainly columnar and, as they grow towards the surface, they become flattened and are then shed.

Non-keratinised stratified epithelium. This is found on wet surfaces that may be subjected to wear and tear but are protected from drying, e.g. the conjunctiva of the eyes, the lining of the mouth, the pharynx, the oesophagus and the vagina.

Figure 3.12 Stratified epithelium.

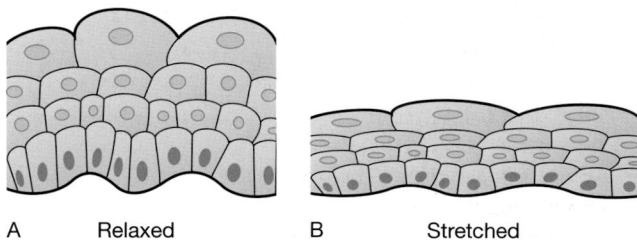

A Relaxed   B Stretched

Figure 3.13 Transitional epithelium: A. Relaxed. B. Stretched.

Keratinised stratified epithelium. This is found on dry surfaces that are subjected to wear and tear, i.e. skin, hair and nails. The surface layer consists of dead epithelial cells to which the protein keratin has been added. This forms a tough, relatively waterproof protective layer that prevents drying of the underlying live cells. The surface layer of skin is rubbed off and is replaced from below (Ch. 14).

Transitional epithelium (Fig. 3.13)

This is composed of several layers of pear-shaped cells and is found lining the urinary bladder. It allows for stretching as the bladder fills.

Connective tissue

Connective tissue is the most abundant tissue in the body. The cells forming the connective tissues are more widely separated from each other than those forming the epithelium, and intercellular substance (matrix) is present in considerably larger amounts. There may or may not be fibres present in the matrix, which may be of a semisolid jelly-like consistency or dense and rigid, depending upon the position and function of the tissue.

Major functions of connective tissue are:

- binding and structural support
- protection
- transport
- insulation.

Cells of connective tissue

Connective tissue, excluding blood (Ch. 4), is found in all organs supporting the specialised tissue. The different types of cell involved include:

- fibroblasts
- fat cells
- macrophages
- leukocytes
- mast cells.

Fibroblasts. Fibroblasts are large flat cells with irregular processes. They produce *collagen* and *elastic fibres* and a matrix of extracellular material. Very fine collagen fibres, sometimes called *reticulin fibres*, are found in very active tissue, such as the liver and lymphoid tissue. Fibroblasts are particularly active in tissue repair (wound healing) where they may bind together the cut surfaces of wounds or form *granulation tissue* following tissue destruction (see p. 367). The collagen fibres formed during healing shrink as they grow old, sometimes interfering with the functions of the organ involved and with adjacent structures.

Fat cells. Also known as *adipocytes* these cells occur singly or in groups in many types of connective tissue and are especially abundant in adipose tissue. They vary in size and shape according to the amount of fat they contain.

Macrophages. These are irregular-shaped cells with granules in the cytoplasm. Some are fixed, i.e. attached to connective tissue fibres, and others are motile. They are an important part of the body's defence mechanisms as they are actively phagocytic, engulfing and digesting cell debris, bacteria and other foreign bodies. Their activities are typical of those of the macrophage/monocyte defence system, e.g. monocytes in blood, phagocytes in the alveoli of the lungs, Kupffer cells in liver sinusoids, fibroblasts in lymph nodes and spleen and microglial cells in the brain.

Leukocytes. White blood cells (p. 64) are normally found in small numbers in healthy connective tissue but migrate in significant numbers during infection when they play an important part in tissue defence. *Lymphocytes* synthesise and secrete specific *antibodies* into the blood in the presence of foreign material, such as microbes (Ch. 15).

Figure 3.14 Loose (areolar) connective tissue.

Mast cells. These cells are similar to basophil leukocytes (see p. 66). They are found in loose connective tissue and under the fibrous capsule of some organs, e.g. liver and spleen, and in considerable numbers round blood vessels. They produce granules containing *heparin*, *histamine* and other substances, which are released when the cells are damaged by disease or injury. Histamine is involved in local and general inflammatory reactions, it stimulates the secretion of gastric juice and is associated with the development of allergies and hypersensitivity states (see p. 383). Heparin prevents coagulation of blood, which may aid the passage of protective substances from blood to affected tissues.

Loose (areolar) connective tissue (Fig. 3.14).

This is the most generalised of all connective tissue. The matrix is described as semisolid with many fibroblasts and some fat cells, mast cells and macrophages widely separated by elastic and collagen fibres. It is found in almost every part of the body providing elasticity and tensile strength. It connects and supports other tissues, for example:

- under the skin
- between muscles
- supporting blood vessels and nerves
- in the alimentary canal
- in glands supporting secretory cells.

Adipose tissue (Fig. 3.15).

Adipose tissue consists of fat cells (adipocytes), containing large fat globules, in a matrix of areolar tissue. There are two types: white and brown.

White adipose tissue. This makes up 20 to 25% of body weight in well-nourished adults. The amount of adipose

Figure 3.15 Adipose tissue.

Figure 3.16 Fibrous tissue.

Figure 3.17 Elastic tissue.

tissue in an individual is determined by the balance between energy intake and expenditure. It is found supporting the kidneys and the eyes, between muscle fibres and under the skin, where it acts as a thermal insulator.

Brown adipose tissue. This is present in the newborn. It has a more extensive capillary network than white adipose tissue. When brown tissue is metabolised, it produces less energy and considerably more heat than other fat, contributing to the maintenance of body temperature. In adults it is present in only small amounts.

Dense connective tissue

Fibrous tissue (Fig. 3.16)
This tissue is made up mainly of closely packed bundles of collagen fibres with very little matrix. Fibrocytes (old and inactive fibroblasts) are few in number and are found lying in rows between the bundles of fibres. Fibrous tissue is found:

- forming the ligaments, which bind bones together
- as an outer protective covering for bone, called *periosteum*

- as an outer protective covering of some organs, e.g. the kidneys, lymph nodes and the brain
- forming muscle sheaths, called *muscle fascia*, which extend beyond the muscle to become the tendon that attaches the muscle to bone.

Elastic tissue (Fig. 3.17)
Elastic tissue is capable of considerable extension and recoil. There are few cells and the matrix consists mainly of masses of *elastic fibres* secreted by fibroblasts. It is found in organs where alteration of shape is required, e.g. in large blood vessel walls, the epiglottis and the outer ears.

Blood

This is a fluid connective tissue and is described in detail in Chapter 4.

Lymphoid tissue (Fig. 3.18)

This tissue has a semisolid matrix with fine branching reticulin fibres. It contains white blood cells (*monocytes* and *lymphocytes*). They are found in blood and in lymphoid tissue in the:

- lymph nodes
- spleen
- palatine and pharyngeal tonsils
- vermiform appendix
- solitary and aggregated nodes in the small intestine
- wall of the large intestine.

Cartilage

Cartilage is a much firmer tissue than any of the other connective tissues; the cells are called *chondrocytes* and are less numerous. They are embedded in matrix reinforced by collagen and elastic fibres. There are three types:

- hyaline cartilage
- fibrocartilage
- elastic fibrocartilage.

Hyaline cartilage (Fig. 3.19)

Hyaline cartilage appears as a smooth bluish-white tissue. The chondrocytes are in small groups within cell nests and the matrix is solid and smooth. Hyaline cartilage is found:

- on the surface of the parts of the bones that form joints
- forming the costal cartilages, which attach the ribs to the sternum
- forming part of the larynx, trachea and bronchi.

Fibrocartilage (Fig. 3.20)

This consists of dense masses of white collagen fibres in a matrix similar to that of hyaline cartilage with the cells widely dispersed. It is a tough, slightly flexible tissue found:

- as pads between the bodies of the vertebrae, called the intervertebral discs
- between the articulating surfaces of the bones of the knee joint, called semilunar cartilages
- on the rim of the bony sockets of the hip and shoulder joints, deepening the cavities without restricting movement
- as ligaments joining bones.

Elastic cartilage (Fig. 3.21)

This flexible tissue consists of yellow elastic fibres lying in a solid matrix. The cells lie between the fibres. It forms the pinna or lobe of the ear, the epiglottis and part of the tunica media of blood vessel walls.

Bone

Bone is a connective tissue with cells (osteocytes) surrounded by a matrix of collagen fibres that is strengthened by inorganic salts, especially calcium and phosphate. This provides bones with their characteristic strength and rigidity. Bone also has considerable capacity for growth in the first two decades of life, and for regeneration throughout life. Two types of bone can be identified by the naked eye:

Figure 3.18 Lymphoid tissue.

Reticular cell
White blood cells
Reticulin fibres
Lymph spaces

Figure 3.20 Fibrocartilage.

Collagen fibre
Chondrocyte

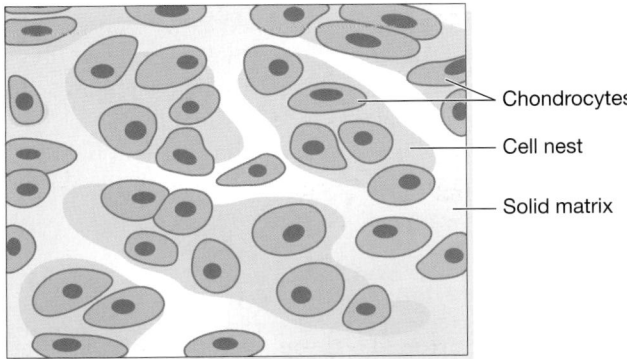

Figure 3.19 Hyaline cartilage.

Chondrocytes
Cell nest
Solid matrix

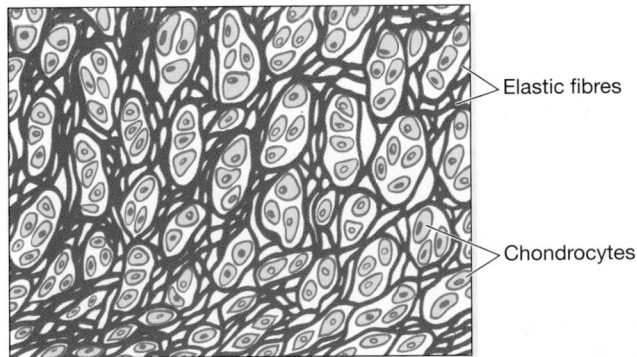

Figure 3.21 Elastic fibrocartilage.

Elastic fibres
Chondrocytes

39

- *compact bone* — solid or dense appearance
- *cancellous or spongy bone* — spongy or fine honeycomb appearance.

These are described in detail in Chapter 16.

Muscle tissue

There are three types of muscle tissue, which consists of specialised contractile cells:

- skeletal muscle
- smooth muscle
- cardiac muscle.

Skeletal muscle tissue (Fig. 3.22)
This may be described as *skeletal, striated, striped* or *voluntary* muscle. It is called voluntary because contraction is under conscious control.

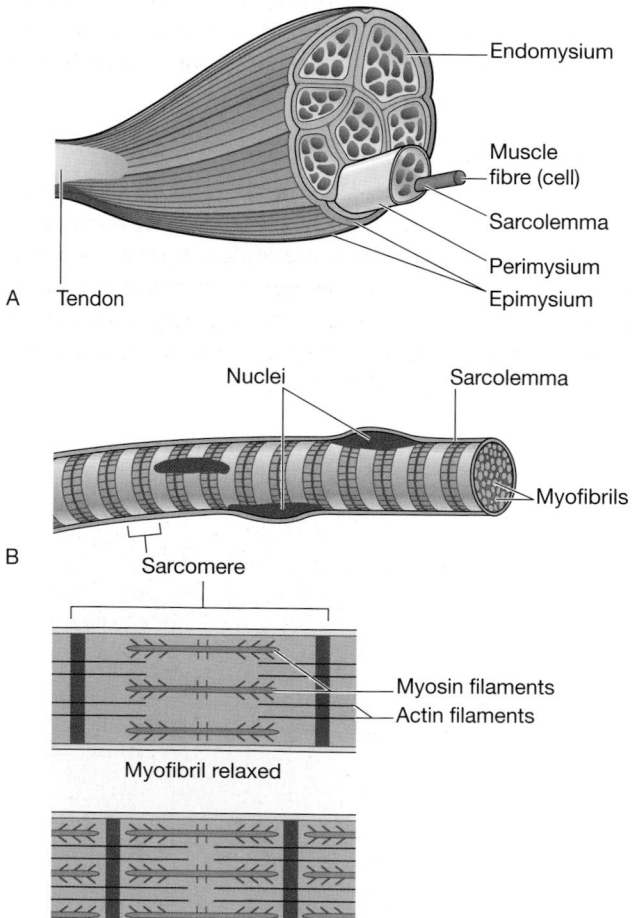

A Tendon
- Endomysium
- Muscle fibre (cell)
- Sarcolemma
- Perimysium
- Epimysium

B
- Nuclei
- Sarcolemma
- Myofibrils
Sarcomere

- Myosin filaments
- Actin filaments
Myofibril relaxed

C   Myofibril contracted

Figure 3.22 Organisation within a skeletal muscle: A. A skeletal muscle and its connective tissue. B. A muscle fibre (cell). C. A myofibril: relaxed and contracted.

When skeletal muscle is examined microscopically the cells are found to be roughly cylindrical in shape and may be as long as 35 cm. Each cell, commonly called a fibre, has several nuclei situated just under the *sarcolemma* or cell membrane of each muscle fibre. The muscle fibres lie parallel to one another and, when viewed under the microscope, they show well-marked transverse dark and light bands, hence the name striated or striped muscle.

Sarcoplasm, the cytoplasm of muscle fibres, contains:

- bundles of *myofibrils*, which consist of filaments of contractile proteins including *actin* and *myosin*
- many mitochondria, which generate chemical energy (ATP) from glucose and oxygen by aerobic respiration
- *glycogen*, a carbohydrate store which is broken down into glucose when required
- *myoglobin*, a unique oxygen-binding protein molecule, similar to haemoglobin in red blood cells, which stores oxygen within muscle cells.

A myofibril has a repeating series of dark and light bands, consisting of units called *sarcomeres*. A sarcomere represents the smallest functional unit of a skeletal muscle fibre and consists of:

- thin filaments of actin
- thick filaments of myosin.

The *sliding filament theory* explains the finding that sarcomeres shorten but the filaments remain the same length when skeletal muscle contracts. The thin actin filaments slide past the thick myosin filaments, increasing the overlap of the filaments when contraction takes place. The movement of filaments occurs as chemical cross-bridges are formed and broken, moving the actin filaments towards the centre of the sarcomere during contraction. As the sarcomeres shorten, so does the skeletal muscle involved. When the muscle relaxes the cross-bridges break, the filaments slide apart and the sarcomeres return to their original length (Fig. 3.22C).

A muscle consists of a large number of muscle fibres. In addition to the sarcolemma mentioned previously, each fibre is enclosed in and attached to fine fibrous connective tissue called *endomysium*. Small bundles of fibres are enclosed in *perimysium*, and the whole muscle in *epimysium*. The fibrous tissue enclosing the fibres, the bundles and the whole muscle extends beyond the muscle fibres to become the *tendon*, which attaches the muscle to bone or skin.

Smooth (visceral) muscle tissue (Fig. 3.23)
Smooth muscle may also be described as *non-striated* or *involuntary*. It is not under conscious control. It is found in the walls of hollow organs:

- regulating the diameter of blood vessels and parts of the respiratory tract
- propelling contents of the ureters, ducts of glands and alimentary tract
- expelling contents of the urinary bladder and uterus.

When examined under a microscope, the cells are seen to be spindle shaped with only one central nucleus. There is no distinct sarcolemma but a very fine membrane surrounds each fibre. Bundles of fibres form sheets of muscle, such as those found in the walls of the above structures.

Cardiac muscle tissue (Fig. 3.24)

This type of muscle tissue is found exclusively in the wall of the heart. It is not under conscious control but, when viewed under a microscope, cross-stripes characteristic of voluntary muscle can be seen. Each fibre (cell) has a nucleus and one or more branches. The ends of the cells and their branches are in very close contact with the ends and branches of adjacent cells. Microscopically these 'joints', or *intercalated discs*, can be seen as lines which are thicker and darker than the ordinary cross-stripes. This arrangement gives cardiac muscle the appearance of a sheet of muscle rather than a very large number of individual fibres. The end-to-end continuity of cardiac muscle cells has significance in relation to the way the heart contracts. A wave of contraction spreads from cell to cell across the intercalated discs which means that cells do not need to be stimulated individually.

Function of muscle tissue

Muscle functions by alternate phases of contraction and relaxation. When the fibres contract they become thicker and shorter. Skeletal muscle fibres are stimulated by *motor nerve impulses* originating in the brain or spinal cord (p. 151 and p. 158) and ending at the *neuromuscular junction* (p. 145). Smooth and cardiac muscle have the intrinsic ability to initiate contraction. In addition,

contraction is stimulated by *autonomic nerve impulses*, some hormones and local metabolites. When muscle fibres contract they follow the *all or none law*; i.e. each fibre contracts to its full capacity or not at all. The *strength* of contraction, e.g. lifting a weight, depends on the *number* of fibres contracting at the same time. When effort is sustained, groups of fibres contract in series. Contraction of smooth muscle is slower and more sustained than skeletal muscle.

In order to contract when it is stimulated, a muscle fibre must have an adequate blood supply to provide sufficient oxygen, calcium and nutritional materials and to remove waste products.

Muscle tone

This is a state of partial contraction of muscles. It is achieved by the contraction of a few muscle fibres at a time. Skeletal muscle tone is essential for maintenance of posture in the sitting and standing positions. The muscle is stimulated to contract through a system of *spinal reflexes*. Stretching of a muscle or its tendon stimulates the reflex action (Ch. 7). A degree of muscle tone is also maintained by smooth and cardiac muscle.

Muscle fatigue

If a muscle is stimulated to contract at very frequent intervals, its response gradually becomes depressed and will in time cease. Fatigue is prevented during sustained muscular effort because the fibres usually contract in series. All the fibres of a muscle rarely contract at the same time but if maximum effort is made it can be sustained, if for only a short time.

Figure 3.23 Smooth muscle fibres.

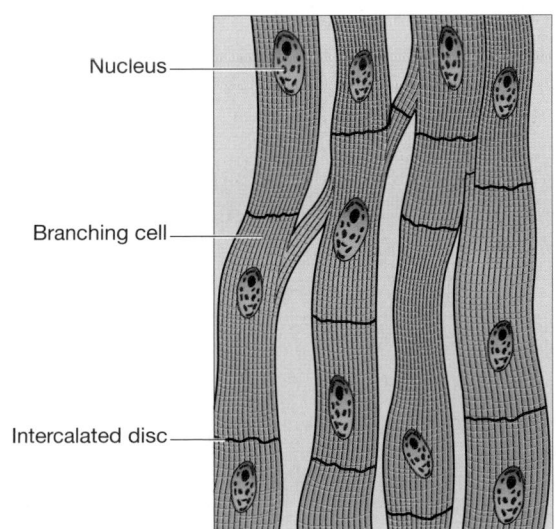

Nucleus

Branching cell

Intercalated disc

Figure 3.24 Cardiac muscle fibres.

Energy source for muscle contraction

The chemical energy (ATP) which muscles require is usually derived from the breakdown (catabolism) of carbohydrate and fat. Protein molecules inside the fibres are used to provide energy when supplies of carbohydrate and fat are deficient. Each molecule undergoes a series of changes and, with each change, small quantities of energy are released. For the complete breakdown of these molecules and the release of all the available energy an adequate supply of oxygen is required. If the individual undertakes excessive exercise, the oxygen supply may be insufficient to meet the metabolic needs of the muscle fibres. This may result in the accumulation of intermediate metabolic products, such as lactic acid. Where the breakdown process and the release of energy are complete, the waste products are carbon dioxide and water (Ch. 12).

Not all the chemical energy (ATP) used by muscle fibres is converted into mechanical energy during contraction. Some is lost as heat.

Further features of skeletal muscle

The skeletal muscles are those which produce body movements. Each muscle consists of a fleshy part made up of striped fibres and tendinous parts consisting of fibrous tissue, usually at both ends of the fleshy part. The muscle is attached to bone or skin by these tendons. When the tendinous attachment of a muscle is broad and flat it is called an *aponeurosis*.

To be able to produce movement at a joint, a muscle or its tendon must stretch across the joint. When a muscle contracts, its fibres shorten and it pulls one bone towards another, e.g. bending the elbow.

The muscles of the skeleton are arranged in groups, some of which are *antagonistic* to each other. To produce movement at a joint, one muscle or group of muscles contracts while the antagonists relax; e.g. to bend the knee the muscles on the back of the thigh contract and those on the front relax. The constant adjustment of the contraction and relaxation of antagonistic groups of muscles is well demonstrated in the maintenance of balance and posture when sitting and standing. These adjustments usually occur without conscious effort.

Individual muscles and groups of muscles have been given names that reflect certain characteristics, e.g.:

- the *shape* of the muscle — the trapezius is shaped like a trapezium
- the *direction* in which the fibres run — the oblique muscles of the abdominal wall
- the *position* of the muscle — the tibialis in the leg is associated with the tibia

- the *movement* produced by contraction of the muscle — flexors, extensors, adductors
- the *number of points of attachment* of a muscle — the biceps muscle has two tendons at one end
- the *names of the bones to which the muscle is attached* — the carpi radialis muscles are attached to the carpal bones in the wrist and to the radius in the forearm.

A more detailed description of skeletal muscles is given in Chapters 17 and 18.

Nervous tissue

Two types of tissue are found in the nervous system:

- *excitable cells* — these are called neurones and they initiate, receive, conduct and transmit information
- *non-excitable cells* — these support the neurones.

These are described in detail in Chapter 7.

Tissue regeneration

When tissue regeneration occurs it is essential that some of the original cells are available to replicate by mitosis. The extent to which regeneration is possible depends on the normal rate of physiological turnover of particular types of cell. Those with a rapid turnover regenerate most effectively. There are three types.

Labile cells. Labile cells are those in which replication is normally a continuous process. They include cells in:

- epithelium of e.g. skin, mucous membrane, secretory glands, ducts, uterus lining
- bone marrow
- blood
- spleen and lymphoid tissue.

Stable cells. Stable cells have retained the ability to replicate but do so infrequently.
They include:

- liver, kidney and pancreatic cells
- fibroblasts
- smooth muscle cells
- osteoblasts and osteoclasts in bone.

Permanent cells. Permanent cells are unable to replicate after normal growth is complete. They include:

- nerve cells (neurones)
- skeletal and cardiac muscle.

Membranes

Membranes are sheets of epithelial tissue and their supporting connective tissue that cover or line internal structures or cavities. The main membranes are:

- mucous
- serous
- synovial.

Mucous membrane

This is the moist lining of the alimentary tract, respiratory tract and genitourinary tracts and is sometimes referred to as the *mucosa*. The membrane consists of epithelial cells, some of which produce a secretion called *mucus*, a slimy tenacious fluid. As it accumulates the cells become distended and finally burst, discharging the mucus on to the free surface. As the cells fill up with mucus they have the appearance of a goblet or flask and are known as *goblet cells* (Fig. 3.25). Organs lined by mucous membrane have a moist slippery surface. Mucus protects the lining membrane from mechanical and chemical injury and in the respiratory tract it traps inhaled foreign particles, preventing them from entering the alveoli of the lungs.

Serous membrane

Serous membranes, or *serosa*, secrete serous watery fluid. They consist of a double layer of loose areolar connective tissue lined by simple squamous epithelium. The *parietal* layer lines a cavity and the *visceral* layer surrounds organs within the cavity. The two layers are separated by *serous fluid* secreted by the epithelium. There are three sites where serous membranes are found:

- the *pleura* lining the thoracic cavity and surrounding the lungs (p. 251)
- the *pericardium* lining the pericardial cavity and surrounding the heart (p. 83)
- the *peritoneum* lining the abdominal cavity and surrounding abdominal organs (p. 284).

The serous fluid between the visceral and parietal layers enables an organ to glide freely within the cavity without being damaged by friction between it and adjacent organs. For example, the heart changes its shape and size during each beat and friction damage is prevented by the arrangement of pericardium and its serous fluid.

Synovial membrane

This membrane is found lining the joint cavities and surrounding tendons, which could be injured by rubbing against bones, e.g. over the wrist joint. It is made up of a layer of fine, flattened epithelial cells on a layer of delicate connective tissue.

Synovial membrane secretes clear, sticky, oily *synovial fluid*, which acts as a lubricant to the joints and helps to maintain their stability (Ch. 17).

Glands

Glands are groups of epithelial cells which produce specialised secretions. Glands that discharge their secretion on to the epithelial surface of an organ, either directly or through a *duct*, are called *exocrine glands*. Exocrine glands vary considerably in size, shape and complexity as shown in Figure 3.26. Other glands discharge their secretions into blood and lymph. These are called *endocrine glands* (ductless glands) and their secretions are *hormones* (see Ch. 9).

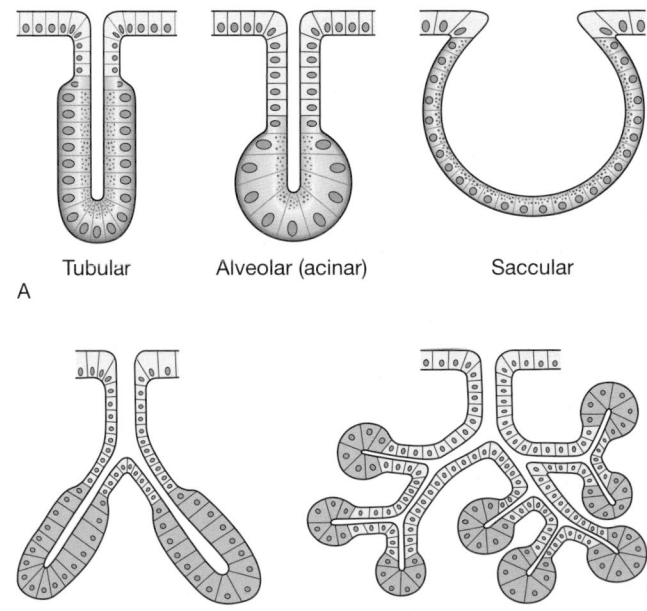

A

Tubular   Alveolar (acinar)   Saccular

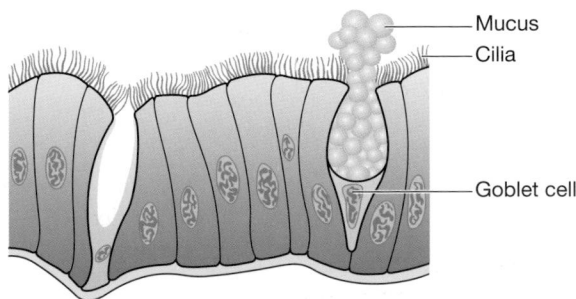

—Mucus
—Cilia
—Goblet cell

Figure 3.25 Ciliated columnar epithelium with goblet cells.

B

Branched tubular   Branched alveolar (acinar)

Figure 3.26 Exocrine glands: A. Simple glands. B. Compound (branching) glands.

ORGANISATION OF THE BODY

Learning outcomes

After studying this section you should be able to:

- define common anatomical terms
- identify the principal bones of the axial skeleton and the appendicular skeleton
- state the boundaries of the four body cavities
- list the contents of the body cavities.

In this part of the chapter a brief account is given of some anatomical terms and the names and positions of bones. A more detailed account of the bones, muscles and joints is given in Chapters 16, 17 and 18.

Anatomical terms

The anatomical position. This is the position assumed in all anatomical descriptions to ensure accuracy and consistency. The body is in the upright position with the head facing forward, the arms at the sides with the palms of the hands facing forward and the feet together.

Median plane. When the body, in the anatomical position, is divided *longitudinally* through the midline into right and left halves it has been divided in the median plane.

Table 3.1 lists the paired directional terms used in anatomy.

The skeleton

The skeleton is the bony framework of the body. It forms the cavities and fossae that protect some structures, forms the joints and gives attachment to muscles. A detailed description of bones is given in Chapter 16. Table 3.2 lists the terminology related to the skeleton.

The skeleton is described in two parts: *axial* and *appendicular* (Fig. 3.27).

The axial skeleton (axis of the body) consists of:

- skull
- vertebral column
- sternum or breast bone
- ribs.

The appendicular skeleton (appendages attached to the axis of the body) consists of:

- the bones of the upper limbs, the two clavicles and the two scapulae
- the bones of the lower limbs and the two innominate bones of the pelvis.

Axial skeleton

Skull

The skull is described in two parts, the *cranium*, which contains the brain, and the *face*. It consists of a number of bones which develop separately but fuse together as they mature. The only movable bone is the mandible or lower jaw. The names and positions of the individual bones of the skull can be seen in Figure 3.28.

Table 3.1 Paired directional terms used in anatomy

Directional term	Meaning
Medial	Structure is nearer to the midline. *The heart is medial to the humerus*
Lateral	Structure is further from the midline or at the side of the body. *The humerus is lateral to the heart*
Proximal	Nearer to a point of attachment of a limb, or origin of a body part. *The femur is proximal to the fibula*
Distal	Further from a point of attachment of a limb, or origin of a body part. *The fibula is distal to the femur*
Anterior or ventral	Part of the body being described is nearer the front of the body. *The sternum is anterior to the vertebrae*
Posterior or dorsal	Part of the body being described is nearer the back of the body. *The vertebrae are posterior to the sternum*
Superior	Structure nearer the head. *The skull is superior to the scapulae*
Inferior	Structure further from the head. *The scapulae are inferior to the skull*

Table 3.2 Terminology related to the skeleton

Term	Meaning
Articulating surface	The part of the bone that enters into the formation of a joint
Articulation	A joint between two or more bones
Bony sinus	A hollow cavity within a bone
Border	A ridge of bone separating two surfaces
Condyle	A smooth rounded projection of bone that forms part of a joint
Facet	A small, generally rather flat, articulating surface
Fissure or cleft	A narrow slit
Foramen (plural: foramina)	A hole in a structure
Fossa (plural: fossae)	A hollow or depression
Meatus	A tube-shaped cavity within a bone
Septum	A partition separating two cavities
Spine, spinous process or crest	A sharp ridge of bone
Styloid process	A sharp downward projection of bone that gives attachment to muscles and ligaments
Suture	An immovable joint, e.g. between the bones of the skull
Trochanter, tuberosity or tubercle	Roughened bony projections, usually for attachment of muscles or ligaments. The different names are used according to the size of the projection. Trochanters are the largest and tubercles the smallest

Functions of the skull

The various parts of the skull have specific and different functions:

- The *cranium* protects the delicate tissues of the brain.
- The *bony eye sockets* provide the eyes with some protection against injury and give attachment to the muscles which move the eyes.
- The *temporal bone* protects the delicate structures of the ear.
- Some bones of the face and the base of the skull give resonance to the voice because they have cavities called *sinuses*, containing air. The sinuses have tiny openings into the nasal cavity.
- The bones of the face form the walls of the posterior part of the nasal cavities. They keep the air passage open, facilitating breathing.
- The *maxilla* and the *mandible* provide alveolar ridges in which the teeth are embedded.

- The mandible is the only movable bone of the skull and chewing food is the result of raising and lowering the mandible by contracting and relaxing some muscles of the face, the muscles of mastication.

Vertebral column

This consists of 24 movable bones (vertebrae) plus the sacrum and coccyx. The bodies of the bones are separated from each other by *intervertebral discs*, consisting of cartilage. The vertebral column is described in five parts and the bones of each part are numbered from above downwards (Figs 3.27 and 3.29):

- 7 cervical
- 12 thoracic
- 5 lumbar
- 1 sacrum (5 fused bones)
- 1 coccyx (4 fused bones).

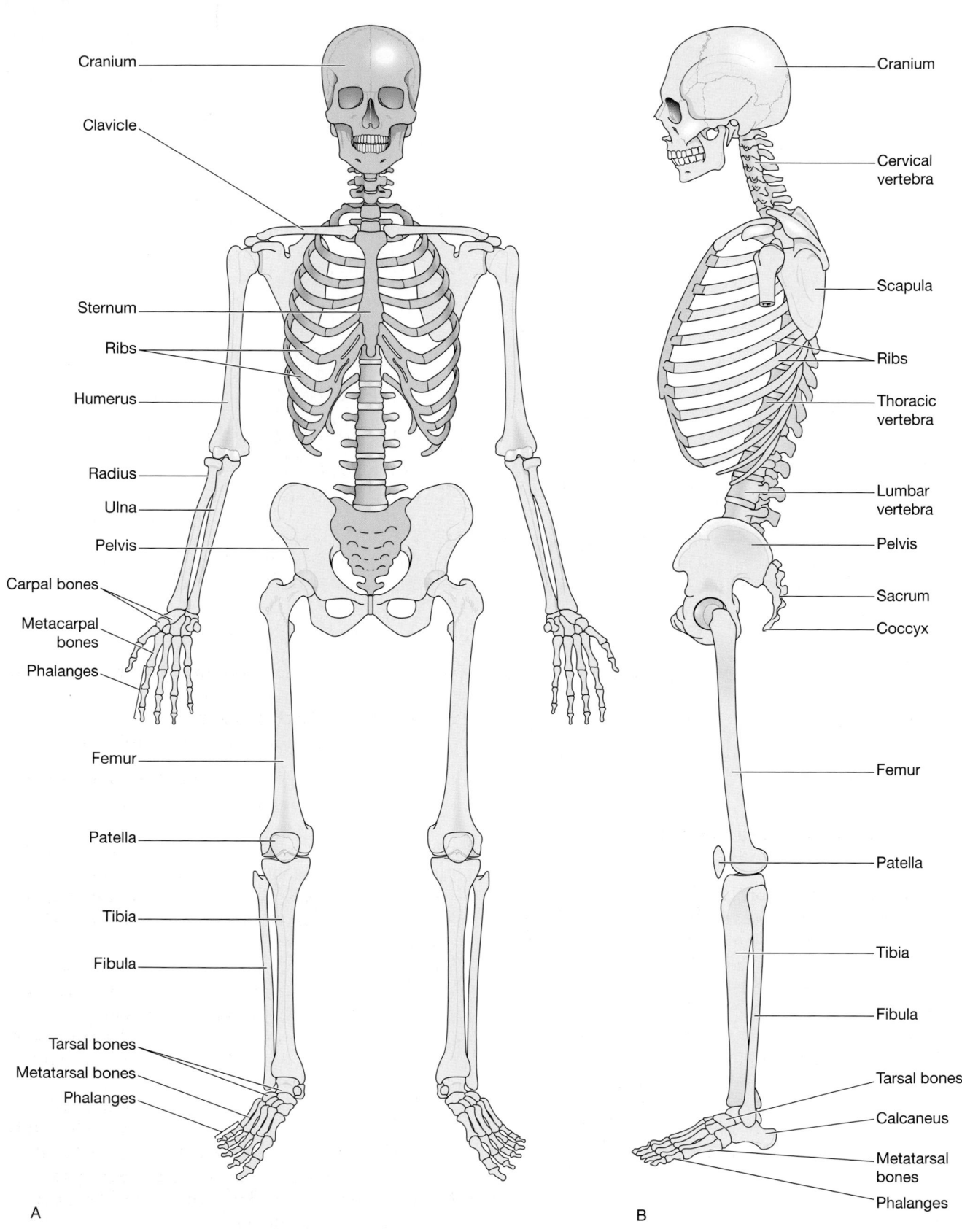

Cranium

Clavicle

Sternum

Ribs

Humerus

Radius

Ulna

Pelvis

Carpal bones

Metacarpal bones

Phalanges

Femur

Patella

Tibia

Fibula

Tarsal bones

Metatarsal bones

Phalanges

Cranium

Cervical vertebra

Scapula

Ribs

Thoracic vertebra

Lumbar vertebra

Pelvis

Sacrum

Coccyx

Femur

Patella

Tibia

Fibula

Tarsal bones

Calcaneus

Metatarsal bones

Phalanges

A

B

46

Figure 3.27 The bony skeleton: A. Anterior view: axial skeleton – gold, appendicular skeleton – brown. B. Lateral view.

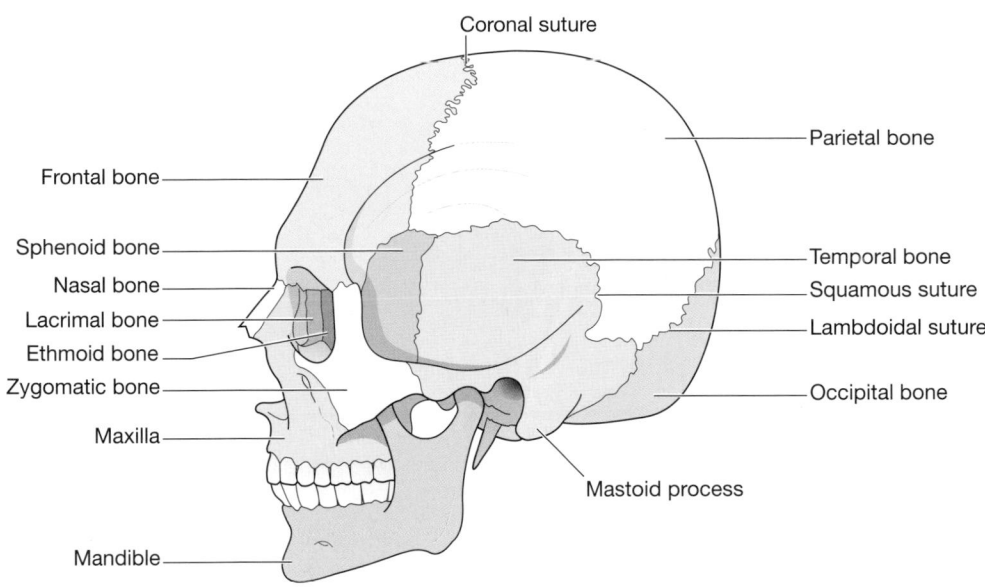

Figure 3.28 The skull: bones of the cranium and face.

The first cervical vertebra, called the *atlas*, articulates with the skull. Thereafter each vertebra forms a joint with the vertebrae immediately above and below. In the cervical and lumbar regions more movement is possible than in the thoracic region.

The *sacrum* consists of five vertebrae fused into one bone which articulates with the fifth lumbar vertebra above, the coccyx below and an innominate (pelvic or hip) bone at each side.

The *coccyx* consists of the four terminal vertebrae fused into a small triangular bone which articulates with the sacrum above.

Functions of the vertebral column

The vertebral column has several important functions:

- It protects the spinal cord. In each bone there is a hole or *foramen* and when the vertebrae are arranged one above the other, as shown in Figure 3.29, the foramina form a canal. The spinal cord, which is an extension of nerve tissue from the brain, lies in this canal (Fig. 3.30).
- Adjacent vertebrae form openings (intervertebral foramina) through which spinal nerves pass from the spinal cord to all parts of the body (Fig. 3.30). There are 31 pairs of spinal nerves.
- In the thoracic region the ribs articulate with the vertebrae forming joints which move during respiration.

Thoracic cage

The thoracic cage is formed by:

- 12 thoracic vertebrae
- 12 pairs of ribs
- 1 sternum or breast bone.

The arrangement of the bones can be seen in Figure 3.31.

Functions of the thoracic cage

The functions of the thoracic cage are as follows:

- It protects the thoracic organs. The bony framework protects the heart, lungs, large blood vessels and other structures.
- It forms joints between the upper limbs and the axial skeleton. The upper part of the sternum, the *manubrium*, articulates with the clavicles forming the only joints between the upper limbs and the axial skeleton.
- It gives attachment to the muscles of respiration:
  - *intercostal muscles* occupy the spaces between the ribs and when they contract the ribs move upwards and outwards, increasing the capacity of the thoracic cage, and inspiration (breathing in) occurs.
  - the *diaphragm* is a dome-shaped muscle which separates the thoracic and abdominal cavities. It is attached to the bones of the thorax and when it contracts it assists with inspiration. Structures which extend from one cavity to the other pass through the diaphragm
- It enables breathing (ventilation) to take place.

47

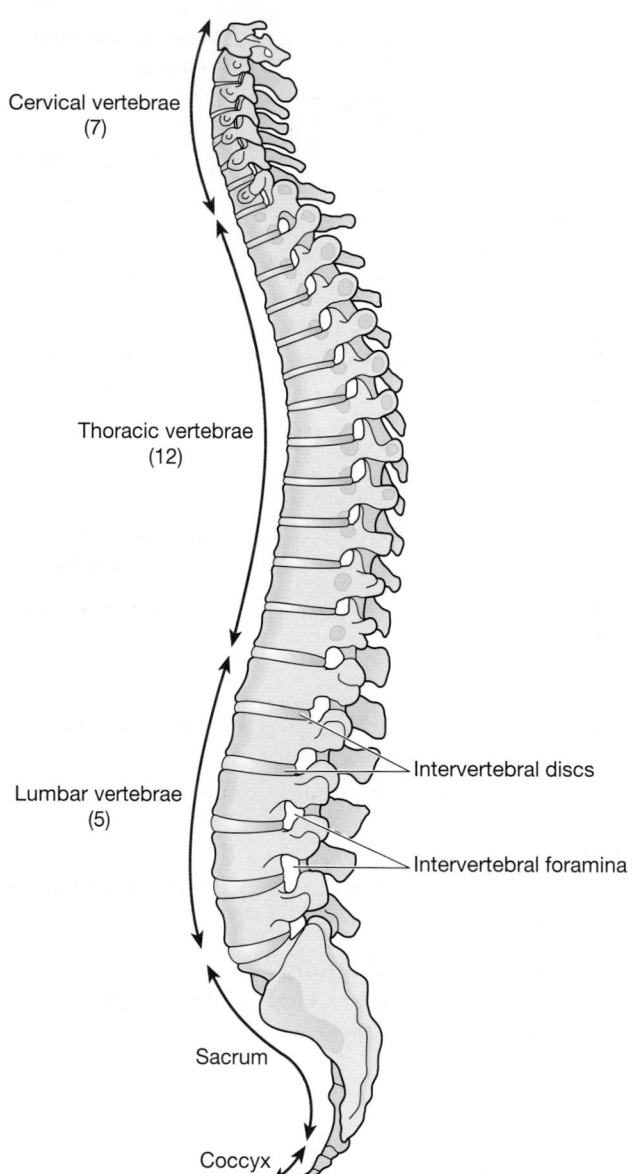

Cervical vertebrae (7)

Thoracic vertebrae (12)

Lumbar vertebrae (5)

Intervertebral discs

Intervertebral foramina

Sacrum

Coccyx

Figure 3.29 The vertebral column – lateral view.

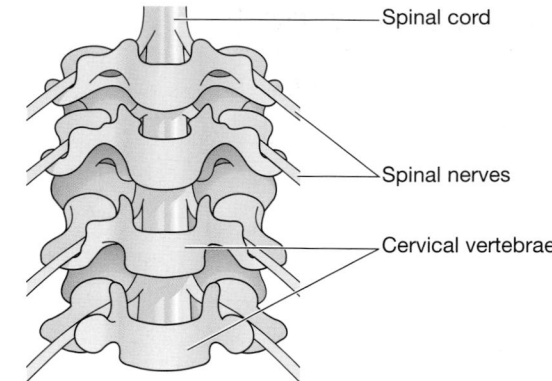

Spinal cord

Spinal nerves

Cervical vertebrae

Figure 3.30 The lower cervical vertebrae separated to show the spinal cord and spinal nerves (in yellow).

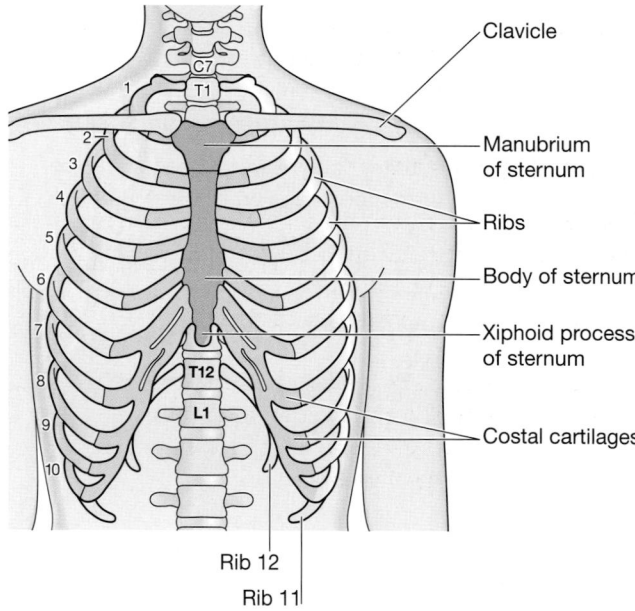

Clavicle

Manubrium of sternum

Ribs

Body of sternum

Xiphoid process of sternum

Costal cartilages

Rib 12

Rib 11

Figure 3.31 The structures forming the walls of the thoracic cage.

Appendicular skeleton

The appendages are:

- the upper limbs and the shoulder girdles
- the lower limbs and the innominate bones of the pelvis.

The names of the bones involved, their position and their relationship to other bones are shown in Figure 3.27.

Functions of the appendicular skeleton
The appendicular skeleton has two functions.

- *Voluntary movement.* The bones, muscles and joints of the limbs are involved in voluntary movement. This may range from the very fine movements of the fingers associated with writing to the coordinated movement of all the limbs associated with running and jumping.
- *Protection of delicate structures.* Structures such as blood vessels and nerves lie along the length of bones of the limbs and are protected from injury by the muscles and skin. These structures are most vulnerable where they cross joints and where bones can be felt near the skin.

Cavities of the body

The organs that make up the systems of the body are contained in four *cavities*:

- cranial
- thoracic
- abdominal
- pelvic.

Cranial cavity

The cranial cavity contains the *brain*, and its boundaries are formed by the bones of the skull (Fig. 3.32):

Anteriorly — 1 frontal bone
Laterally — 2 temporal bones
Posteriorly — 1 occipital bone
Superiorly — 2 parietal bones
Inferiorly — 1 sphenoid and 1 ethmoid bone and parts of the frontal, temporal and occipital bones.

Thoracic cavity

This cavity is situated in the upper part of the trunk. Its boundaries are formed by a bony framework and supporting muscles (Fig. 3.33):

Anteriorly — the sternum and costal cartilages of the ribs
Laterally — 12 pairs of ribs and the intercostal muscles
Posteriorly — the thoracic vertebrae and the intervertebral discs between the bodies of the vertebrae

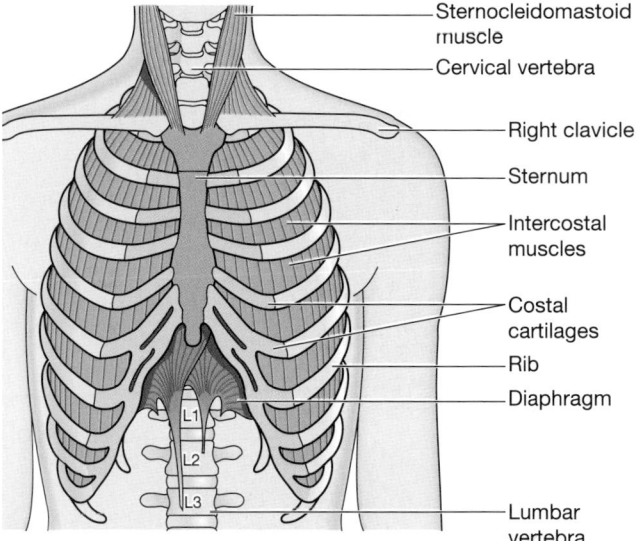

Figure 3.33 Structures forming the walls of the thoracic cavity and associated structures.

Superiorly — the structures forming the root of the neck
Inferiorly — the diaphragm, a dome-shaped muscle.

Contents

The main organs and structures contained in the thoracic cavity are (Fig. 3.34):

- the trachea, 2 bronchi, 2 lungs
- the heart, aorta, superior and inferior vena cava, numerous other blood vessels
- the oesophagus

49

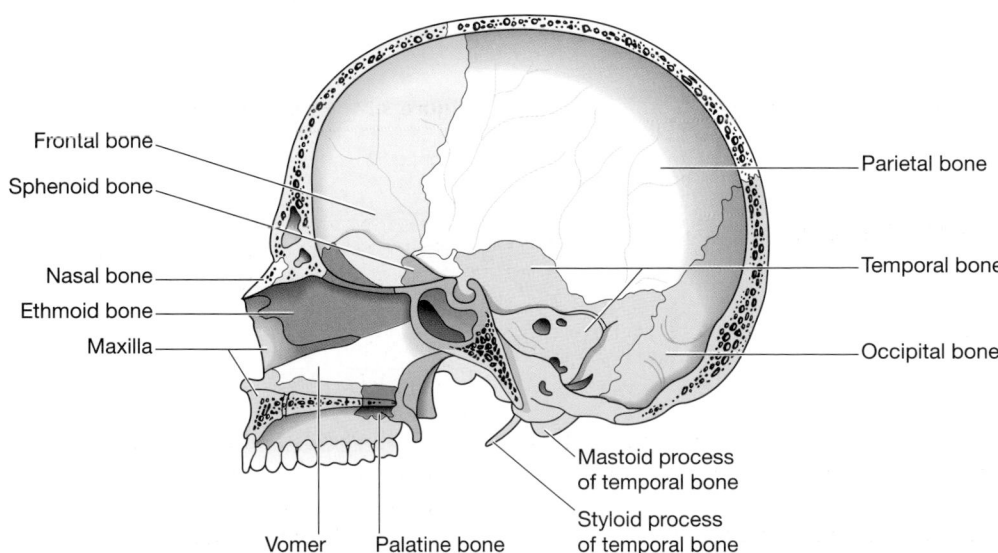

Figure 3.32 Bones forming the right half of the cranium and the face – viewed from the left.

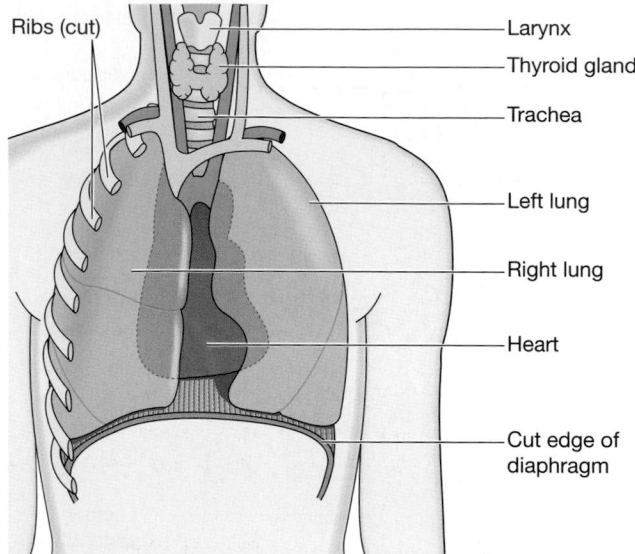

Ribs (cut) —
Larynx —
Thyroid gland —
Trachea —
Left lung —
Right lung —
Heart —
Cut edge of diaphragm —

Figure 3.34 Some of the main structures in the thoracic cavity and the root of the neck.

- lymph vessels and lymph nodes
- nerves.

The *mediastinum* is the name given to the space between the lungs including the structures found there, such as the heart, oesophagus and blood vessels.

Abdominal cavity

This is the largest cavity in the body and is oval in shape (Figs 3.35 and 3.36). It is situated in the main part of the trunk and its boundaries are:

Superiorly — the diaphragm, which separates it from the thoracic cavity
Anteriorly — the muscles forming the anterior abdominal wall
Posteriorly — the lumbar vertebrae and muscles forming the posterior abdominal wall
Laterally — the lower ribs and parts of the muscles of the abdominal wall
Inferiorly — the pelvic cavity with which it is continuous.

By convention, the abdominal cavity is divided into the nine regions shown in Figure 3.37. This facilitates the description of the positions of the organs and structures it contains.

Contents

Most of the space in the abdominal cavity is occupied by the organs and glands involved in the digestion and absorption of food (Figs 3.35 and 3.36). These are:

- the stomach, small intestine and most of the large intestine
- the liver, gall bladder, bile ducts and pancreas.

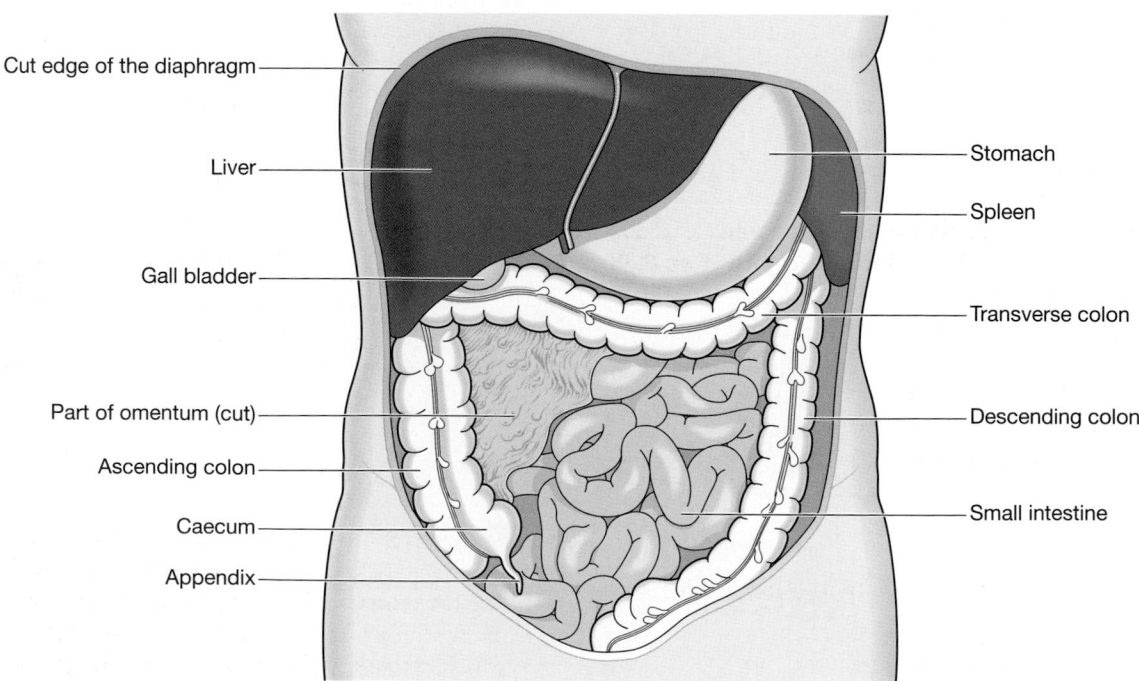

Cut edge of the diaphragm —
Liver —
Gall bladder —
Part of omentum (cut) —
Ascending colon —
Caecum —
Appendix —
Stomach —
Spleen —
Transverse colon —
Descending colon —
Small intestine —

Figure 3.35 Organs occupying the anterior part of the abdominal cavity and the diaphragm (cut).

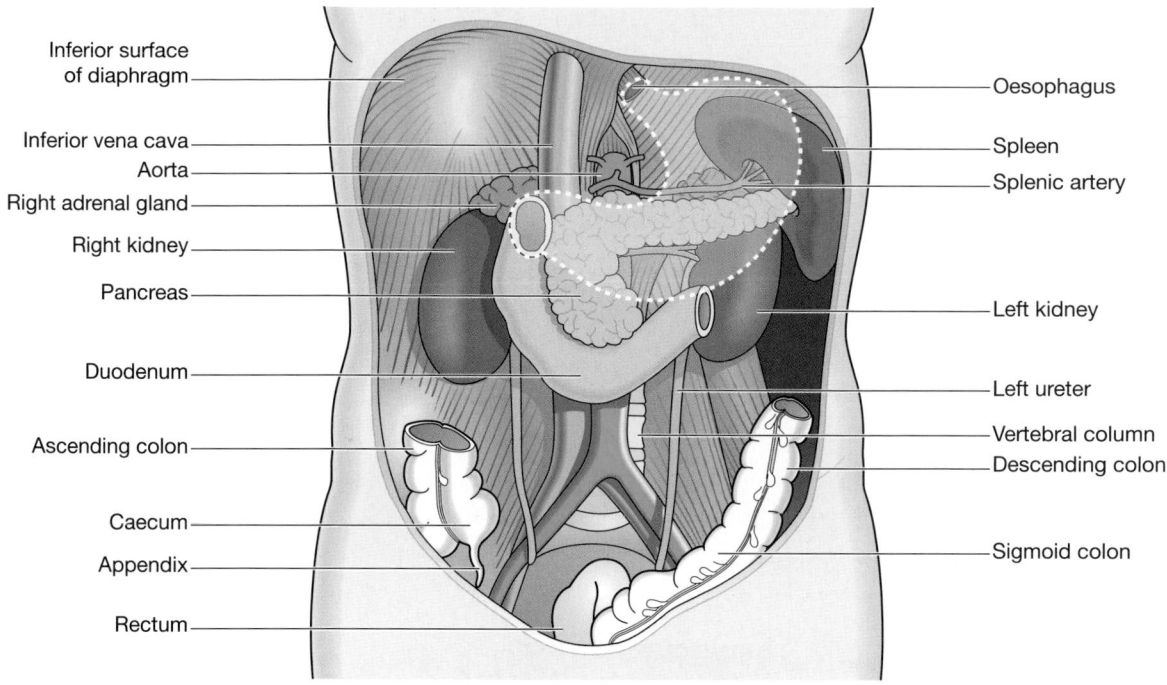

Figure 3.36 Organs occupying the posterior part of the abdominal cavity and the diaphragm (cut). The broken line shows the position of the stomach.

Other structures include:

- the spleen
- 2 kidneys and the upper part of the ureters
- 2 adrenal (suprarenal) glands
- numerous blood vessels, lymph vessels, nerves
- lymph nodes.

Pelvic cavity

The pelvic cavity is roughly funnel shaped and extends from the lower end of the abdominal cavity (Figs 3.38 and 3.39). The boundaries are:

Superiorly — it is continuous with the abdominal cavity
Anteriorly — the pubic bones
Posteriorly — the sacrum and coccyx
Laterally — the innominate bones
Inferiorly — the muscles of the pelvic floor.

Contents

The pelvic cavity contains the following structures:

- sigmoid colon, rectum and anus
- some loops of the small intestine
- urinary bladder, lower parts of the ureters and the urethra

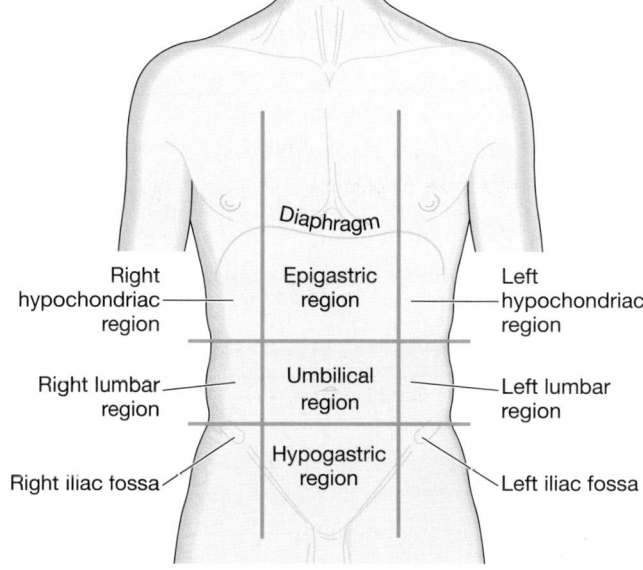

Figure 3.37 Regions of the abdominal cavity.

51

- in the female, the organs of the reproductive system: the uterus, uterine tubes, ovaries and vagina (Fig. 3.38)
- in the male, some of the organs of the reproductive system: the prostate gland, seminal vesicles, spermatic cords, deferent ducts (vas deferens), ejaculatory ducts and the urethra (common to the reproductive and urinary systems) (Fig. 3.39).

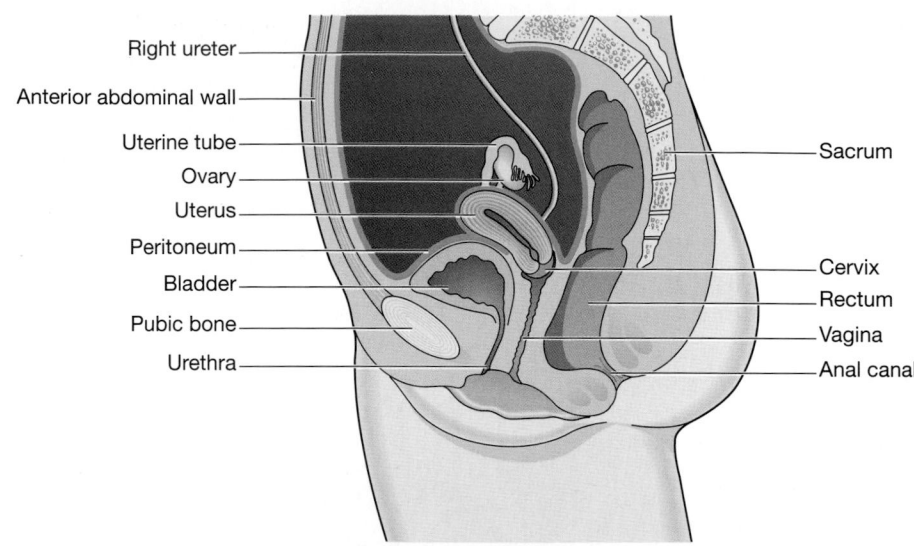

Figure 3.38 Female reproductive organs and other structures in the pelvic cavity.

Figure 3.39 Male reproductive organs and other structures in the pelvic cavity.

DISORDERS OF CELLS AND TISSUES

Learning outcomes

After studying this section you should be able to:

- outline the common causes of tumours
- explain the terms 'well differentiated' and 'poorly differentiated'
- outline causes of death in malignant disease
- compare and contrast the effects of benign and malignant tumours.

Table 3.3 Differences between benign and malignant tumours

Benign	Malignant
Slow growth	Rapid growth
Cells well differentiated	Cells poorly differentiated
Usually encapsulated	Not encapsulated
Does not spread	Spreads: – by local infiltration – via lymph – via blood – via body cavities
Recurrence is rare	Recurrence is common

Neoplasms or tumours

A tumour or *neoplasm* (literally meaning 'new growth') is a mass of tissue that grows faster than normal in an uncoordinated manner, and continues to grow after the initial stimulus has ceased.

Tumours are classified as benign or malignant although a clear distinction is not always possible (see Table 3.3). Benign tumours only rarely change their character and become malignant.

Causes of neoplasms

Some factors are known to precipitate the changes found in tumour cells but the reasons for the uncontrolled cell multiplication are not known. The process of change is *carcinogenesis* and the agents precipitating the change are *carcinogens*. Carcinogenesis may be of genetic and/or environmental origin and a clear-cut distinction is not always possible.

Carcinogens

Environmental agents known to cause malignant changes in cells do so by progressive irreversible disorganisation and modification of the chromosomes and genes. It is impossible to specify a maximum 'safe dose' of a carcinogen. A small dose may initiate change but this may not be enough to cause malignancy unless there are repeated doses within a limited period of time that have a cumulative effect. In addition there are widely varying latent periods between exposure and evidence of malignancy.

There may also be other unknown factors. Environmental carcinogens include chemicals, irradiations and oncogenic viruses.

Chemical carcinogens

Some chemicals are carcinogens when absorbed; others are modified after absorption and become carcinogenic. Some known chemical carcinogens are:

- aniline dyes
- arsenic compounds
- asbestos
- benzene derivatives
- cigarette smoke
- nickel compounds
- some fuel oils
- vinyl chloride.

Radiation carcinogens

Exposure to ionising radiation including X-rays, radioactive isotopes, environmental radiations and ultraviolet rays in sunlight may cause malignant changes in some cells and kill others. The cells are affected during mitosis so those normally undergoing continuous controlled division are most susceptible. These labile tissues include skin, mucous membrane, bone marrow, lymphoid tissue and gametes in the ovaries and testes.

Oncogenic viruses

Viruses, some consisting of DNA and some of RNA, are known to cause malignant changes in animals and there are indications of similar involvement in humans. Viruses enter cells and the addition of DNA or RNA to the host cell's nucleus causes mutation. The mutant cells may be malignant.

53

Host factors

Internal body factors of the host can influence susceptibility to tumours. These include:

- race
- diet
- age
- inherited factors.

Tumours of individual structures are described in the appropriate chapters.

Growth of tumours

Normally cells divide in an orderly manner. Neoplastic cells have escaped from the normal controls and they multiply in a disorderly manner forming a tumour. Blood vessels grow with the proliferating cells, but in some malignant tumours the blood supply does not keep pace with growth and *ischaemia* (lack of blood supply) leads to tumour cell death, called *necrosis*. If the tumour is near the surface, this may result in skin ulceration and infection. In deeper tissues there is fibrosis; e.g. retraction of the nipple in breast cancer is due to the shrinkage of fibrous tissue in a necrotic tumour. The mechanisms controlling the life span of tumour cells are poorly understood.

Cell differentiation

Differentiation of cells into types with particular structural and functional characteristics occurs at an early stage in fetal development; e.g. epithelial cells develop different characteristics from lymphocytes. Later, when cell replacement occurs, daughter cells have the same appearance, functions and genetic make-up as the parent cell. In benign tumours the cells from which they originate are easily recognised; i.e. tumour cells are *well differentiated*. Tumours with well-differentiated cells are usually benign but some may be malignant. Malignant tumours grow beyond their normal boundaries and show varying levels of differentiation:

- *mild dysplasia* — this means the tumour cells have retained most of their normal features and their parent cells can usually be identified
- *anaplasia* — this means the tumour cells have lost most of their normal features and their parent cells cannot be identified.

Encapsulation and spread of tumours

Most benign tumours are contained within a fibrous capsule derived partly from the surrounding tissues and partly from the tumour. They neither infiltrate local tissues nor spread to other parts of the body, even when they are not encapsulated.

Malignant tumours are not encapsulated. They spread locally by infiltration, and tumour fragments may spread to other parts of the body in blood or lymph. Some spreading cells may be phagocytosed but others lodge in tissues away from the primary site and grow into *secondary tumours* (metastases).

Local spread

Benign tumours enlarge and may cause pressure damage to local structures. They do not spread to other parts of the body.

Benign or malignant tumours may:

- damage nerves, causing pain and loss of nerve control of other tissues and organs supplied by the damaged nerves
- compress adjacent structures causing e.g. ischaemia (lack of blood), necrosis (death of tissue), blockage of ducts, organ dysfunction or displacement, or pain due to pressure on nerves.

Additionally *malignant tumours* grow into and infiltrate surrounding tissues and they may:

- erode blood and lymph vessel walls, causing spread of tumour cells to other parts of the body.

Lymphatic spread

This occurs when malignant tumours grow into lymph vessels. Groups of tumour cells break off and are carried to lymph nodes where they lodge and may grow into secondary tumours. There may be further spread through the lymphatic system, and to blood because lymph eventually enters the subclavian veins.

Blood spread

This occurs when the walls of a blood vessel are eroded by a malignant tumour. A *thrombus* (blood clot) may form at the site and *emboli* consisting of fragments of tumour and blood clot enter the bloodstream. These emboli block small blood vessels, cause *infarcts* (areas of dead tissue) and metastatic tumours develop. Phagocytosis of tumour cells in the emboli is unlikely to occur because these are protected by the blood clot. Single tumour cells can also lodge in the capillaries of other body organs. Division and subsequent growth of secondary tumours, or *metastases*, may then occur. The sites of blood-spread metastases depend on the site of the original tumour and the anatomy of the circulatory system, although the reasons why some organs develop metastases more frequently than others are not always clear.

Table 3.4 **Common sites of primary tumours and their metastases**	
Primary tumour	Metastatic tumours
Bronchi	Adrenal glands, brain
Alimentary tract	Abdominal and pelvic structures, especially liver
Prostate gland	Pelvic bones, vertebrae
Thyroid gland	Pelvic bones, vertebrae
Breast	Vertebrae, brain
Many organs	Lungs

Body cavities spread

This occurs when a tumour penetrates the wall of a cavity. The peritoneal cavity is most frequently involved. If, for example, a malignant tumour in an abdominal organ penetrates the visceral peritoneum, tumour cells may metastasise to folds of peritoneum or any abdominal or pelvic organ. Where there is less scope for the movement of fragments within a cavity the tumour tends to bind layers of tissue together; e.g. a pleural tumour binds the visceral and parietal layers together, limiting expansion of the lung.

Table 3.4 shows common sites of primary tumours and their metastases.

Effects of tumours

Pressure effects

Both benign and malignant tumours may cause pressure damage to adjacent structures, especially if in a confined space. The effects depend on the site of the tumour but are most marked in areas where there is little space for expansion, e.g. inside the skull, under the periosteum of bones, in bony sinuses and respiratory passages. Compression of adjacent structures may cause ischaemia, necrosis, blockage of ducts, organ dysfunction or displacement, pain due to invasion of nerves or pressure on nerves.

Hormonal effects

Tumours of endocrine glands may secrete hormones, producing the effects of hypersecretion. The extent of cell dysplasia is an important factor. Well-differentiated benign tumours are more likely to secrete hormones than are markedly dysplastic malignant tumours. High levels of hormones are found in the bloodstream as secretion occurs in the absence of the normal stimulus and homeostatic control mechanism. Some malignant tumours produce *uncharacteristic hormones*. The cells of the tumour do not appear to originate from the appropriate endocrine gland. There is evidence of this phenomenon but the reasons for it are unclear. Endocrine glands may be destroyed by invading tumours, causing hormone deficiency.

Cachexia

This is the severe weight loss accompanied by progressive weakness, loss of appetite, wasting and anaemia that is usually associated with advanced cancer. The severity is usually indicative of the stage of development of the disease. The causes are not clear.

Causes of death in malignant disease

Infection

Acute infection is a common cause of death when superimposed on advanced malignancy. Predisposition to infection is increased by prolonged bedrest, and by depression of the immune system by cytotoxic drugs and irradiation by X-rays or radioactive isotopes used in treatment. The most commonly occurring infections are pneumonia, septicaemia, peritonitis and pyelonephritis.

Organ failure

A tumour may destroy so much tissue that an organ cannot function. Severe damage to vital organs, such as lungs, brain, liver and kidneys, are common causes of death.

Carcinomatosis

When there is widespread metastatic disease associated with cachexia, severe physiological and biochemical disruption follows. In time, this results in loss of the homeostatic control mechanisms necessary to maintain life.

Haemorrhage

This may occur when a tumour grows into and ruptures the wall of a vein or artery. The most common sites are the gastrointestinal tract, brain, lungs and the peritoneal cavity.

Communication

2

4

The blood

Blood is a connective tissue. It provides one of the means of communication between the cells of different parts of the body and the external environment, e.g. it carries:

- oxygen from the lungs to the tissues and carbon dioxide from the tissues to the lungs for excretion
- nutrients from the alimentary tract to the tissues and cell wastes to the excretory organs, principally the kidneys
- hormones secreted by endocrine glands to their target glands and tissues
- heat produced in active tissues to other less active tissues
- protective substances, e.g. antibodies, to areas of infection
- clotting factors that coagulate blood, minimising its loss from ruptured blood vessels.

Blood makes up about 7% of body weight (about 5.6 litres in a 70 kg man). This proportion is less in women and considerably greater in children, gradually decreasing until the adult level is reached.

Blood in the blood vessels is always in motion. The continual flow maintains a fairly constant environment for the body cells.

Blood volume and the concentration of its many constituents are kept within narrow limits by homeostatic mechanisms.

COMPOSITION OF BLOOD

Learning outcomes

After studying this section, you should be able to:

- describe the chemical composition of plasma
- discuss the structure, function and formation of red blood cells, including the systems used in medicine to classify the different types
- discuss the functions and formation of the different types of white blood cell
- outline the role of platelets in blood clotting.

Blood is composed of a straw-coloured transparent fluid, *plasma*, in which different types of cells are suspended. Plasma constitutes about 55% and cells about 45% of blood volume (Fig. 4.1A).

Figure 4.1 A. The proportions of blood cells and plasma in whole blood separated by gravity. B. A blood clot in serum.

Plasma

The constituents of plasma are water (90 to 92%) and dissolved substances, including:

- plasma proteins: albumins, globulins (including *antibodies*), fibrinogen, clotting factors
- inorganic salts (mineral salts): sodium chloride, sodium bicarbonate, potassium, magnesium, phosphate, iron, calcium, copper, iodine, cobalt
- nutrients, principally from digested foods, e.g. monosaccharides (mainly glucose), amino acids, fatty acids, glycerol and vitamins
- organic waste materials, e.g. urea, uric acid, creatinine
- hormones
- enzymes, e.g. certain clotting factors
- gases, e.g. oxygen, carbon dioxide, nitrogen.

Plasma proteins

Plasma proteins, which make up about 7% of plasma, are normally retained within the blood, because they are too big to escape through the capillary pores into the tissues. They are largely responsible for creating the osmotic pressure of blood (normally 25 mmHg or 3.3 kPa*), which keeps plasma fluid within the circulation. If plasma protein levels fall, because of either reduced production or loss from the blood vessels, osmotic pressure is also reduced, and fluid moves into the tissues (oedema) and body cavities.

---

*1 kilopascal (kPa) = 7.5 millimetres of mercury (mmHg)
1 mmHg = 133.3 Pa = 0.133 kPa

Albumins. These are formed in the liver. They are the most abundant plasma proteins and their main function is to maintain a normal plasma osmotic pressure. Albumins also act as carrier molecules for lipids and steroid hormones.

Globulins. Most are formed in the liver and the remainder in lymphoid tissue. Their main functions are:

- as antibodies (immunoglobulins), which are complex proteins produced by lymphocytes that play an important part in immunity. They bind to, and neutralise, foreign materials (antigens) such as micro-organisms (see also p. 380).
- transportation of some hormones and mineral salts; e.g. thyroglobulin carries the hormone thyroxine and transferrin carries the mineral iron
- inhibition of some proteolytic enzymes, e.g. α_2 macroglobulin inhibits trypsin activity.

Clotting factors. These are substances essential for coagulation of blood (p. 67). *Serum* is plasma from which clotting factors have been removed (Fig. 4.1B).

Fibrinogen. This is synthesised in the liver and is essential for blood coagulation.

Plasma viscosity (thickness) is due to plasma proteins, mainly albumin and fibrinogen. Viscosity is used as a measure of the body's response to some diseases.

Inorganic salts (mineral salts)

These are involved in a wide variety of activities, including cell formation, contraction of muscles, transmission of nerve impulses, formation of secretions and maintenance of the balance between acids and alkalis. In health the blood is slightly alkaline. Alkalinity and acidity are expressed in terms of pH, which is a measure of hydrogen ion concentration, or $[H^+]$ (p. 21 and Fig. 2.6). The pH of blood is maintained between 7.35 and 7.45 by an ongoing complicated series of chemical activities, involving buffering systems.

Nutrients

Food is digested in the alimentary tract and the resultant nutrients are absorbed, e.g. monosaccharides, amino acids, fatty acids, glycerol and vitamins. Together with mineral salts they are required by all body cells to provide energy, heat, materials for repair and replacement, and for the synthesis of other blood components and body secretions.

Organic waste products

Urea, creatinine and uric acid are the waste products of protein metabolism. They are formed in the liver and conveyed in blood to the kidneys for excretion. Carbon dioxide, released by all cells, is conveyed to the lungs for excretion.

Hormones (Ch. 8)

These are chemical compounds synthesised by endocrine glands. Hormones pass directly from the cells of the glands into the blood which transports them to their target tissues and organs elsewhere in the body, where they influence cellular activity.

Gases

Oxygen, carbon dioxide and nitrogen are transported round the body in solution in plasma. Oxygen and carbon dioxide are also transported in combination with haemoglobin in red blood cells (p. 256). Most oxygen is carried in combination with haemoglobin and most carbon dioxide as bicarbonate ions dissolved in plasma. Atmospheric nitrogen enters the body in the same way as other gases and is present in plasma but it has no physiological function (p. 255).

Cellular content of blood

There are three types of blood cells (see Fig. 1.5, p. 8).

- erythrocytes or red cells
- thrombocytes or platelets
- leukocytes or white cells.

All blood cells originate from *pluripotent stem cells* and go through several developmental stages before entering the blood. Different types of blood cells follow separate lines of development. The process of blood cell formation is called *haemopoiesis* (Fig. 4.2) and takes place within red bone marrow. For the first few years of life, red marrow occupies the entire bone capacity and, over the next 20 years, is gradually replaced by fatty yellow marrow that has no erythropoietic function. In adults, erythropoiesis is confined to flat bones, irregular bones and the ends (*epiphyses*) of long bones, the main sites being the sternum, ribs, pelvis and skull.

Erythrocytes (red blood cells)

These are circular biconcave non-nucleated discs with a diameter of about 7 microns. Measurements of red cell numbers, volume and haemoglobin content are routine and useful assessments made in clinical practice (Table 4.1). The symbols in brackets are the abbreviations commonly used in laboratory reports.

Erythrocyte count. This is the number of erythrocytes per litre (l) or per cubic millimetre (mm^3) of blood.

Packed cell volume or haematocrit. This is the volume of red cells in 1 litre or 1 mm^3 of whole blood.

61

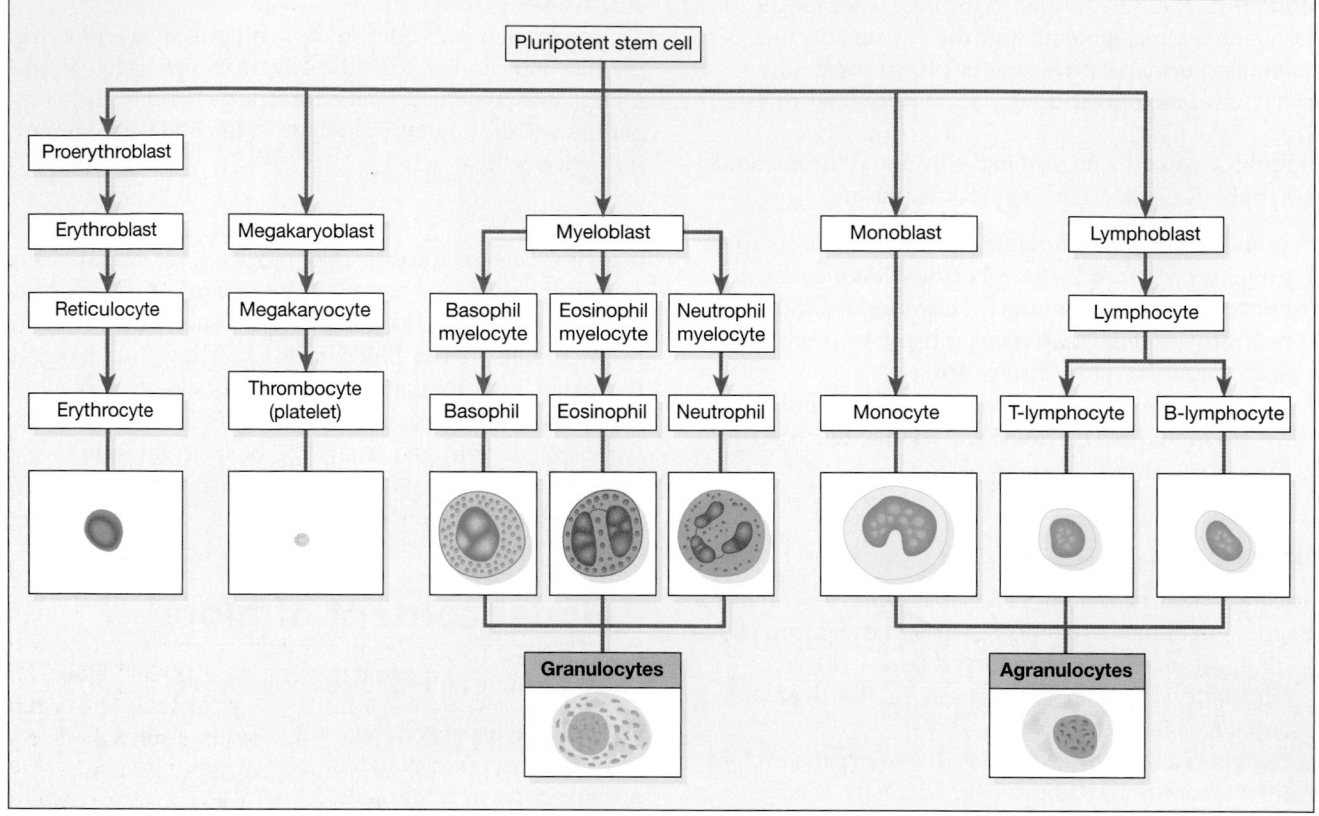

Figure 4.2 Haemopoiesis: stages in the development of blood cells.

Mean cell volume. This is the average volume of cells, measured in femtolitres ($fl = 10^{-15}$ litre).

Haemoglobin. This is the weight of haemoglobin in whole blood, measured in grams per 100 ml.

Mean cell haemoglobin. This is the average amount of haemoglobin in each cell, measured in picograms ($pg = 10^{-12}$ gram).

Mean cell haemoglobin concentration. This is the amount of haemoglobin in 100 ml of red cells.

Development and life span of erythrocytes

Erythrocytes are formed in red bone marrow, which is present in the ends of long bones and in flat and irregular bones. They pass through several stages of development before entering the blood. Their life span in the circulation is about 120 days.

Table 4.1 Erythrocytes – normal values

Measure	Normal values
Erythrocyte count	
Male	$4.5 \times 10^{12}/l$ to $6.5 \times 10^{12}/l$ (4.5 to 6.5 million/mm³)
Female	$4.5 \times 10^{12}/l$ to $5 \times 10^{12}/l$ (4.5 to 5 million/mm³)
Packed cell volume (PCV)	0.4 to 0.5 l/l (40 to 50/mm³)
Mean cell volume (MCV)	80 to 96 fl
Haemoglobin (Hb)	
Male	13 to 18 g/100 ml
Female	11.5 to 16.5 g/100 ml
Mean cell haemoglobin (MCH)	27 to 32 pg/cell
Mean cell haemoglobin concentration (MCHC)	30 to 35 g/100 ml of cells

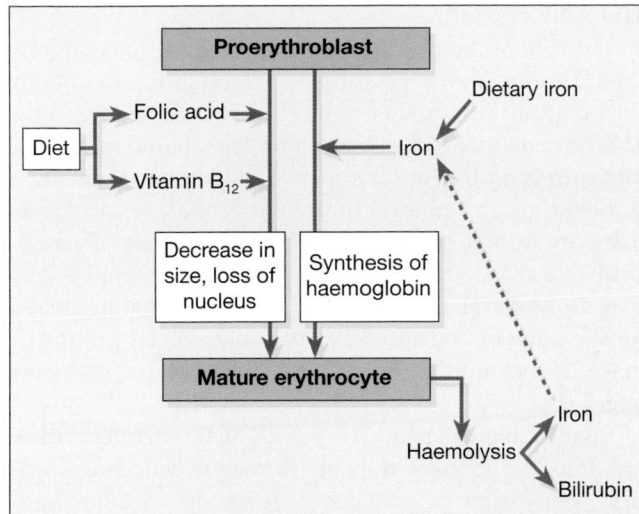

Figure 4.3 Maturation of the erythrocyte.

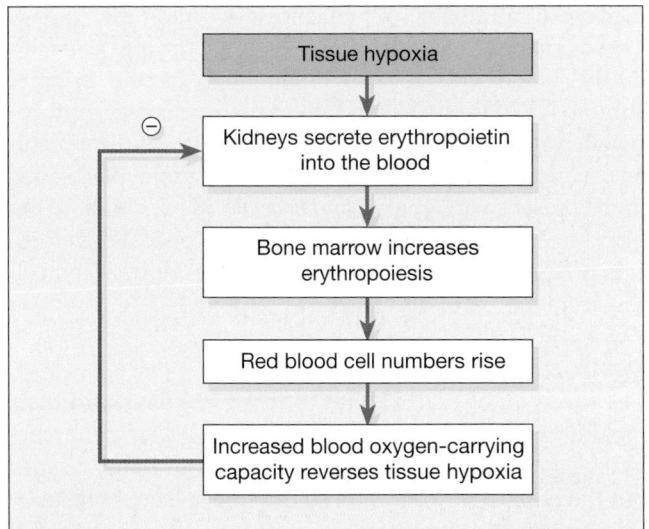

Figure 4.4 Control of erythropoiesis: the role of erythropoietin.

The process of development of red blood cells from pluripotent stem cells takes about 7 days and is called *erythropoiesis* (Fig. 4.2). It is characterised by two main features:

- maturation of the cell
- formation of haemoglobin inside the cell (Fig. 4.3).

Maturation of the cell. During this process the cell decreases in size and loses its nucleus. These changes depend on a number of factors, especially the presence of vitamin B_{12} and folic acid. These are present in sufficient quantity in a normal diet containing dairy products, meat and green vegetables. If the diet contains more than is needed, they are stored in the liver. Absorption of vitamin B_{12} depends on a glycoprotein called *intrinsic factor* secreted by parietal cells in the gastric glands. Together they form the *intrinsic factor–vitamin B_{12}* complex (IF–B_{12}). During its passage through the intestines, the bound vitamin is protected from enzymatic digestion, and is absorbed in the terminal ileum.

The effects of deficient intake of vitamin B_{12} do not appear for several years because there are large stores in the liver.

Folic acid is absorbed in the duodenum and jejunum where it undergoes change before entering the blood. Signs of deficiency are apparent within a few months.

Deficiency of either vitamin B_{12} or folic acid leads to impaired red cell production.

Formation of haemoglobin. Haemoglobin is a complex protein, consisting of *globin* and an iron-containing substance called *haem*, and is synthesised inside developing erythrocytes in red bone marrow.

Haemoglobin in mature erythrocytes combines with oxygen to form *oxyhaemoglobin*, giving arterial blood its characteristic red colour. In this way the bulk of oxygen absorbed from the lungs is transported around the body to maintain a continuous oxygen supply to all cells. Haemoglobin is also involved, to a lesser extent, in the transport of carbon dioxide from the body cells to the lungs for excretion.

Each haemoglobin molecule contains four atoms of iron. Each atom can carry one molecule of oxygen, therefore one haemoglobin molecule can carry up to four molecules of oxygen. Haemoglobin is said to be saturated when all its available binding sites for oxygen are filled. When oxygen levels are low, only partial saturation is possible.

Control of erythropoiesis

The number of red cells remains fairly constant, which means that the bone marrow produces erythrocytes at the rate at which they are destroyed. This is due to a homeostatic negative feedback mechanism (Fig. 4.4).

The primary stimulus to increased erythropoiesis is *hypoxia*, i.e. deficient oxygen supply to body cells. This occurs when:

- the oxygen-carrying power of blood is reduced by e.g. haemorrhage or excessive erythrocyte breakdown (*haemolysis*) due to disease
- the oxygen tension in the air is reduced, as at high altitudes.

Hypoxia increases erythrocyte formation by stimulating the production of the hormone *erythropoietin*, mainly by the kidneys. Erythropoietin stimulates an increase in the production of proerythroblasts and the release of increased numbers of reticulocytes into the blood. These changes increase the oxygen-carrying capacity of the blood and reverse tissue hypoxia, the original stimulus. When the tissue hypoxia is overcome, erythropoietin production declines (Fig. 4.4). When erythropoietin levels are low, red cell formation does not take place even in the presence of hypoxia, and *anaemia* (the inability of the blood to carry adequate oxygen for body needs) develops. It is believed that erythropoietin regulates normal red cell replacement, i.e. in the absence of hypoxia.

Destruction of erythrocytes

The life span of erythrocytes is about 120 days and their breakdown, or *haemolysis*, is carried out by *phagocytic reticuloendothelial cells*. These cells are found in many tissues but the main sites of haemolysis are the spleen, bone marrow and liver. As erythrocytes age, changes in their cell membranes make them more susceptible to haemolysis. Iron released by haemolysis is retained in the body and reused in the bone marrow to form haemoglobin (Fig. 4.3). *Biliverdin* is formed from the protein part of the erythrocytes. It is almost completely reduced to the yellow pigment *bilirubin*, before it is bound to plasma globulin and transported to the liver (see Fig. 12.41, p. 310). In the liver it is changed from a fat-soluble to a water-soluble form before it is excreted as a constituent of bile.

Blood groups

Individuals have different types of antigen on the surfaces of their red blood cells. These antigens, which are inherited, determine the individual's *blood group*. In addition, individuals make antibodies to these antigens, but not to their own type of antigen, since if they did the antigens and antibodies would react causing a *transfusion reaction*. The main signs are clumping of red blood cells, haemolysis, shock and kidney failure. These antibodies circulate in the bloodstream and the ability to make them, like the antigens, is genetically determined and not associated with acquired immunity (see also Ch. 15).

If individuals are transfused with blood of the same group, i.e. possessing the same antigens on the surface of the cells, their immune system will not recognise them as foreign and will not reject them. However, if they are given blood from an individual of a different blood type, i.e. with a different type of antigen on the red cells, their immune system will mount an attack upon them and destroy the transfused cells. This is the basis of the transfusion reaction; the two blood types, the donor and the recipient, are *incompatible*.

There are many different collections of red cell surface antigens, but the most important are the ABO and the Rhesus systems.

The ABO system

About 55% of the population has either A-type antigens (blood group A), B-type antigens (blood group B) or both (blood group AB) on their red cell surface. The remaining 45% have neither A nor B type antigens (blood group O). The corresponding antibodies are called anti-A and anti-B. Blood group A individuals cannot make anti-A (and therefore do not have these antibodies in their plasma), since otherwise a reaction to their own cells would occur; they do, however, make anti-B. Blood group B individuals, for the same reasons, make only anti-A. Blood group AB make neither, and blood group O make both anti-A and anti-B (Fig. 4.5).

Because blood group AB people make neither anti-A nor anti-B antibodies, they are known as *universal recipients*: transfusion of either type A or type B blood into these individuals is safe, since there are no antibodies to react with them. Conversely, group O people have neither A nor B antigens on their red cell membranes, and their blood may be safely transfused into A, B, AB or O types; group O is known as the *universal donor*.

The Rhesus system

The red blood cell membrane antigen important here is the Rhesus (Rh) antigen, or Rhesus factor. About 85% of people have this antigen; they are Rhesus positive (Rh$^+$) and do not therefore make anti-Rhesus antibodies. The remaining 15% have no Rhesus antigen (they are Rhesus negative, or Rh$^-$). Rh$^-$ individuals are capable of making anti-Rhesus antibodies, but are stimulated to do so only in certain circumstances, e.g. in pregnancy (p. 71), or as the result of an incompatible blood transfusion.

Leukocytes (white blood cells)

These cells have an important function in defending the body against microbes and other foreign materials. Leukocytes are the largest blood cells and they account for about 1% of the blood volume. They contain nuclei and some have granules in their cytoplasm. There are two main types (Table 4.2):

- granulocytes (polymorphonuclear leukocytes)
  - neutrophils, eosinophils and basophils
- agranulocytes
  - monocytes and lymphocytes.

Granulocytes (polymorphonuclear leukocytes)

During their formation, *granulopoiesis*, they follow a common line of development through *myeloblast* to *myelocyte* before differentiating into the three types (Figs 4.2 and

Blood group	Antigen + antibody(ies) present	As donor, is	As recipient, is
A	Antigen A — Makes anti-B	Compatible with: A and AB. Incompatible with: B and O, because both make anti-A antibodies that will react with A antigens	Compatible with: A and O. Incompatible with: B and AB, because type A makes anti-B antibodies that will react with B antigens
B	Antigen B — Makes anti-A	Compatible with: B and AB. Incompatible with: A and O, because both make anti-B antibodies that will react with B antigens	Compatible with: B and O. Incompatible with: A and AB, because type B makes anti-A antibodies that will react with A antigens
AB	Antigens A and B — Makes neither anti-A nor anti-B	Compatible with: AB only. Incompatible with: A, B and O, because all three make antibodies that will react with AB antigens	Compatible with all groups **UNIVERSAL RECIPIENT**. AB makes no antibodies and therefore will not react with any type of donated blood
O	Neither A nor B antigen — Makes both anti-A and anti-B	Compatible with all groups **UNIVERSAL DONOR**. O red cells have no antigens, and will therefore not stimulate anti-A or anti-B antibodies	Compatible with: O only. Incompatible with: A, AB and B, because type O makes anti-A and anti-B antibodies

Figure 4.5 The ABO system of blood grouping: antigens, antibodies and compatibility.

65

4.6). All granulocytes have multilobed nuclei in their cytoplasm. Their names represent the dyes they take up when stained in the laboratory. Eosinophils take up the red acid dye, eosin; basophils take up alkaline methylene blue; and neutrophils are purple because they take up both dyes.

Neutrophils

Their main function is to protect against any foreign material that gains entry to the body, mainly microbes, and to remove waste materials, e.g. cell debris. They are attracted in large numbers to any area of infection by chemical substances, released by damaged cells, called *chemotaxins*. Neutrophils pass through the capillary walls in the affected area by *amoeboid movement* (Fig. 4.7). Thereafter they engulf and kill the microbes by *phagocytosis* (Fig. 4.8). Their granules are *lysosomes* that contain enzymes that digest the engulfed material. The pus that may form in the affected area consists of dead tissue cells, dead and live microbes, and phagocytes killed by microbes.

There is a physiological increase in circulating neutrophils following strenuous exercise and in the later stages of normal pregnancy. Numbers are also increased in:

Table 4.2 Numbers of different types of leukocyte in adult blood

Type of cell	Number × 10⁹/l	Percentage of total
Granulocytes		
Neutrophils	2.5 to 7.5	40 to 75
Eosinophils	0.04 to 0.44	1 to 6
Basophils	0.015 to 0.1	<1
Agranulocytes		
Monocytes	0.2 to 0.8	2 to 10
Lymphocytes	1.5 to 3.5	20 to 50
Total	5 to 9	100

- microbial infection
- tissue damage, e.g. inflammation, myocardial infarction, burns, crush injuries
- metabolic disorders, e.g. diabetic ketoacidosis, acute gout
- leukaemia
- heavy smoking
- use of oral contraceptives.

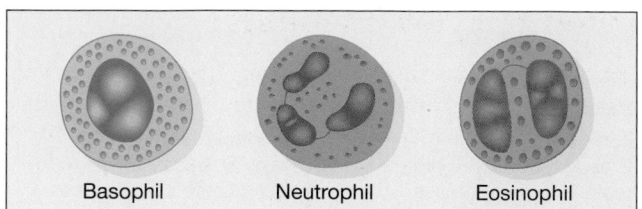

Figure 4.6 The granulocytes (granular leukocytes).

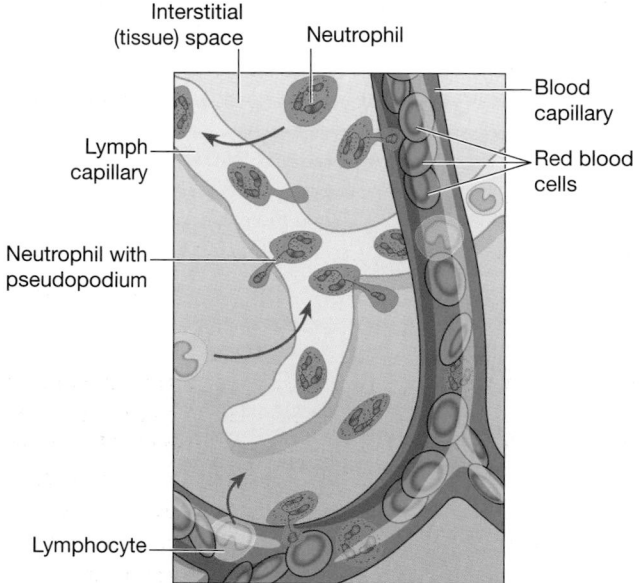

Figure 4.7 Amoeboid movement of leukocytes.

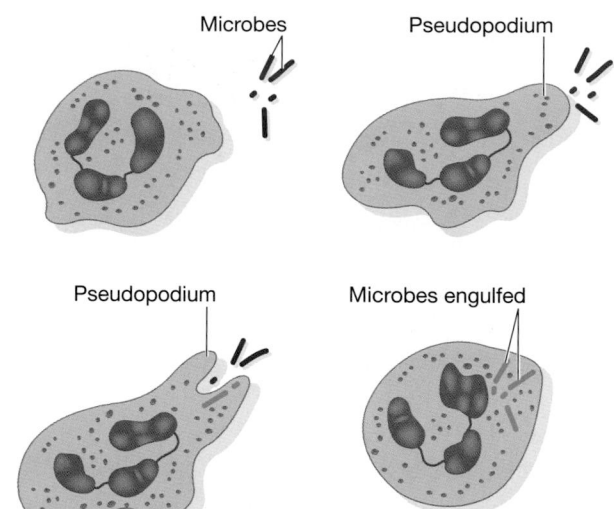

Figure 4.8 Phagocytic action of neutrophils.

Eosinophils

Eosinophils, although capable of phagocytosis, are less active in this than neutrophils; their specialised role appears to be in the elimination of parasites, such as worms, which are too big to be phagocytosed. They are equipped with certain toxic chemicals, stored in their granules, which they release when the eosinophil binds an infecting organism.

Eosinophils are often found at sites of allergic inflammation, such as the asthmatic airway and skin allergies. There, they promote tissue inflammation by releasing their array of toxic chemicals, but they may also dampen down the inflammatory process through the release of other chemicals, such as an enzyme that breaks down histamine (p. 376).

Basophils

Basophils, which are closely associated with allergic reactions, contain cytoplasmic granules packed with *heparin* (an anticoagulant), *histamine* (an inflammatory agent) and other substances that promote inflammation. Usually the stimulus that causes basophils to release the contents of

their granules is an *allergen* (an antigen that causes allergy) of some type. This binds to antibody-type receptors on the basophil membrane. A cell type very similar to basophils, except that it is found in the tissues, not in the circulation, is the *mast cell*. Mast cells release their granule contents within seconds of binding an allergen, which accounts for the rapid onset of allergic symptoms following exposure to, for example, pollen in hay fever.

Agranulocytes

The types of leukocyte with a large nucleus and no granules in their cytoplasm are *monocytes* and *lymphocytes* and they make up 25% to 50% of all leukocytes (Figs 4.2 and 4.9).

Monocytes

These are large mononuclear cells that originate in red bone marrow. Some circulate in the blood and are actively motile and phagocytic while others migrate into the tissues where they develop into *macrophages*. Both types of cell produce *interleukin 1* which:

- acts on the hypothalamus, causing the rise in body temperature associated with microbial infections
- stimulates the production of some globulins by the liver
- enhances the production of activated T-lymphocytes.

Macrophages have important functions in inflammation (p. 375) and immunity.

The monocyte–macrophage system. This system, which is sometimes called the *reticuloendothelial system*, consists of the body's complement of monocytes and

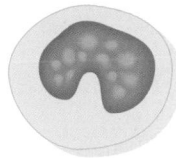

Lymphocyte   Monocyte

Figure 4.9 The agranulocytes.

macrophages. Some macrophages are mobile whereas others are fixed. These include:

- *histiocytes* in connective tissues
- *microglia* in the brain
- *Kupffer cells* in the liver
- *alveolar macrophages* in the lungs
- *sinus-lining macrophages* (reticular cells) in the spleen, lymph nodes and thymus gland
- *mesangial cells* in the glomerulus of nephrons in the kidney
- *osteoclasts* in bone.

Macrophages function in close association with monocytes in the blood and with lymphocytes which influence their activity. They are actively phagocytic and if they encounter large amounts of foreign or waste material, they tend to multiply at the site and 'wall off' the area, isolating the material, e.g. in the lungs when foreign material has been inhaled. Their numbers are increased in microbial infections, collagen diseases and some non-infective bowel conditions.

Lymphocytes

Lymphocytes are smaller than monocytes and have large nuclei. They circulate in the blood and are present in great numbers in lymphatic tissue such as lymph nodes and the spleen. Lymphocytes develop from pluripotent stem cells in red bone marrow, then travel in the blood to lymphoid tissue elsewhere in the body where they are *activated*, i.e. they become immunocompetent which means they are able to respond to *antigens* (foreign material). Examples of antigens include:

- cells regarded by lymphocytes as abnormal, e.g. those that have been invaded by viruses, cancer cells, tissue transplant cells
- pollen from flowers and plants
- fungi
- bacteria
- some large molecule drugs, e.g. penicillin, aspirin.

Although all lymphocytes originate from one type of stem cell, when they are activated in lymphatic tissue, two distinct types of lymphocyte are produced — *T-lymphocytes* and *B-lymphocytes*. The specific functions of these two types are discussed in Chapter 15.

Thrombocytes (platelets)

These are very small non-nucleated discs, 2 to 4 μm in diameter, derived from the cytoplasm of megakaryocytes in red bone marrow (Fig. 4.2). They contain a variety of substances that promote blood clotting, which causes *haemostasis* (cessation of bleeding).

The normal blood platelet count is between $200 \times 10^9/l$ and $350 \times 10^9/l$ (200 000 to 350 000/mm³). The control of platelet production is not yet entirely clear but it is believed that one stimulus is a fall in platelet count and that a substance called *thrombopoietin* is involved. The life span of platelets is between 8 and 11 days and those not used in haemostasis are destroyed by macrophages, mainly in the spleen.

Haemostasis

When a blood vessel is damaged, loss of blood is stopped and healing occurs in a series of overlapping processes, in which platelets play a vital part.

1. Vasoconstriction. When platelets come in contact with a damaged blood vessel, their surface becomes sticky and they adhere to the damaged wall. They then release *serotonin* (5-hydroxytryptamine), which constricts (narrows) the vessel, reducing blood flow through it. Other chemicals that cause vasoconstriction, e.g. thromboxanes, are released by the damaged vessel itself.

2. Platelet plug formation. The adherent platelets clump to each other and release other substances, including *adenosine diphosphate* (ADP), which attract more platelets to the site. Passing platelets stick to those already at the damaged vessel and they too release their chemicals. This is a positive feedback system by which many platelets rapidly arrive at the site of vascular damage and quickly form a temporary seal — the *platelet plug*.

3. Coagulation (blood clotting). This is a complex process that also involves a positive feedback system and only a few stages are included here. The factors involved are listed in Table 4.3. Their numbers represent the order in which they were discovered and not the order of participation in the clotting process. Blood clotting results in formation of an insoluble thread-like mesh of *fibrin* which traps blood cells and is much stronger than the rapidly formed platelet plug. In the final stages of this process *prothrombin activator* acts on the plasma protein *prothrombin* converting it to thrombin.

Thrombin then acts on another plasma protein *fibrinogen* and converts it to fibrin (Fig. 4.10).

Prothrombin activator can be formed by two processes which often occur together: the extrinsic and intrinsic

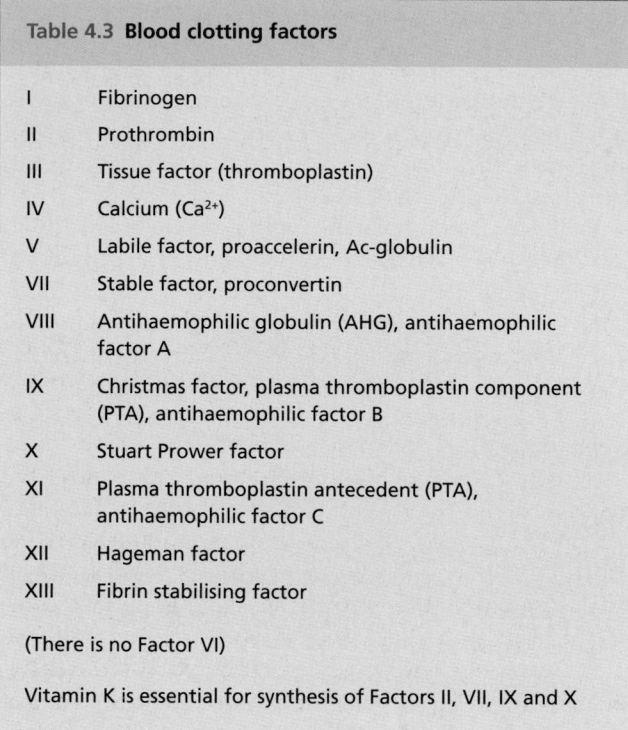

Table 4.3 Blood clotting factors

I	Fibrinogen
II	Prothrombin
III	Tissue factor (thromboplastin)
IV	Calcium (Ca^{2+})
V	Labile factor, proaccelerin, Ac-globulin
VII	Stable factor, proconvertin
VIII	Antihaemophilic globulin (AHG), antihaemophilic factor A
IX	Christmas factor, plasma thromboplastin component (PTA), antihaemophilic factor B
X	Stuart Prower factor
XI	Plasma thromboplastin antecedent (PTA), antihaemophilic factor C
XII	Hageman factor
XIII	Fibrin stabilising factor

(There is no Factor VI)

Vitamin K is essential for synthesis of Factors II, VII, IX and X

Figure 4.10 Stages of blood clotting (coagulation).

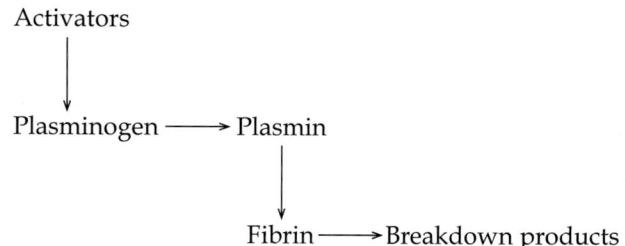

pathways (Fig. 4.10). The *extrinsic pathway* occurs rapidly (within seconds) when there is tissue damage outside the circulation. Damaged tissue releases a complex of chemicals called *thromboplastin* or tissue factor, which initiates coagulation. The *intrinsic pathway* is slower (3–6 minutes) and is confined to the circulation. It is triggered by damage to a blood vessel lining (endothelium) and the effects of platelets adhering to it. After a time the clot shrinks, squeezing out *serum*, a clear sticky fluid that consists of plasma from which clotting factors have been removed.

4. Fibrinolysis. After the clot has formed the process of removing it and healing the damaged blood vessel begins. The breakdown of the clot, or fibrinolysis, is the first stage. An inactive substance called *plasminogen* is present in the clot and is converted to the enzyme *plasmin* by activators released from the damaged endothelial cells. Plasmin initiates the breakdown of fibrin to soluble products that are treated as waste material and removed by phagocytosis. As the clot is removed, the healing process restores the integrity of the blood vessel wall.

Control of coagulation

The process of blood clotting relies heavily on several processes that are self-perpetuating—that is, once started, a positive feedback mechanism promotes their continuation. For example, thrombin is a powerful stimulator of its own production. The body therefore possesses several mechanisms to control and limit the coagulation cascade; otherwise once started the clotting process would spread throughout the circulatory system, far beyond requirements. The main controls are:

- the perfect smoothness of normal blood vessel lining; platelets do not adhere to this surface
- the binding of thrombin to a special thrombin receptor on the cells lining blood vessels; once bound, thrombin is inactivated
- the presence of natural anticoagulants, e.g. heparin, in the blood, which inactivate clotting factors.

ERYTHROCYTE DISORDERS

Learning outcomes

After studying this section, you should be able to:

- define the term anaemia
- compare and contrast the causes and effects of iron deficiency, megaloblastic, aplastic, hypoplastic and haemolytic anaemias
- explain why polycythaemia occurs.

Anaemias

In anaemia there is not enough haemoglobin available to carry sufficient oxygen from the lungs to supply the needs of the tissues. It occurs when the rate of production of mature cells entering the blood from the red bone marrow does not keep pace with the rate of haemolysis. The classification of anaemia is based on the cause:

- impaired erythrocyte production
  - iron deficiency
  - megaloblastic anaemias
  - hypoplastic anaemia
- increased erythrocyte loss
  - haemolytic anaemias
  - normocytic anaemia.

Red cells may appear abnormal when examined microscopically. Characteristic changes are listed in Table 4.4. Signs and symptoms of anaemia relate to the inability of the blood to supply body cells with enough oxygen, and may represent adaptive measures. Examples include:

- tachycardia; the heart rate increases to improve blood supply and speed circulation

- palpitations (an awareness of the heartbeat), or angina pectoris (p. 121); these are caused by the increased effort of the overworked heart muscle
- breathlessness on exertion; when oxygen requirements increase, respiratory rate and effort rise in an effort to meet the greater demand.

Iron deficiency anaemia

This is the most common form of anaemia in many parts of the world. The normal daily requirement of iron intake in men is about 1 to 2 mg derived from meat and highly coloured vegetables. The normal daily requirement in women is 3 mg. The increase is necessary to compensate for loss of blood during menstruation and to meet the needs of the growing fetus during pregnancy. Children, during their period of rapid growth, require more than adults.

The amount of haemoglobin in each cell is regarded as below normal when the MCH is less than 27 pg/cell. The anaemia is regarded as severe when the haemoglobin level is below 9 g/dl blood. It is caused by deficiency of iron in the bone marrow and may be due to dietary deficiency, excessively high requirement or malabsorption. Usually more than one factor is involved, e.g. loss of blood and malabsorption.

In this type of anaemia erythrocytes are microcytic and hypochromic because their haemoglobin content is low.

Normal requirements, deficient intake

Because of the relative inefficiency of iron absorption, deficiency occurs frequently, even in individuals whose requirements are normal. The likelihood of deficiency increases if the daily diet is restricted in some way, as in poorly planned vegetarian diets, or in calorie-controlled diets where the range of foods eaten is small. Babies dependent on milk may also suffer mild iron deficiency anaemia if weaning on to a mixed diet is delayed much past the first year, since the liver carries only a few months' store and milk is a poor source of iron.

Table 4.4 Terms used to describe changes in red blood cells		
Term	**Definition**	**Example**
Normocytic	Cells normal sized	Acute haemorrhage
Microcytic	Cells smaller than normal	Iron deficiency
Macrocytic	Cells bigger than normal	Vitamin B_{12} or folic acid deficiency
Hypochromic	Cells paler than normal	Iron deficiency anaemia
Haemolytic	Rate of cell destruction raised	Autoimmune disease
		Sickle cell anaemia

High requirements, normal or deficient intake

This type of anaemia occurs in pregnancy, when iron requirements are increased both for fetal growth and to support the additional load on the mother's cardiovascular system. It may also occur as a result of chronic blood loss, the causes of which include:

- chronic peptic ulcers
- menorrhagia
- intestinal ulceration
- haemorrhoids
- carcinoma.

Malabsorption

Iron absorption is usually increased following haemorrhage but may be reduced in abnormalities of the stomach, duodenum or jejunum including:

- resection of stomach or upper part of the small intestine
- hypochlorhydria, e.g. in malignant disease, Addisonian pernicious anaemia.

Megaloblastic anaemias

Maturation of erythrocytes is impaired when deficiency of vitamin B_{12} and/or folic acid occurs (Fig. 4.3) and abnormally large erythrocytes (megaloblasts) are found in the blood. During normal erythropoiesis (Fig. 4.2) several cell divisions occur and the daughter cells at each stage are smaller than the parent cell because there is not much time for cell enlargement between divisions. When deficiency of vitamin B_{12} and/or folic acid occurs, the rate of DNA and RNA synthesis is reduced, delaying cell division. The cells can therefore grow larger than normal between divisions. Circulating cells are immature, larger than normal and some are nucleated (MCV >94 fl). The haemoglobin content of each cell is normal or raised. The cells are fragile and their life span is reduced to between 40 and 50 days. Depressed production and early lysis cause anaemia.

Vitamin B_{12} deficiency anaemia

Pernicious anaemia

This is the most common form of vitamin B_{12} deficiency anaemia. It occurs more often in females than males, usually between 45 and 65 years of age. It is an autoimmune disease in which auto-antibodies destroy intrinsic factor (IF) and parietal cells in the stomach.

Dietary deficiency of vitamin B_{12}

This is rare, except in true vegans, i.e. when no animal products are included in the diet. The store of vitamin B_{12} is such that deficiency takes several years to appear.

Other causes of vitamin B_{12} deficiency

These include the following.

- *Gastrectomy* — this leaves fewer cells available to produce IF after partial resection of the stomach.
- *Chronic gastritis, malignant disease and ionising radiation* — these damage the gastric mucosa including the parietal cells that produce IF.
- *Blind loop syndrome* — this occurs when the contents of the small intestine are slow moving or static, allowing microbes to colonise the small intestine and use or destroy the intrinsic factor–vitamin B_{12} (IF–B_{12}) complex before it reaches the terminal ileum where it is absorbed. Blind loops of bowel occur in diverticular disease (p. 328) and are left after some surgical procedures.
- *Malabsorption of intrinsic factor–vitamin B_{12} complex* — this may follow resection of terminal ileum or inflammation of the terminal ileum, e.g. Crohn's disease or tropical sprue.

Complications of vitamin B_{12} deficiency anaemia

These may appear before the signs of anaemia. They include:

- subacute combined degeneration of the spinal cord in which nerve fibres in the posterior and lateral columns of white matter become demyelinated. Vitamin B_{12} is essential for the secretion and maintenance of myelin (p. 142 and p. 186).
- ulceration of the tongue and glossitis.

Folic acid deficiency anaemia

Deficiency in the bone marrow causes a form of megaloblastic anaemia not associated with degeneration of the spinal cord. It may be due to:

- dietary deficiency, e.g. in infants if there is delay in establishing a mixed diet, in alcoholics, in anorexia and in pregnancy when the requirement is raised
- malabsorption from the jejunum caused by e.g. coeliac disease, tropical sprue or anticonvulsant drugs
- interference with use by e.g. cytotoxic and anticonvulsant drugs.

Hypoplastic and aplastic anaemias

Hypoplastic and aplastic anaemias are due to varying degrees of bone marrow failure. Bone marrow function is reduced in hypoplastic anaemia, and absent in aplastic anaemia. Since the bone marrow produces leukocytes and platelets as well as erythrocytes, *leukopenia* (low white cell count) and *thrombocytopenia* (low platelet count) are likely to accompany diminished red cell numbers. When all three cell types are low, the condition is called *pancytopenia*, and is accompanied by anaemia, diminished immunity and a tendency to bleed. The condition is often idiopathic, but the known causes include:

- drugs, e.g. cytotoxic drugs, some anti-inflammatory and anticonvulsant drugs, some sulphonamides and antibiotics
- ionising radiation
- some chemicals, e.g. benzene and its derivatives
- chronic nephritis
- viral disease, including hepatitis
- invasion of bone marrow by, e.g., malignant disease, leukaemia or fibrosis.

Haemolytic anaemias

These occur when red cells are destroyed while in circulation or are removed prematurely from the circulation because the cells are abnormal or the spleen is overactive.

Congenital haemolytic anaemias

In these diseases genetic abnormality leads to the synthesis of abnormal haemoglobin and increased red cell membrane friability, reducing cell oxygen-carrying capacity and life span. The most common forms are sickle cell anaemia and thalassaemia.

Sickle cell anaemia

The abnormal haemoglobin molecules become misshapen when deoxygenated, making the erythrocytes sickle shaped. A high proportion of abnormal molecules makes the sickling permanent. The life span of cells is reduced by early haemolysis. Sickle cells do not move smoothly through the small blood vessels. This tends to increase the viscosity of the blood, reducing the rate of blood flow and leading to intravascular clotting, ischaemia and infarction. The anaemia is due to early haemolysis of irreversibly sickled cells.

Blacks are more affected than other races. Some affected individuals have a degree of immunity to malaria because the life span of the sickled cells is less than the time needed for the malaria parasite to mature inside the cells.

Complications. Pregnancy, infection and dehydration predispose to the development of 'crises' due to intravascular clotting and ischaemia, causing severe pain in long bones, chest or the abdomen. The formation of gallstones (*cholelithiasis*) and inflammation of the gall bladder (*cholecystitis*) also occurs (p. 336).

Thalassaemia

There is reduced globin synthesis with resultant reduced haemoglobin production and increased friability of the cell membrane, leading to early haemolysis. Severe cases may cause death in infants or young children. This condition is most common in Mediterranean countries.

Haemolytic disease of the newborn

In this disorder, the mother's immune system makes antibodies to the baby's red blood cells, causing haemolysis and phagocytosis of fetal erythrocytes. The antigen system involved is usually (but not always) the Rhesus (Rh) antigen.

A Rh$^-$ mother carries no Rh antigen on her red blood cells, but she has the capacity to produce anti-Rh antibodies. If she conceives a child fathered by a Rh$^+$ man, and the baby inherits the Rh antigen from him, the baby may also be Rh$^+$, i.e. different from the mother. During pregnancy, the placenta protects the baby from the mother's immune system, but at delivery a few fetal red blood cells may enter the maternal circulation. Because they carry an antigen (the Rh antigen) foreign to the mother, her immune system will be stimulated to produce neutralising antibodies to it. The red cells of second and subsequent Rh$^+$ babies are attacked by these maternal antibodies, which can cross the placenta and enter the fetal circulation (Fig. 4.11). In the most severe cases, the baby dies in the womb from profound anaemia. In less serious circumstances, the baby is born with some degree of anaemia, which is corrected with blood transfusions.

The disease is much less common than it used to be, because it was discovered that if a Rh$^-$ mother is given an injection of anti-Rh antibodies within 72 hours of the delivery of a Rh$^+$ baby, her immune system does not make its own anti-Rh antibodies to the fetal red cells. Subsequent pregnancies are therefore not affected. The anti-Rh antibodies given to the mother bind to, and neutralise, any fetal red cells present in her circulation before her immune system becomes sensitised to them.

Acquired haemolytic anaemias

In this context acquired means haemolytic anaemia in which no familial or racial factors have been identified. There are several causes.

Chemical agents

These substances cause early or excessive haemolysis, e.g.:

- some drugs, especially when taken long term in large doses, e.g. phenacetin, primaquine, sulphonamides
- chemicals encountered in the general or work environment, e.g. lead, arsenic compounds

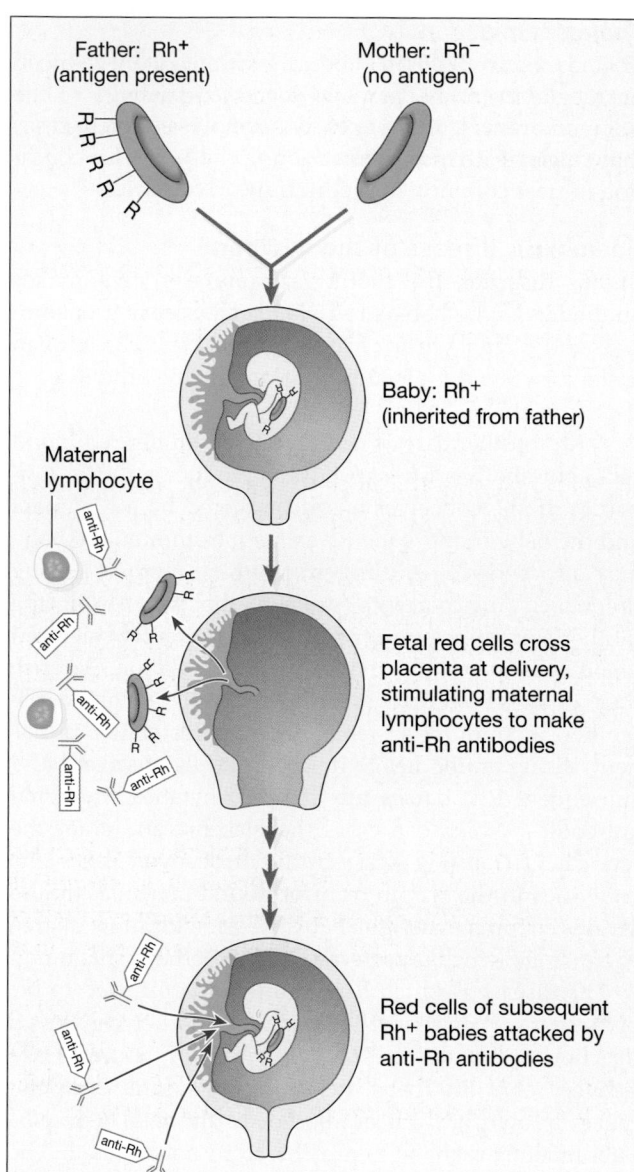

Figure 4.11 The immune processes involved in haemolytic disease of the newborn.

- toxins produced by microbes, e.g. *Streptococcus pyogenes, Clostridium welchii*.

Autoimmunity

In this disease individuals make antibodies to their own red cell antigens, causing haemolysis. It may be acute or chronic and primary or secondary to other diseases, e.g. carcinoma, viral infection or other autoimmune diseases.

Blood transfusion reactions

Individuals do not normally produce antibodies to their own red blood cell antigens; if they did, the antigens and antibodies would react, causing clumping and lysis of the erythrocytes (see Fig. 4.5, p. 65). However, if individuals receive a transfusion of blood possessing antigens different from their own, their immune system will recognise them as foreign, make antibodies to them and destroy them (transfusion reaction). This adverse reaction between the blood of incompatible recipients and donors leads to haemolysis within the recipient's cardiovascular system. The breakdown products of haemolysis lodge in, and block, the filtering mechanism of the nephron, impairing kidney function. Other principal signs of a transfusion reaction include fever, chills, lumbar pain and shock.

Other causes of haemolytic anaemia

These include:

- parasitic diseases, e.g. malaria
- ionising radiation, e.g. X-rays, radioactive isotopes
- destruction of blood trapped in tissues in, e.g., severe burns, crushing injuries
- physical damage to cells by, e.g., artificial heart valves, kidney dialysis machines.

Normocytic normochromic anaemia

In this type the cells are normal but the numbers are reduced and the proportion of reticulocytes in the blood may be increased as the body tries to restore erythrocyte numbers to normal. This occurs:

- in many chronic disease conditions, e.g. in chronic inflammation
- following severe haemorrhage
- in haemolytic disease.

Polycythaemia

There are an abnormally large number of erythrocytes in the blood. This increases blood viscosity, slows the rate of flow and increases the risk of intravascular clotting, ischaemia and infarction.

Relative increase in erythrocyte count

This occurs when the erythrocyte count is normal but the blood volume is reduced by fluid loss, e.g. excessive serum exudate from extensive superficial burns.

True increase in erythrocyte count

Physiological. Prolonged hypoxia stimulates erythropoiesis and the number of cells released into the normal volume of blood is increased. This occurs in people living at high altitudes where the oxygen tension in the air is low and the partial pressure of oxygen in the alveoli of the lungs is correspondingly low. Each cell carries less oxygen so more cells are needed to meet the body's oxygen needs.

Pathological. The reason for this increase in circulating red cells, sometimes to twice the normal number, is not known. It may be secondary to other factors that cause hypoxia of the red bone marrow, e.g. cigarette smoking, pulmonary disease, bone marrow cancer.

Polycythaemia rubra vera

In this primary condition of unknown cause there is abnormal excessive production of the erythrocyte precursors, i.e. *myeloproliferation*. This raises the haemoglobin level and the haematocrit (relative proportion of cells to plasma). The blood viscosity is increased and may lead to hypertension and cerebral, coronary or mesenteric thrombosis. Aplastic anaemia and leukaemia may also be present.

LEUKOCYTE DISORDERS

Learning outcomes

After studying this section, you should be able to:

■ define the terms leukopenia and leukocytosis

■ review the physiological importance of abnormally increased and decreased leukocyte numbers in the blood

■ discuss the main forms of leukaemia, including the causes, signs and symptoms of the disease.

Leukopenia

This is the name of the condition in which the total blood leukocyte count is less than $4 \times 10^9/1$ (4000/mm^3).

Granulocytopenia (neutropenia)

This is a general term used to indicate an abnormal reduction in the numbers of circulating granulocytes (polymorphonuclear leukocytes), commonly called neutropenia because 40 to 75% of granulocytes are neutrophils. A reduction in the number of circulating granulocytes occurs when production does not keep pace with the normal removal of cells or when the life span of the cells is reduced. Extreme shortage or the absence of granulocytes is called *agranulocytosis*. A temporary reduction occurs in response to inflammation but the numbers are usually quickly restored. Inadequate granulopoiesis may be caused by:

■ drugs, e.g. cytotoxic drugs, phenylbutazone, phenothiazines, some sulphonamides and antibiotics
■ irradiation damage to granulocyte precursors in the bone marrow by, e.g., X-rays, radioactive isotopes
■ diseases of red bone marrow, e.g. leukaemias, some anaemias
■ severe microbial infections.

In conditions where the spleen is enlarged, excessive numbers of granulocytes are trapped, reducing the number in circulation. Neutropenia predisposes to severe infections that can lead to tissue necrosis, septicaemia and death. Septicaemia is the presence of significant numbers of active pathogens in the blood. The pathogens are commonly *commensals*, i.e. microbes that are normally present in the body but do not usually cause infection, such as those in the bowel.

Leukocytosis

An increase in the number of circulating leukocytes occurs as a normal protective reaction in a variety of pathological conditions, especially in response to infections. When the infection subsides the leukocyte count returns to normal.

Pathological leukocytosis exists when a blood leukocyte count of more than $11 \times 10^9/1$ (11 000/mm^3) is sustained and is not consistent with the normal protective function. One or more of the different types of cell is involved.

Leukaemia

Leukaemia is a malignant proliferation of white blood cell precursors by the bone marrow. It results in the uncontrolled increase in the production of leukocytes and/or their precursors. As the tumour cells enter the blood the total leukocyte count is usually raised but in some cases it may be normal or even low. The proliferation of immature leukaemic blast cells crowds out other blood cells formed in bone marrow, causing anaemia, thrombocytopenia and leukopenia (pancytopenia).

Causes of leukaemia

Some causes of leukaemia are known but many cases cannot be accounted for. Some people may have a genetic predisposition that is triggered by environmental factors. Known causes include:

73

Ionising radiation. Radiation such as that produced by X-rays and radioactive isotopes causes malignant changes in the precursors of white blood cells. The DNA of the cells may be damaged and some cells die while others reproduce at an abnormally rapid rate. Leukaemia may develop at any time after irradiation, even 20 or more years later.

Chemicals. Some chemicals encountered in the general or work environment alter the DNA of the white cell precursors in the bone marrow. These include benzene and its derivatives, asbestos, cytotoxic drugs, chloramphenicol.

Viral infections.

Genetic factors. Identical twins of leukaemia sufferers have a much higher risk than normal of developing the disease, suggesting involvement of genetic factors.

Types of leukaemia

Leukaemias are usually classified according to the type of cell involved, the maturity of the cells and the rate at which the disease develops (Fig. 4.2 and Table 4.5).

Acute leukaemias

These types usually have a sudden onset and affect the poorly differentiated and immature 'blast' cells (Fig. 4.2). They are aggressive tumours that reach a climax within a few weeks or months. The rapid progress of bone marrow invasion impairs its function and culminates in anaemia, haemorrhage and susceptibility to infection. The mucous membranes of the mouth and upper gastrointestinal tract are most commonly affected.

Acute myeloblastic leukaemia. This occurs at any age, but most commonly between 25 and 60 years.

Acute lymphoblastic leukaemia. This disease is most common in children under 10 years, although a number of cases may occur up to about 40 years of age.

Chronic leukaemias

These conditions are less aggressive than the acute forms and the leukocytes are more differentiated, i.e. at the 'cyte' stage (Fig. 4.2).

Chronic granulocytic leukaemia. There is a gradual increase in the number of immature granulocytes in the blood. In the later stages, anaemia, secondary haemorrhages, infections and fever become increasingly severe. It is slightly more common in men than women and

Table 4.5 Types of leukaemia and the cells involved	
Type of leukaemia	**Type of cell involved**
Myeloid (myelogenous myeloblastic)	Granulocytes, myelocytes, myeloblasts
Lymphocytic	Lymphocytes, lymphoblasts
Monocytic	Monocytes

usually occurs between the ages of 20 and 40 years. Although treatment may appear to be successful, death usually occurs within about 5 years.

Chronic lymphocytic leukaemia. There is enlargement of the lymph nodes and hyperplasia of lymphoid tissue throughout the body. The lymphocyte count is considerably higher than normal. Lymphocytes accumulate in the bone marrow and there is progressive anaemia and thrombocytopenia. It is three times more common in males than females and it occurs mainly between the ages of 50 and 70 years. Death is usually due to repeated infections of increasing severity, with great variations in survival times.

HAEMORRHAGIC DISEASES

Learning outcomes

After studying this section, you should be able to:

- indicate the main causes and effects of thrombocytopenia
- relate levels of vitamin K to clotting disorders
- explain the term disseminated intravascular coagulation, including its principal causes
- describe the physiological deficiencies present in the haemophilias
- explain the pattern of inheritance of haemophilia.

Thrombocytopenia

This is defined as a blood platelet count below $150 \times 10^9/l$ (150 000/mm³) but spontaneous capillary bleeding does not usually occur unless the count falls below $30 \times 10^9/l$ (30 000/mm³). It may be due to a reduced rate of platelet production or increased rate of destruction.

Reduced platelet production

This is usually due to bone marrow deficiencies, and therefore production of erythrocytes and leukocytes is also reduced, giving rise to pancytopenia. It is often due to:

- platelets being crowded out of the bone marrow in bone marrow diseases, e.g. leukaemias, pernicious anaemia, malignant tumours
- ionising radiation, e.g. X-rays or radioactive isotopes, that damage the rapidly dividing precursor cells in the bone marrow
- drugs, e.g. cytotoxic drugs, chloramphenicol, chlorpromazine, phenylbutazone, sulphonamides.

Increased platelet destruction

A reduced platelet count occurs when production of new cells does not keep pace with destruction of damaged and worn out cells. This occurs in disseminated intravascular coagulation (see below) and autoimmune thrombocytopenic purpura.

Autoimmune thrombocytopenic purpura. This condition, which usually affects children and young adults, may be triggered by a viral infection such as measles. Antiplatelet antibodies are formed that coat platelets, leading to platelet destruction and their removal from the circulation. A significant feature of this disease is the presence of *purpura*, which are haemorrhages into the skin ranging in size from pinpoints to large blotches. The severity of the disease varies from mild bleeding into the skin to severe haemorrhage. When the platelet count is very low there may be severe bruising, haematuria, gastrointestinal or cranial haemorrhages.

Secondary thrombocytopenic purpura. This may occur in association with red bone marrow diseases, excessive irradiation and some drugs, e.g. digoxin, chlorthiazides, quinine, sulphonamides.

Vitamin K deficiency

Vitamin K is required by the liver for the synthesis of many clotting factors and therefore deficiency predisposes to impairment of haemostasis (p. 67).

Haemorrhagic disease of the newborn

Spontaneous haemorrhage from the umbilical cord and intestinal mucosa occurs in babies when the stored vitamin K obtained from the mother before birth has been used up and the intestinal bacteria needed for its synthesis in the infant's bowel are not yet established. This is most likely to occur when the baby is premature.

Deficient absorption in adults

Vitamin K is fat soluble and bile salts are required in the colon for its absorption. Deficiency may occur when there is liver disease, prolonged obstruction to the biliary tract or in any other disease where fat absorption is impaired, e.g. coeliac disease.

Dietary deficiency

This is rare because a sufficient supply of vitamin K is usually synthesised in the intestine by bacterial action. However, deficiency may occur during treatment with drugs that sterilise the bowel.

Disseminated intravascular coagulation (DIC)

DIC is a common complication of a number of other disorders. The coagulation system is activated within the blood vessels, leading to formation of intravascular clots and deposition of fibrin within the tissues. Because of this consumption of clotting factors and platelets there is a consequent tendency to haemorrhage. The causes of DIC include:

- severe shock, especially when due to microbial infection
- septicaemia when endotoxins are released by Gram-negative bacteria
- severe trauma
- premature separation of placenta when amniotic fluid enters maternal blood
- acute pancreatitis when digestive enzymes are released into the blood
- malignant tumours with widely dispersed metastases.

Congenital disorders

The haemophilias

In each body cell, except gametes, there are 46 chromosomes arranged in 23 pairs, of which one pair are sex chromosomes. In the female, the two sex chromosomes are identical and are called X chromosomes. In the male, each cell has one X chromosome and one Y chromosome.

> Female—XX
> Male—XY

Each gamete (ovum and spermatozoon) has only 23 chromosomes, one from each of the 23 pairs. This means that each ovum has an X chromosome and each spermatozoon has either an X *or* a Y chromosome.

Fusion of an ovum with a spermatozoon carrying an X chromosome results in the conception of a female child, whereas if the spermatozoon bears a Y chromosome the child is male.

The Y chromosome is shorter than, and therefore carries fewer genes than, the X chromosome. Traits coded for on the section of the X chromosome that has no corresponding material on the Y are said to be *sex linked*. The gene that codes for the synthesis of clotting factors VIII and IX is one example, and is therefore carried on X chromosomes only. If the gene is abnormal on one of a female's two X chromosomes, she is most likely to have a normal gene on her other X chromosome, which ensures production of normal clotting factors. A female who carries the faulty gene, even though the disease is not expressed in her, may pass the faulty gene on to her children and is said to be a *carrier*. If the gene is abnormal in a male, who has only one copy of the gene since he has only one X chromosome, he will therefore have haemophilia. Haemophilia is inherited as shown in Figure 4.12. This illustrates the possible genetic combinations of the children of a carrier mother (one normal gene and one faulty gene) and a normal father (one normal gene).

Sufferers from haemophilia experience repeated episodes of severe and prolonged bleeding at any site, with little evidence of trauma. Recurrent bleeding into joints is common, causing severe pain and, in the long term, cartilage is damaged.

The two main forms of haemophilia differ only in the clotting factor involved; the clinical picture in both is identical.

Haemophilia A. In this disease, factor VIII is abnormal and is less biologically active.

Haemophilia B (Christmas disease). This is the less common sex-linked genetic haemorrhagic disease. Factor IX is deficient, resulting in deficiency of thromboplastin.

von Willebrand's disease. In this disease a deficiency in the von Willebrand factor causes low levels of factor VIII. As the inheritance is not sex-linked, haemorrhages due to defective clotting occur equally in males and females.

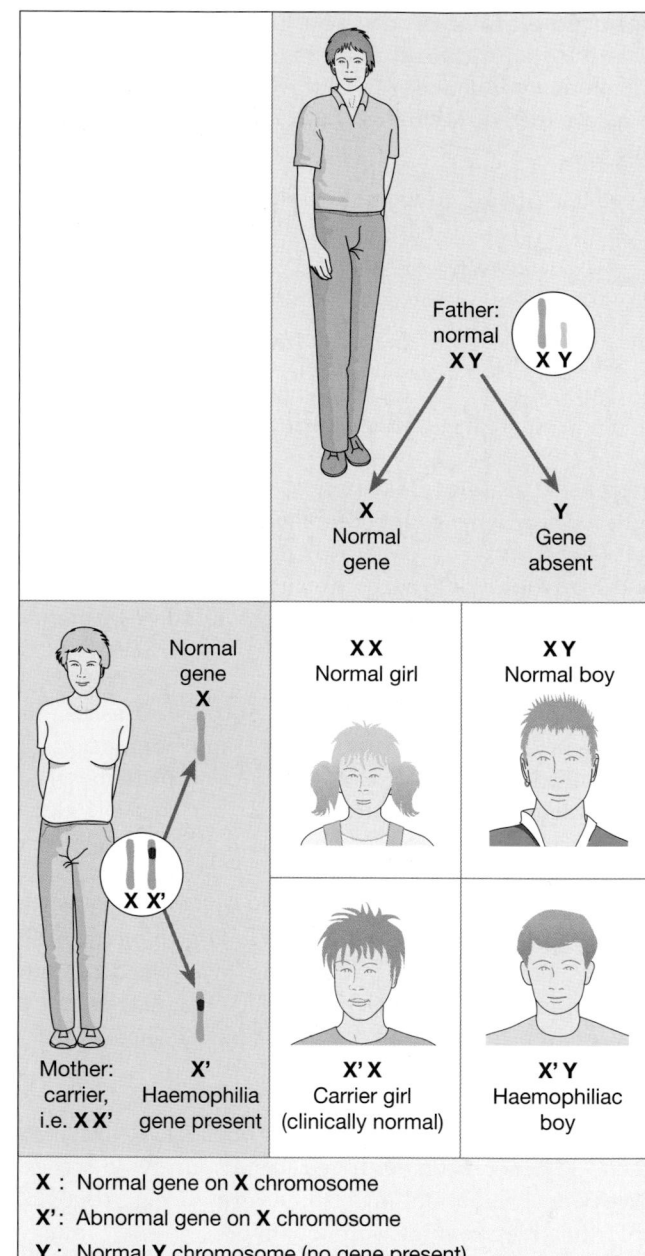

Figure 4.12 Transmission of the sex-linked haemophilia gene between generations.

5 The cardiovascular system

The cardiovascular system is divided for descriptive purposes into two main parts.

1. The *circulatory system*, consisting of the *heart*, which acts as a pump, and the *blood vessels* through which the *blood* circulates
2. The *lymphatic system*, consisting of *lymph nodes* and *lymph vessels*, through which colourless *lymph* flows.

The two systems communicate with one another and are intimately associated.

The heart pumps blood into two anatomically separate systems of blood vessels (Fig. 5.1).

- the pulmonary circulation
- the systemic circulation.

The right side of the heart pumps blood to the lungs (the pulmonary circulation) where gas exchange occurs; i.e. CO_2 leaves the blood and enters the lungs, and O_2 leaves the lungs and enters the blood. The left side of the heart pumps blood into the systemic circulation, which supplies the rest of the body. Here, tissue wastes are passed into the blood for excretion, and body cells extract nutrients and O_2.

The circulatory system ensures a continuous flow of blood to all body cells, and its function is subject to continual physiological adjustments in order to maintain an adequate blood supply. Should the supply of oxygen and nutrients to body cells become inadequate, tissue damage occurs and cell death may follow.

BLOOD VESSELS

Learning outcomes

After studying this section, you should be able to:

- describe the structures and functions of arteries, veins and capillaries
- explain the relationship between the different types of blood vessel
- indicate the main factors controlling blood vessel diameter
- explain the mechanisms by which exchange of nutrients, gases and wastes occurs between the blood and the tissues.

The heart pumps blood into vessels that vary in structure, size and function, and there are several types: arteries, arterioles, capillaries, venules and veins (Fig. 5.2).

Arteries and arterioles

These are the blood vessels that transport blood away from the heart. They vary considerably in size and their walls consist of three layers of tissue (Fig. 5.3):

Figure 5.1 The relationship between the pulmonary and the systemic circulations.

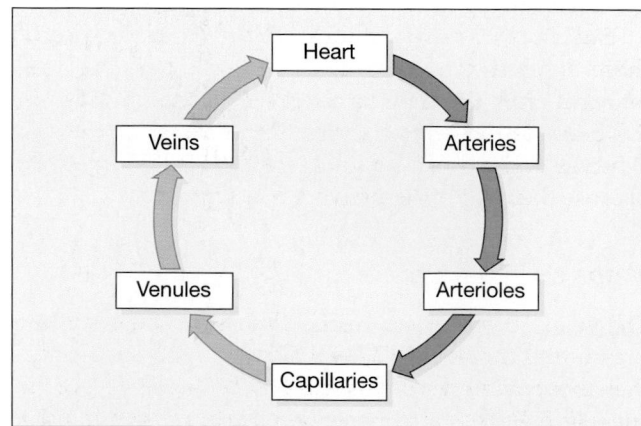

Figure 5.2 The relationship between the heart and the different types of blood vessel.

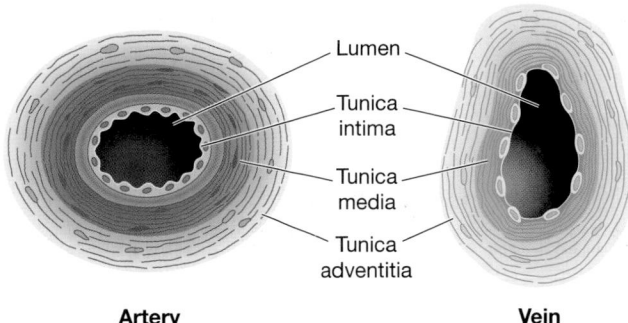

Figure 5.3 Structures of an artery and a vein.

- *tunica adventitia* or outer layer of fibrous tissue
- *tunica media* or middle layer of smooth muscle and elastic tissue
- *tunica intima* or inner lining of squamous epithelium called *endothelium*.

The amount of muscular and elastic tissue varies in the arteries depending upon their size. In the large arteries, sometimes called elastic arteries, the tunica media consists of more elastic tissue and less smooth muscle. These proportions gradually change as the arteries branch many times and become smaller until in the *arterioles* (the smallest arteries) the tunica media consists almost entirely of smooth muscle. Arteries have thicker walls than veins and this enables them to withstand the high pressure of arterial blood.

Anastomoses and end-arteries

Anastomoses are arteries that form a link between main arteries supplying an area, e.g. the arterial supply to the palms of the hand (p. 102) and soles of the feet, the brain, the joints and, to a limited extent, the heart muscle. If one artery supplying the area is occluded anastomotic arteries provide a *collateral circulation*. This is most likely to provide an adequate blood supply when the occlusion occurs gradually, giving the anastomotic arteries time to dilate.

End-arteries are the arteries with no anastomoses or those beyond the most distal anastomosis, e.g. the branches from the circulus arteriosus (circle of Willis) in the brain or the central artery to the retina of the eye. When an end-artery is occluded the tissues it supplies die because there is no alternative blood supply.

Veins and venules

The veins are the blood vessels that return blood at low pressure to the heart. The walls of the veins are thinner than those of arteries but have the same three layers of tissue (Fig. 5.3). They are thinner because there is less muscle and elastic tissue in the tunica media. When cut, the veins collapse while the thicker-walled arteries remain open.

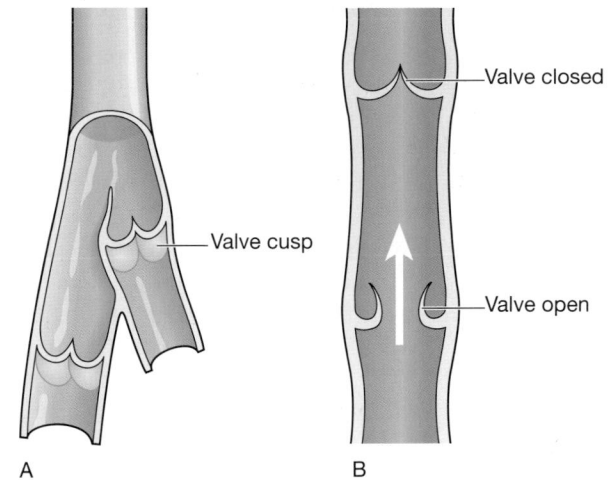

Figure 5.4 Interior of a vein: A. The valves and cusps. B. The direction of blood flow through a valve.

When an artery is cut blood spurts at high pressure while a slower, steady flow of blood escapes from a vein.

Some veins possess *valves*, which prevent backflow of blood, ensuring that it flows towards the heart (Fig. 5.4). Valves are abundant in the veins of the limbs, especially the lower limbs where blood must travel a considerable distance against gravity when the individual is standing. Valves are absent in very small and very large veins in the thorax and abdomen. They are formed by a fold of tunica intima strengthened by connective tissue. The cusps are *semilunar* in shape with the concavity towards the heart.

The smallest veins are called *venules*.

Capillaries and sinusoids

The smallest arterioles break up into a number of minute vessels called *capillaries*. Capillary walls consist of a single layer of endothelial cells through which water and other small-molecule substances can pass. Blood cells and large-molecule substances such as plasma proteins do not normally pass through capillary walls. The capillaries form a vast network of tiny vessels which link the smallest arterioles to the smallest venules. Their diameter is approximately that of an erythrocyte (7 µm). The capillary bed is the site of exchange of substances between the blood and the tissue fluid, which bathes the body cells.

Sinusoids are wider than capillaries and have extremely thin walls separating blood from the neighbouring cells. In some there are distinct spaces between the endothelial cells. Among the endothelial cells there may be many phagocytic macrophages, e.g. Kupffer cells in the liver. Sinusoids are found in bone marrow, endocrine glands, spleen and liver. Because of their larger lumen the blood pressure in sinusoids is lower than in capillaries and there is a slower rate of blood flow.

Control of blood vessel diameter

All blood vessels except capillaries have smooth muscle fibres in the tunica media which are supplied by nerves of the *autonomic nervous system*. These nerves arise from the *vasomotor centre* in the *medulla oblongata* and they change the diameter of the lumen of blood vessels, controlling the volume of blood they contain. Medium-sized and small arteries have more muscle than elastic tissue in their walls. In large arteries, such as the aorta, the middle layer is almost entirely elastic tissue. This means that small arteries and arterioles respond to nerve stimulation whereas the diameter of large arteries varies according to the amount of blood they contain.

Vasodilatation and vasoconstriction

Sympathetic nerves supply the smooth muscle of the tunica media of blood vessels. There is no parasympathetic nerve supply to most blood vessels and therefore the diameter of the vessel lumen and the tone of the smooth muscle is determined by the degree of sympathetic nerve stimulation. There is always some nerve input to the smooth muscle in the vessel walls which can then be increased or decreased (Fig. 5.5). Decreased nerve stimulation causes the smooth muscle to relax, thinning the vessel wall and enlarging the lumen. This process is called *vasodilatation* and results in increased blood flow under less resistance. Conversely, when nervous activity is increased the smooth muscle of the tunica media contracts and thickens; this process is called *vasoconstriction*.

The blood vessels primarily responsible for providing resistance to blood flow are the small arterioles, the walls of which consist mainly of smooth muscle. A small change in their lumen results in considerable alteration in blood flow to the part of the body they supply. Arterioles provide the *peripheral resistance* to the flow of blood and are therefore called resistance vessels. This is important in maintaining homeostasis of blood pressure (p. 91).

Resistance to flow of fluids along a tube is determined by three factors: the diameter of the tube; the length of the tube; and the viscosity of the fluid involved. The most important factor in relation to flow of blood along vessels is peripheral resistance. The length of the vessels and viscosity of blood could also contribute but in health these are constant and are therefore not significant determinants of changes in blood flow.

Autoregulation

The accumulation of metabolites in local tissues also influences the degree of dilatation of arterioles. This mechanism ensures that local blood flow is increased or decreased in response to tissue need. For example in:

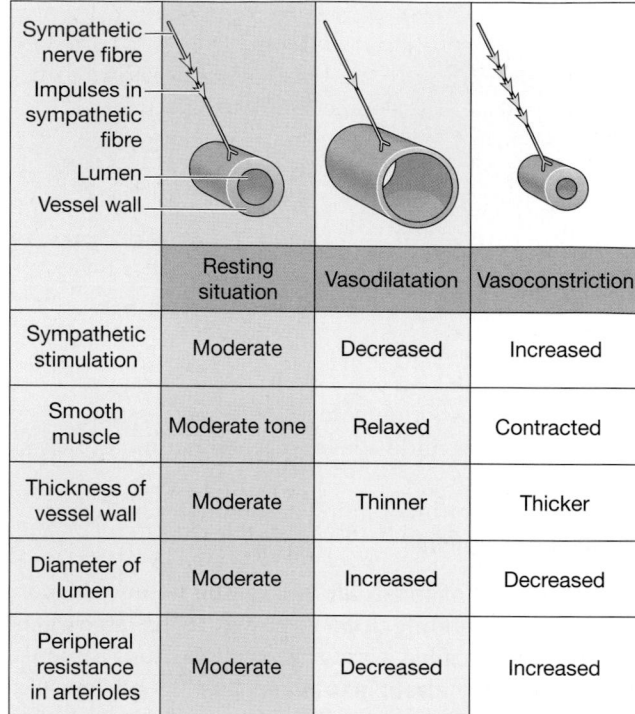

	Resting situation	Vasodilatation	Vasoconstriction
Sympathetic stimulation	Moderate	Decreased	Increased
Smooth muscle	Moderate tone	Relaxed	Contracted
Thickness of vessel wall	Moderate	Thinner	Thicker
Diameter of lumen	Moderate	Increased	Decreased
Peripheral resistance in arterioles	Moderate	Decreased	Increased

Figure 5.5 The relationship between sympathetic stimulation and blood vessel diameter.

- exercise; e.g. lactic acid accumulation in muscle causes vasodilatation
- hypoxia; vasodilatation follows an episode of reduced tissue blood flow
- tissue damage; e.g. in inflammation, mediators such as histamine, prostaglandins and bradykinin lead to vasodilatation (p. 376),
- situations where the circulation to vital organs, such as the brain and heart, is threatened.

Blood supply

The outer layers of tissue of thick-walled blood vessels receive their blood supply via a network of blood vessels called the *vasa vasorum*. Vessels with thin walls and the endothelium of the others receive oxygen and nutrients by diffusion from the blood passing through them.

Internal respiration

Internal respiration (Fig. 5.6) is the exchange of gases between capillary blood and local body cells.

Oxygen is carried from the lungs to the tissues in chemical combination with haemoglobin as *oxyhaemoglobin*. The exchange in the tissues takes place between blood at the arterial end of the capillaries and the tissue fluid and then between the tissue fluid and the cells. The process involved is that of diffusion from a higher concentration of oxygen in the blood to a lower concentration in the cells, i.e. down the concentration gradient.

Oxyhaemoglobin is an unstable compound and breaks up (dissociates) easily to liberate oxygen. Factors that increase dissociation include raised carbon dioxide content of tissue fluid, raised temperature and 2,3 diphosphoglycerate (DPG), a substance present in red blood cells. In active tissues there is an increased production of carbon dioxide and heat which leads to an increased availability of oxygen. In this way oxygen is available to the tissues in greatest need.

DPG is produced in red blood cells and causes haemoglobin to give up its oxygen more readily. Erythrocyte production of DPG increases in anaemia and other conditions, promoting oxygen release to the tissues.

Carbon dioxide is one of the waste products of cell metabolism and, towards the venous end of the capillary, it diffuses into the blood down the concentration gradient. Blood transports carbon dioxide to the lungs for excretion by three different mechanisms:

- dissolved in the water of the blood plasma—7%
- in chemical combination with sodium in the form of sodium bicarbonate—70%
- remainder in combination with haemoglobin—23%.

Cell nutrition

The nutrients required by the cells of the body are transported round the body in the blood plasma. In passing from the blood to the cells, the nutrients pass through the semipermeable capillary walls into the tissue fluid which bathes the cells, then through the cell membrane into the cell. The mechanism of the transfer of water and other substances from the blood capillaries depends mainly upon diffusion, osmosis and active transport.

Diffusion (p. 26)

The capillary walls consist of a single layer of epithelial cells that constitutes a *semipermeable membrane* which allows substances with small molecules to pass through into tissue fluid, and retains large molecules in the blood. Diffusible substances include dissolved oxygen and carbon dioxide, glucose, amino acids, fatty acids, glycerol, vitamins, mineral salts and water.

Osmosis (p. 27)

Osmotic pressure across a semipermeable membrane draws water from a dilute to a more concentrated solution in an attempt to establish a state of equilibrium. The force of the osmotic pressure depends on the *number of non-diffusible* particles in the solutions separated by the membrane. The main substances responsible for the osmotic pressure between blood and tissue fluid are the plasma proteins, especially albumin.

Capillary fluid dynamics

At the arterial end the capillary blood pressure, i.e. *hydrostatic pressure*, is about 35 mmHg (5 kPa). This causes the forward movement of blood and forces some water and solutes of small enough molecular size to pass out of the capillaries into the tissue spaces. The *osmotic pressure* in the capillaries is about 25 mmHg (3 kPa). This pressure draws water into the capillaries and is exerted mainly by plasma proteins of molecular size too large to pass through the capillary walls. The net outward pressure of 10 mmHg is the difference between the hydrostatic and osmotic pressures (Figs 5.7 and 5.8).

At the venous end of the capillaries hydrostatic pressure is reduced to about 15 mmHg (2 kPa) and the osmotic pressure remains the same, at 25 mmHg (3 kPa). The net

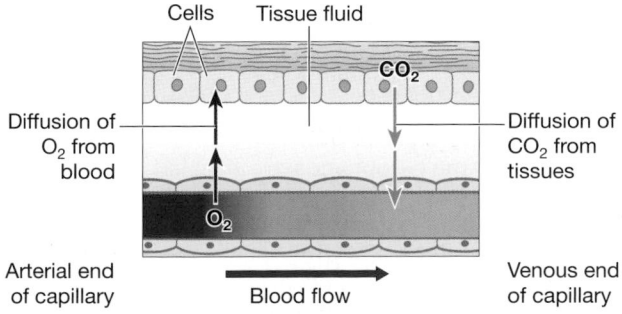

Figure 5.6 The exchange of gases in internal respiration.

Figure 5.7 Diffusion of nutrients and waste products between capillaries and cells.

Figure 5.8 Effect of capillary pressures on water movement between capillaries and cells.

force moving water and solvents into the capillaries is again the difference between the two pressures, i.e. 10 mmHg.

This transfer of substances, including water, to the tissue spaces is a dynamic process. As blood flows slowly through the large network of capillaries from the arterial to the venous end, there is constant change. Not all the water and cell waste products return to the blood capillaries. The excess is drained away from the tissue spaces in the minute *lymph capillaries* which originate as blind-end tubes with walls similar to, but more permeable than, those of the blood capillaries (Fig. 5.7). Extra tissue fluid and some cell waste materials enter the lymph capillaries and are eventually returned to the bloodstream (Ch. 6).

HEART

Learning outcomes

After studying this section, you should be able to:

- describe the structure of the heart and its position within the thorax

- trace the circulation of the blood through the heart and the blood vessels of the body

- outline the conducting system of the heart

- relate the electrical activity of the cardiac conduction system to the cardiac cycle

- describe the main factors determining heart rate and cardiac output.

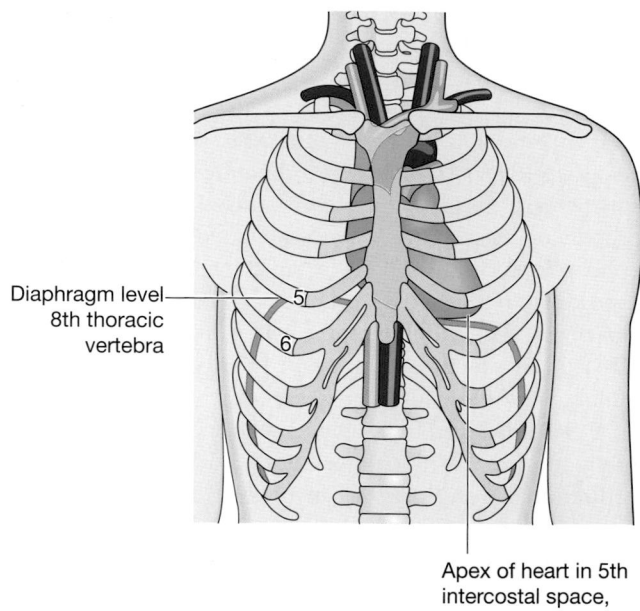

Figure 5.9 Position of the heart in the thorax.

The heart is a roughly cone-shaped hollow muscular organ. It is about 10 cm long and is about the size of the owner's fist. It weighs about 225 g in women and is heavier in men (about 310 g).

Position

The heart lies in the thoracic cavity in the mediastinum between the lungs (Fig. 5.9). It lies obliquely, a little more to the left than the right, and presents a *base* above, and an *apex* below. The apex is about 9 cm to the left of the midline at the level of the 5th intercostal space, i.e. a little below the nipple and slightly nearer the midline. The base extends to the level of the 2nd rib.

Organs associated with the heart (Fig. 5.10)

Inferiorly — the apex rests on the central tendon of the diaphragm

Superiorly — the great blood vessels, i.e. the aorta, superior vena cava, pulmonary artery and pulmonary veins

Posteriorly — the oesophagus, trachea, left and right bronchus, descending aorta, inferior vena cava and thoracic vertebrae

Laterally — the lungs — the left lung overlaps the left side of the heart

Anteriorly — the sternum, ribs and intercostal muscles

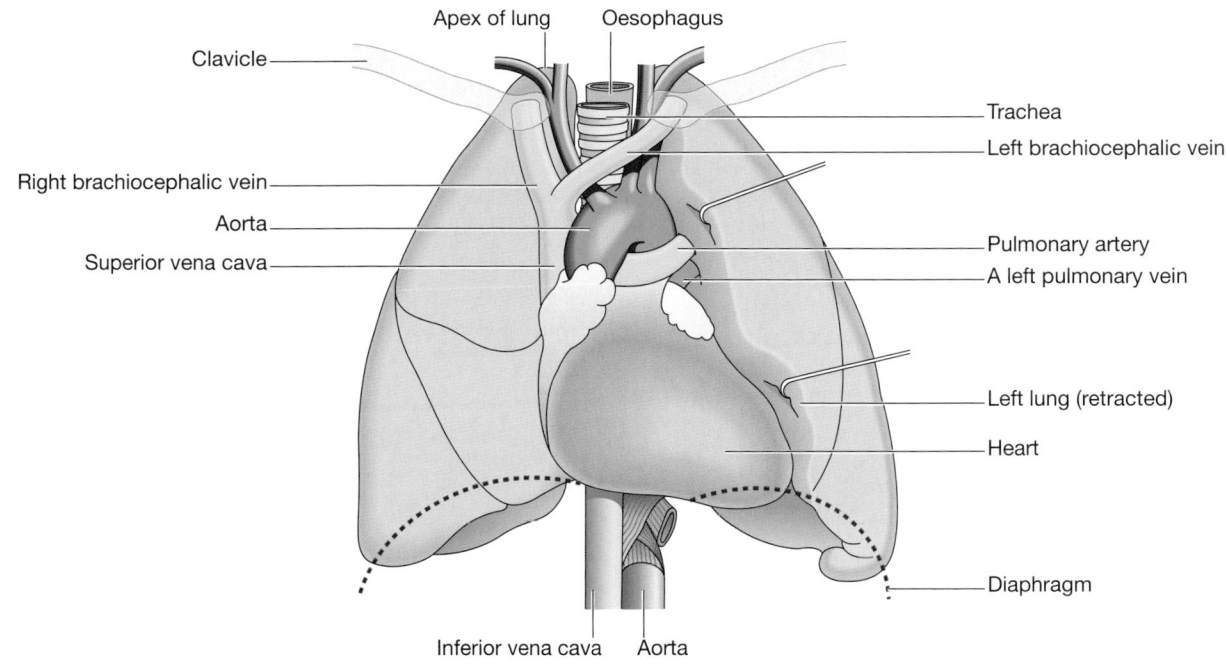

Figure 5.10 Organs associated with the heart.

Structure

The heart is composed of three layers of tissue (Fig. 5.11): pericardium, myocardium and endocardium.

Pericardium

The pericardium is made up of two sacs. The outer sac consists of fibrous tissue and the inner of a continuous double layer of serous membrane.

The outer fibrous sac is continuous with the tunica adventitia of the great blood vessels above and is adherent to the diaphragm below. Its inelastic, fibrous nature prevents overdistension of the heart.

The outer layer of the serous membrane, the *parietal pericardium*, lines the fibrous sac. The inner layer, the *visceral pericardium*, or epicardium, which is continuous with the parietal pericardium, is adherent to the heart muscle. A similar arrangement of a double membrane forming a closed space is seen also with the pleura, the membrane enclosing the lungs (see Fig. 10.16, p. 251).

The serous membrane consists of flattened epithelial cells. It secretes serous fluid into the space between the visceral and parietal layers which allows smooth movement between them when the heart beats. The space between the parietal and visceral pericardium is only a *potential space*. In health the two layers are in close association, with only the thin film of serous fluid between them.

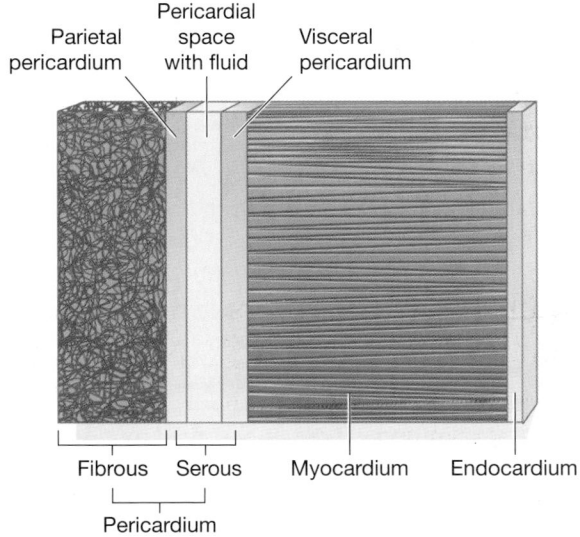

Figure 5.11 Layers of the heart wall.

Myocardium

The myocardium is composed of specialised cardiac muscle found only in the heart (Fig. 5.12). It is not under voluntary control but, like skeletal muscle, cross-stripes are seen on microscopic examination. Each fibre (cell) has a nucleus and one or more branches. The ends of the cells and their branches are in very close contact with the ends and branches of adjacent cells. Microscopically these

83

Figure 5.12 Cardiac muscle, with fibres separated.

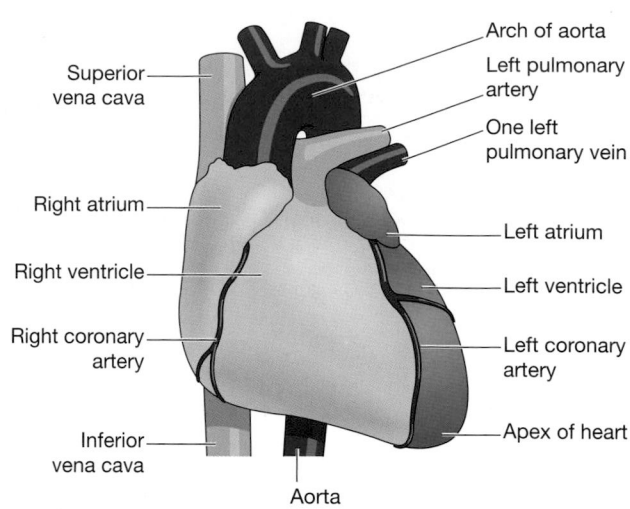

Figure 5.13 The heart and the great vessels, viewed from the front.

'joints', or *intercalated discs*, can be seen as thicker, darker lines than the ordinary cross-stripes. This arrangement gives cardiac muscle the appearance of being a sheet of muscle rather than a very large number of individual cells. Because of the end-to-end continuity of the fibres, each one does not need to have a separate nerve supply. When an impulse is initiated it spreads from cell to cell via the branches and intercalated discs over the whole 'sheet' of muscle, causing contraction. The 'sheet' arrangement of the myocardium enables the atria and ventricles to contract in a coordinated and efficient manner.

The myocardium is thickest at the apex and thins out towards the base (Fig. 5.15). This reflects the amount of work each chamber contributes to the pumping of blood. It is thickest in the left ventricle.

The atria and the ventricles are separated by a *ring of fibrous tissue* that does not conduct electrical impulses. Consequently, when a wave of electrical activity passes over the atrial muscle, it can only spread to the ventricles through the conducting system which bridges the fibrous ring from atria to ventricles (p. 87).

Endocardium

This forms the lining of the myocardium and the heart valves. It is a thin, smooth, glistening membrane which permits smooth flow of blood inside the heart. It consists of flattened epithelial cells, continuous with the endothelium that lines the blood vessels.

Interior of the heart

The heart is divided into a right and left side by the *septum* (Fig. 5.14), a partition consisting of myocardium

Figure 5.14 The left atrioventricular valve: A. Valve open. B. Valve closed.

covered by endocardium. After birth blood cannot cross the septum from one side to the other. Each side is divided by an *atrioventricular valve* into an upper chamber, the *atrium*, and a lower chamber, the *ventricle* (Fig. 5.15). The atrioventricular valves are formed by double folds of endocardium strengthened by a little fibrous tissue. The *right atrioventricular valve* (tricuspid valve) has three flaps or *cusps* and the *left atrioventricular valve* (mitral valve) has two cusps.

The valves between the atria and ventricles open and close passively according to changes in pressure in the chambers. They open when the pressure in the atria is greater than that in the ventricles. During *ventricular systole* (contraction) the pressure in the ventricles rises above that in the atria and the valves snap shut preventing backward flow of blood. The valves are prevented

Figure 5.15 Interior of the heart.

from opening upwards into the atria by tendinous cords, called *chordae tendineae*, which extend from the inferior surface of the cusps to little projections of myocardium covered with endothelium, called *papillary muscles* (Fig. 5.14).

Flow of blood through the heart

(Fig. 5.16)

The two largest veins of the body, the *superior* and *inferior venae cavae*, empty their contents into the right atrium. This blood passes via the right atrioventricular valve into the right ventricle, and from there it is pumped into the *pulmonary artery* or *trunk* (the only artery in the body which carries deoxygenated blood). The opening of the pulmonary artery is guarded by the *pulmonary valve*, formed by three *semilunar cusps*. This valve prevents the back flow of blood into the right ventricle when the ventricular muscle relaxes. After leaving the heart the pulmonary artery divides into *left* and *right pulmonary arteries*, which carry the venous blood to the lungs where exchange of gases takes place: carbon dioxide is excreted and oxygen is absorbed.

Two *pulmonary veins* from each lung carry *oxygenated blood* back to the *left atrium*. Blood then passes through the left atrioventricular valve into the left ventricle, and from there it is pumped into the aorta, the first artery of

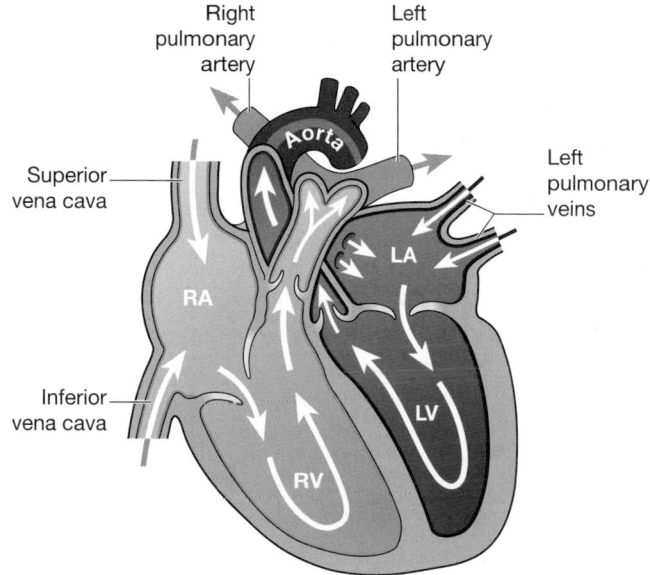

Figure 5.16 Direction of blood flow through the heart.

the general circulation. The opening of the aorta is guarded by the *aortic valve*, formed by three *semilunar cusps* (Fig. 5.17).

From this sequence of events it can be seen that the blood passes from the right to the left side of the heart via the lungs, or pulmonary circulation (Fig. 5.18). However, it should be noted that both atria contract at the same

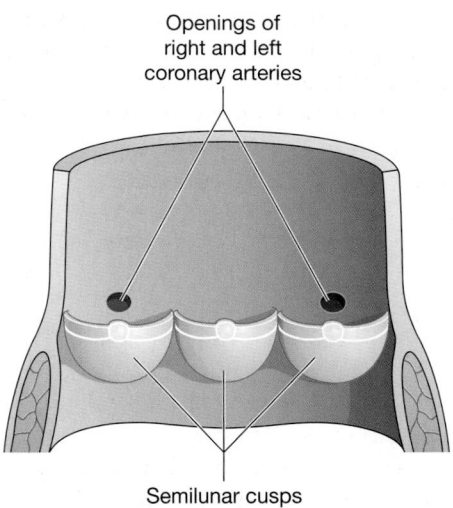

Figure 5.17 The aorta cut open to show the semilunar cusps of the aortic valve.

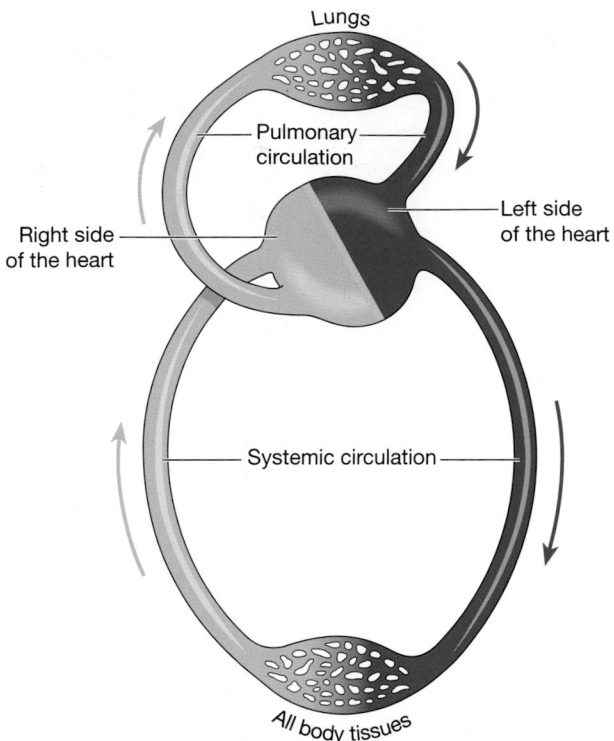

Figure 5.18 The relationship between the systemic and pulmonary circulations.

time and this is followed by the simultaneous contraction of both ventricles.

The muscle layer of the walls of the atria is very thin in comparison with that of the ventricles (Fig. 5.16). This is consistent with the amount of work it does. The atria, usually assisted by gravity, only propel the blood through the atrioventricular valves into the ventricles, whereas the ventricles actively pump the blood to the lungs and round the whole body. The muscle layer is thickest in the wall of the left ventricle.

The pulmonary trunk leaves the heart from the upper part of the right ventricle, and the aorta leaves from the upper part of the left ventricle.

Blood supply to the heart

Arterial supply (Fig. 5.19). The heart is supplied with arterial blood by the *right and left coronary arteries* which branch from the aorta immediately distal to the aortic valve (Figs 5.17 and 5.19). The coronary arteries receive about 5% of the blood pumped from the heart, although the heart comprises a small proportion of body weight. This large blood supply, especially to the left ventricle, highlights the importance of the heart to body function. The coronary arteries traverse the heart, eventually forming a vast network of capillaries.

Venous drainage. Most of the venous blood is collected into several small veins that join to form the *coronary sinus* which opens into the right atrium. The remainder passes directly into the heart chambers through little venous channels.

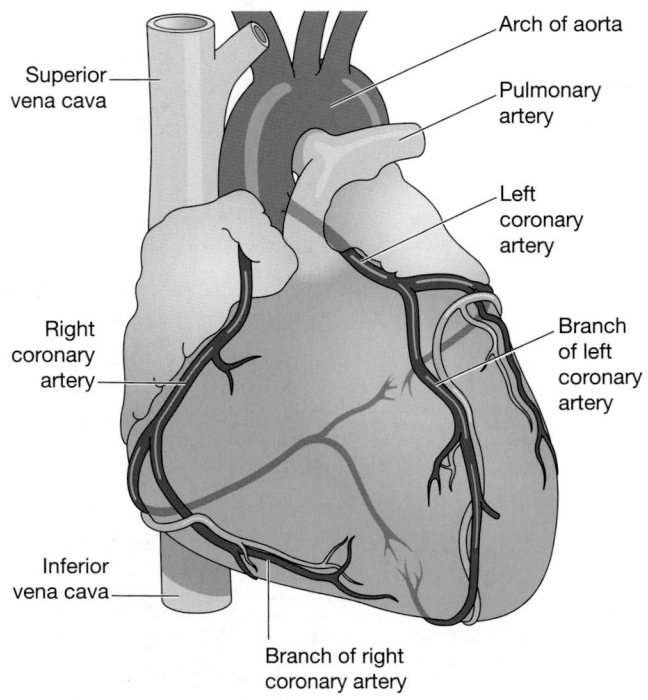

Figure 5.19 The coronary arteries.

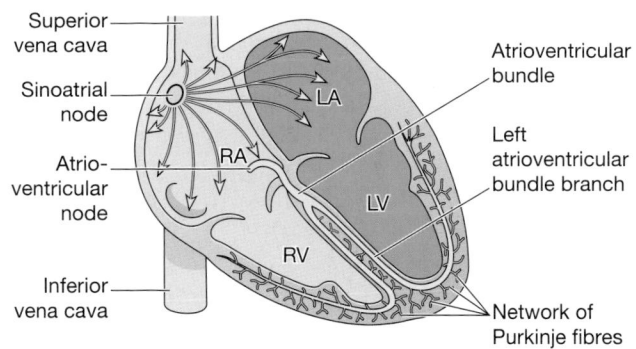

Figure 5.20 The conducting system of the heart.

Conducting system of the heart

The heart has an intrinsic system whereby the cardiac muscle is automatically stimulated to contract without the need for a nerve supply from the brain (Fig. 5.20). However, the intrinsic system can be stimulated or depressed by nerve impulses initiated in the brain and by circulating chemicals including hormones.

There are small groups of specialised neuromuscular cells in the myocardium which initiate and conduct impulses causing coordinated and synchronised contraction of the heart muscle.

Sinoatrial node (SA node)

This small mass of specialised cells is in the wall of the right atrium near the opening of the superior vena cava. The SA node is the '*pace-maker*' of the heart because it normally initiates impulses more rapidly than other groups of neuromuscular cells.

Atrioventricular node (AV node)

This small mass of neuromuscular tissue is situated in the wall of the atrial septum near the atrioventricular valves. Normally the AV node is stimulated by impulses that sweep over the atrial myocardium. However, it too is capable of initiating impulses that cause contraction but at a slower rate than the SA node.

Atrioventricular bundle (AV bundle or bundle of His)
This is a mass of specialised fibres that originate from the AV node. The AV bundle crosses the fibrous ring that separates atria and ventricles then, at the upper end of the ventricular septum, it divides into *right and left bundle branches*. Within the ventricular myocardium the branches break up into fine fibres, called the *Purkinje fibres*. The AV bundle, bundle branches and Purkinje fibres convey electrical impulses from the AV node to the apex of the myocardium where the wave of ventricular contraction begins, then sweeps upwards and outwards, pumping blood into the pulmonary artery and the aorta.

Nerve supply to the heart

In addition to the intrinsic impulses generated within the conducting system described above, the heart is influenced by autonomic nerves originating in the *cardiovascular centre* in the *medulla oblongata* which reach it through the autonomic nervous system. These consist of *parasympathetic* and *sympathetic nerves* and their actions are antagonistic to one another.

The *vagus nerves* (parasympathetic) supply mainly the SA and AV nodes and atrial muscle. Parasympathetic stimulation reduces the rate at which impulses are produced, decreasing the rate and force of the heart beat.

The *sympathetic nerves* supply the SA and AV nodes and the myocardium of atria and ventricles. Sympathetic stimulation *increases* the rate and force of the heart beat.

Factors affecting heart rate

Autonomic nervous system. As described above, the rate at which the heart beats is a balance of sympathetic and parasympathetic activity and this is the most important factor in determining heart rate.

Circulating chemicals. The hormones adrenaline and noradrenaline, secreted by the adrenal medulla, have the same effect as sympathetic stimulation, i.e. they increase the heart rate. Other hormones including thyroxine increase heart rate by their metabolic effect. Some drugs, dissolved gases and electrolytes in the blood may either increase or decrease the heart rate.

Position. When the person is upright, the heart rate is usually faster than when lying down.

Exercise. Active muscles need more blood than resting muscles and this is achieved by an increased heart rate and selective vasodilatation.

Emotional states. During excitement, fear or anxiety the heart rate is increased. Other effects mediated by the sympathetic nervous system may be present (see Fig. 7.43, p. 171).

Gender. The heart rate is faster in women than men.

Age. In babies and small children the heart rate is more rapid than in older children and adults.

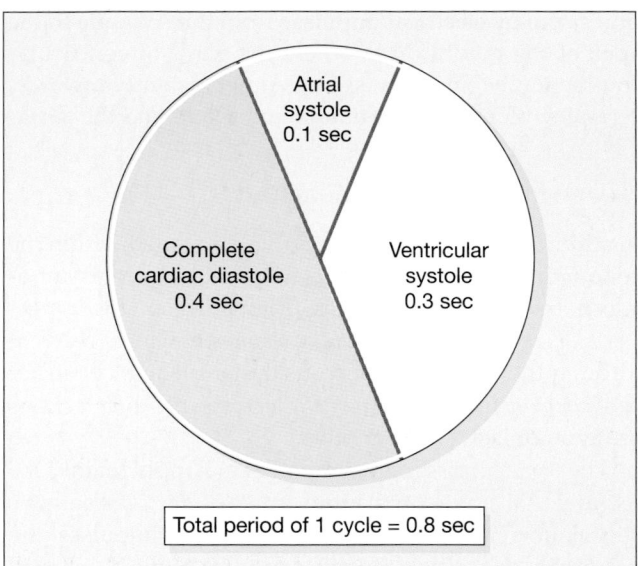

Figure 5.21 The stages of one cardiac cycle.

Temperature. The heart rate rises and falls with body temperature.

Baroreceptor reflex. See page 92.

The cardiac cycle

The function of the heart is to maintain a constant circulation of blood throughout the body. The heart acts as a pump and its action consists of a series of events known as the *cardiac cycle* (Fig. 5.21).

During each heartbeat, or cardiac cycle, the heart contracts and then relaxes. The period of contraction is called *systole* and that of relaxation, *diastole*.

Stages of the cardiac cycle

The normal number of cardiac cycles per minute ranges from 60 to 80. Taking 74 as an example each cycle lasts about *0.8 of a second* and consists of:

- *atrial systole*—contraction of the atria
- *ventricular systole*—contraction of the ventricles
- *complete cardiac diastole*—relaxation of the atria and ventricles.

It does not matter at which stage of the cardiac cycle a description starts. For convenience the period when the atria are filling has been chosen.

The superior vena cava and the inferior vena cava transport deoxygenated blood into the right atrium *at the same time* as the four pulmonary veins convey oxygenated blood into the left atrium. The atrioventricular valves are open and blood flows through to the ventricles. The SA node triggers a wave of contraction that spreads over the myocardium of both atria, emptying the atria and completing ventricular filling (atrial systole 0.1 s). When the wave of contraction reaches the AV node it is stimulated to emit an impulse which quickly spreads to the ventricular muscle via the AV bundle, the bundle branches and Purkinje fibres. This results in a wave of contraction which sweeps upwards from the apex of the heart and across the walls of both ventricles pumping the blood into the pulmonary artery and the aorta (ventricular systole 0.3 s). The high pressure generated during ventricular contraction is greater than that in the aorta and forces the atrioventricular valves to close, preventing backflow of blood into the atria.

After contraction of the ventricles there is *complete cardiac diastole*, a period of *0.4 seconds*, when atria and ventricles are relaxed. During this time the myocardium recovers until it is able to contract again, and the atria refill in preparation for the next cycle.

The valves of the heart and of the great vessels open and close according to the pressure within the chambers of the heart. The AV valves are open while the ventricular muscle is relaxed during atrial filling and systole. When the ventricles contract there is a gradual increase in the pressure in these chambers, and when it rises above atrial pressure the atrioventricular valves close. When the ventricular pressure rises above that in the pulmonary artery and in the aorta, the pulmonary and aortic valves open and blood flows into these vessels. When the ventricles relax and the pressure within them falls, the reverse process occurs. First the pulmonary and aortic valves close, then the atrioventricular valves open and the cycle begins again. This sequence of opening and closing valves ensures that the blood flows in only one direction (Fig. 5.22). This figure also shows how the walls of the aorta and other elastic arteries stretch and recoil in response to blood pumped into them.

Heart sounds

The individual is not usually conscious of his heartbeat, but if the ear or the diaphragm of a stethoscope is placed on the chest wall a little below the left nipple and slightly nearer the midline the heartbeat can be heard.

Two sounds, separated by a short pause, can be clearly distinguished. They are described in words as 'lub dup'. The first sound, 'lub', is fairly loud and is due to the closure of the atrioventricular valves. This corresponds with ventricular systole. The second sound, 'dup', is softer and is due to the closure of the aortic and pulmonary valves. This corresponds with atrial systole.

Ventricular systole   **Ventricular diastole**

Figure 5.22 Diagram showing the elasticity of the walls of the aorta.

Figure 5.23 Electrocardiogram of one cardiac cycle.

Electrical changes in the heart

As the body fluids and tissues are good conductors of electricity, the electrical activity within the heart can be detected by attaching electrodes to the surface of the body. The pattern of electrical activity may be displayed on an oscilloscope screen or traced on paper. The apparatus used is an *electrocardiograph* and the tracing is an *electrocardiogram* (ECG).

The normal ECG tracing shows five waves which, by convention, have been named P, Q, R, S and T (Fig. 5.23).

The P wave arises when the impulse from the SA node sweeps over the atria.

The QRS complex represents the very rapid spread of the impulse from the AV node through the AV bundle and the Purkinje fibres and the electrical activity of the ventricular muscle.

The T wave represents the relaxation of the ventricular muscle.

The ECG described above originates from the SA node and is known as *sinus rhythm*. The rate of sinus rhythm is 60 to 100 beats per minute. A faster heart rate is called *tachycardia* and a slower heart rate, *bradycardia*.

By examining the pattern of waves and the time interval between cycles and parts of cycles, information about the state of the myocardium and the cardiac conduction system is obtained.

Cardiac output

The cardiac output is the amount of blood ejected from the heart. The amount expelled by each contraction of the ventricles is the *stroke volume*. Cardiac output is expressed in litres per minute (l/min) and is calculated by multiplying the stroke volume by the heart rate (measured in beats per minute):

Cardiac output = Stroke volume × Heart rate.

In a healthy adult at rest, the stroke volume is approximately 70 ml and if the heart rate is 72 per minute, the cardiac output is 5 l/minute. This can be greatly increased to meet the demands of exercise to around 25 l/minute, and in athletes up to 35 l/minute. This increase during exercise is called the *cardiac reserve*.

When increased blood supply is needed to meet increased tissue requirements of oxygen and nutrients, heart rate and/or stroke volume can be increased.

Stroke volume

The stroke volume is determined by the volume of blood in the ventricles immediately before they contract, i.e. the ventricular end-diastolic volume (VEDV), sometimes called *preload*. This depends on the amount of blood returning to the heart through the superior and inferior venae cavae (the *venous return*). Increased VEDV leads to stronger myocardial contraction, and more blood is expelled. In turn the stroke volume and cardiac output rise. This capacity to increase the stroke volume with increasing VEDV is finite, and when the limit is reached, i.e. the cardiac output cannot match the venous return, the cardiac output decreases and the heart begins to fail (p. 119). Other factors that increase myocardial contraction include:

- increased stimulation of the sympathetic nerves innervating the heart
- hormones, e.g. adrenaline, noradrenaline, thyroxine.

Arterial blood pressure. This affects the stroke volume as it creates resistance to blood being pumped from the ventricles into the great arteries. This resistance (sometimes called *afterload*) is determined by the distensibility, or *elasticity*, of the large arteries and the *peripheral resistance* of arterioles.

Blood volume. This is normally kept constant by the kidneys and if deficient the stroke volume, cardiac output and venous return decrease.

Venous return

Venous return is the major determinant of cardiac output and, normally, the heart pumps out all blood returned to it. The force of contraction of the left ventricle ejecting blood into the aorta is not sufficient to return the blood through the veins and back to the heart. Other factors are involved.

The position of the body. Gravity assists the venous return from the head and neck when standing or sitting and offers less resistance to venous return from the lower parts of the body when an individual is lying flat.

Muscular contraction. Back flow of blood in veins of the limbs, especially when standing, is prevented by valves. The contraction of skeletal muscles surrounding the deep veins puts pressure on them, pushing blood towards the heart (Fig. 5.24). In the lower limbs, this is called the *skeletal muscle pump*. When the pressure in deep veins is lowered during muscle relaxation, blood flows into them from superficial veins through *communicating veins*.

The respiratory pump. During inspiration the expansion of the chest creates a negative pressure within the thorax, assisting flow of blood towards the heart. In addition, when the diaphragm descends during inspiration, the increased intra-abdominal pressure pushes blood towards the heart.

A summary of the factors that alter cardiac output is given in Box 5.1.

Valves open

Proximal valve open, distal valve closed

Figure 5.24 The flow of blood through a vein, aided by the contraction of skeletal muscle.

Box 5.1 Summary of factors affecting cardiac output

| **Cardiac output = Stroke volume × Heart rate** |

Factors affecting stroke volume:

- VEDV (ventricular end-diastolic volume)
- Venous return
  - position of the body
  - skeletal muscle pump
  - respiratory pump
- Strength of myocardial contraction
- Blood volume.

Factors affecting heart rate:

- Autonomic nerve stimulation
- Circulating chemicals
- Activity and exercise
- Emotional states
- Gender
- Age
- Body temperature
- Baroreceptor reflex.

BLOOD PRESSURE

Learning outcomes

After studying this section, you should be able to:

- define the term blood pressure
- describe the main control mechanisms for regulation of blood pressure.

Blood pressure is the force or pressure which the blood exerts on the walls of the blood vessels.

The systemic arterial blood pressure, usually called simply arterial blood pressure, is the result of the discharge of blood from the left ventricle into the already full aorta.

When the left ventricle contracts and pushes blood into the aorta the pressure produced within the arterial system is called the *systolic blood pressure*. In adults it is about 120 mmHg (millimetres of mercury) or 16 kPa (kilopascals).

When *complete cardiac diastole* occurs and the heart is resting following the ejection of blood, the pressure within the arteries is called *diastolic blood pressure*. In an adult this is about 80 mmHg or 11 kPa. The difference between systolic and diastolic blood pressures is the *pulse pressure*.

These figures vary according to the time of day, the posture, gender and age of the individual. During bedrest at night the blood pressure tends to be lower. It increases with age and is usually higher in women than in men.

Arterial blood pressure is measured with a *sphygmomanometer* and is usually expressed in the following manner:

$$BP = \frac{120}{80} \text{ mmHg or } BP = \frac{16}{11} \text{ kPa}$$

The elasticity of the artery walls. There is a considerable amount of elastic tissue in the arterial walls, especially in large arteries. Therefore, when the left ventricle ejects blood into the already full aorta, it distends, then the elastic recoil pushes the blood onwards. This distension and recoil occurs throughout the arterial system. During cardiac diastole the elastic recoil of the arteries maintains the diastolic pressure (Fig. 5.22).

Systemic arterial blood pressure maintains the essential flow of substances into and out of the organs of the body. Control of blood pressure especially to the vital organs is essential to maintain homeostasis.

The blood pressure is maintained within normal limits by fine adjustments. Blood pressure is determined by cardiac output and peripheral resistance:

$$\text{Blood pressure} = \frac{\text{Cardiac}}{\text{output}} \times \frac{\text{Peripheral}}{\text{resistance}}$$

Cardiac output

The cardiac output is determined by the stroke volume and the heart rate. Factors that affect the heart rate and stroke volume are described above, and they may increase or decrease cardiac output and, in turn, blood pressure. An increase in cardiac output raises both the systolic and diastolic pressure. An increase in stroke volume increases systolic pressure more than it does diastolic pressure.

Peripheral or arteriolar resistance

Arterioles are the smallest arteries and they have a tunica media composed almost entirely of smooth muscle which responds to nerve and chemical stimulation. Constriction and dilatation of the arterioles are the main determinants of peripheral resistance (p. 80). Vasoconstriction causes blood pressure to rise and vasodilatation causes it to fall.

When elastic tissue in the tunica media is replaced by inelastic fibrous tissue as part of the ageing process, blood pressure rises.

Dilatation and constriction of arterioles occurs selectively around the body, resulting in changes in the blood flow through organs according to their needs. The highest priorities are the blood supply to the brain and the heart muscle, and in an emergency, supplies to other parts of the body are reduced in order to ensure an adequate supply to these organs. Generally, changes in the amount of blood flowing to any organ depend on how active it is. A very active organ needs more oxygen and nutrients than a resting organ and it produces more waste materials for excretion.

Control of blood pressure (BP)

Blood pressure is controlled in two ways:

- short-term control, on a moment-to-moment basis, which mainly involves the baroreceptor reflex, to be discussed below, and also chemoreceptors and circulating hormones
- long-term control, which involves regulation of blood volume by the kidneys and the renin—angiotensin—aldosterone system (p. 223).

The cardiovascular centre (CVC) is a collection of interconnected neurones in the brain and is situated

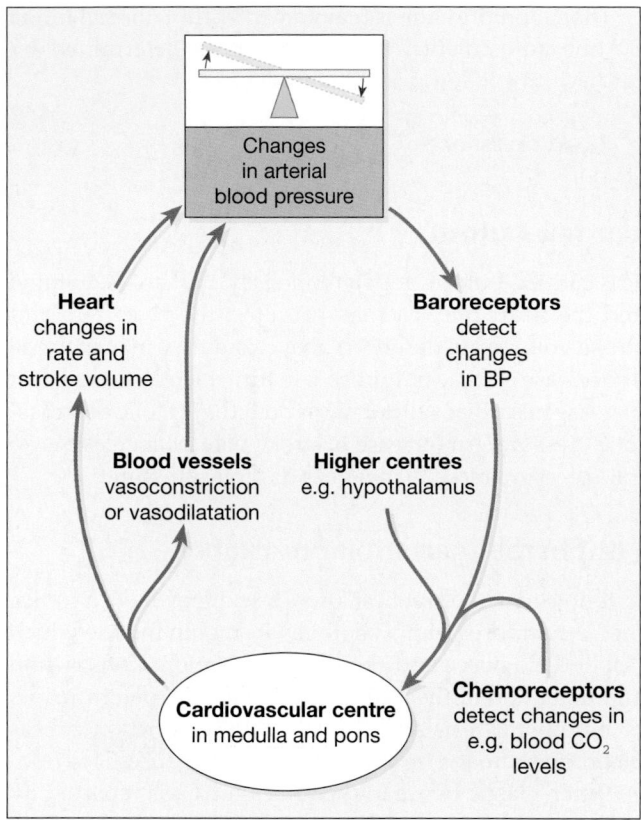

Figure 5.25 Summary of the main mechanisms in blood pressure control.

Table 5.1 **The sympathetic and parasympathetic nervous systems**		
	Sympathetic stimulation	Parasympathetic stimulation
Heart	↑Rate ↑Strength of contraction	↓Rate ↓Strength of contraction
Blood vessels	Most constrict	There is little parasympathetic innervation to most blood vessels

the body's principal moment-to-moment regulatory mechanism for controlling blood pressure. A rise in blood pressure in these arteries stimulates the baroreceptors, increasing their input to the CVC. The CVC responds by increasing parasympathetic nerve activity to the heart; this slows the heart down. At the same time, sympathetic stimulation to the blood vessels is inhibited, causing vasodilatation. The net result is a fall in systemic blood pressure. Conversely, if pressure within the aortic arch and carotid sinuses falls, the rate of baroreceptor discharge also falls. The CVC responds by increasing sympathetic drive to the heart to speed it up. Sympathetic activity in blood vessels is also increased, leading to vasoconstriction. Both these measures counteract the falling blood pressure. Baroreceptor control of blood pressure is also called the *baroreceptor reflex* (Fig. 5.26).

Chemoreceptors

These are nerve endings situated in the carotid and aortic bodies. They are primarily involved in control of respiration (p. 256). They are sensitive to changes in the levels of carbon dioxide, oxygen and the acidity of the blood (pH). Their input to the CVC influences its output only when severe disruption of respiratory function occurs or when arterial BP falls to less than 80 mmHg. The effects are outlined in Figure 5.27.

Higher centres in the brain

Input to the CVC from the higher centres is influenced by emotional states such as fear, anxiety, pain and anger that may stimulate changes in blood pressure.

The hypothalamus in the brain controls body temperature and influences the CVC which responds by adjusting the diameter of blood vessels in the skin—an important mechanism in determining heat loss and retention (p. 365).

within the medulla and pons. The CVC receives, integrates and coordinates inputs from:

- baroreceptors (pressure receptors)
- chemoreceptors
- higher centres in the brain.

The CVC sends autonomic nerves (both sympathetic and parasympathetic) to the heart and blood vessels. It controls BP by slowing down or speeding up the heart rate and by dilating or constricting blood vessels. Activity in these fibres is essential for control of blood pressure (Fig. 5.25). The two divisions of the autonomic nervous system, the sympathetic and the parasympathetic systems, are described more fully in Chapter 7. Their actions relating to the heart and blood vessels are summarised in Table 5.1.

Baroreceptors

These are nerve endings sensitive to pressure changes (stretch) within the vessel, situated in the arch of the aorta and in the carotid sinuses (Fig. 5.26) and are

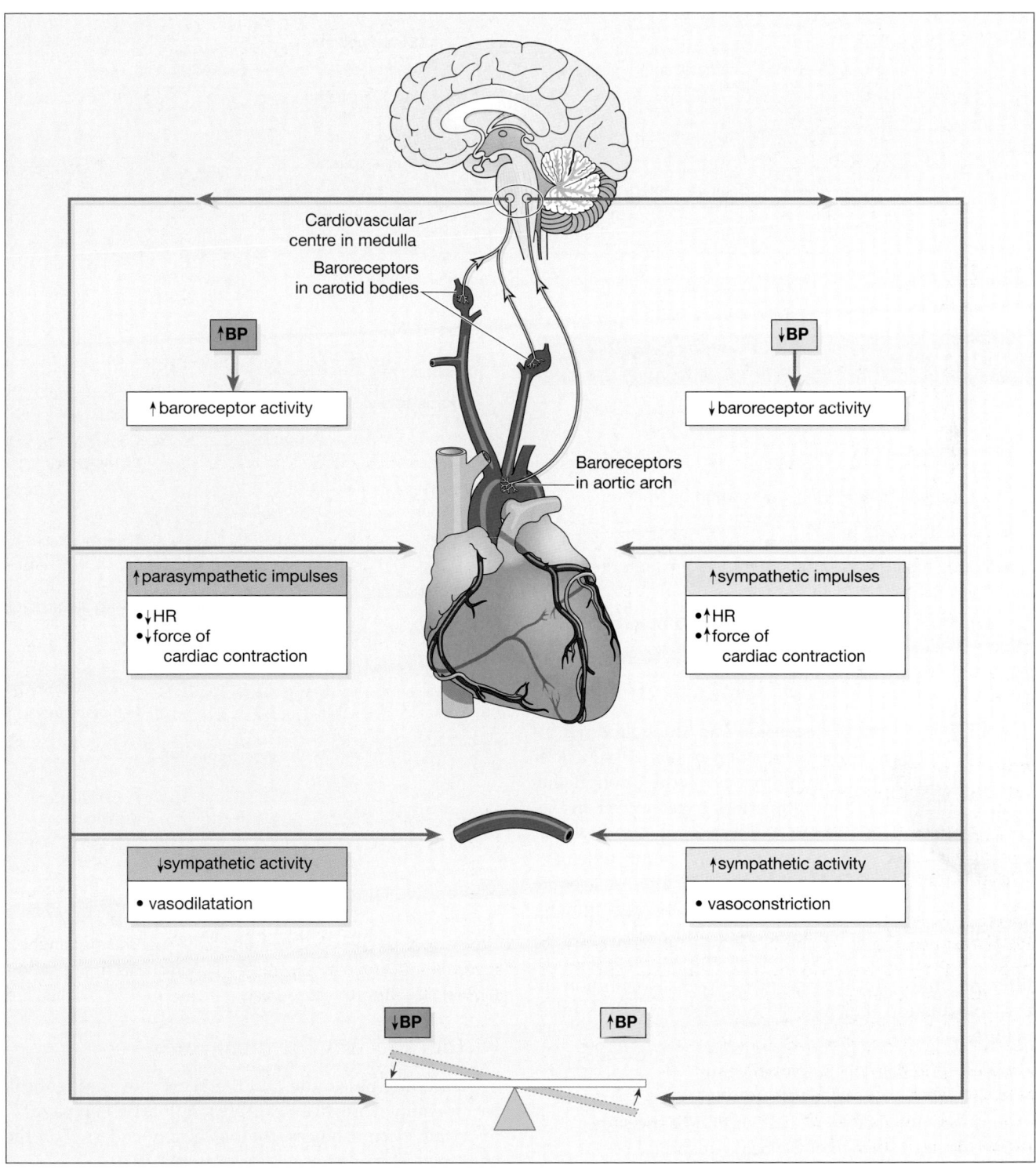

Figure 5.26 The baroreceptor reflex.

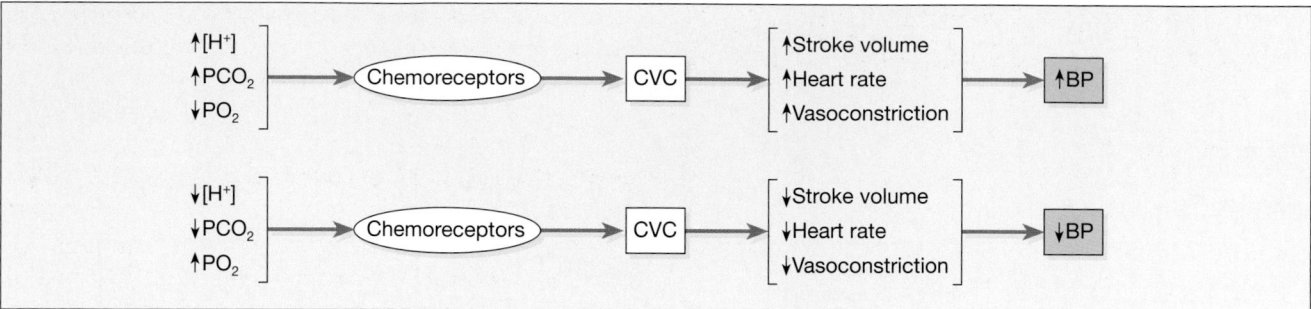

Figure 5.27 The relationship between stimulation of chemoreceptors and arterial blood pressure.

PULSE

Learning outcomes

After studying this section, you should be able to:

- define the term pulse
- list the main sites on the body surface where the pulse is detected
- describe the main factors affecting the pulse rate.

94

The pulse is a wave of distension and elongation felt in an artery wall due to the contraction of the left ventricle forcing about 60 to 80 millilitres of blood through the already full aorta and into the arterial system. When the aorta is distended, a wave passes along the walls of the arteries and can be felt at any point where a superficial artery can be pressed gently against a bone (Fig. 5.28). The number of pulse beats per minute normally represents the heart rate and varies considerably in different people and in the same person at different times. An average of 60 to 80 is common at rest. Information that may be obtained from the pulse includes:

- *the rate* at which the heart is beating
- *the regularity* with which the heartbeats occur, i.e. the length of time between beats should be the same
- *the volume or strength* of the beat—it should be possible to compress the artery with moderate pressure, stopping the flow of blood; the compressibility of the blood vessel gives some indication of the blood pressure and the state of the blood vessel wall
- *the tension* — the artery wall should feel soft and pliant under the fingers.

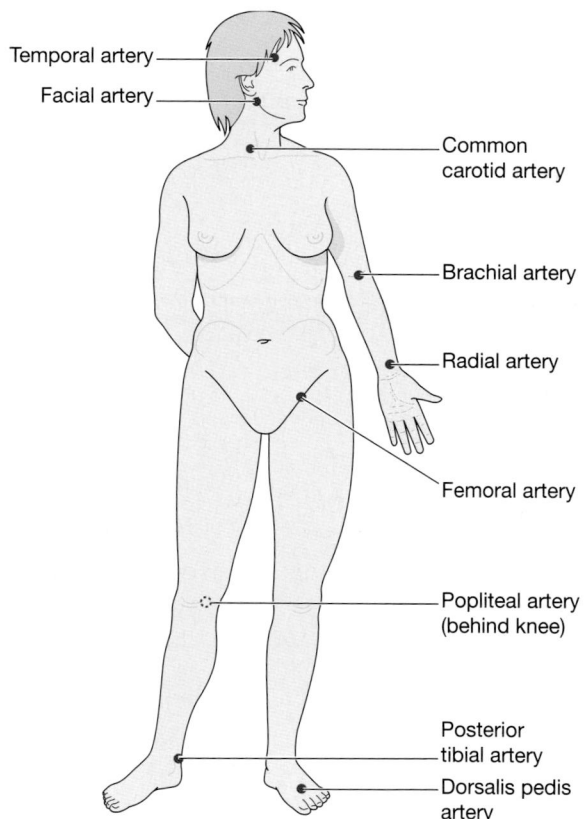

Figure 5.28 The main pulse points.

Factors affecting the pulse rate

In health, the pulse rate and the heart rate are identical. Factors influencing heart rate are summarised on page 87. In certain circumstances, the pulse may be less than the heart rate. This may occur, for example, if:

- the arteries supplying the peripheral tissues are narrowed or blocked and the blood therefore is not pumped through them with each heartbeat
- the heart is diseased or failing, and is unable to generate enough force, with each contraction, to circulate blood to the peripheral arteries.

CIRCULATION OF THE BLOOD

Learning outcomes

After studying this section, you should be able to:

■ describe the circulation of the blood through the lungs, naming the main vessels involved

■ list the arteries supplying blood to all major body structures, including the heart itself

■ describe the venous drainage involved in returning blood to the heart from the body

■ describe the arrangement of blood vessels relating to the portal circulation

■ explain the physiological importance of the portal circulation.

Although circulation of blood round the body is continuous (Fig. 5.18) it is convenient to describe it in two parts:

■ pulmonary circulation
■ systemic or general circulation.

Pulmonary circulation

This consists of the circulation of blood from the right ventricle of the heart to the lungs and back to the left atrium. In the lungs, carbon dioxide is excreted and oxygen is absorbed.

The pulmonary artery or trunk, carrying *deoxygenated blood*, leaves the upper part of the right ventricle of the heart. It passes upwards and divides into left and right pulmonary arteries at the level of the 5th thoracic vertebra.

The left pulmonary artery runs to the root of the left lung where it divides into two branches, one passing into each lobe.

The right pulmonary artery passes to the root of the right lung and divides into two branches. The larger branch carries blood to the middle and lower lobes, and the smaller branch to the upper lobe.

Within the lung these arteries divide and subdivide into smaller arteries, arterioles and capillaries. The interchange of gases takes place between capillary blood and air in the alveoli of the lungs (p. 255). In each lung the capillaries containing oxygenated blood join up and eventually form two veins.

Two pulmonary veins leave each lung, returning oxygenated blood to the left atrium of the heart. During atrial systole this blood passes into the left ventricle, and during ventricular systole it is forced into the aorta, the first artery of the general circulation.

Systemic or general circulation

The blood pumped out from the left ventricle is carried by the *branches of the aorta* around the body and is returned to the right atrium of the heart by the *superior* and *inferior venae cavae*. Figure 5.32 shows the general positions of the aorta and the main arteries of the limbs. Figure 5.33 provides an overview of the venae cavae and the veins of the limbs.

The circulation of blood to the different parts of the body will be described in the order in which their arteries branch off the aorta.

Aorta

The aorta (Fig. 5.29) begins at the upper part of the left ventricle and, after passing upwards for a short way, it arches backwards and to the left. It then descends behind the heart through the thoracic cavity a little to the left of the thoracic vertebrae. At the level of the 12th thoracic vertebra it passes behind the diaphragm then downwards in the abdominal cavity to the level of the 4th lumbar vertebra, where it divides into the *right* and *left common iliac arteries*.

Throughout its length the aorta gives off numerous branches. Some of the branches are *paired*, i.e. there is a right and left branch of the same name, for instance, the right and left renal arteries supplying the kidneys, and some are single or *unpaired*, e.g. the coeliac artery.

Thoracic aorta

This part of the aorta is above the diaphragm and is described in three parts:

■ ascending aorta
■ arch of the aorta
■ descending aorta in the thorax.

Ascending aorta

This is about 5 cm long and lies behind the sternum.

The right and left coronary arteries are its only branches and they arise from the aorta just above the level of the aortic valve (Fig. 5.17).

Arch of the aorta

The arch of the aorta is a continuation of the ascending aorta. It begins behind the manubrium of the sternum

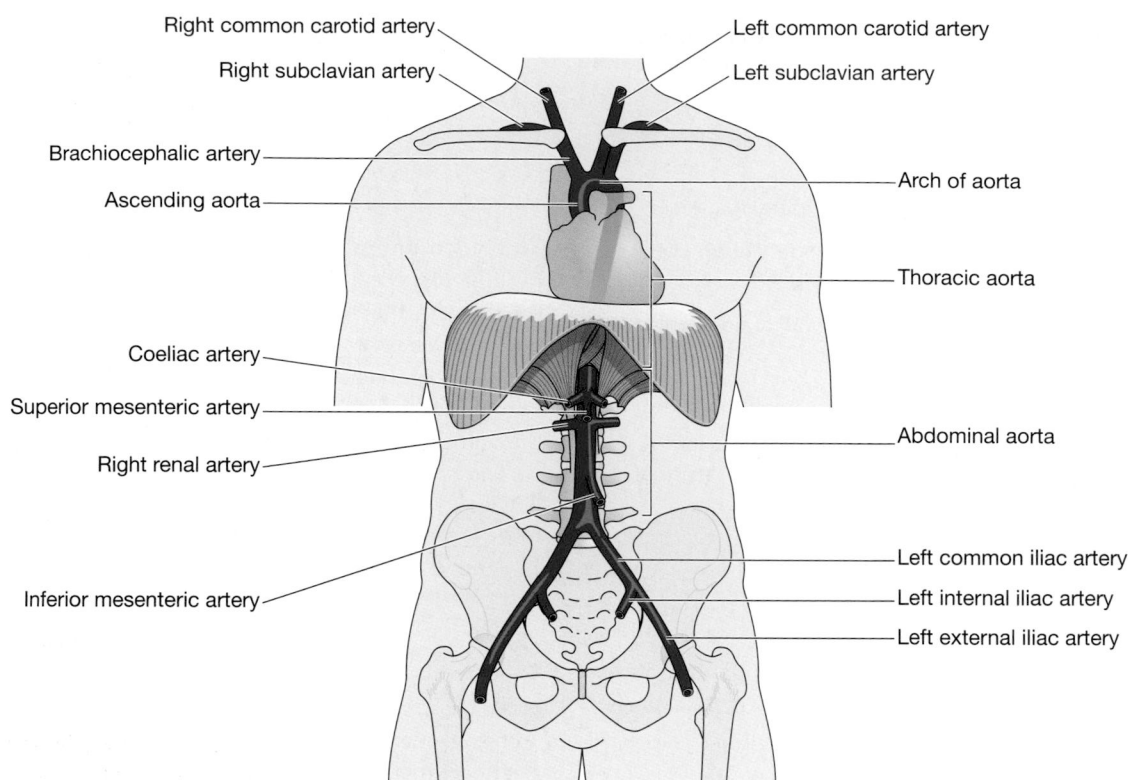

Right common carotid artery

Right subclavian artery

Brachiocephalic artery

Ascending aorta

Coeliac artery

Superior mesenteric artery

Right renal artery

Inferior mesenteric artery

Left common carotid artery

Left subclavian artery

Arch of aorta

Thoracic aorta

Abdominal aorta

Left common iliac artery

Left internal iliac artery

Left external iliac artery

Figure 5.29 The aorta and its main branches.

and runs upwards, backwards and to the left in front of the trachea. It then passes downwards to the left of the trachea and is continuous with the descending aorta.

Three branches are given off from its upper aspect (Fig. 5.30):

- brachiocephalic artery or trunk
- left common carotid artery
- left subclavian artery.

The brachiocephalic artery is about 4 to 5 cm long and passes obliquely upwards, backwards and to the right. At the level of the sternoclavicular joint it divides into the *right common carotid artery* and the *right subclavian artery.*

Circulation of blood to the head and neck

Arterial supply

The paired arteries supplying the head and neck are the *common carotid arteries* and the *vertebral arteries* (Fig. 5.31).

Carotid arteries. The *right common carotid artery* is a branch of the brachiocephalic artery. The *left common carotid artery* arises directly from the arch of the aorta. They pass upwards on either side of the neck and have the same distribution on each side. The common carotid arteries are

embedded in fascia, called the *carotid sheath*. At the level of the upper border of the thyroid cartilage they divide into:

- external carotid artery.
- internal carotid artery.

The carotid sinuses are slight dilatations at the point of division (bifurcation) of the common carotid arteries into their internal and external branches. The walls of the sinuses are thin and contain numerous nerve endings of the glossopharyngeal nerves. These nerve endings, or *baroreceptors*, are stimulated by changes in blood pressure in the carotid sinuses. The resultant nerve impulses initiate reflex adjustments of blood pressure through the vasomotor centre in the medulla oblongata (p. 92).

The carotid bodies are two small groups of specialised cells, called *chemoreceptors*, one lying in close association with each common carotid artery at its bifurcation. They are supplied by the glossopharyngeal nerves and their cells are stimulated by changes in the carbon dioxide and oxygen content of blood. The resultant nerve impulses initiate reflex adjustments of respiration through the respiratory centre in the medulla oblongata.

External carotid artery (Fig. 5.31). This artery supplies the superficial tissues of the head and neck, via a number of branches.

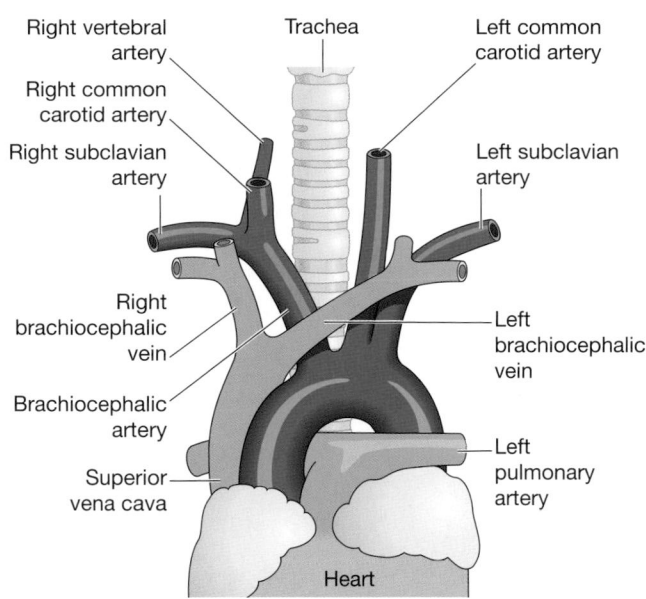

Figure 5.30 The arch of the aorta and its branches.

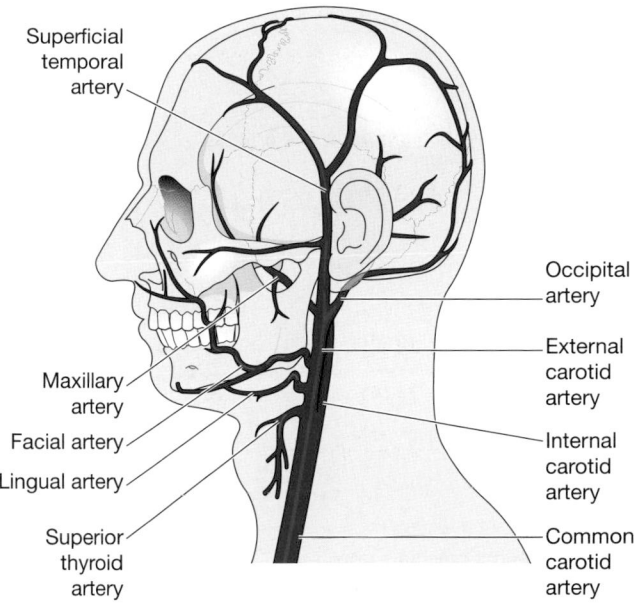

Figure 5.31 Main arteries of the left side of the head and neck.

- The *superior thyroid artery* supplies the thyroid gland and adjacent muscles.
- The *lingual artery* supplies the tongue, the lining membrane of the mouth, the structures in the floor of the mouth, the tonsil and the epiglottis.
- The *facial artery* passes outwards over the mandible just in front of the angle of the jaw and supplies the muscles of facial expression and structures in the mouth. The pulse may be felt where the artery crosses the jaw bone.
- The *occipital artery* supplies the posterior part of the scalp.
- The *temporal artery* passes upwards over the zygomatic process in front of the ear and supplies the frontal, temporal and parietal parts of the scalp. The pulse may be felt in front of the upper part of the ear.
- The *maxillary artery* supplies the muscles of mastication and a branch of this artery, the *middle meningeal artery*, runs deeply to supply structures in the interior of the skull.

Internal carotid artery. The internal carotid artery is a major contributor to the circulus arteriosus (circle of Willis) (Fig. 5.34) which supplies the greater part of the brain. It also has branches that supply the eyes, forehead and nose. It ascends to the base of the skull and passes through the carotid foramen in the temporal bone.

Circulus arteriosus (circle of Willis). The greater part of the brain is supplied with arterial blood by an arrangement of arteries called the *circulus arteriosus* or the *circle of*

Willis (Fig. 5.34). Four large arteries contribute to its formation: two *internal carotid arteries* and two *vertebral arteries* (Fig. 5.35). The vertebral arteries arise from the subclavian arteries, pass upwards through the foramina in the transverse processes of the cervical vertebrae, enter the skull through the foramen magnum, then join to form the *basilar artery*. The arrangement in the circulus arteriosus (circle of Willis) is such that the brain as a whole receives an adequate blood supply when a contributing artery is damaged and during extreme movements of the head and neck.

Anteriorly, *two anterior cerebral arteries* arise from the internal carotid arteries and are joined by the *anterior communicating artery*.

Posteriorly, *two vertebral arteries* join to form the *basilar artery*. After travelling for a short distance the basilar artery divides to form *two posterior cerebral arteries*, each of which is joined to the corresponding internal carotid artery by a *posterior communicating artery*, completing the circle. The *circulus arteriosus* is therefore formed by:

- 2 anterior cerebral arteries
- 2 internal carotid arteries
- 1 anterior communicating artery
- 2 posterior communicating arteries
- 2 posterior cerebral arteries
- 1 basilar artery.

From this circle, the *anterior cerebral arteries* pass forward to supply the anterior part of the brain, the *middle cerebral arteries* pass laterally to supply the sides of the

97

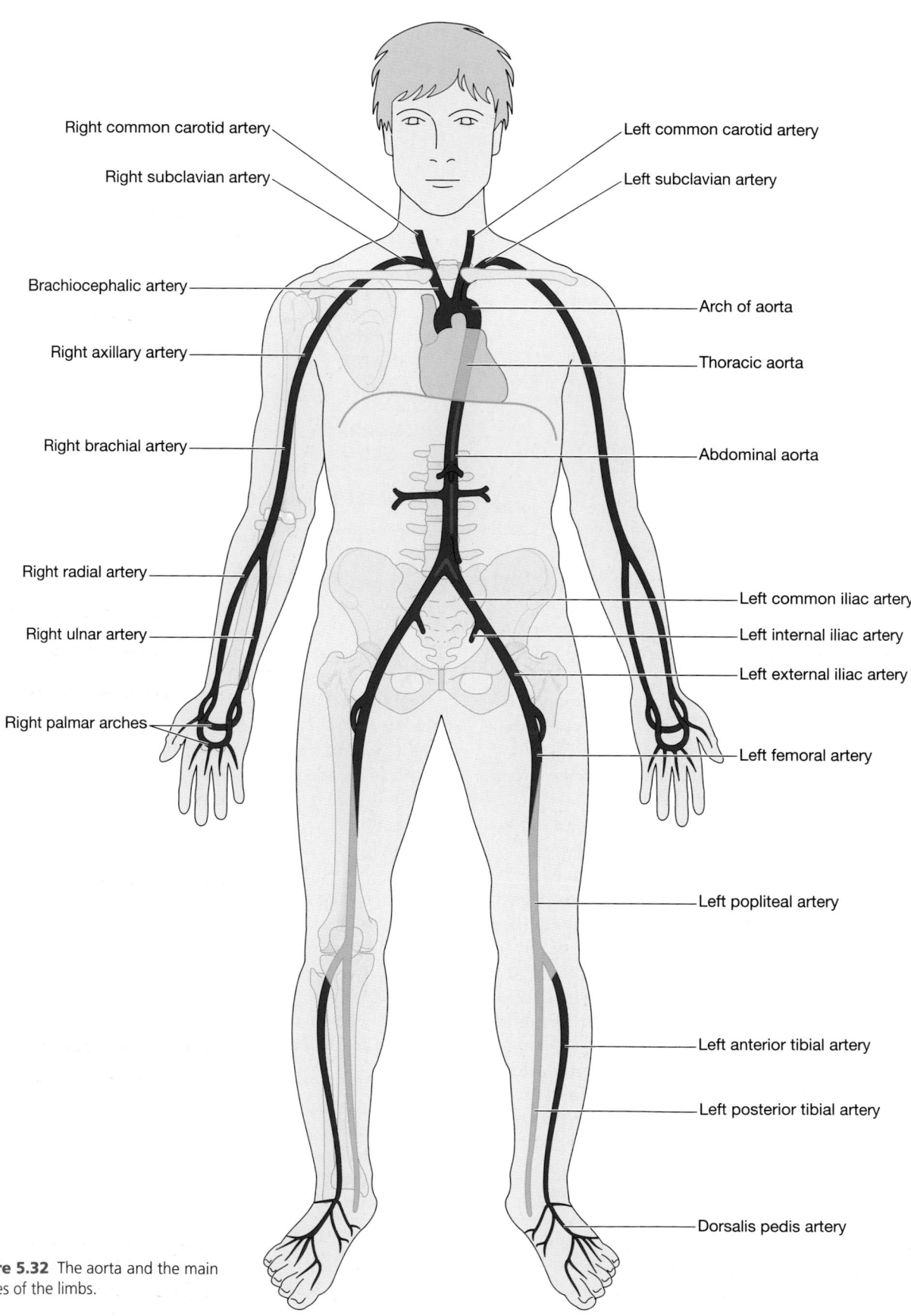

Figure 5.32 The aorta and the main arteries of the limbs.

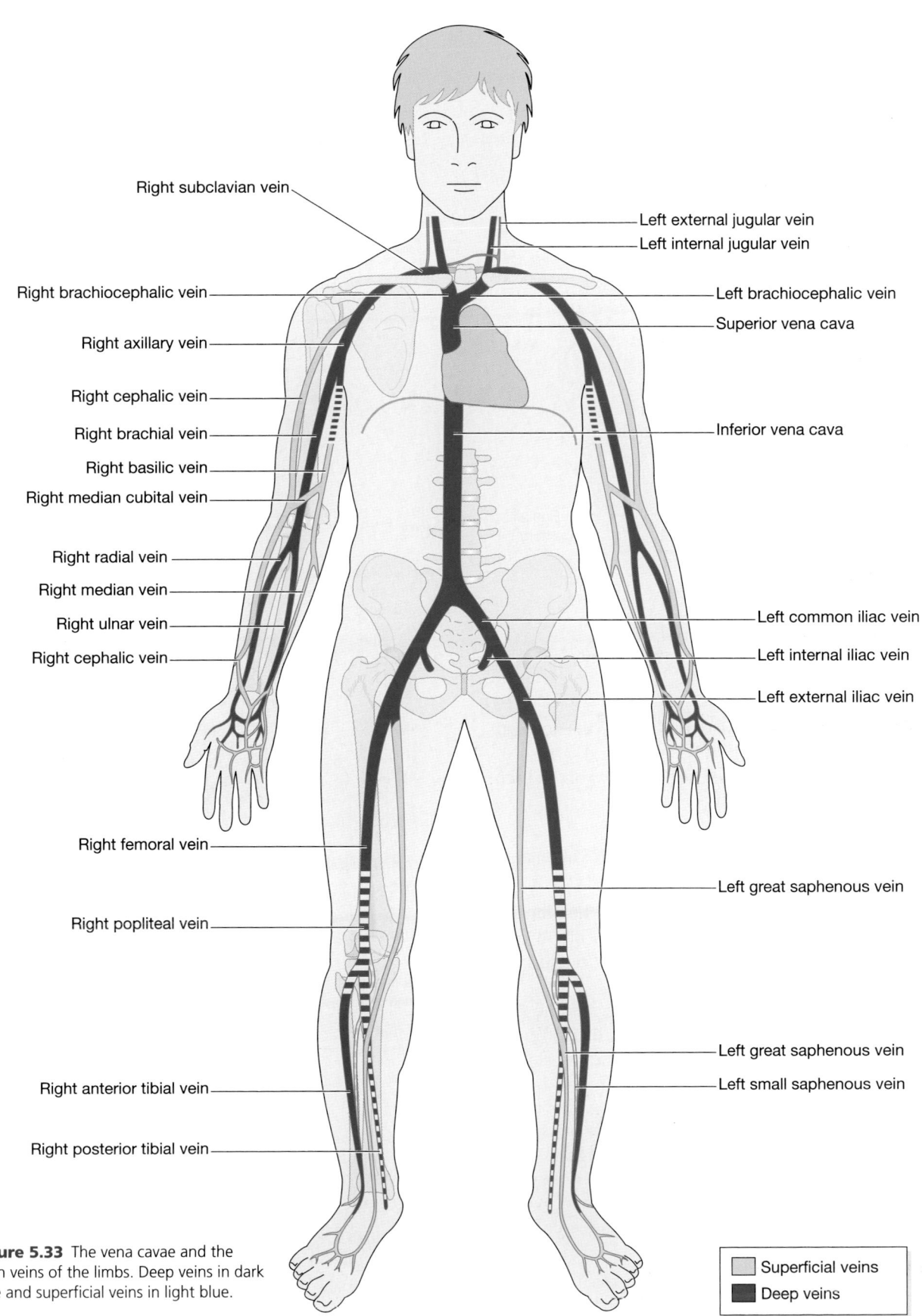

Right subclavian vein

Right brachiocephalic vein

Right axillary vein

Right cephalic vein

Right brachial vein

Right basilic vein

Right median cubital vein

Right radial vein

Right median vein

Right ulnar vein

Right cephalic vein

Right femoral vein

Right popliteal vein

Right anterior tibial vein

Right posterior tibial vein

Left external jugular vein

Left internal jugular vein

Left brachiocephalic vein

Superior vena cava

Inferior vena cava

Left common iliac vein

Left internal iliac vein

Left external iliac vein

Left great saphenous vein

Left great saphenous vein

Left small saphenous vein

Figure 5.33 The vena cavae and the main veins of the limbs. Deep veins in dark blue and superficial veins in light blue.

| | Superficial veins |
| | Deep veins |

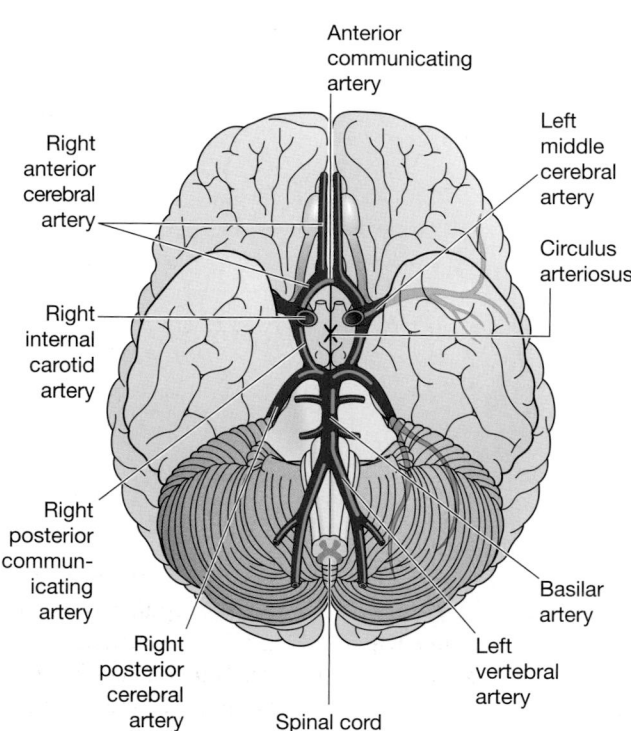

Figure 5.34 Arteries forming the circulus arteriosus (circle of Willis) and its main branches to the brain.

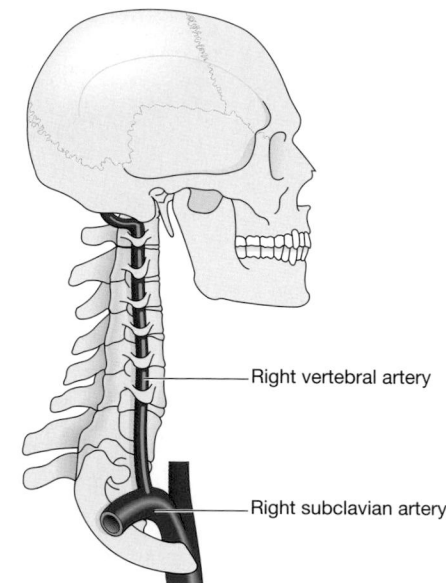

Figure 5.35 The right vertebral artery.

brain, and the *posterior cerebral arteries* supply the posterior part of the brain.

Branches of the basilar artery supply parts of the brain stem.

Venous return from the head and neck

The venous blood from the head and neck is returned by *deep and superficial veins*.

Superficial veins with the same names as the branches of the external carotid artery return venous blood from the superficial structures of the face and scalp and unite to form the external jugular vein (Fig. 5.36).

The *external jugular vein* begins in the neck at the level of the angle of the jaw. It passes downwards in front of the sternocleidomastoid muscle, then behind the clavicle before entering the *subclavian vein*.

The venous blood from the deep areas of the brain is collected into channels called the *dural venous sinuses*.

The dural venous sinuses of the brain (Figs 5.37 and 5.38) are formed by layers of dura mater lined with endothelium. The dura mater is the outer protective covering of the brain (p. 147). The main venous sinuses are:

- 1 superior sagittal sinus
- 1 inferior sagittal sinus

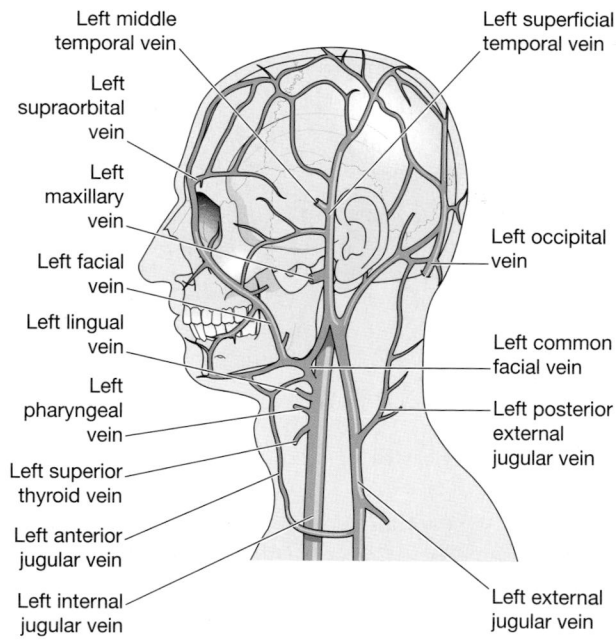

Figure 5.36 Veins of the left side of the head and neck.

- 1 straight sinus
- 2 transverse or lateral sinuses
- 2 sigmoid sinuses.

The *superior sagittal sinus* carries the venous blood from the superior part of the brain. It begins in the frontal region and passes directly backwards in the midline of

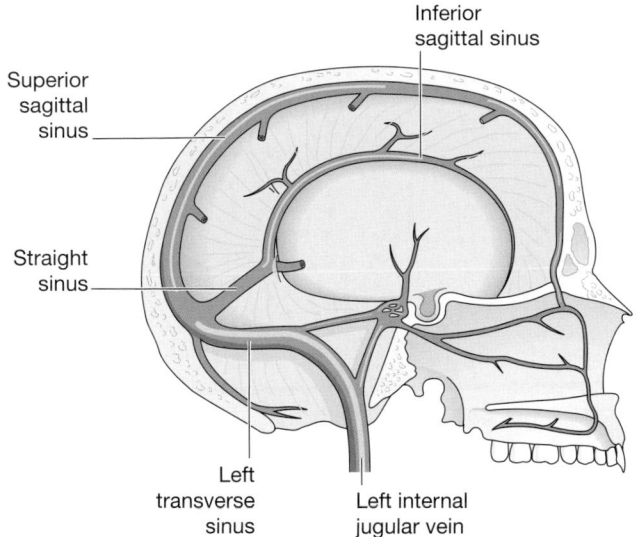

Figure 5.37 Venous sinuses of the brain viewed from the right.

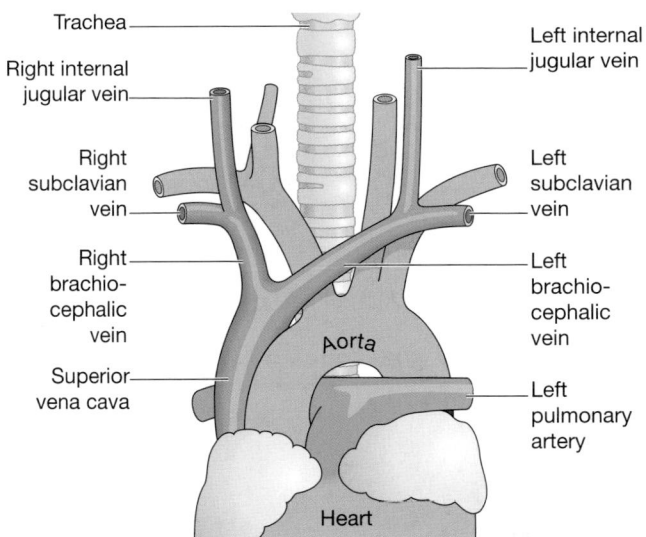

Figure 5.39 The superior vena cava and the veins which form it.

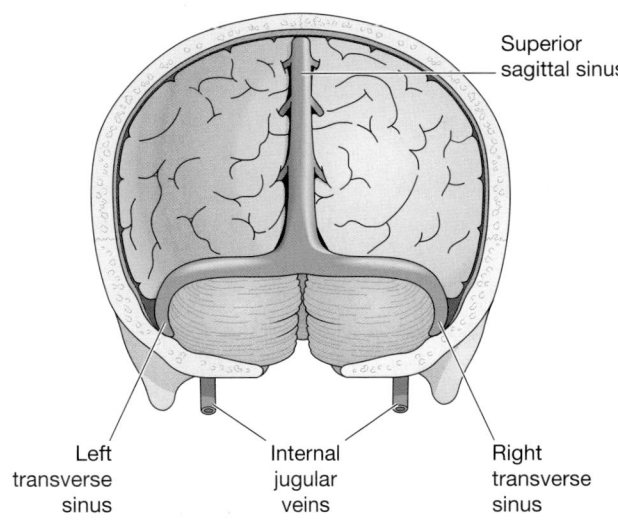

Figure 5.38 Venous sinuses of the brain viewed from above.

the skull to the occipital region where it turns to the right side and continues as the *right transverse sinus*.

The *inferior sagittal sinus* lies deep within the brain and passes backwards to form the *straight sinus*.

The *straight sinus* runs backwards and downwards to become the *left transverse sinus*.

The *transverse sinuses* begin in the occipital region. They run forward and medially in a curved groove of the skull, to become continuous with the *sigmoid sinuses*.

The *sigmoid sinuses* are a continuation of the transverse sinuses. Each curves downwards and medially and lies in a groove in the mastoid process of the temporal bone. Anteriorly only a thin plate of bone separates the sinus from the air cells in the mastoid process of the temporal

bone. Inferiorly it continues as the internal jugular vein.

The *internal jugular veins* begin at the jugular foramina in the middle cranial fossa and each is the continuation of a sigmoid sinus. They run downwards in the neck behind the sternocleidomastoid muscles. Behind the clavicle they unite with the *subclavian veins*, carrying blood from the upper limbs, to form the *brachiocephalic veins*.

The *brachiocephalic veins* are situated one on each side in the root of the neck. Each is formed by the union of the internal jugular and the subclavian veins. The left brachiocephalic vein is longer than the right and passes obliquely behind the manubrium of the sternum, where it joins the right brachiocephalic vein to form the *superior vena cava* (Fig. 5.39).

The *superior vena cava*, which drains all the venous blood from the head, neck and upper limbs, is about 7 cm long. It passes downwards along the right border of the sternum and ends in the right atrium of the heart.

Circulation of blood to the upper limb

Arterial supply

The subclavian arteries. The right subclavian artery arises from the brachiocephalic artery; the left branches from the arch of the aorta. They are slightly arched and pass behind the clavicles and over the first ribs before entering the axillae, where they continue as the *axillary arteries* (Fig. 5.40).

Before entering the axilla each subclavian artery gives off two branches: the *vertebral artery*, which passes upwards to supply the brain, and the *internal thoracic artery*, which supplies the breast and a number of structures in the thoracic cavity.

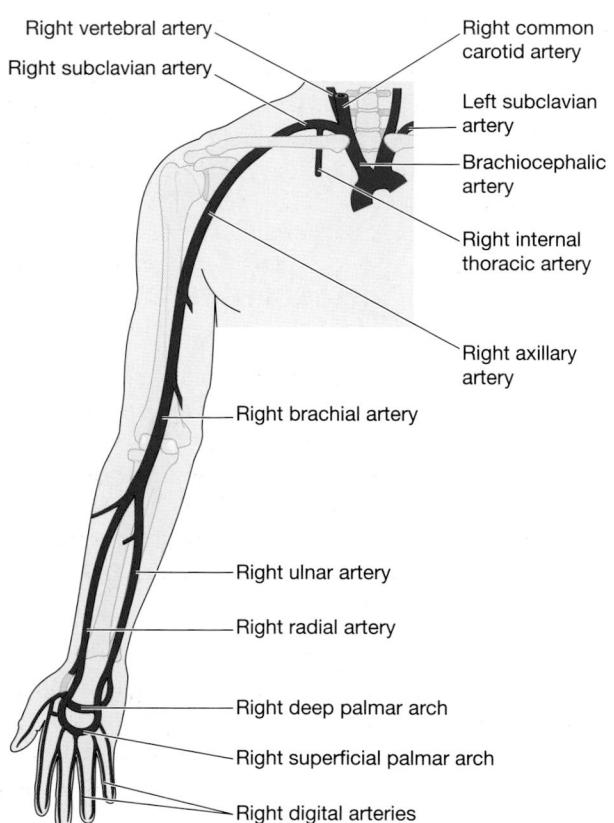

Figure 5.40 The main arteries of the right arm.

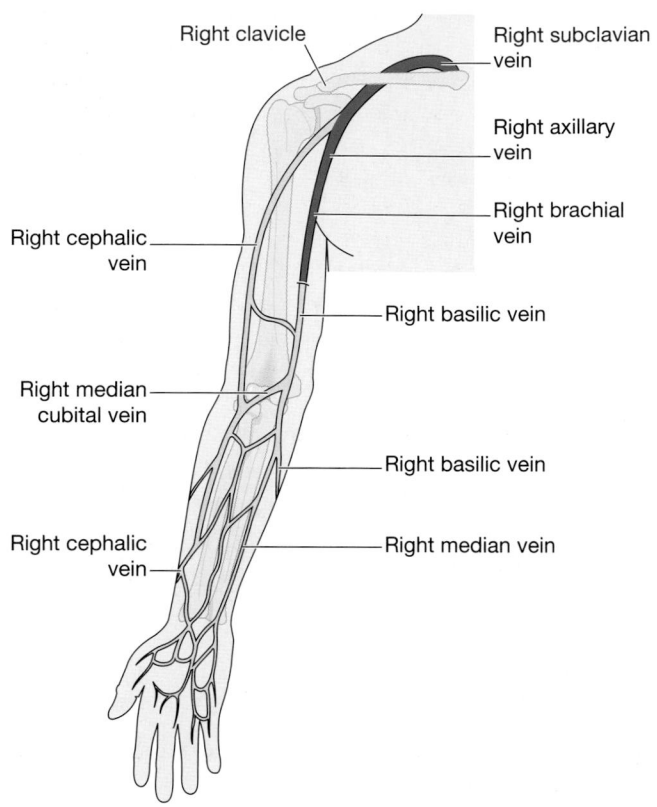

Figure 5.41 The main veins of the right arm. Dark blue indicates deep veins.

The *axillary artery* is a continuation of the subclavian artery and lies in the axilla. The first part lies deeply; then it runs more superficially to become the *brachial artery*.

The *brachial artery* is a continuation of the axillary artery. It runs down the medial aspect of the upper arm, passes to the front of the elbow and extends to about 1 cm below the joint, where it divides into *radial* and *ulnar arteries*.

The *radial artery* passes down the radial or lateral side of the forearm to the wrist. Just above the wrist it lies superficially and can be felt in front of the radius, where the radial pulse is palpable. The artery then passes between the first and second metacarpal bones and enters the palm of the hand.

The *ulnar artery* runs downwards on the ulnar or medial aspect of the forearm to cross the wrist and pass into the hand.

There are anastomoses between the radial and ulnar arteries, called the *deep* and *superficial palmar arches*, from which *palmar metacarpal* and *palmar digital arteries* arise to supply the structures in the hand and fingers.

Branches from the axillary, brachial, radial and ulnar arteries supply all the structures in the upper limb.

Venous return from the upper limb

The veins of the upper limb are divided into two groups: deep and superficial veins (Fig. 5.41).

The *deep veins* follows the course of the arteries and have the same names:

- palmar metacarpal veins
- deep palmar venous arch
- ulnar and radial veins
- brachial vein
- axillary vein
- subclavian vein.

The *superficial veins* begin in the hand and consist of the following:

- cephalic vein
- basilic vein
- median vein
- median cubital vein.

The *cephalic vein* begins at the back of the hand where it collects blood from a complex of superficial veins, many of which can be easily seen. It then winds round the radial side to the anterior aspect of the forearm.

In front of the elbow it gives off a large branch, the *median cubital vein*, which slants upwards and medially to join the *basilic vein*. After crossing the elbow joint the cephalic vein passes up the lateral aspect of the arm and in front of the shoulder joint to end in the axillary vein. Throughout its length it receives blood from the superficial tissues on the lateral aspects of the hand, forearm and arm.

The *basilic vein* begins at the back of the hand on the ulnar aspect. It ascends on the medial side of the forearm and upper arm then joins the axillary vein. It receives blood from the medial aspect of the hand, forearm and arm. There are many small veins which link the cephalic and basilic veins.

The *median vein* is a small vein that is not always present. It begins at the palmar surface of the hand, ascends on the front of the forearm and ends in the basilic vein or the median cubital vein.

The *brachiocephalic vein* is formed when the subclavian and internal jugular veins unite. There is one on each side.

The *superior vena cava* is formed when the two brachiocephalic veins unite. It drains all the venous blood from the head, neck and upper limbs and terminates in the right atrium. It is about 7 cm long and passes downwards along the right border of the sternum.

Descending aorta in the thorax

This part of the aorta is continuous with the arch of the aorta and begins at the level of the 4th thoracic vertebra. It extends downwards on the anterior surface of the bodies of the thoracic vertebrae (Fig. 5.42) to the level of the 12th thoracic vertebra, where it passes behind the diaphragm to become the abdominal aorta.

The descending aorta in the thorax gives off many *paired branches* which supply the walls of the thoracic cavity and the organs within the cavity, including:

- *bronchial arteries* that supply the bronchi and their branches, connective tissue in the lungs and the lymph nodes at the root of the lungs
- *oesophageal arteries* that supply the oesophagus
- *intercostal arteries* that run along the inferior border of the ribs and supply the intercostal muscles, some muscles of the thorax, the ribs, the skin and its underlying connective tissues.

Venous return from the thoracic cavity

Most of the venous blood from the organs in the thoracic cavity is drained into the *azygos vein* and the *hemiazygos vein* (Fig. 5.43). Some of the main veins which join them are the *bronchial, oesophageal* and *intercostal veins*. The azygos

Figure 5.42 The aorta and its main branches in the thorax.

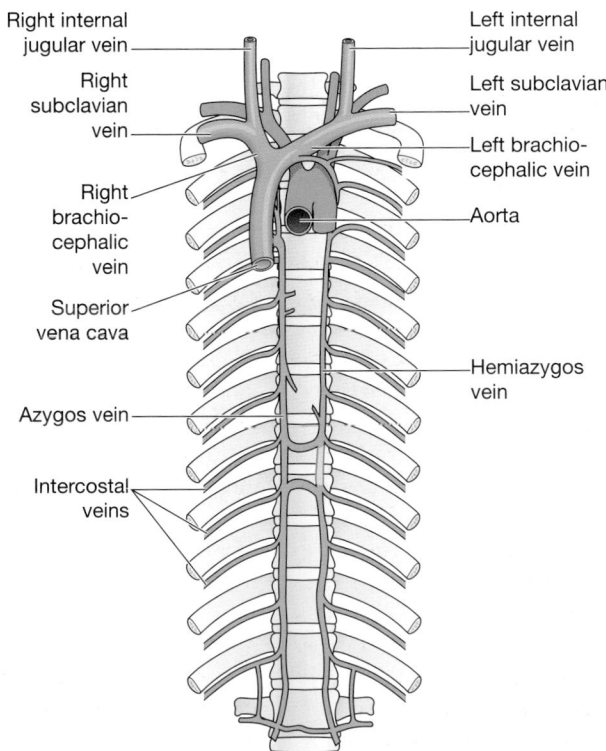

Figure 5.43 The superior vena cava and the main veins of the thorax.

vein joins the superior vena cava and the hemiazygos vein joins the left brachiocephalic vein. At the distal end of the oesophagus some oesophageal veins join the azygos vein and others, the left gastric vein. A venous plexus is formed by anastomoses between the veins joining the azygos vein and those joining the left gastric veins, linking the general and portal circulations (see Fig. 12.50, p. 321).

Abdominal aorta

The abdominal aorta is a continuation of the thoracic aorta. The name changes when the aorta enters the abdominal cavity by passing behind the diaphragm at the level of the 12th thoracic vertebra. It descends in front of the bodies of the vertebrae to the level of the 4th lumbar vertebra, where it divides into the *right* and *left common iliac arteries* (Fig. 5.44).

When a branch of the abdominal aorta supplies an organ it is only named here and is described in more detail in association with the organ. However, illustrations showing the distribution of blood from the coeliac, superior and inferior mesenteric arteries are presented here (Figs 5.45 and 5.46).

Many branches arise from the abdominal aorta, some of which are *paired* and some *unpaired*.

Paired branches

- *Inferior phrenic arteries* supply the diaphragm.
- *Renal arteries* supply the kidneys and give off branches, the *suprarenal arteries*, to supply the adrenal glands.
- *Testicular arteries* supply the testes in the male.
- *Ovarian arteries* supply the ovaries in the female.

The testicular and ovarian arteries are much longer than the other paired branches. This is because the testes and the ovaries begin their development in the region of the kidneys. As they grow they descend into the scrotum and the pelvis respectively and are accompanied by their blood vessels.

Unpaired branches

The *coeliac artery* (Fig. 5.44) is a short thick artery about 1.25 cm long. It arises immediately below the diaphragm and divides into three branches:

- *left gastric artery*: supplies the stomach
- *splenic artery*: supplies the pancreas and the spleen
- *hepatic artery*: supplies the liver, gall bladder and parts of the stomach, duodenum and pancreas.

Figure 5.44 The abdominal aorta and its branches.

The *superior mesenteric artery* (Fig. 5.44) branches from the aorta between the coeliac artery and the renal arteries. It supplies the whole of the small intestine and the proximal half of the large intestine.

The *inferior mesenteric artery* (Fig. 5.44) arises from the aorta about 4 cm above its division into the common iliac arteries. It supplies the distal half of the large intestine and part of the rectum.

Venous return from the abdominal organs

The *inferior vena cava* is formed when *right* and *left common iliac veins* join at the level of the body of the 5th lumbar vertebra. This is the largest vein in the body and it conveys blood from all parts of the body below the diaphragm to the right atrium of the heart. It passes through the central tendon of the diaphragm at the level of the 8th thoracic vertebra.

Paired testicular, ovarian, renal and adrenal veins join the inferior vena cava.

Blood from the remaining organs in the abdominal cavity passes through the liver via the *portal circulation* before entering the inferior vena cava (Fig. 5.45).

Portal circulation

In all the parts of the circulation which have been described previously, venous blood passes from the tissues to the heart by the most direct route through only one capillary bed. In the portal circulation, venous blood passes from the capillary beds of the abdominal part of the digestive system, the spleen and pancreas to the liver.

It passes through a second capillary bed, the hepatic sinusoids, in the liver before entering the general circulation via the inferior vena cava. In this way blood with a high concentration of nutrients, absorbed from the stomach and intestines, goes to the liver first. In the liver certain modifications take place, including the regulation of nutrient supply to other parts of the body.

Portal vein

This is formed by the union of the following veins (Figs 5.47 and 5.48), each of which drains blood from the area supplied by the corresponding artery:

- splenic vein
- inferior mesenteric vein
- superior mesenteric vein
- gastric veins
- cystic vein.

The *splenic vein* drains blood from the spleen, the pancreas and part of the stomach.

The *inferior mesenteric vein* returns the venous blood from the rectum, pelvic and descending colon of the large intestine. It joins the splenic vein.

The *superior mesenteric vein* returns venous blood from the small intestine and the proximal parts of the large intestine, i.e. the caecum, ascending and transverse colon. It unites with the *splenic vein* to form the *portal vein*.

The *gastric veins* drain blood from the stomach and the distal end of the oesophagus, then join the portal vein.

The *cystic vein* which drains venous blood from the gall bladder joins the portal vein.

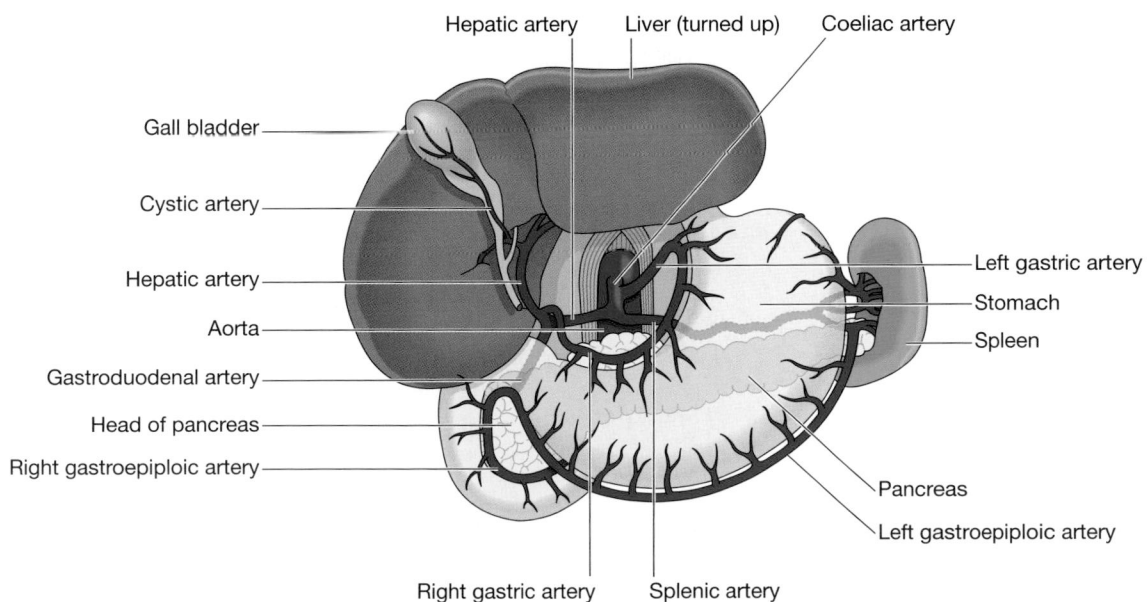

Figure 5.45 The coeliac artery and its branches, and the inferior phrenic arteries.

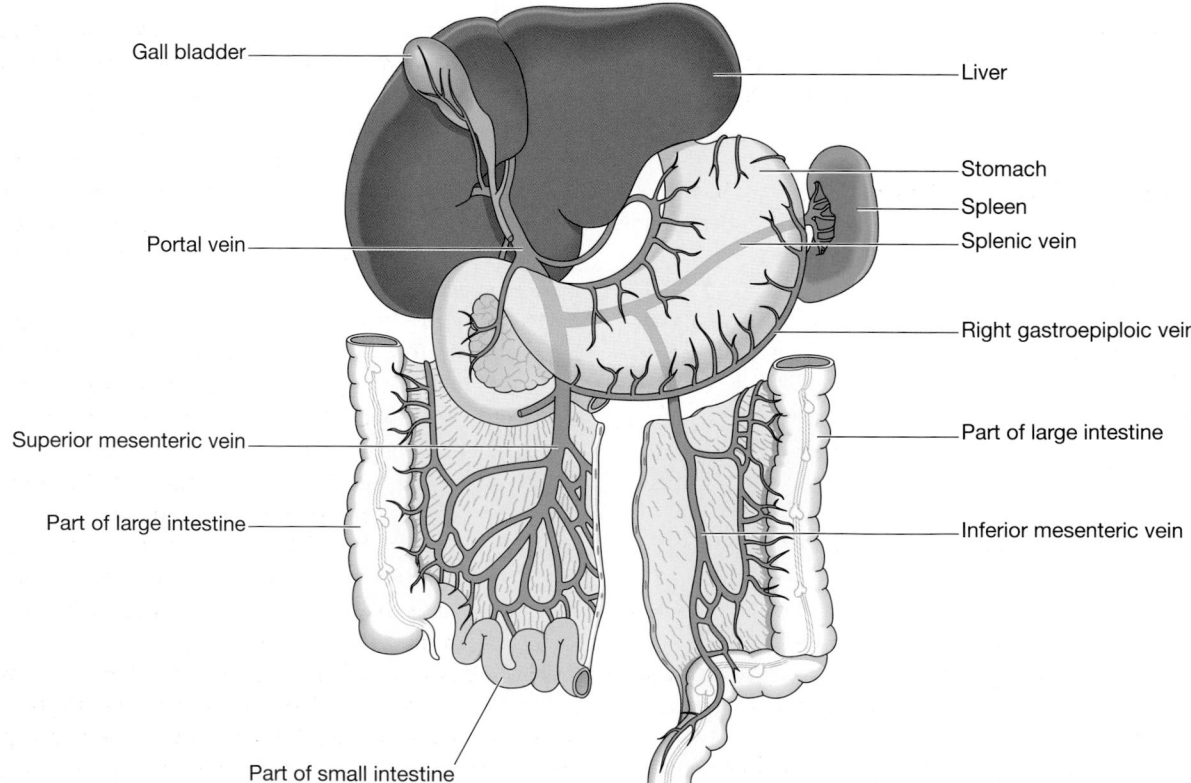

Figure 5.46 The superior and inferior mesenteric arteries and their branches.

Figure 5.47 Venous drainage from the abdominal organs and the formation of the portal vein.

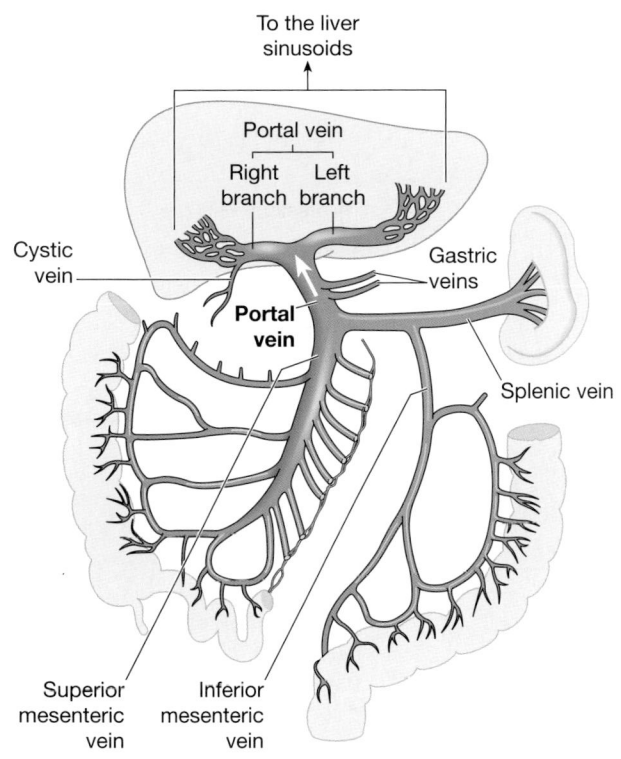

Figure 5.48 The portal vein – formation and termination.

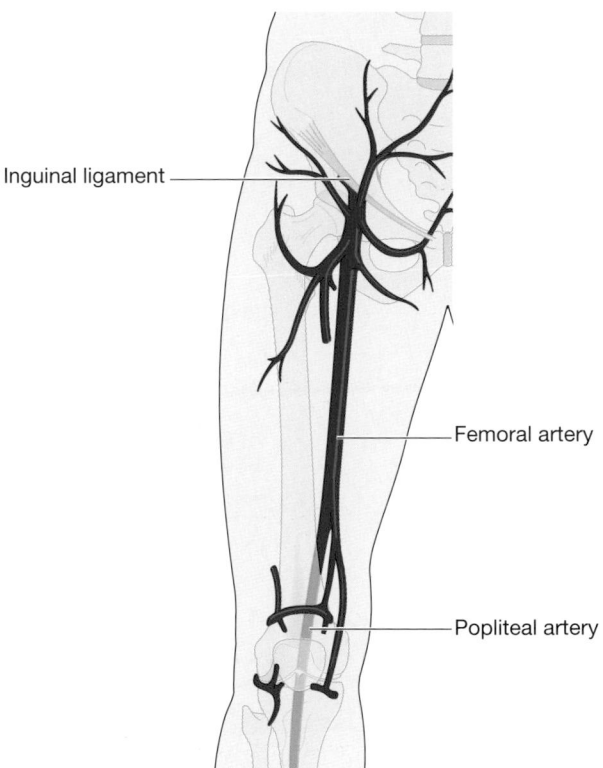

Figure 5.49 The femoral artery and its main branches.

Hepatic veins

These are very short veins that leave the posterior surface of the liver and, almost immediately, enter the inferior vena cava.

Circulation of blood to the pelvis and lower limb

Arterial supply

Common iliac arteries. The right and left common iliac arteries are formed when the abdominal aorta divides at the level of the 4th lumbar vertebra (Fig. 5.32). In front of the sacroiliac joint each divides into:

- internal iliac artery
- external iliac artery.

The *internal iliac artery* runs medially to supply the organs within the pelvic cavity. In the female, one of the largest branches is the *uterine artery* which provides the main arterial blood supply to the reproductive organs.

The *external iliac artery* runs obliquely downwards and passes behind the inguinal ligament into the thigh where it becomes the *femoral artery*.

The *femoral artery* (Fig. 5.49) begins at the midpoint of the inguinal ligament and extends downwards in front of the thigh; then it turns medially and eventually passes

round the medial aspect of the femur to enter the popliteal space where it becomes the *popliteal artery*. It supplies blood to the structures of the thigh and some superficial pelvic and inguinal structures.

The *popliteal artery* (Fig. 5.50) passes through the popliteal fossa behind the knee. It supplies the structures in this area, including the knee joint. At the lower border of the popliteal fossa it divides into the anterior and posterior tibial arteries.

The *anterior tibial artery* (Fig. 5.50) passes forwards between the tibia and fibula and supplies the structures in the front of the leg. It lies on the tibia, runs in front of the ankle joint and continues over the dorsum (top) of the foot as the *dorsalis pedis artery*.

The *dorsalis pedis artery* is a continuation of the anterior tibial artery and passes over the dorsum of the foot, supplying arterial blood to the structures in this area. It ends by passing between the first and second metatarsal bones into the sole of the foot where it contributes to the formation of the plantar arch.

The *posterior tibial artery* (Fig. 5.50) runs downwards and medially on the back of the leg. Near its origin it gives off a large branch called the *peroneal artery* which supplies the lateral aspect of the leg. In the lower part it becomes superficial and passes medial to the ankle joint to reach the sole of the foot where it continues as the *plantar artery*.

Posterior view

Inferior view **Anterior view**

Figure 5.50 The right popliteal artery and its main branches.

The *plantar artery* supplies the structures in the sole of the foot. This artery, its branches and the dorsalis pedis artery form the *plantar arch* from which the digital branches arise to supply the toes.

Venous return

There are both deep and superficial veins in the lower limb (Fig. 5.31). Blood entering the superficial veins passes to the deep veins through *communicating veins*. Movement of blood towards the heart is partly dependent on contraction of skeletal muscles. Backward flow is prevented by a large number of valves. Superficial veins receive less support by surrounding tissues than deep veins.

Deep veins. The deep veins accompany the arteries and their branches and have the same names. They are:

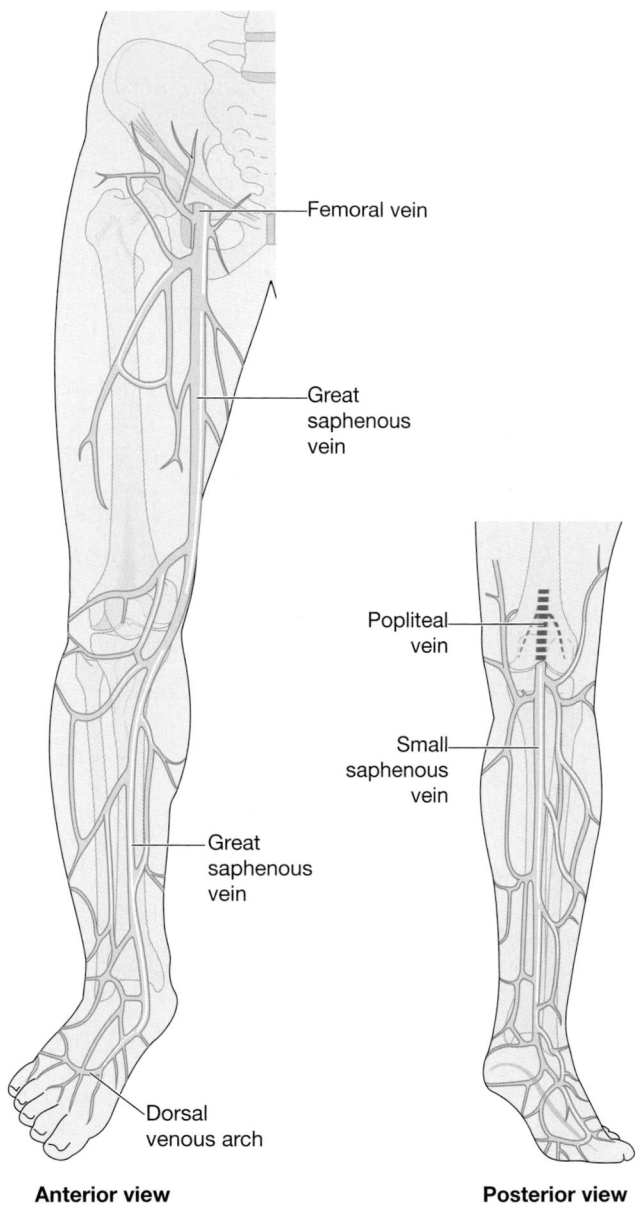

Anterior view **Posterior view**

Figure 5.51 Superficial veins of the leg.

- digital veins
- plantar venous arch
- posterior tibial vein
- anterior tibial vein
- popliteal vein
- femoral vein
- external iliac vein
- internal iliac vein
- common iliac vein.

The *femoral vein* ascends in the thigh to the level of the inguinal ligament where it becomes the external iliac vein.

The *external iliac vein* is the continuation of the femoral vein where it enters the pelvis lying close to the femoral artery. It passes along the brim of the pelvis and at the level of the sacroiliac joint it is joined by the *internal iliac vein* to form the *common iliac vein*.

The *internal iliac vein* receives tributaries from several veins which drain the organs of the pelvic cavity.

The *two common iliac veins* begin at the level of the sacroiliac joints. They ascend obliquely and end a little to the right of the body of the 5th lumbar vertebra by uniting to form the *inferior vena cava*.

Superficial veins (Fig. 5.51). The two main superficial veins draining blood from the lower limbs are:

- small saphenous vein
- great saphenous vein.

The *small saphenous vein* begins behind the ankle joint where many small veins which drain the dorsum of the

foot join together. It ascends superficially along the back of the leg and in the popliteal space it joins the *popliteal vein* — a deep vein.

The *great saphenous vein* is the longest vein in the body. It begins at the medial half of the dorsum of the foot and runs upwards, crossing the medial aspect of the tibia and up the inner side of the thigh. Just below the inguinal ligament it joins the *femoral vein*.

Many *communicating veins* join the superficial veins, and the superficial and deep veins of the lower limb.

SUMMARY OF THE MAIN BLOOD VESSELS

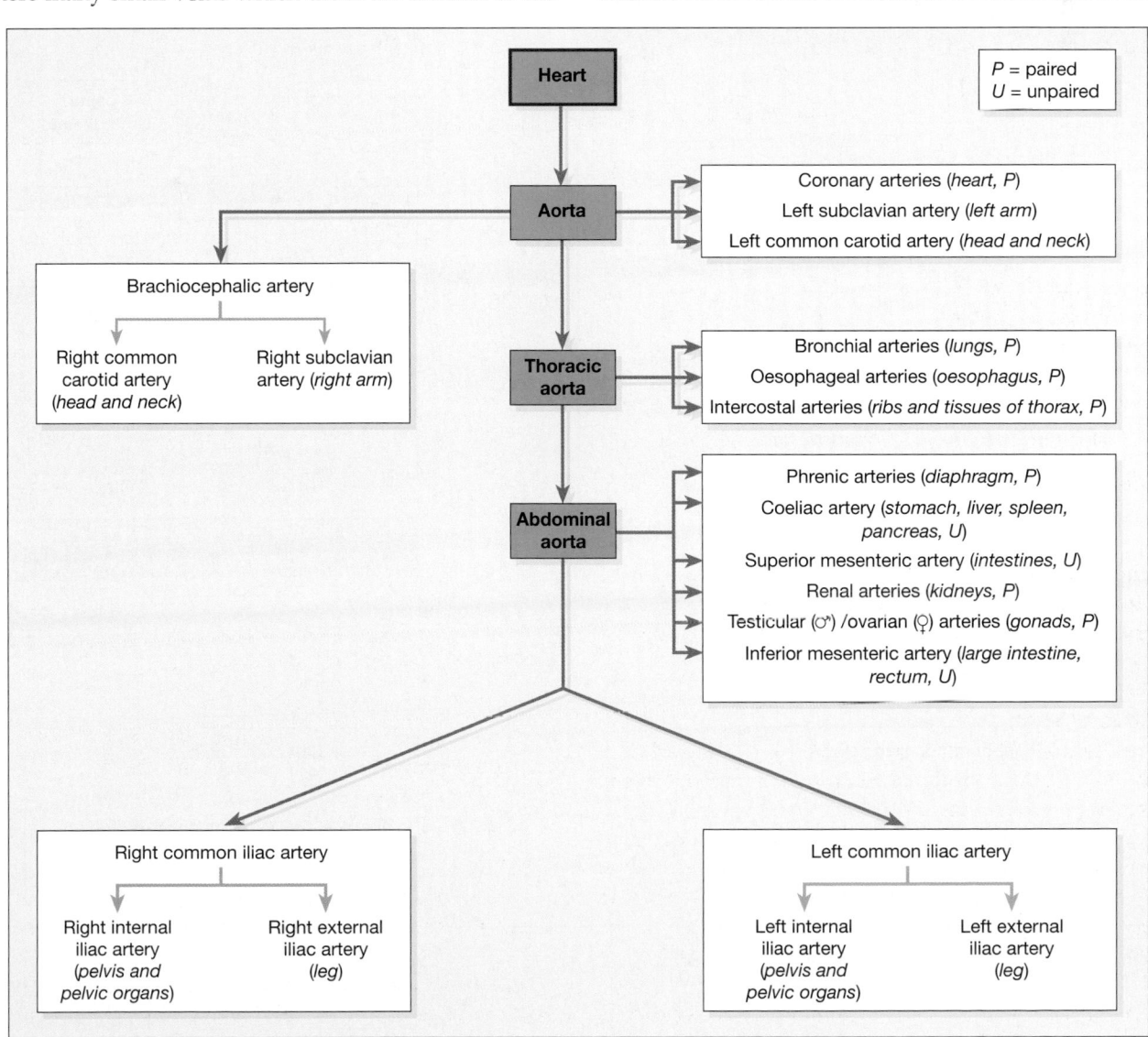

Figure 5.52 A. The aorta and main arteries of the body.

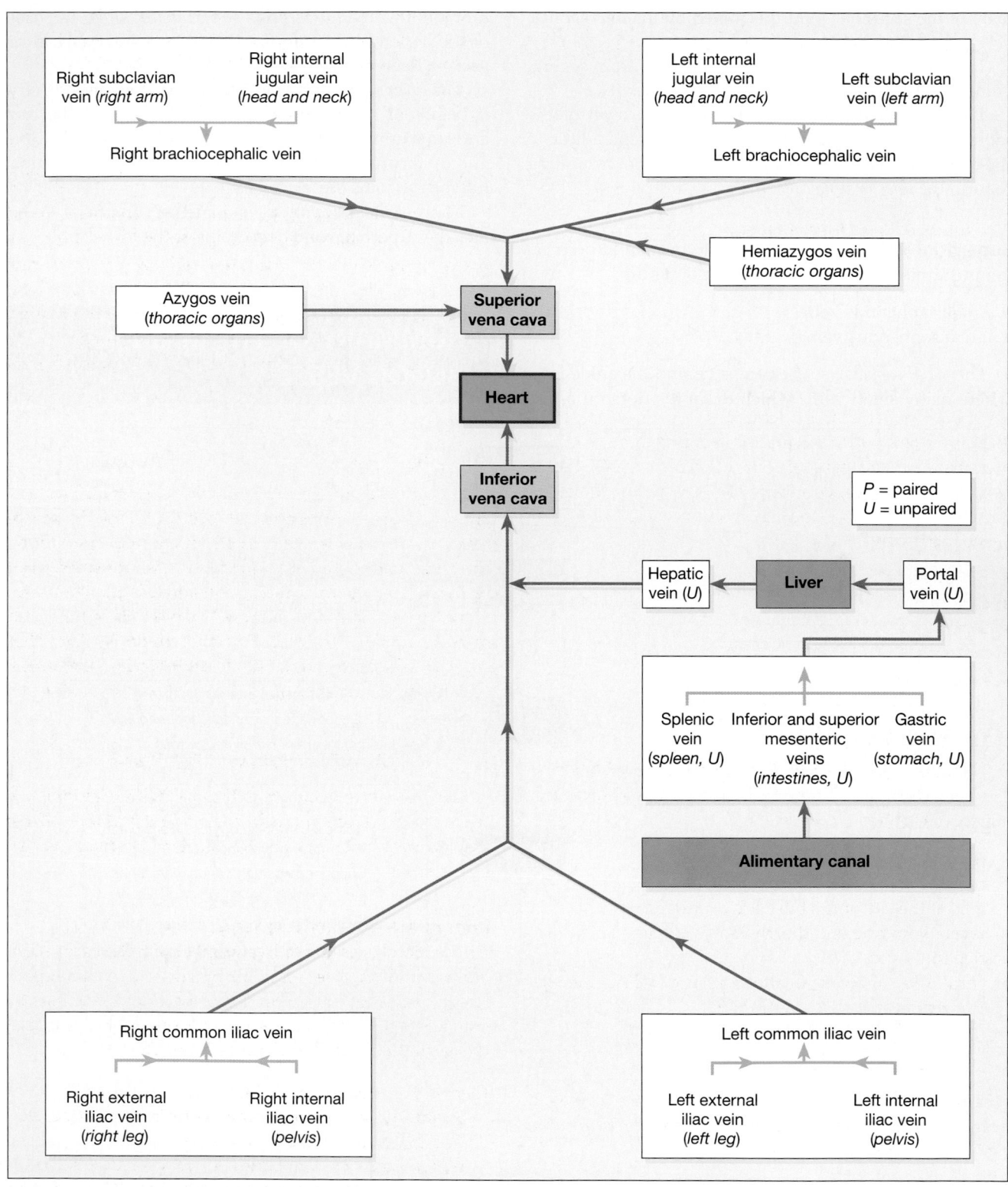

Figure 5.52 B. The venae cavae and main veins of the body.

SHOCK

Learning outcomes

After studying this section, you should be able to:

- define the term shock
- describe the main physiological changes that occur during shock
- explain the underlying pathophysiology of the main causes of shock.

Shock occurs when the metabolic needs of cells are not being met because of inadequate blood flow. In effect, there is a reduction in circulating blood volume, in blood pressure and in cardiac output. This causes tissue hypoxia, an inadequate supply of nutrients and the accumulation of waste products. A number of different types of shock are described:

- hypovolaemic
- cardiogenic
- septic
- neurogenic
- anaphylactic.

Hypovolaemic shock

This occurs when the blood volume is reduced by 15 to 25%. Reduced venous return and in turn cardiac output may occur following:

- severe haemorrhage—whole blood is lost
- extensive superficial burns—serum is lost and blood cells at the site of the burn are destroyed
- severe vomiting and diarrhoea—water and electrolytes are lost
- perforation of an organ allowing its contents to enter the peritoneal cavity (peritonitis).

Cardiogenic shock

This occurs in acute heart disease when the damaged heart muscle cannot maintain an adequate cardiac output, e.g. in myocardial infarction.

Septic shock (bacteraemic, endotoxic)

This is caused by severe infections in which endotoxins are released into the circulation from dead Gram-negative bacteria, e.g. *Enterobacteria, Pseudomonas*.

The mode of action of the toxins is not clearly understood. It may be that they cause an apparent reduction in the blood volume because of vasodilatation and pooling of blood in the large veins. This reduces the venous return to the heart and the cardiac output.

Neurogenic shock (vasovagal attack, fainting)

The causes include sudden acute pain, severe emotional experience, spinal anaesthesia and spinal cord damage. Parasympathetic nerve impulses reduce the heart rate, and in turn, the cardiac output. The venous return may also be reduced by the pooling of blood in dilated veins. These changes effectively reduce the blood supply to the brain, causing fainting. The period of unconsciousness is usually of short duration.

Anaphylactic shock

In allergic reactions an antigen interacts with an antibody and a variety of responses can occur (p. 383). In severe cases, the chemicals released, e.g. histamine, bradykinin, produce widespread vasodilatation and constriction of bronchiolar smooth muscle (bronchospasm). The vasodilatation profoundly reduces the venous return and cardiac output resulting in tissue hypoxia. Bronchospasm reduces the amount of air entering the lungs, increasing tissue hypoxia.

Physiological changes during shock

In the short term these are associated with physiological attempts to restore an adequate blood circulation. If the state of shock persists, the longer-term changes may be irreversible.

Immediate or reactive changes

As the blood pressure falls, a number of reflexes are stimulated and hormone secretions increased in an attempt to restore homeostasis. These raise the blood pressure by increasing peripheral resistance, the blood volume and the cardiac output. The changes include:

1. vasoconstriction, following:
   a. stimulation of the baroreceptors in the aortic arch and carotid sinuses
   b. sympathetic stimulation of the adrenal glands which causes increased secretion of adrenaline and noradrenaline
   c. stimulation of the renin—angiotensin—aldosterone system by diminished blood flow to the kidneys (p. 223)

111

2. increased heart rate, following sympathetic stimulation
3. water retention by the kidney, following increased release of antidiuretic hormone by the posterior lobe of the pituitary gland, increasing salt and water retention.

In shock of moderate severity the circulation to the heart and brain is maintained, in the short term. Restlessness, confusion and coma occur as circulation to the brain is impaired. If shock is very severe there may not be time for the above changes to be effective. The severe hypoxia that occurs disrupts cell metabolism. In the absence of adequate oxygen, cellular metabolism switches to less efficient anaerobic pathways, large amounts of lactic acid are formed and hydrogen ions accumulate, reaching dangerous levels in a few minutes. These are the changes that lead to the severe metabolic acidosis which occurs immediately prior to and following cardiac arrest.

Long-term changes associated with shock

If the state of shock is not reversed, hypoxia and low blood pressure cause irreversible brain damage and capillary dilatation and a vicious circle of events is established.

Hypoxia. When this persists there is cell damage and a release of chemical substances that increase the permeability of the capillaries. More fluid enters the interstitial spaces, leading to further hypovolaemia, further reduction in blood pressure and increased hypoxia.

Low blood pressure. As the blood pressure continues to fall, cerebral and myocardial hypoxia becomes progressively more marked and the reduced blood flow encourages the formation of thrombi and infarcts. There is acute renal failure and a marked reduction in the secretion of urine, leading to the retention of damaging metabolic waste products. If effective treatment is not possible these irreversible changes become progressively more severe and eventually may cause death.

DISEASES OF BLOOD VESSELS

Learning outcomes

After studying this section, you should be able to:

- discuss the main causes, effects and complications of arterial disease, including atheroma, arteriosclerosis and aneurysm

- explain the main causes of venous thrombosis

- discuss the underlying abnormality in varicose veins

- list the predisposing factors and the common sites of occurrence of varicose veins

- describe the main tumours that affect blood vessels.

Atheroma

Pathological changes

Patchy changes (*atheromatous plaques*) develop in the tunica intima of large and medium-sized arteries. These consist of accumulations of cholesterol and other lipid compounds, excess smooth muscle and fat-filled monocytes (foam cells). The plaque is covered with a fibrous cap. As plaques grow they spread along the artery wall forming swellings that protrude into the lumen. Eventually the whole thickness of the wall and long sections of the vessel may be affected (Fig. 5.53). Plaques may rupture, exposing subintimal materials to the blood. This may cause thrombosis and vasospasm and will compromise blood flow.

Arteries most commonly involved are those in the heart, brain, kidneys, small intestine and lower limbs.

Causes of atheroma

The origin of atheromatous plaques is uncertain. *Fatty streaks* present in artery walls of infants are usually absorbed but their incomplete absorption may be the origin of atheromatous plaques in later life.

Atherosclerosis is considered to be a disease of older people because it is usually in these age groups that clinical signs appear. Plaques, however, start to form in childhood in developed countries.

The incidence of atheroma is widespread in developed countries. Why atheromatous plaques develop is not yet clearly understood but the predisposing factors appear to exert their effects over a long period. This may mean that the development of atheroma can be delayed or even

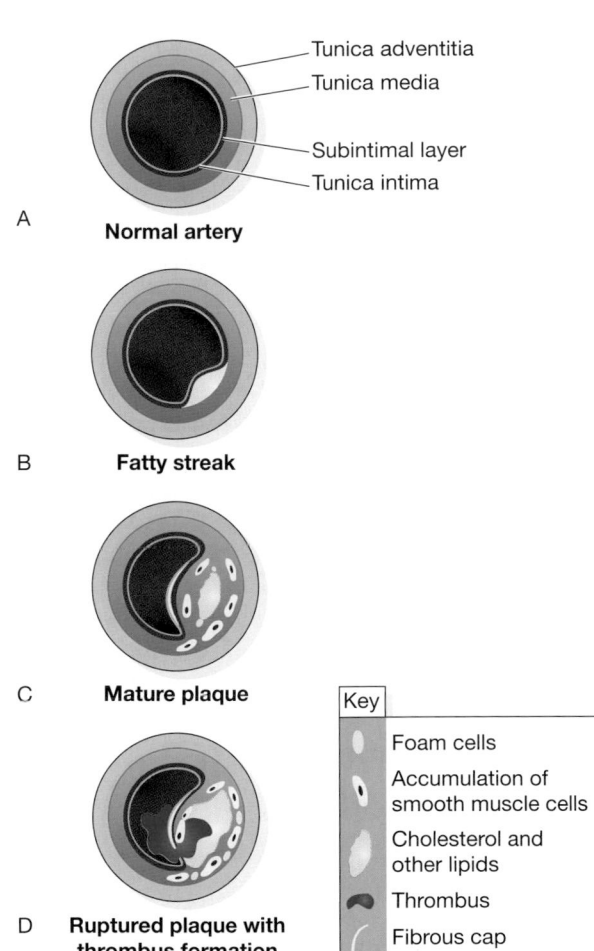

A **Normal artery**
- Tunica adventitia
- Tunica media
- Subintimal layer
- Tunica intima

B **Fatty streak**

C **Mature plaque**

D **Ruptured plaque with thrombus formation**

Key
- Foam cells
- Accumulation of smooth muscle cells
- Cholesterol and other lipids
- Thrombus
- Fibrous cap

Figure 5.53 Stages in the development of an atheromatous plaque.

arrested by a change in lifestyle. Predisposing factors include:

- heredity—family history
- gender—males are more susceptible than females until after the menopause
- increasing age
- hypertension
- diabetes mellitus
- smoking, especially cigarettes
- excessive emotional stress in work or home environment
- diet, e.g. high intake of refined carbohydrates and/or cholesterol and saturated fatty acids (from animal fats)
- obesity
- sedentary lifestyle
- excessive alcohol consumption.

Effects of atheroma

Arteries may be partially or completely blocked by atheromatous plaques alone, or by plaques combined with a thrombus. This may reduce or completely block the blood supply. The effects depend on the site and size of the artery involved and the extent of collateral circulation. Commonly the arteries affected are those in the heart, abdomen and pelvis.

Narrowing of an artery

The tissues distal to the narrow point become ischaemic. The cells may receive enough blood to meet their minimum needs, but not enough to cope with an increase in metabolic rate, e.g. when muscle activity is increased. This causes acute cramp-like ischaemic pain. Cardiac muscle and skeletal muscles of the lower limb are most commonly affected. Ischaemic pain in the heart is called *angina pectoris* (p. 121), and in the lower limbs, *intermittent claudication*.

Occlusion of an artery

When an artery is completely blocked, the tissues it supplies rapidly undergo degeneration and die from *ischaemia* which leads to *infarction*. The extent of tissue damage depends on:

- the size of the artery occluded
- the amount and type of tissue involved
- the extent of collateral circulation, e.g. in the brain the circulus arteriosus (circle of Willis) provides extensive collateral blood vessels while in the heart there are very few.

When a coronary artery is occluded *myocardial infarction* (p. 121) occurs. Occlusion of arteries in the brain causes cerebral ischaemia and this leads to *cerebral infarction* (stroke).

Complications of atheroma

Thrombosis and infarction

If the fibrous cap overlying a plaque breaks down, platelets are activated by the damaged cells and a blood clot (thrombus) forms, blocking the artery and causing ischaemia and infarction. Pieces of the clot (emboli) may break off, travel in the bloodstream and lodge in small arteries distal to the clot, causing small infarcts (areas of dead tissue).

Haemorrhage

When calcium salts are deposited in the plaques, the artery walls become brittle, rigid and unresponsive to rises in blood pressure and may rupture, causing haemorrhage.

Aneurysm formation

When the arterial wall is weakened by spread of the plaque between the layers of tissue, a local dilatation

113

(aneurysm) may develop (see below). This may lead to thrombosis and embolism, or the aneurysm may rupture causing severe haemorrhage. The most common sites affected are the aorta and the abdominal and pelvic arteries.

Arteriosclerosis

This is a progressive degeneration of arterial walls, associated with ageing and accompanied by hypertension.

Large and medium arteries
The tunica media is infiltrated with fibrous tissue and calcium. This causes the vessels to lose their elasticity. The lumen dilates and they become tortuous (Fig. 5.54). Loss of elasticity increases systolic blood pressure, and the *pulse pressure* (the difference between systolic and diastolic pressure).

Small arteries and arterioles
Hyaline thickening of the tunica media and tunica intima causes narrowing of the lumen and they become tortuous (Fig. 5.54). These arteries are the main determinants of peripheral resistance (p. 80) and narrowing of their lumens increases peripheral resistance and blood pressure. Ischaemia of tissues supplied by affected arteries may occur. In the limbs, the resultant ischaemia predisposes to gangrene which is particularly serious in people with diabetes mellitus.

Epithelium
Muscle and fibroelastic tissue
Normal

Fibrous tissue and calcium deposits
Dilated lumen
Large artery

Hyaline material
Narrow lumen
Small artery

Tortuous artery

Figure 5.54 Arteriosclerotic arteries.

Senile arteriosclerosis. This is a condition affecting elderly people in which the progressive loss of elasticity and reduced arterial lumen leads to cerebral ischaemia and loss of mental function. There may or may not be evidence of hypertension.

Thromboangiitis obliterans (Buerger's disease)

In this condition there is acute inflammation with thrombosis of the small arteries mainly in the lower limbs. It occurs most commonly in men between the ages of 20 and 40 years and is associated with heavy cigarette smoking. The condition may be caused by an immune response to an antigen, possibly a tobacco protein. The condition may become chronic and the vessel walls become fibrosed, lose their elasticity and do not dilate during exercise. The individual suffers from acute ischaemic pain and, as the disease progresses, the distance walked with comfort is gradually reduced. In the long term the skin may ulcerate and, in extreme cases, gangrene may develop.

Polyarteritis nodosa

This is a connective tissue disorder associated with inflammation of the tunica media of medium-sized arteries in any part of the body. The most common sites are the heart, kidneys, alimentary tract, liver, pancreas and nervous system. It is acute at first but frequently becomes chronic. Necrosis and rupture of blood vessels may occur in the acute phase followed by thrombosis, ischaemia, infarction and death. It is believed to be caused by an immune reaction. In most cases the antigen is not known but it may be a virus or drug such as a sulphonamide or antibiotic.

Aneurysms

Aneurysms are abnormal local dilatations of arteries which vary considerably in size (Fig. 5.55). The causes are not clear but predisposing factors include atheroma, hypertension and defective formation of collagen in the arterial wall.

Fusiform or spindle-shaped distensions occur mainly in the abdominal aorta and less commonly in the iliac arteries. They are usually associated with atheromatous changes.

Saccular aneurysms bulge out on one side of the artery. When they occur in the relatively thin-walled arteries of the circulus arteriosus (circle of Willis) in the brain they are sometimes called 'berry' aneurysms. They may be associated with defective collagen production, with atheromatous changes or be congenital.

Dissecting aneurysms occur mainly in the arch of the aorta due to infiltration of blood between the endothelium and tunica media, beginning at a site of endothelial damage.

Microaneurysms are fusiform or saccular aneurysms, occurring in small arteries and arterioles in the brain. They are associated with hypertension. Recurring small strokes (transient ischaemic attacks) are commonly due to thrombosis in the aneurysm or to haemorrhage when an aneurysm ruptures.

Complications of aneurysms

Haemorrhage

A ruptured aneurysm may cause sudden death or disability of varying severity, depending on the size and site of the artery.

Pressure

Localised swelling may cause pressure affecting adjacent tissues including organs, blood vessels and nerves.

Thrombosis and embolism

A blood clot (thrombus) may form in an artery where the endothelium has been damaged by an aneurysm. A piece of clot (embolus) may break off and travel in the bloodstream until it lodges in a small artery distal to the aneurysm and obstructs the blood flow, causing ischaemia and infarction.

Venous thrombosis

This may be *superficial thrombophlebitis* or *deep vein thrombosis*.

Superficial thrombophlebitis

In this acute inflammatory condition a thrombus forms in a superficial vein and the tissue around the affected vein becomes red and painful. The most common causes are:

- intravenous infusion
- varicosities in the saphenous vein.

Deep vein thrombosis (DVT)

A thrombus forms in a deep vein commonly in the lower limb, pelvic or iliac veins, but occasionally in an upper limb. The thrombus may affect a long section of the vein and, after some days, fibrinolysis (p. 68) may enable recanalisation through the blockage. Deep vein throm-

Saccular

Fusiform

Dissecting

Figure 5.55 Types of aneurysm.

bosis may be accompanied by pain and swelling, but is often asymptomatic. There are several predisposing factors.

Reduced rate of blood flow. This may be caused by:

- immobility associated with prolonged bedrest
- pressure on veins in the popliteal region by, e.g., a pillow under the knees in bed or sitting in a chair for long periods, as in long journeys
- pressure on a vein by an adjacent tumour
- prolonged low blood pressure, as in shock.

Changes in the blood. These may trigger intravascular clotting, e.g.:

- increased blood viscosity in, e.g., dehydration, polycythaemia (p. 72)
- increased adhesiveness of platelets, e.g. associated with the use of some oral contraceptive drugs, and in some malignant diseases.

Damage to the blood vessel wall. This can result in intravascular clotting, e.g.:

- accidental injury
- surgery.

The most common complication of DVT is *pulmonary embolism*, which occurs when a large piece or several small fragments of a venous thrombus become detached and travel through the heart to lodge in the pulmonary artery or one of its branches. It causes infarction of lung tissue. A massive pulmonary embolism usually causes sudden collapse and death.

Varicose veins

A varicosed vein is one which is so dilated that the valves do not close to prevent backward flow of blood. Such veins lose their elasticity, become elongated and tortuous and fibrous tissue replaces the tunica media.

Predisposing factors

Heredity. There appears to be a familial tendency but no abnormal genetic factor has been identified.

Gender. Females are affected more than males, especially following pregnancy.

Age. There is progressive loss of elasticity in the vein walls with increasing age so that elastic recoil is less efficient.

Obesity. Superficial veins in the limbs are supported by subcutaneous areolar tissue. Excess adipose tissue may not provide sufficient support.

Gravity. Standing for long periods with little muscle contraction tends to cause pooling of blood in the lower limbs and pelvis.

Pressure. Because of their thin walls, veins are easily compressed by surrounding structures, leading to increased venous pressure distal to the site of compression.

Sites and effects of varicose veins

Varicose veins of the legs
When valves in the anastomosing veins between the deep and superficial veins in the legs become incompetent the venous pressure in the superficial veins rises. In the long term they stretch and become chronically dilated because the superficial veins are not supported by much tissue. Such areas are seen externally as *varicosities* (Fig. 5.56). The great and small saphenous veins and the anterior tibial veins are most commonly affected causing aching and fatigue of the legs especially during long periods of standing. These dilated, inelastic veins rupture easily if injured, and haemorrhage occurs.

The skin over a varicose vein may become poorly nourished due to stasis of blood, leading to the formation of *varicose ulcers* usually on the medial aspects of the leg just above the ankle.

Haemorrhoids
Sustained pressure on the veins at the junction of the rectum and anus leads to increased venous pressure, valvular incompetence and the development of haemorrhoids (Fig. 5.56). The most common causes are chronic constipation, and the increased pressure in the pelvis towards the end of pregnancy. Slight bleeding may occur each time stools are passed and, in time, may cause anaemia. Severe haemorrhage is rare.

Normal	Varicosed
A vein	vein

B

Figure 5.56 A. Normal and varicosed veins. B. Common sites for varicosities – the leg, scrotum (varicocele) and anus (haemorrhoids).

Scrotal varicocele

Each spermatic cord is surrounded by a plexus of veins that may become varicosed (Fig. 5.56), especially in men whose work necessitates standing for long periods. If the varicocele is bilateral the increased temperature due to venous congestion may cause depressed spermatogenesis and result in infertility.

Oesophageal varices

The veins involved are at the lower end of the oesophagus. When the venous pressure in the liver rises, there is a rise in pressure in the anastomosing veins between the left gastric vein and the azygos vein. Sustained pressure causes varicosities to develop in the oesophagus (see Fig. 12.50, p. 321). The commonest causes of increased portal vein pressure are cirrhosis of the liver and right-sided cardiac failure. If the pressure continues to rise, inelastic varicosed veins may rupture causing severe haemorrhage, and possibly death.

Tumours of blood and lymph vessels

Angiomas

Angiomas are benign tumours of either blood vessels (haemangiomas) or lymph vessels (lymphangiomas). The latter rarely occur, so angioma is usually taken to mean haemangioma.

Haemangiomas. These are not true tumours but are sufficiently similar to be classified as such. They consist of an excessive growth of blood vessels arranged in an uncharacteristic manner and interspersed with collagen fibres.

Capillary haemangiomas. Excess capillary growth interspersed with collagen in a localised area makes a dense, plexus-like network of tissue. Each haemangioma is supplied by only one blood vessel and if it thromboses the haemangioma atrophies and disappears.

Capillary haemangiomas are usually present at birth and are seen as a purple or red mole or birthmark. They may be quite small at birth but grow at an alarming rate in the first few months, keeping pace with the growth of the child. After 1 to 3 years, atrophy may begin and by the end of 5 years in about 80% of cases the tumours have disappeared.

Cavernous haemangiomas. Blood vessels larger than capillaries grow in excess of normal needs in a localised area and are interspersed with collagen fibres. They are dark red in colour and may be present in the skin, though more commonly in the liver. They grow slowly, do not regress and may become large and unsightly.

THROMBOSIS, EMBOLISM AND INFARCTION

Learning outcomes

After studying this section, you should be able to:

- define the terms thrombosis, embolism and infarction
- explain, in general terms, the effects of the above on the body.

A *thrombus* is an intravascular blood clot, causing *thrombosis*. It may partially or completely occlude an artery or vein, interfering with the circulation of blood.

Factors which predispose to thrombus formation include:

- an abnormality of the normally smooth endothelium, e.g. ruptured atheromatous plaque
- abnormal blood flow in a vessel, especially venous stasis
- increased coagulability of the blood.

If a fragment of thrombus, called an *embolus*, becomes detached, it travels in the bloodstream until it lodges in and blocks a smaller vessel. The tissue supplied by the vessel becomes ischaemic and dies; this is *infarction*.

An *embolus* is a mass of any material carried in the bloodstream and large enough to block a blood vessel. Most emboli consist of fragments of thrombi but other materials include:

- fragments of atheromatous plaques
- fragments of vegetations from heart valves, e.g. infective endocarditis
- tumour fragments that may cause metastases
- amniotic fluid, during childbirth
- fat, from extensive bone fractures
- air, iatrogenic or following puncture of a blood vessel in the lung by a broken rib
- nitrogen in decompression sickness — 'the bends'
- pus from an abscess
- clumps of platelets with adherent microbes.

Emboli in veins move towards the heart and lodge in the smaller vessels of the lungs or the liver (an important cause of metastases in tumours of the alimentary tract). Those in arteries travel away from the heart and lodge in smaller arteries or arterioles.

117

The effects of an embolus are determined by the site and size of the blood vessel occluded, not its composition. Common serious consequences include:

- myocardial infarction (p. 121)
- cerebral infarction (p. 180)
- pulmonary embolism (p. 116).

OEDEMA

Learning outcomes

After studying this section, you should be able to:

- define the term oedema

- describe the main causes of oedema

- relate the causes of oedema to relevant clinical problems

- explain the causes and consequences of excess fluid collecting in body cavities.

In oedema there is excess tissue fluid, which causes swelling. It may occur in internal organs or in superficial tissues when there is disruption of the mechanisms that maintain homeostasis (p. 81).

Sites of oedema

When oedema is present in the superficial tissues *pitting* of the surface may be observed, i.e. an indentation in the skin remains after firm finger pressure has been applied. The sites at which superficial oedema is observed may be influenced by gravity and the position of the individual. When the individual is in the standing or sitting position the oedema is observed in the lower limbs, beginning in the feet and ankles. Patients on bedrest tend to develop oedema in the sacral area. This may be described as *dependent oedema*.

In *pulmonary oedema*, venous congestion in the lungs, or increased vessel permeability results in accumulation of fluid in the tissue spaces and in the alveoli. This reduces the area available for gaseous exchange and results in *dyspnoea* (breathlessness), cyanosis and expectoration of frothy sputum. The most common causes of pulmonary oedema are:

- cardiac failure
- inhalation of irritating gases

- inflammation
- intravenous infusion of excess fluid.

Causes of oedema

Increased venous hydrostatic pressure

Congestion of the venous circulation increases venous hydrostatic pressure, reducing the effect of osmotic pressure that draws fluid back into the capillary at the venous end. Excess fluid then remains in the tissues. This may be caused by:

- heart failure
- kidney disease
- external pressure on a limb due to, e.g., prolonged sitting or tight garments.

Decreased plasma osmotic pressure

When there is depletion of plasma proteins, less fluid returns to the circulation at the venous end of the capillary (Fig. 5.57B). Causes include:

- acute nephritis when the kidneys excrete protein
- nephrotic syndrome (p. 352)
- liver failure (p. 335)
- malnourishment where protein intake is very low.

Impaired lymphatic drainage

Some fluid returns to the circulation via the lymphatic system and when flow is impaired, oedema develops (Fig. 5.57C). Causes include:

- malignancy causing blockage of lymph nodes
- surgical removal of lymph nodes
- destruction of lymph nodes by chronic inflammation.

Increased small vessel permeability

In inflammation (p. 375), chemical mediators increase small vessel permeability in the affected area. Plasma proteins then leave the circulation (Fig. 5.57D) and the increased tissue osmotic pressure draws fluid into the area causing swelling of the affected tissue. This type of oedema also occurs in allergic reactions, e.g. anaphylaxis, asthma, hay fever.

Ascites and effusions

Ascites. This is the name given to the accumulation of excess fluid in the peritoneal cavity. The most common causes are:

- liver disease (p. 333)
- obstruction of lymph vessels in the abdominal cavity
- acute inflammation.

Pleural effusion. This is excess serous fluid in the pleural cavity. The most common causes are:

- heart failure due to increased blood pressure in the pulmonary circulation
- inflammation of the pleural membrane.

Figure 5.57 Mechanisms of oedema formation: A. Normal distribution of tissue fluid. B, C and D. Different mechanisms of oedema formation. Arrows indicate direction of movement of water.

DISEASES OF THE HEART

Learning outcomes

After studying this section, you should be able to:

- describe the consequences of failure of either or both sides of the heart
- explain the physiological compensatory mechanisms that occur in heart failure
- explain the causes and consequences of faulty heart valve function
- define the term ischaemic heart disease
- discuss the main conditions associated with ischaemic heart disease
- outline rheumatic heart disease and its effects on cardiac function
- explain the underlying pathophysiology of pericarditis
- describe, with reference to standard ECG trace, the main cardiac arrhythmias
- describe the principal congenital abnormalities of the heart.

Cardiac failure

The heart is described as failing when the cardiac output is unable to maintain the circulation of sufficient blood to meet the needs of the body. In mild cases, cardiac output is adequate at rest and becomes inadequate only when increased cardiac output is required, e.g. in exercise. Heart failure may affect either side of the heart, but since both sides of the heart are part of one circuit, when one half of the pump begins to fail it frequently leads to increased strain on, and eventual failure of, the other half. The main clinical manifestations depend on which side of the heart is most affected.

Compensatory mechanisms in heart failure

When heart failure happens acutely, the body has little time to make compensatory changes, but if the heart fails over a period of time the following changes are likely to occur in an attempt to maintain cardiac output and tissue perfusion, especially of vital organs.

- the cardiac muscle fibres enlarge and increase in number, which makes the walls of the chambers thicker
- the heart chambers enlarge
- decreased renal blood flow activates the renin–angiotensin–aldosterone system (p. 223), which leads to salt and water retention. This increases blood volume and cardiac workload. The direct vasoconstrictor action of angiotensin 2 increases peripheral resistance and puts further strain on the failing heart.

Acute cardiac failure

A sudden decrease in output of blood from both ventricles causes acute reduction in the oxygen supply to all the tissues. Recovery from the acute phase may be followed by chronic failure, or death may occur due to anoxia of vital centres in the brain. The commonest causes are:

- severe damage to an area of cardiac muscle due to ischaemia caused by sudden occlusion of one of the larger coronary arteries by atheroma or atheroma with thrombosis
- pulmonary embolism
- acute toxic myocarditis
- severe cardiac arrhythmia
- rupture of a heart chamber or valve cusp
- severe malignant hypertension.

Chronic cardiac failure

This develops gradually and in the early stages there may be no symptoms because certain compensatory changes occur as described above. When further compensation is not possible there is a gradual decline in myocardial efficiency. Underlying causes include:

- chronic hypertension, myocardial fibrosis, valvular disease, lung diseases, anaemia
- previous acute cardiac failure
- degenerative changes of old age.

Right-sided (congestive) cardiac failure

The right ventricle fails when pressure developed within it by the contracting myocardium is less than the force needed to push blood through the lungs.

When compensation has reached its limit, and the ventricle is not emptying completely, the right atrium and venae cavae become congested with blood and this is

followed by congestion throughout the venous system. The organs affected first are the liver, spleen and kidneys. *Oedema* (p. 118) of the limbs and *ascites* (excess fluid in the peritoneal cavity) usually follow.

This problem may be caused by increased vascular resistance in the lungs, weakness of the myocardium and/or stenosis and incompetence of valves in the heart or great vessels.

Resistance to blood flow through the lungs

When this is increased the right ventricle has more work to do. It may be caused by:

- the formation of fibrous tissue following inflammation or chronic disease of the lungs
- back pressure of blood from the left side of the heart, e.g. in left ventricular failure, when the mitral valve is stenosed and/or incompetent.

Weakness of the myocardium

This may be caused by ischaemia following numerous small myocardial infarcts.

Left-sided or left ventricular failure

This occurs when the pressure developed in the left ventricle by the contracting myocardium is less than the pressure in the aorta and the ventricle cannot then pump out all the blood it receives. Causes include:

- excessively high systemic (aortic) blood pressure
- incompetence of the mitral and/or the aortic valve
- aortic valve stenosis
- myocardial weakness.

Failure of the left ventricle leads to dilatation of the atrium and an increase in pulmonary blood pressure. This is followed by a rise in the blood pressure in the right side of the heart and eventually systemic venous congestion.

Congestion in the lungs leads to pulmonary oedema and dyspnoea, often most severe at night. This *paroxysmal nocturnal dyspnoea* may be due to raised blood volume as fluid from peripheral oedema is reabsorbed when the patient slips down in bed during sleep.

Disorders of heart valves

The heart valves prevent backflow of blood in the heart during the cardiac cycle. The left atrioventricular and aortic valves are subject to greater pressures than those on the right side and are therefore more susceptible to damage.

Distinctive heart sounds arise when the valves close during the cardiac cycle (p. 88). Damaged valves generate abnormal heart sounds called *murmurs*. A severe valve disorder results in heart failure. The most common causes of valve defects are rheumatic fever, fibrosis following inflammation and congenital abnormalities.

Stenosis

This is the narrowing of a valve opening, impeding blood flow through the valve. It occurs when inflammation and encrustations roughen the edges of the cusps so that they stick together, narrowing the valve opening. When healing occurs fibrous tissue is formed which shrinks as it ages, increasing the stenosis and leading to incompetence.

Incompetence

Sometimes called *regurgitation*, this is a functional defect caused by failure of a valve to close completely, allowing blood to flow back into the ventricle when it relaxes.

Ischaemic heart disease

Ischaemic heart disease is due to the effects of atheroma, causing narrowing or occlusion of one or more branches of the coronary arteries. The narrowing is caused by atheromatous plaques (p. 112). Occlusion may be by plaques alone, or plaques complicated by thrombosis. The overall effect depends on the size of the coronary artery involved and whether it is narrowed or occluded. Narrowing of an artery leads to *angina pectoris*, and occlusion to *myocardial infarction*, i.e. an area of dead tissue.

When atheroma develops slowly, a *collateral arterial blood supply* may have time to develop and effectively supplement or replace the original. This consists of the dilatation of normally occurring anastomotic arteries joining adjacent branch arteries. When sudden severe narrowing or occlusion of an artery occurs the anastomotic arteries dilate but may not be able to supply enough blood to meet the needs of the myocardium.

Angina pectoris

This is sometimes called *angina of effort* because increased cardiac output required during extra physical effort causes severe ischaemic pain in the chest. The pain may also radiate to the arms, neck and jaw. Other factors which may precipitate angina include:

- cold weather
- exercising after a heavy meal
- strong emotions.

A narrowed coronary artery may supply sufficient blood to the myocardium to meet its needs during rest or moderate exercise but not when greatly increased cardiac output is needed, e.g. walking may be tolerated but not running. The thick, inflexible atheromatous artery wall is unable to dilate to allow for the increased blood flow needed by the more active myocardium which then becomes ischaemic. In the early stages of development of the disease the chest pain stops when the cardiac output returns to its resting level soon after the extra effort stops.

Myocardial infarction

An *infarct* is an area of tissue that has died because of lack of oxygenated blood (p. 117). The myocardium is affected when a branch of a coronary artery is occluded. The commonest cause is an atheromatous plaque complicated by thrombosis. The extent of myocardial damage depends on the size of the blood vessel and site of the infarct. The damage is permanent because cardiac muscle cannot regenerate and the dead tissue is replaced with non-functional fibrous tissue. Speedy restoration of blood flow through the blocked artery using clot-dissolving (thrombolytic) drugs can greatly reduce the extent of the permanent damage and improve prognosis, but treatment must be started within a few hours of the infarction occurring. The effects and complications are greatest when the left ventricle is involved.

Myocardial infarction is usually accompanied by very severe crushing chest pain behind the sternum which, unlike angina pectoris, continues even when the individual is at rest.

Complications

These may be fatal and include:

- severe arrhythmias, especially *ventricular fibrillation*, due to disruption of the cardiac conducting system
- cardiac failure, caused by impaired contraction of the damaged myocardium and, in severe cases, cardiogenic shock
- rupture of a ventricle wall, usually within 2 weeks of the original episode
- pulmonary or cerebral embolism originating from a mural clot within a ventricle, i.e. a clot that forms inside the heart over the area of dead tissue
- pericarditis
- angina pectoris
- recurrence.

Rheumatic heart disease

Rheumatic fever

This autoimmune disease occurs 2 to 4 weeks after a throat infection, caused by *Streptococcus pyogenes* (beta-haemolytic Group A). The antibodies developed to combat the infection damage the heart. The microbes are not present in the heart lesion and the same infection in other parts of the body is very rarely followed by rheumatic fever. How the antibodies damage the heart is not yet understood. Children and young adults are most commonly affected.

Death rarely occurs in the acute phase but after recovery there may be permanent damage to the heart valves, eventually leading to disability and possibly cardiac failure.

Effects on the endocardium

The endocardium becomes inflamed and oedematous and tiny pale areas called *Aschoff's bodies* appear which, when they heal, leave thick fibrous tissue. Thrombotic fibrous nodules consisting of platelets and fibrin form on the free borders of the cusps of the heart valves. When healing occurs the fibrous tissue formed shrinks as it ages, distorting the shape of the cusps and causing stenosis and incompetence of the valve. The mitral and aortic valves are commonly affected, the tricuspid valve sometimes and the pulmonary valve rarely.

Effects on the myocardium

Aschoff's bodies form on the connective tissue between the cardiac muscle fibres. As in the endocardium, healing is accompanied by fibrosis which may interfere with myocardial contraction.

Effects on the pericardium

Inflammation leads to the accumulation of exudate in the pericardial cavity. Healing is accompanied by fibrous thickening of the pericardium and adhesions form between the two layers. In severe cases the layers may fuse, obliterating the cavity. Within this inelastic pericardium the heart may not be able to expand fully during diastole, leading to reduced cardiac output, generalised venous congestion and oedema.

Sydenham's chorea

This usually occurs between the ages of 5 and 15 years. The causes are unknown but it is commonly associated with streptococcal throat infection, rheumatic fever or endocarditis. There are rapid, uncoordinated, involuntary muscle movements. In mild cases recovery takes place within about 4 weeks. In some cases the initial recovery may be followed by recurrences.

Choreiform movements may occasionally occur during pregnancy, in women taking contraceptive pills and following cerebrovascular lesions, especially in the elderly.

Subclinical rheumatic heart disease

Valvular incompetence developing in older people who have a history of rheumatic fever many years previously is believed to be due to repeated subclinical attacks. These attacks are not associated with repeated episodes of sore throat so it is assumed that the original disease has remained active in a subclinical form. In some cases there is no history of rheumatic fever.

Infective endocarditis

Pathogenic organisms in the blood may colonise any part of the endocardium but the most common sites are on or near the heart valves and round the margins of congenital heart defects. These areas are susceptible to infection because they are exposed to fast-flowing blood that may cause mild trauma.

The main predisposing factors are bacteraemia, depressed immune response and heart abnormalities.

Bacteraemia

Microbes may or may not multiply while in the bloodstream and, if not destroyed by phagocytes or antibodies, they tend to adhere to platelets and form tiny infected emboli. Inside the heart the emboli are most likely to settle on already damaged endocardium. Vegetations consisting of platelets and fibrin surround the microbes and seem to protect them from normal body defences and antibiotics. Because of this, infection may be caused by a wide range of microbes, including some of low pathogenicity, e.g.:

- non-haemolytic streptococci, e.g. following tooth extraction, tonsillectomy
- *Escherichia coli* and other normal bowel inhabitants, e.g. following intestinal surgery
- *Staphylococcus aureus*, e.g. from boils and carbuncles
- microbes from infections of, e.g., the biliary, urinary, respiratory tracts
- microbes accidentally introduced during medical and nursing procedures, e.g. cystoscopy, bladder catheterisation, arterial and venous cannulation, surgery, wound dressing
- low-virulence microbes that cause infection in people with reduced immune response.

Depressed immune response

This enables low-virulence bacteria, viruses, yeasts and fungi to become established and cause infection. These are organisms always present in the body and the environment. Depression of the immune systems may be caused by:

- cytotoxic drugs
- ionising radiation, e.g. X-rays used in cancer treatment
- anti-inflammatory drugs, e.g. corticosteroids
- malignant diseases, e.g. leukaemia, tumours of lymphoid tissue
- sharing of syringes by drug addicts, spreading human immunodeficiency virus (HIV).

Heart abnormalities

The sites most commonly infected are already abnormal in some way, e.g. valve cusps damaged by earlier attacks of rheumatic fever, endothelium damaged by the fast flow of blood through a narrow opening, such as a stenosed valve or congenital septal defect.

Acute infective endocarditis

This is a severe febrile illness usually caused by high-virulence microbes, commonly *Staphylococcus aureus*. Vegetations grow rapidly and pieces may break off, becoming infected emboli. These settle in other organs where the microbes grow, destroying tissue and forming pus. The effects depend on the organ involved, e.g. brain or kidney infection may cause death in a few days. The causative microbes rapidly destroy heart valves, impairing their function and resulting in acute heart failure.

Subacute infective endocarditis

This endocarditis is usually caused by low-virulence microbes, e.g. non-haemolytic streptococci or some staphylococci. Infected emboli may settle in any organ but do not cause suppuration and rarely cause death. Microbes in the vegetations seem to be protected by surrounding platelets and fibrin from normal body defences and antibiotics. Healing by fibrosis further distorts the shape of the valve cusps, increasing the original stenosis and incompetence. Heart failure may develop later.

Cardiac arrhythmias

The heart rate is normally initiated by intrinsic impulses generated in the SA node. The rhythm is determined by the route of impulse transmission through the conducting system. The heart rate is usually measured as the pulse, but to determine the rhythm, an electrocardiogram (ECG) is required (Fig. 5.58A). A *cardiac arrhythmia* is any disorder of heart rate or rhythm, and is the result of abnormal generation or conduction of impulses. The normal cardiac cycle (p. 88) gives rise to *normal sinus rhythm* which has a rate between 60 and 100 beats per minute.

Sinus bradycardia. This is sinus rhythm below 60 beats per minute. This may occur during sleep and is common in athletes. It is an abnormality when it follows myocardial infarction or accompanies raised intracranial pressure (p. 177).

Sinus tachycardia. This is sinus rhythm above 100 beats per minute when the individual is at rest. This accompanies exercise and anxiety; but is an indicator of some disorders, e.g. fever, hyperthyroidism, some cardiac conditions.

Asystole

This occurs when there is no electrical activity in the ventricles and therefore no cardiac output. The ECG shows a flat line (Fig. 5.58B). Ventricular fibrillation and asystole cause sudden and complete loss of cardiac output, i.e. *cardiac arrest* and death.

123

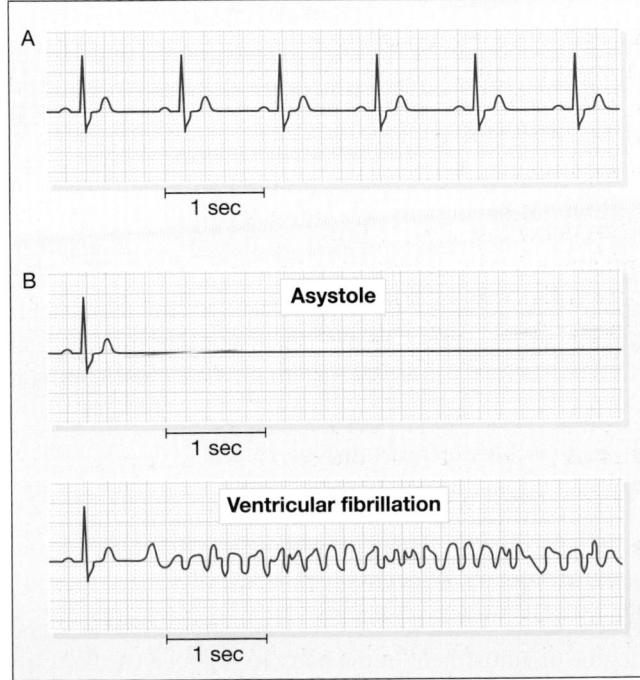

Figure 5.58 ECG traces: A. Normal sinus rhythm. B. Life-threatening arrhythmias.

Fibrillation

This is the contraction of the cardiac muscle fibres in a disorderly sequence. The chambers do not contract as a whole and the pumping action is disrupted.

In *atrial fibrillation* contraction of the atria is uncoordinated and rapid, pumping is ineffective and stimulation of the AV node is disorderly. Ventricular contraction becomes rapid and rhythm and force irregular; although an adequate cardiac output and blood pressure may be maintained, the pulse is irregular. The causes of increased excitability and disorganised activity are not always clear but predisposing conditions include:

- ischaemic heart disease
- degenerative changes in the heart due to old age
- thyrotoxicosis
- rheumatic heart disease.

In *ventricular fibrillation* there is disorganised and very rapid contraction causing disruption of ventricular function. Blood is not pumped from the heart into either the pulmonary or the systemic circulation. No pulses can be felt, consciousness is lost and breathing stops. The ECG shows an irregular chaotic trace with no recognisable wave pattern (Fig. 5.58B). If normal heart action cannot be restored quickly, death follows due to cerebral anoxia.

Heart block

Heart block occurs when impulse formation is impaired or conduction is prevented, and the delay between atrial and ventricular contraction is increased. The severity depends on the extent of loss of stimulation of the AV node.

In *complete heart block*, ventricular contraction is entirely independent of impulses initiated by the SA node. Impulses generated by the AV node result in slow, regular ventricular contractions and a heart rate of about 30 to 40 beats per minute. In this state the heart is unable to respond quickly to a sudden increase in demand by, e.g., muscular exercise. The most common causes are:

- acute ischaemic heart disease
- myocardial fibrosis following repeated infarctions or myocarditis
- drugs used to treat heart disease, e.g. digitalis, propranolol.

When heart block develops gradually there is some degree of adjustment in the body to reduced cardiac output but, if progressive, it eventually leads to death from cardiac failure and cerebral anoxia.

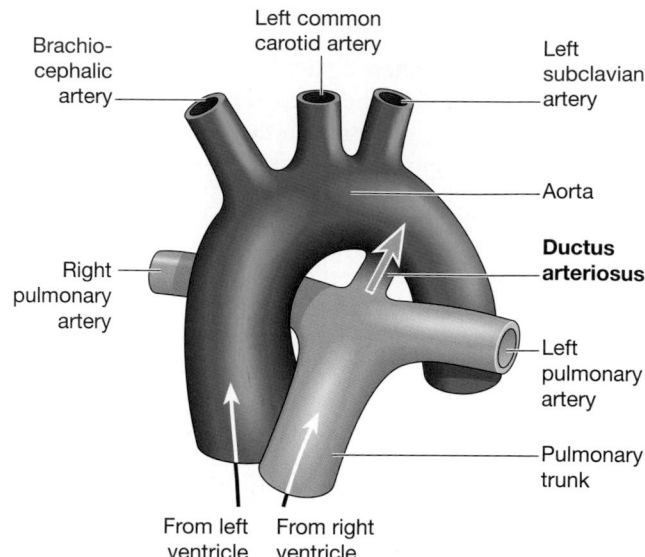

Figure 5.59 The position of the ductus arteriosus in the fetus. The arrow indicates the direction of flow of blood from the pulmonary circulation into the aorta.

Congenital abnormalities

Abnormalities in the heart and great vessels at birth may be due to intrauterine developmental errors or to the failure of the heart and blood vessels to adapt to extrauterine life. Sometimes, there are no symptoms in early life and the abnormality is recognised only when complications appear.

Patent ductus arteriosus

Before birth the ductus arteriosus, joining the arch of the aorta and the pulmonary artery, allows blood to pass from the pulmonary artery to the aorta (Fig. 5.59). It carries blood pumped into the pulmonary trunk by the right ventricle into the aorta, bypassing the pulmonary circulation. At birth, when the pulmonary circulation is established, the ductus arteriosus should close completely. If it remains patent, blood regurgitates from the aorta to the pulmonary artery where the pressure is lower, reducing the volume entering the systemic circulation and increasing the volume of blood in the pulmonary circulation. This leads to pulmonary congestion and eventually cardiac failure.

Atrial septal defect

Before birth most oxygenated blood from the placenta enters the left atrium from the right atrium through the

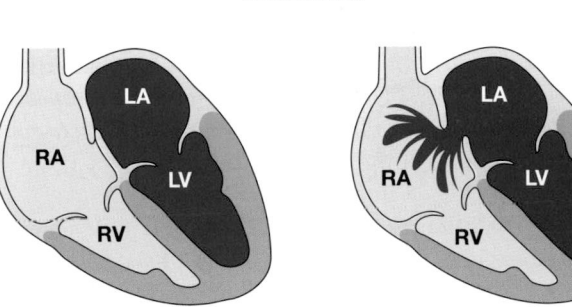

Figure 5.60 Atrioseptal valve: normal and defective closure after birth.

foramen ovale in the septum. There is a valve-like structure across the opening consisting of two partly overlapping membranes. The 'valve' is open when the pressure in the right atrium is higher than in the left. This diverts blood flow from the right to the left side of the heart, bypassing the pulmonary circulation. After birth, when the pulmonary circulation is established and the pressure in the left atrium is the higher, the two membranes come in contact, closing the 'valve'. Later the closure becomes permanent due to fibrosis (Fig. 5.60).

When the membranes do not overlap an opening between the atria remains patent after birth. In many cases it is too small to cause symptoms in early life but they may appear later. In severe cases blood flows back to the right atrium from the left. This increases the right ventricular and pulmonary pressure, causing hypertrophy of the myocardium and eventually cardiac failure. As pressure in the right atrium rises, blood flow through the defect may be reversed, but this is not an improvement because deoxygenated blood gains access to the general circulation.

Coarctation of the aorta

The most common site of coarctation (narrowing) of the aorta is between the left subclavian artery and ductus arteriosus. This leads to hypertension in the upper body (which is supplied by arteries arising from the aorta proximal to the narrowing) because increased force of contraction of the heart is needed to push the blood through the coarctation. There is hypotension in the rest of the body.

Fallot's tetralogy

A characteristic combination of four congenital cardiac abnormalities, called the tetralogy of Fallot, causes cyanosis, growth retardation and exercise intolerance in babies and young children. The four abnormalities are:

- stenosis of the pulmonary artery at its point of origin, which increases right ventricular workload
- ventricular septal defect, i.e. an abnormal communicating hole between the two ventricles, just below the atrioventricular valves
- aortic misplacement, i.e. the origin of the aorta is displaced to the right so that it is immediately above the septal defect
- right ventricular hypertrophy to counteract the pulmonary stenosis.

Cardiac function is inadequate to meet the needs of the growing child; surgical correction carries a good prognosis.

125

DISORDERS OF BLOOD PRESSURE

Learning outcomes

After studying this section, you should be able to:

- define the term hypertension
- identify normal and abnormal blood pressure recordings, taking into account the age of the individual
- define essential and secondary hypertension and list the main causes of the latter
- discuss the effects of prolonged hypertension on the body, including elevated blood pressure in the lungs
- describe the term hypotension.

Hypertension

The term hypertension is used to describe blood pressure that is sustained at a higher than the generally accepted 'normal' maximum level for a particular age group, e.g.:

- at 20 years — 140/90 mmHg
- at 50 years — 160/95 mmHg
- at 75 years — 170/105 mmHg.

Arteriosclerosis (p. 114) contributes to increasing blood pressure with age but is not the only factor involved.

Hypertension is described as *essential* (primary, idiopathic) or *secondary to other diseases*. Irrespective of the cause, hypertension commonly affects the kidneys (p. 353).

Essential hypertension

This means hypertension of unknown cause. It accounts for 85 to 90% of all cases and is subdivided according to the rate at which the disease progresses.

Benign (chronic) hypertension

The rise in blood pressure is usually slight to moderate and continues to rise slowly over many years. Sometimes complications are the first indication of hypertension, e.g. heart failure, cerebrovascular accident, myocardial infarction. Occasionally the rate of progress increases and the hypertension becomes malignant. Predisposing factors include:

- inherited tendency
- obesity
- excessive alcohol intake
- cigarette smoking
- lack of exercise.

Malignant (accelerated) hypertension

The blood pressure is already elevated and continues to rise rapidly over a few months. Diastolic pressure in excess of 120 mmHg is common. The effects are serious and quickly become apparent, e.g. haemorrhages into the retina, papilloedema (oedema around the optic disc), encephalopathy (cerebral oedema) and progressive renal disease, leading to cardiac failure.

Secondary hypertension

Hypertension resulting from other diseases accounts for 10 to 15% of all cases.

Kidney diseases

Raised blood pressure is a complication of many kidney diseases. The vasoconstrictor effect of excess *renin* released by damaged kidneys is one causative factor but there may be others, as yet unknown.

Endocrine disorders

Adrenal cortex. Secretion of excess *aldosterone* and *cortisol* stimulates the retention of excess sodium and water by the kidneys, raising the blood volume and pressure. Oversecretion of aldosterone (Conn's syndrome) is due to a hormone-secreting tumour. Oversecretion of cortisol may be due to overstimulation of the gland by *adrenocorticotrophic hormone* secreted by the pituitary gland, or to a hormone-secreting tumour.

Adrenal medulla. Secretion of excess *adrenaline* and *noradrenaline* raises blood pressure, e.g. phaeochromocytoma (p. 234).

Stricture of the aorta

Hypertension develops in branching arteries proximal to the site of a stricture. In *congenital coarctation* the stricture is between the ductus arteriosus and the left subclavian artery causing hypertension in the head, neck and right arm. Compression of the aorta by an adjacent tumour may cause hypertension proximal to the stricture.

Hypertension may be a complication of some drug treatment, e.g.:

- corticosteroids
- non-steroidal anti-inflammatory drugs
- oral contraceptives.

Effects and complications of hypertension

The effects of long-standing and progressively rising blood pressure are serious. Hypertension predisposes to atherosclerosis and has specific effects on particular organs.

Heart

The rate and force of cardiac contraction are increased to maintain the cardiac output against a sustained rise in arterial pressure. The left ventricle hypertrophies and begins to fail when compensation has reached its limit. This is followed by back pressure and accumulation of blood in the lungs (pulmonary congestion), hypertrophy of the right ventricle and eventually to right ventricular failure. Hypertension also predisposes to ischaemic heart disease (p. 121) and aneurysm formation (p. 114).

Brain

Stroke, caused by cerebral haemorrhage, is common, the effects depending on the position and size of the ruptured vessel. When a series of small blood vessels rupture, e.g. microaneurysms, at different times, there is progressive disability. Rupture of a large vessel causes extensive loss of function or possibly death.

Hypertensive encephalopathy. Hypertensive encephalopathy is a rare condition in which hypertension is accompanied by neurological disturbance, e.g. papilloedema, difficulty with speech, paraesthesia, convulsions and loss of consciousness. It is usually reversed when hypertension is controlled.

Kidneys

Essential hypertension causes kidney damage. If sustained for only a short time recovery may be complete. Otherwise the kidney damage causes further hypertension owing to activation of the renin–angiotensin–aldosterone system (p. 223), progressive loss of kidney function and kidney failure.

Pulmonary hypertension

Raised blood pressure in the pulmonary circulation is secondary to:

- changes in blood vessels, described above
- chronic diseases of the respiratory system
- diseases of the heart, e.g. congenital defects of the septum, stenosis and incompetence of the mitral or aortic valve, heart failure
- diseases of other organs that cause raised pressure in the left side of the heart, e.g. cirrhosis of the liver, thrombosis of the portal vein.

Hypotension

This usually occurs as a complication of other conditions, e.g.:

- shock (p. 111)
- Addison's disease (p. 233).

Low blood pressure leads to inadequate blood supply to the brain. Depending on the cause, unconsciousness may be brief (fainting) or more prolonged, possibly causing death.

Postural hypotension syncope (fainting) is due to sudden reduction in blood pressure on standing up quickly from a sitting or lying position. It occurs most commonly in the elderly. It may be caused by delay in response of the baroreceptors in the carotid sinuses to the gravitational effects of standing up. It may also occur when patients are being treated with antihypertensive drugs, especially when the most appropriate dose is being established.

6 The lymphatic system

All body tissues are bathed in tissue fluid, consisting of the diffusible constituents of blood and waste materials from cells. Some tissue fluid returns to the capillaries at their venous end and the remainder diffuses through the more permeable walls of the lymph capillaries and becomes lymph.

Lymph passes through vessels of increasing size and a varying number of *lymph nodes* before returning to the blood. The lymphatic system (Fig. 6.1) consists of:

- lymph
- lymph vessels
- lymph nodes
- lymph organs, e.g. spleen and thymus

- diffuse lymphoid tissue, e.g. tonsils
- bone marrow.

Functions of the lymphatic system include the following.

- *Tissue drainage*. Every day, around 21 litres of plasma fluid, carrying dissolved substances and some plasma protein, escape from the arterial end of the capillaries and into the tissues. Most of this fluid is returned directly to the bloodstream via the capillary at its venous end, but 3–4 litres of fluid are drained away by the lymphatic vessels. Without this, the tissues would rapidly become waterlogged, and the cardiovascular system would begin to fail as the blood volume falls.

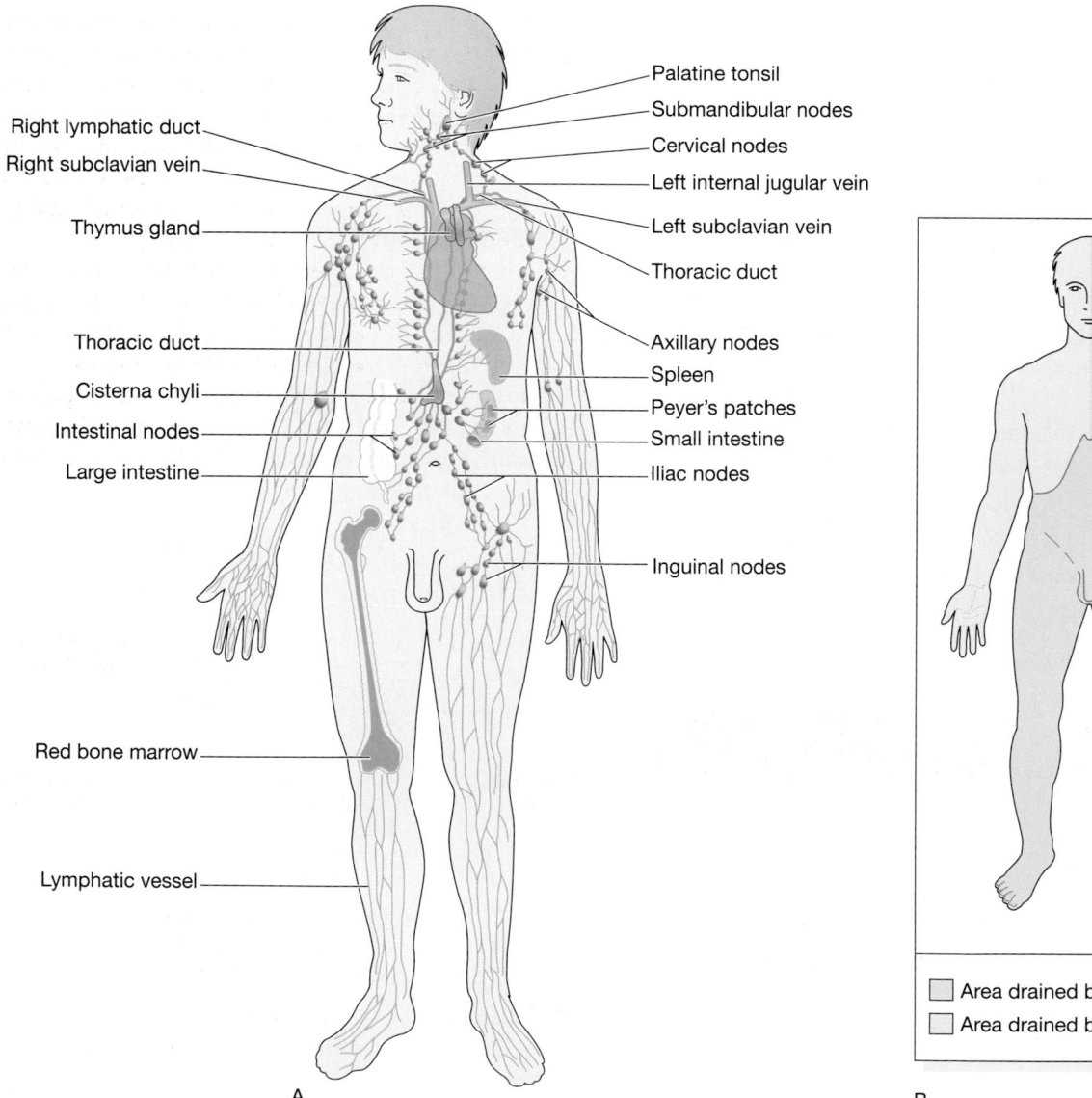

A   B

Figure 6.1 A. The lymphatic system. B. Lymph drainage. Green area drained by the thoracic duct; gold area drained by the right lymphatic duct.

■ *Absorption in the small intestine.* Fat and fat-soluble materials, e.g. the fat-soluble vitamins, are absorbed into the central lacteals (lymphatic vessels) of the villi.

■ *Immunity.* The lymphatic organs are concerned with the production and maturation of lymphocytes, the white blood cells that are primarily responsible for provision of immunity. Bone marrow is therefore considered to be lymphatic tissue, since lymphocytes are produced there.

LYMPH

Learning outcome

After studying this section, you should be able to:

■ describe the composition and the main functions of lymph.

Lymph is a clear watery fluid, similar in composition to plasma, with the important exception of plasma proteins, and identical in composition to interstitial fluid. Lymph transports the plasma proteins that seep out of the capillary beds back to the bloodstream. It also carries away larger particles, e.g. bacteria and cell debris from damaged tissues, which can then be filtered out and destroyed by the lymph nodes. Lymph contains lymphocytes, which circulate in the lymphatic system allowing them to patrol the different regions of the body. In the lacteals of the small intestine, fats absorbed into the lymphatics give the lymph (now called *chyle*), a milky appearance.

LYMPH VESSELS

Learning outcome

After studying this section, you should be able to:

■ identify the locations and functions of the main lymphatic vessels of the body.

Lymph capillaries

These originate as blind-end tubes in the interstitial spaces (Fig. 6.2). They have the same structure as blood capillaries, i.e. a single layer of endothelial cells, but their walls are more permeable to all interstitial fluid constituents, including proteins and cell debris. The tiny capillaries join up to form larger lymph vessels.

All tissues of the body have a network of lymphatic vessels, with the exception of the central nervous system, the bones and the most superficial layers of the skin.

Larger lymph vessels

The walls of lymph vessels are about the same thickness as those of small veins and have the same layers of tissue, i.e. a fibrous covering, a middle layer of smooth muscle and elastic tissue and an inner lining of endothelium. Lymph vessels have numerous cup-shaped valves which ensure that lymph flows in one way only, i.e. towards the thorax (Fig. 6.3). There is no 'pump', like the heart, involved in the onward movement of lymph but the muscle tissue in the walls of the large lymph vessels has an intrinsic ability to contract rhythmically (the lymphatic pump).

In addition, any structure that periodically compresses the lymphatic vessels can assist in the movement of lymph along the vessels, commonly including the contraction of adjacent muscles and the pulsation of large arteries.

Lymph vessels become larger as they join together, eventually forming two large ducts, the *thoracic duct* and *right lymphatic duct*, that empty lymph into the subclavian veins.

131

Figure 6.2 The origin of a lymph capillary.

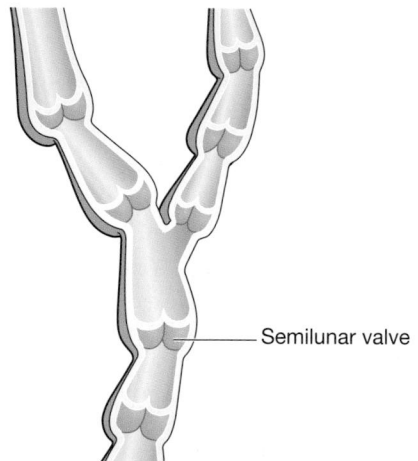

Figure 6.3 A lymph vessel cut open to show valves.

Thoracic duct

This duct begins at the *cisterna chyli*, which is a dilated lymph channel situated in front of the bodies of the first two lumbar vertebrae. The duct is about 40 cm long and opens into the left subclavian vein in the root of the neck. It drains lymph from both legs, the pelvic and abdominal cavities, the left half of the thorax, head and neck and the left arm (Fig. 6.1A and B).

Right lymphatic duct

This is a dilated lymph vessel about 1 cm long. It lies in the root of the neck and opens into the right subclavian vein. It drains lymph from the right half of the thorax, head and neck and the right arm (Fig. 6.1A and B).

LYMPHATIC ORGANS AND TISSUES

Learning outcomes

After studying this section, you should be able to:

- compare and contrast the structure and functions of a typical lymph node with that of the spleen

- describe the location, structure and function of the thymus gland

- describe the location, structure and function of mucosa-associated lymphatic tissue (MALT).

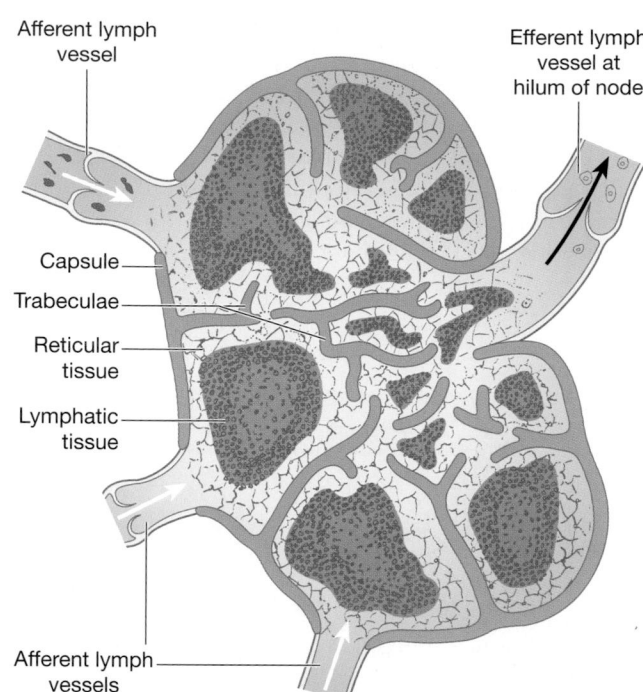

Figure 6.4 Section of a lymph node. Arrows indicate the direction of lymph flow.

Lymph nodes

Lymph nodes are oval or bean-shaped organs that lie, often in groups, along the length of lymph vessels. The lymph drains through a number of nodes, usually 8 to 10, before returning to the venous circulation. These nodes vary considerably in size: some are as small as a pin head and the largest are about the size of an almond.

Structure of lymph nodes

Lymph nodes (Fig. 6.4) have an outer capsule of fibrous tissue which dips down into the node substance forming partitions, or *trabeculae*. The main substance of the node consists of *reticular and lymphatic tissue* containing many lymphocytes and macrophages.

As many as four or five *afferent* lymph vessels may enter a lymph node while only one *efferent* vessel carries lymph away from the node. Each node has a concave surface called the hilum where an artery enters and a vein and the efferent lymph vessel leave.

The large numbers of lymph nodes situated in strategic positions throughout the body are arranged in deep and superficial groups.

Lymph from the head and neck passes through deep and superficial *cervical nodes* (Fig. 6.5).

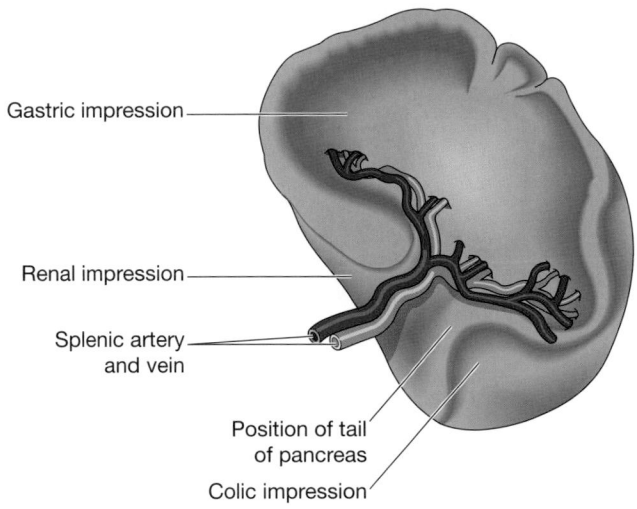

Gastric impression

Renal impression

Splenic artery
and vein

Position of tail
of pancreas

Colic impression

Figure 6.6 The spleen.

Occipital
nodes

Submandibular nodes

Deep cervical nodes

Superficial
cervical nodes

• Lymph nodes

Figure 6.5 Some lymph nodes of the face and neck.

Lymph from the upper limbs passes through nodes situated in the elbow region then through the deep and superficial *axillary nodes*.

Lymph from organs and tissues in the thoracic cavity drains through groups of nodes that are situated close to the mediastinum, large airways, oesophagus and chest wall. Most of the lymph from the breast passes through the axillary nodes.

Lymph from the pelvic and abdominal cavities passes through many lymph nodes before entering the cisterna chyli. The abdominal and pelvic nodes are situated mainly in association with the blood vessels supplying the organs and close to the main arteries, i.e. the aorta and the external and internal iliac arteries.

The lymph from the lower limbs drains through deep and superficial nodes including groups of nodes behind the knee and in the groin (inguinal nodes).

Functions of lymph nodes

Filtering and phagocytosis

Lymph is filtered by the reticular and lymphoid tissue as it passes through lymph nodes. Particulate matter may include microbes, dead and live phagocytes containing ingested microbes, cells from malignant tumours, worn-out and damaged tissue cells and inhaled particles. Organic material is destroyed in lymph nodes by macrophages and antibodies. Some inorganic inhaled particles cannot be destroyed by phagocytosis. These

remain inside the macrophages, either causing no damage or killing the cell. Material not filtered off and dealt with in one lymph node passes on to successive nodes and by the time lymph enters the blood it has usually been cleared of foreign matter and cell debris. In some cases where phagocytosis of microbes is incomplete they may stimulate inflammation and enlargement of the node (*lymphadenopathy*).

Proliferation of lymphocytes

Activated T- and B-lymphocytes multiply in lymph nodes. Antibodies produced by sensitised B-lymphocytes enter lymph and blood draining the node.

Spleen

The spleen (Fig. 6.6) is formed by reticular and lymphatic tissue and is the largest lymph organ.

The spleen lies in the left hypochondriac region of the abdominal cavity between the fundus of the stomach and the diaphragm. It is purplish in colour and varies in size in different individuals, but is usually about 12 cm long, 7 cm wide and 2.5 cm thick. It weighs about 200 g.

Organs associated with the spleen

Superiorly and
posteriorly —diaphragm
Inferiorly —left colic flexure of the large intestine
Anteriorly —fundus of the stomach
Medially —pancreas and the left kidney
Laterally —separated from the 9th, 10th and 11th ribs and the intercostal muscles by the diaphragm

133

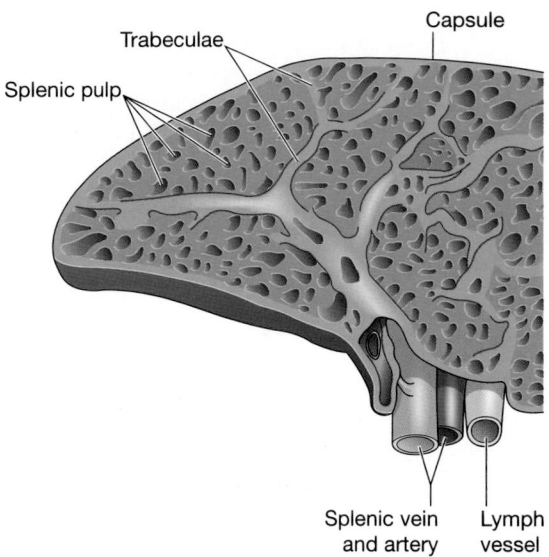

Labels: Trabeculae, Splenic pulp, Capsule, Splenic vein and artery, Lymph vessel

Figure 6.7 A section of the spleen.

Structure (Fig. 6.7)

The spleen is slightly oval in shape with the hilum on the lower medial border. The anterior surface is covered with peritoneum. It is enclosed in a fibroelastic capsule that dips into the organ, forming *trabeculae*. The cellular material, consisting of lymphocytes and macrophages, is called *splenic pulp*, and it lies between the trabeculae. *Red pulp* is the part suffused with blood and *white pulp* consists of areas of lymphatic tissue where there are sleeves of lymphocytes and macrophages around blood vessels.

The structures entering and leaving the spleen at the hilum are:

- splenic artery, a branch of the coeliac artery
- splenic vein, a branch of the portal vein
- lymph vessels (efferent only)
- nerves.

Blood passing through the spleen flows in sinuses which have distinct pores between the endothelial cells, allowing it to come into close association with splenic pulp.

Functions

Phagocytosis

As described previously (p. 64), old and abnormal erythrocytes are destroyed in the spleen and the breakdown products, bilirubin and iron, are passed to the liver via the splenic and portal veins. Other cellular material, e.g. leukocytes, platelets and microbes, are phagocytosed in the spleen. Unlike lymph nodes, the spleen has no afferent lymphatics entering it, so it is not exposed to diseases spread by lymph.

Storage of blood

The spleen contains up to 350 ml of blood, and in response to sympathetic stimulation can rapidly return a large part of this volume to the circulation, e.g. in haemorrhage.

Immune response

The spleen contains T- and B-lymphocytes, which are activated by the presence of antigens, e.g. in infection. Lymphocyte proliferation during serious infection can cause enlargement of the spleen (*splenomegaly*).

Erythropoiesis

The spleen and liver are important sites of fetal blood cell production, and the spleen can also fulfil this function in adults in times of great need.

Thymus gland

The thymus gland lies in the upper part of the mediastinum behind the sternum and extends upwards into the root of the neck (Fig. 6.8). It weighs about 10 to 15 g at birth and grows until the individual reaches puberty, when it begins to atrophy. Its maximum weight, at puberty, is between 30 and 40 g and by middle age it has returned to approximately its weight at birth.

Organs associated with the thymus

Anteriorly — sternum and upper four costal cartilages
Posteriorly — aortic arch and its branches, brachiocephalic veins, trachea
Laterally — lungs
Superiorly — structures in the root of the neck
Inferiorly — heart

Structure

The thymus consists of two lobes joined by areolar tissue. The lobes are enclosed by a fibrous capsule which dips into their substance, dividing them into lobules that consist of an irregular branching framework of epithelial cells and lymphocytes.

Function

Lymphocytes originate from pluripotent stem cells in red bone marrow. Those that enter the thymus develop into activated T-lymphocytes (p. 379).

Thymic processing produces mature T-lymphocytes that can distinguish 'self' tissue from foreign tissue, and also provides each T-lymphocyte with the ability to react to only one specific antigen from the millions it will

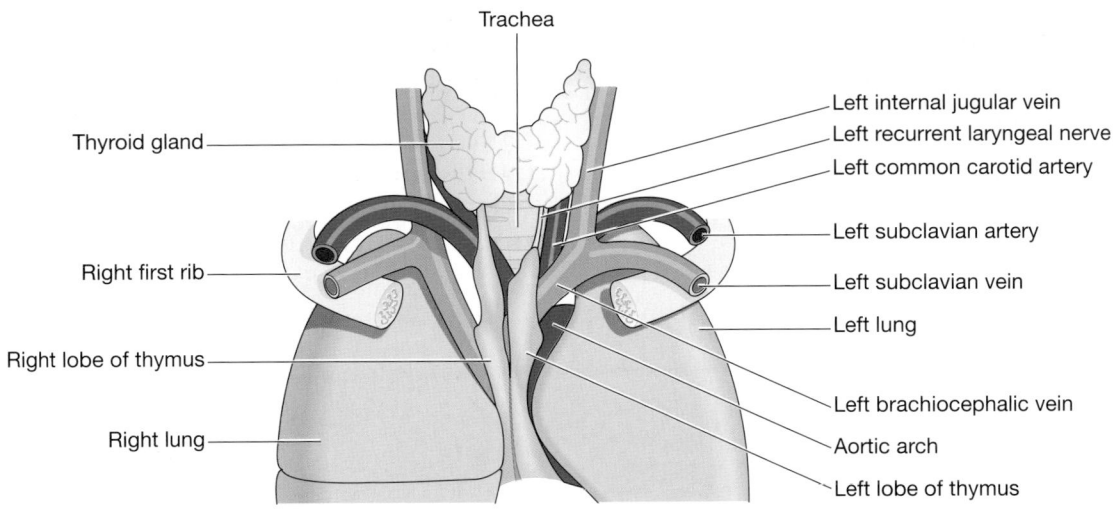

Figure 6.8 The thymus gland in the adult, and related structures.

encounter (p. 374). T-lymphocytes then leave the thymus and enter the blood. Some enter lymphoid tissues and others circulate in the bloodstream. T-lymphocyte production, although most prolific in youth, continues probably throughout life from a resident population of thymic stem cells.

The maturation of the thymus and other lymphoid tissue is stimulated by *thymosin*, a hormone secreted by the epithelial cells that form the framework of the thymus gland. Involution of the gland begins in adolescence and, with increasing age, the effectiveness of the T-lymphocyte response to antigens declines.

Mucosa-associated lymphoid tissue (MALT)

Throughout the body, at strategically placed locations, are collections of lymphoid tissue which, unlike the spleen and thymus, are not enclosed in a capsule. They contain B- and T-lymphocytes, which have migrated from bone marrow and the thymus, and are important in the early detection of invaders. However, as they have no afferent lymphatic vessels, they do not filter lymph, and are therefore not exposed to diseases spread by lymph. MALT is found throughout the gastrointestinal tract, in the respiratory tract and in the genitourinary tract, all systems of the body exposed to the external environment.

The main groups of MALT are the tonsils and Peyer's patches.

Tonsils. These are located in the mouth and throat, and will therefore destroy swallowed and inhaled antigens (see also p. 243).

Peyer's patches. These large collections of lymphoid tissue are found in the small intestine, and intercept swallowed antigens.

PATHOLOGY ASSOCIATED WITH LYMPH VESSELS

Learning outcomes

After studying this section, you should be able to:

- explain the role of lymphatic vessels in the spread of infectious and malignant disease

- discuss the main causes and consequences of lymphatic obstruction.

The main involvements of lymph vessels are in relation to:

- the spread of disease in the body
- the effects of lymphatic obstruction.

Spread of disease

The materials most commonly spread via the lymph vessels from their original site to the circulating blood are fragments of tumours and infected material.

Fragments of tumours

Tumour cells may enter a lymph capillary draining a tumour, or a larger vessel when a tumour has eroded its wall. Cells from a malignant tumour, if not phagocytosed, settle and multiply in the first lymph node they encounter. Later, there may be further spread to other lymph nodes, to the blood and to other parts of the body via the blood. In this sequence of events, each new metastatic tumour becomes a source of malignant cells that may spread by the same routes.

Infected material

Infected material may enter lymph vessels either at their origin in the interstitial spaces, or through the walls of larger vessels invaded by microbes when infection spreads locally. If phagocytosis is not effective the infection may spread from node to node, and eventually reach the bloodstream.

Lymphangitis (infection of lymph vessel walls). This occurs in some acute pyogenic infections in which the microbes in the lymph draining from the area infect and spread along the walls of lymph vessels, e.g. in acute *Streptococcus pyogenes* infection of the hand, a red line may be seen extending from the hand to the axilla. This is caused by an inflamed superficial lymph vessel and

adjacent tissues. The infection may be stopped at the first lymph node or spread through the lymph drainage network to the blood.

Lymphatic obstruction

When a lymph vessel is obstructed there is an accumulation of lymph distal to the obstruction, called *lymphoedema*. The amount of resultant swelling and the size of the area affected depend on the size of the vessel involved. Lymphoedema usually leads to low-grade inflammation and fibrosis of the lymph vessel and further lymphoedema. The most common causes are tumours and surgery.

Tumours

A tumour may grow into, and block, a lymph vessel or node, obstructing the flow of lymph. A large tumour outside the lymphatic system may cause sufficient pressure to stop the flow of lymph.

Surgery

In some surgical procedures lymph nodes are removed because cancer cells may have already spread to them. This is done to prevent growth of secondary tumours in local lymph nodes and further spread of the disease via the lymphatic system, e.g. axillary nodes may be removed during mastectomy.

DISEASES OF LYMPH NODES

Learning outcomes

After studying this section, you should be able to:

- describe the term lymphadenitis, listing its primary causes

- describe the effects of the two main forms of lymphoma on the body

- explain why secondary disease of the lymph nodes in commonly found in individuals with cancer.

Lymphadenitis

Acute lymphadenitis (acute infection of lymph nodes) is usually caused by microbes transported in lymph from other areas of infection. The nodes become inflamed, enlarged and congested with blood, and chemotaxis attracts large numbers of phagocytes. If lymph node defences (phagocytes and antibody production) are overwhelmed, the infection may cause abscess formation within the node. Adjacent tissues may become involved, and infected materials may be transported through other nodes and into the blood.

Acute lymphadenitis is secondary to a number of conditions.

Infectious mononucleosis (glandular fever)

This is a highly contagious viral infection, usually of young adults, spread by direct contact. During the incubation period of 7 to 10 days, viruses multiply in the epithelial cells of the pharynx. They subsequently spread to cervical nodes, then to lymphoid tissue throughout the body.

Clinical features include tonsillitis, lymphadenopathy and splenomegaly. A common complication is myalgic encephalitis (chronic fatigue syndrome, p. 184). Clinical or subclinical infection confers life-long immunity.

Other diseases

Minor lymphadenitis accompanies many infections and indicates the mobilisation of normal protective resources. More serious infection occurs in:

- measles
- anthrax
- typhoid fever
- wound and skin infections
- cat-scratch fever.

Chronic lymphadenitis occurs following unresolved acute infections, in tuberculosis, syphilis and some low-grade infections.

Lymphomas

These are malignant tumours of lymphoid tissue and are classified as either Hodgkin's or non-Hodgkin lymphomas.

Hodgkin's disease

In this disease there is progressive, painless enlargement of lymph nodes throughout the body, as lymphoid tissue within them proliferates. The superficial lymph nodes in the neck are often the first to be noticed. The disease is malignant and the cause is unknown. The rate of progress varies considerably but the pattern of spread is predictable because the disease spreads to adjacent nodes and to other tissues in a consistent way. The effectiveness of treatment depends largely on the stage of the disease at which it begins. The disease leads to reduced immunity, because lymphocyte function is depressed, and

recurrent infection is therefore common. As lymph nodes enlarge, they may compress adjacent tissues and organs. Anaemia and changes in leukocyte numbers occur if the bone marrow is involved.

Non-Hodgkin lymphomas

These tumours, e.g. *multiple myeloma* and *Burkitt's lymphoma*, may occur in any lymphoid tissue and in bone marrow. They are classified according to the type of cell involved and the degree of malignancy, i.e. low, intermediate or high grade. Low-grade tumours consist of well-differentiated cells and slow progress of the disease, death occurring after a period of years. High-grade lymphomas consist of poorly differentiated cells and rapid progress of the disease, death occurring in weeks or months. Some low- or intermediate-grade tumours change their status to high grade with increased rate of progress.

The expanding lymph nodes may compress adjacent tissues and organs. Immunological deficiency leads to increased incidence of infections, and if the bone marrow and/or spleen is involved there may be varying degrees of anaemia and leukopenia.

Malignant neoplastic metastases

Metastatic tumours develop in lymph nodes in any part of the body. Lymph from a tumour may contain cancer cells that are filtered off by the lymph nodes. If not phagocytosed they multiply, forming metastatic tumours. Nodes nearest the primary tumour are affected first but there may be further spread through the sequence of nodes, eventually reaching the bloodstream.

DISORDERS OF THE SPLEEN

Learning outcome

After studying this section, you should be able to:

- identify the main causes of splenomegaly.

Splenomegaly (enlargement of the spleen)

Enlargement of the spleen is usually secondary to other conditions, e.g. infections, circulatory disorders, blood diseases, malignant neoplasms.

Infections

The spleen may be infected by blood-borne microbes or by local spread of infection. The red pulp becomes congested with blood and there is an accumulation of phagocytes and plasma cells. Acute infections are rare.

Chronic infections. Some chronic non-pyogenic infections cause splenomegaly, but this is usually less severe than in the case of acute infections. The most commonly occurring primary infections include:

- tuberculosis
- typhoid fever
- malaria
- brucellosis (undulant fever)
- infectious mononucleosis.

Circulatory disorders

Splenomegaly due to congestion of blood occurs when the flow of blood through the liver is impeded by, e.g., fibrosis in cirrhosis of liver, portal venous congestion in right-sided heart failure.

Blood diseases

Splenomegaly may be caused by blood diseases. The spleen enlarges to deal with the extra workload associated with removing damaged, worn out and abnormal blood cells in, e.g., haemolytic and macrocytic anaemia, polycythaemia and chronic myeloid leukaemia.

Splenomegaly may cause blood disease. When the spleen is enlarged for any reason, especially in portal hypertension, excessive and premature haemolysis of red cells or phagocytosis of normal white cells and platelets leads to marked anaemia, leukopenia and thrombocytopenia.

Tumours

Benign and primary malignant tumours of the spleen are rare but blood-spread tumour fragments from elsewhere in the body may cause metastatic tumours. Splenomegaly caused by infiltration of malignant cells is characteristic of some conditions, especially chronic leukaemia, Hodgkin's disease and non-Hodgkin lymphoma.

DISEASES OF THE THYMUS GLAND

Learning outcome

After studying this section, you should be able to:

- describe the principal disorders of the thymus gland.

Enlargement of the gland is associated with some autoimmune diseases, such as thyrotoxicosis and Addison's disease. Autoimmune conditions are those in which the immune system treats normal body cells or secretions as antigens and destroys them (p. 385).

Tumours are rare and seldom metastasise. Pressure caused by enlargement of the gland may damage or interfere with the functions of adjacent structures, e.g. the trachea, oesophagus or veins in the neck.

In myasthenia gravis, an autoimmune disease in which there is skeletal muscle weakness (p. 385), most patients have either thymic hyperplasia (majority) or thymoma (minority).

7

The nervous system

The nervous system detects and responds to changes inside and outside the body. Together with the endocrine system it controls important aspects of body function and maintains homeostasis. Nervous system stimulation provides an immediate response while endocrine activity is, in the main, slower and more prolonged (Ch. 8).

The nervous system consists of the brain, the spinal cord and peripheral nerves. Organisation of nervous tissue within the body enables rapid communication between different parts of the body.

Response to changes in the internal environment maintains homeostasis and regulates involuntary functions, e.g. blood pressure and digestive activity. Response to changes in the external environment maintains posture and other voluntary activities.

For descriptive purposes the parts of the nervous system are grouped as follows:

- *the central nervous system* (CNS), consisting of the brain and the spinal cord

- *the peripheral nervous system* (PNS) consisting of all the nerves outside the brain and spinal cord.

The PNS comprises paired cranial and sacral nerves— some of these are sensory (afferent), some are motor (efferent) and some mixed. It is useful to consider two functional parts within the PNS:

- the sensory division
- the motor division (Fig. 7.1).

In turn the motor division is involved in activities that are:

- *voluntary*—the somatic nervous system (movement of voluntary muscles)
- *involuntary*—the autonomic nervous system (functioning of smooth and cardiac muscle and glands). The autonomic nervous system has two parts: *sympathetic* and *parasympathetic*.

Figure 7.1 Functional components of the nervous system.

NEURONES

Learning outcomes

After studying this section you should be able to:

■ describe the structure of a myelinated neurone

■ compare and contrast the transmission of impulses in myelinated and unmyelinated neurones

■ state the functions of sensory and motor nerves

■ describe the events that occur following release of a neurotransmitter at a synapse

■ identify the common neurotransmitters in the peripheral nervous system.

The nervous system consists of a vast number of cells called *neurones* (Fig. 7.2), supported by a special type of connective tissue, *neuroglia*. Each neurone consists of a *cell body* and its processes, one *axon* and many *dendrites*. Neurones are commonly referred to simply as nerve cells. Bundles of axons bound together are called *nerves*. Neurones cannot divide and for survival they need a continuous supply of oxygen and glucose. Unlike many other cells, neurones can synthesise chemical energy (ATP) only from glucose. The effects of damage to neurones are described on page 175.

The physiological 'units' of the nervous system are *nerve impulses*, or *action potentials*, which are akin to tiny electrical charges. However, unlike ordinary electrical wires, the neurones are actively involved in conducting nerve impulses. In effect the strength of the impulse is maintained throughout the length of the neurone.

Some neurones initiate nerve impulses while others act as 'relay stations' where impulses are passed on and sometimes redirected.

Properties of neurones

Neurones have the characteristics of *irritability* and *conductivity*.

Irritability is the ability to initiate nerve impulses in response to stimuli from:

■ outside the body, e.g. touch, light waves
■ inside the body, e.g. a change in the concentration of carbon dioxide in the blood alters respiration; a thought may result in voluntary movement.

In the body this stimulation may be described as partly electrical and partly chemical—electrical in that motor

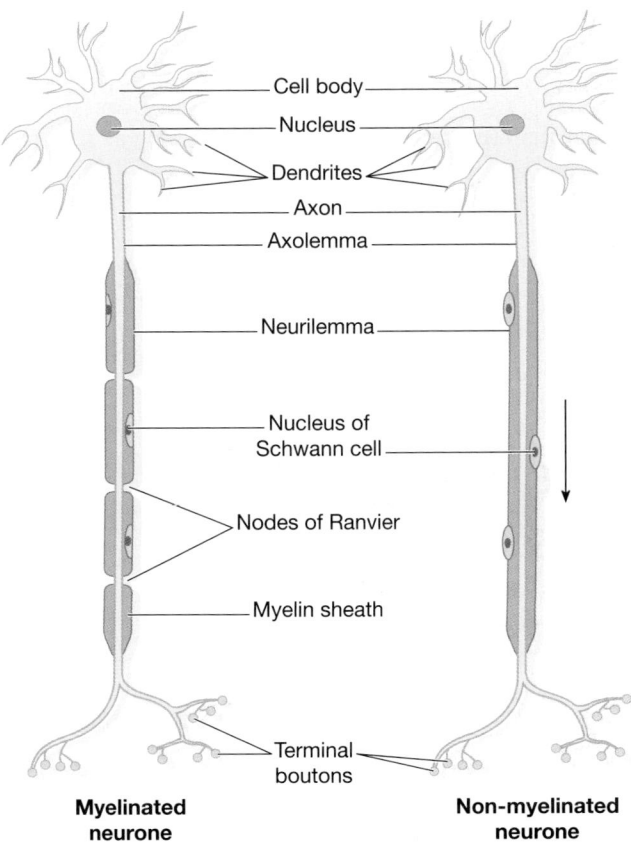

Figure 7.2 The structure of neurones. (Arrow indicates direction of impulse conduction.)

141

neurones and sensory nerve endings initiate nerve impulses, and chemical in the transmission of impulses between one neurone and the next or between a neurone and an effector organ.

Conductivity means the ability to transmit an impulse.

Cell bodies

Nerve cells vary considerably in size and shape but they are all too small to be seen by the naked eye. Cell bodies form the *grey matter* of the nervous system and are found at the periphery of the brain and in the centre of the spinal cord. Groups of cell bodies are called *nuclei* in the central nervous system and *ganglia* in the peripheral nervous system.

Axons and dendrites

Axons and dendrites are extensions of cell bodies and form the *white matter* of the nervous system. Axons are found deep in the brain and in groups, called *tracts*, at the periphery of the spinal cord. They are referred to as *nerves* or *nerve fibres* outside the brain and spinal cord.

Axons

Each nerve cell has only one axon, carrying nerve impulses away from the cell body. They are usually longer than the dendrites, sometimes as long as 100 cm.

Structure of an axon

The membrane of the axon is called *axolemma* and it encloses the cytoplasmic extension of the cell body.

Large axons and those of peripheral nerves are surrounded by a *myelin sheath* (Fig. 7.3A). This consists of a series of *Schwann cells* arranged along the length of the axon. Each one is wrapped around the axon so that it is covered by a number of concentric layers of Schwann cell plasma membrane. Between the layers of plasma membrane there is a small amount of fatty substance called *myelin*. The outermost layer of Schwann cell plasma membrane is sometimes called *neurilemma*. There are tiny areas of exposed axolemma between adjacent Schwann cells, called *nodes of Ranvier*, which assist the rapid transmission of nerve impulses.

Postganglionic fibres and some small fibres in the central nervous system are *non-myelinated*. In this type a number of axons are embedded in Schwann cell plasma membranes (Fig. 7.3B). The adjacent Schwann cells are in close association and there is no exposed axolemma. The speed of transmission of nerve impulses is significantly slower in non-myelinated fibres.

Dendrites

The dendrites are the many short processes that receive and carry incoming impulses towards cell bodies. They have the same structure as axons but they are usually shorter and branching. In motor neurones they form part of synapses (Fig. 7.8A) and in sensory neurones they form the sensory receptors that respond to stimuli.

The nerve impulse (action potential)

An impulse is initiated by stimulation of sensory nerve endings or by the passage of an impulse from another nerve. Transmission of the impulse, or action potential, is due to movement of ions across the nerve cell membrane. In the resting state the nerve cell membrane is *polarised* due to differences in the concentrations of ions across the plasma membrane. This means that there is a different electrical charge on each side of the membrane that is called the *resting membrane potential*. At rest the charge on the outside is positive and inside it is negative. The principal ions involved are:

- sodium (Na^+) the main extracellular cation
- potassium (K^+) the main intracellular cation.

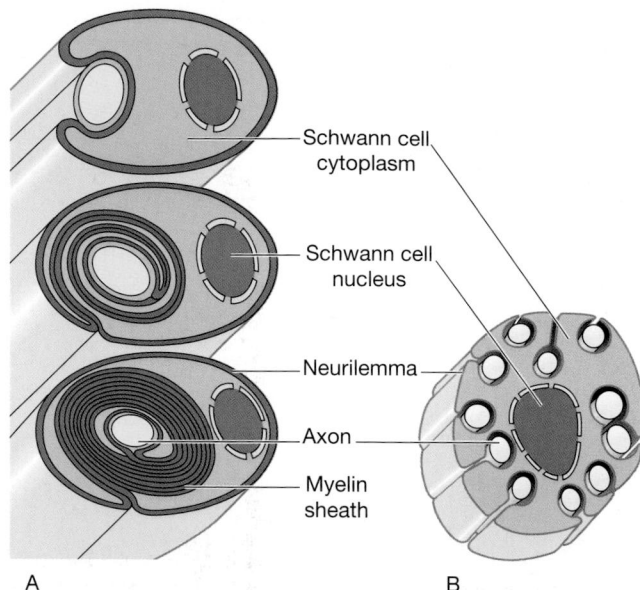

Figure 7.3 Nerve fibres: A. Myelinated. B. Non-myelinated.

Labels: Schwann cell cytoplasm; Schwann cell nucleus; Neurilemma; Axon; Myelin sheath

In the *resting state* there is a continual tendency for these ions to diffuse along their concentration gradients, i.e. K^+ outwards and Na^+ into cells. When stimulated, the permeability of the nerve cell membrane to these ions changes. Initially Na^+ floods into the neurone from the ECF causing *depolarisation*, creating a *nerve impulse* or *action potential*. Depolarisation is very rapid, enabling the conduction of a nerve impulse along the entire length of a neurone in a few milliseconds (ms). It passes from the point of stimulation in one direction only, i.e. away from the point of stimulation towards the area of resting potential. The one-way direction of transmission is ensured because following depolarisation it takes time for *repolarisation* to occur.

During this process K^+ floods out of the neurone and the movement of these ions returns the membrane potential to its resting state. This is called the *refractory period* during which restimulation is not possible. As the neurone returns to its original resting state, the action of the *sodium pump* expels Na^+ from the cell in exchange for K^+ (p. 34).

In myelinated neurones, the insulating properties of the myelin sheath prevent the movement of ions. Therefore electrical changes across the membrane can only occur at the gaps in the myelin sheath, i.e. at the nodes of Ranvier. When an impulse occurs at one node, depolarisation passes along the myelin sheath to the next node so that the flow of current appears to 'leap' from one node to the next. This is called *saltatory conduction* (Fig. 7.4).

The speed of conduction depends on the diameter of the neurone: the larger the diameter, the faster the conduction. Myelinated fibres conduct impulses faster

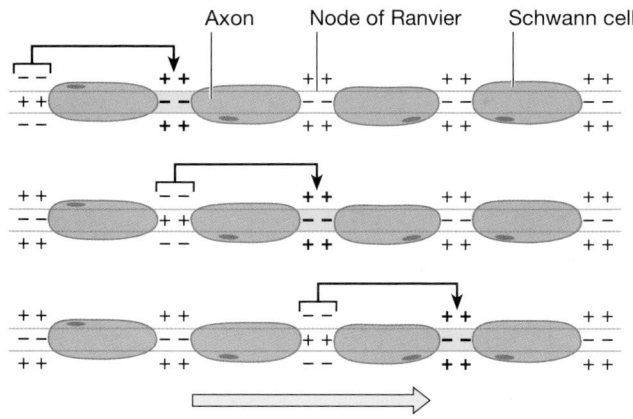

Axon   Node of Ranvier   Schwann cell

Direction of transmission of nerve impulse

Figure 7.4 Saltatory conduction of an impulse in a myelinated nerve fibre.

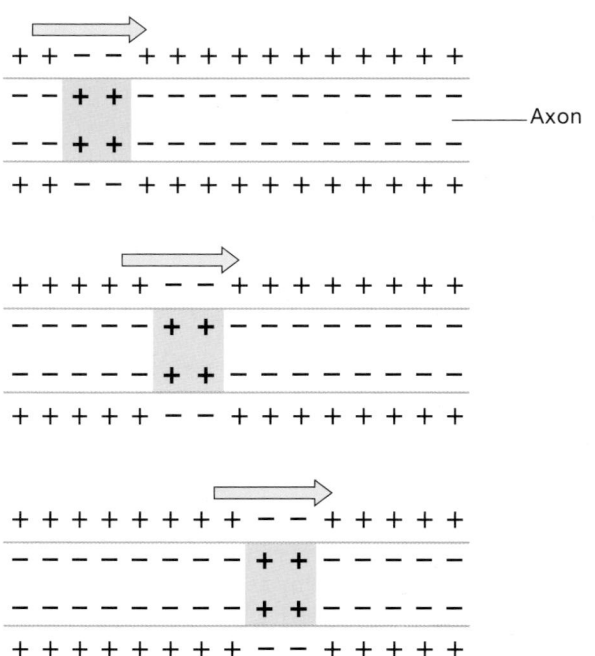

Axon

Figure 7.5 Simple propagation of an impulse in a non-myelinated nerve fibre. (Arrows indicate the direction of impulse transmission.)

than unmyelinated fibres because saltatory conduction is faster than the complete conduction, or *simple propagation* (Fig. 7.5). The fastest fibres can conduct impulses to, e.g., skeletal muscles at a rate of 130 metres per second while the slowest impulses travel at 0.5 metres per second.

Types of nerves (Fig. 7.6)

Sensory or afferent nerves

When action potentials are generated by sensory receptors on the dendrites of these neurones, they are transmitted to the spinal cord by the sensory nerve fibres. The impulses may then pass to the brain or to connector neurones of reflex arcs in the spinal cord (p. 159).

Sensory receptors

Specialised endings of sensory neurones respond to different stimuli (changes) inside and outside the body.

Somatic, cutaneous or *common senses*. These originate in the skin. They are: pain, touch, heat and cold. Sensory nerve endings in the skin are fine branching filaments without myelin sheaths (Fig. 7.7). When stimulated, an impulse is generated and transmitted by the sensory nerves to the brain where the sensation is perceived.

Proprioceptor senses. These originate in muscles and joints and contribute to the maintenance of balance and posture.

Special senses. These are sight, hearing, smell, touch and taste (Ch. 8).

Autonomic afferent nerves. These originate in internal organs, glands and tissues, e.g. baroreceptors, chemoreceptors, and are associated with reflex regulation of involuntary activity and visceral pain.

Motor or efferent nerves

Motor nerves originate in the brain, spinal cord and autonomic ganglia. They transmit impulses to the effector organs: muscles and glands. There are two types:

- *somatic nerves* — involved in voluntary and reflex skeletal muscle contraction
- *autonomic nerves* (sympathetic and parasympathetic) — involved in cardiac and smooth muscle contraction and glandular secretion.

Mixed nerves

In the spinal cord, sensory and motor nerves are arranged in separate groups, or *tracts*. Outside the spinal cord, when sensory and motor nerves are enclosed within the same sheath of connective tissue they are called *mixed nerves*.

The synapse and neurotransmitters

There is always more than one neurone involved in the transmission of a nerve impulse from its origin to its destination, whether it is sensory or motor. There is no physical contact between these neurones. The point at which the nerve impulse passes from one to another is the *synapse* (Fig. 7.8). At its free end the axon of the

143

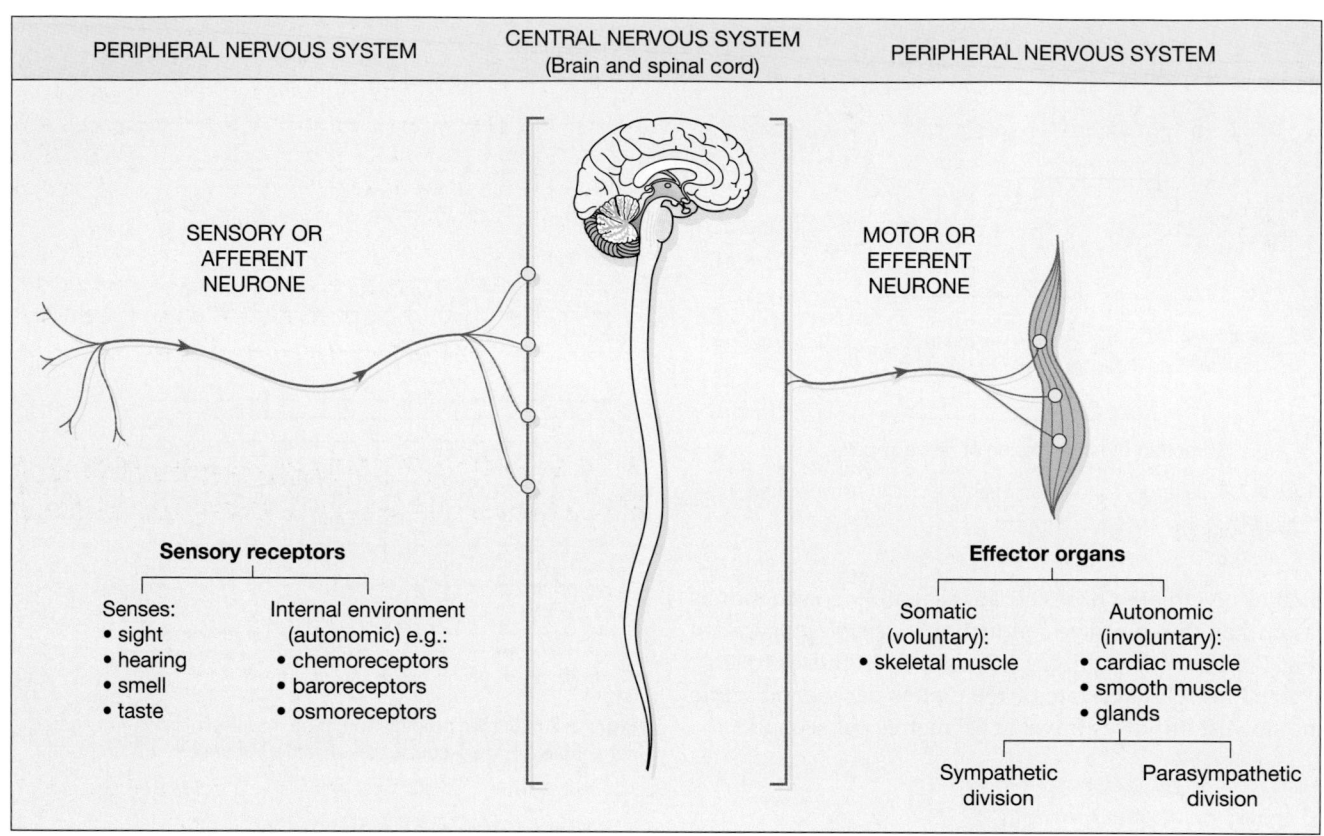

Figure 7.6 Functional components of the nervous system.

presynaptic neurone breaks up into minute branches which terminate in small swellings called *synaptic knobs*, or terminal boutons. These are in close proximity to the dendrites and the cell body of the *postsynaptic neurone*. The space between them is the *synaptic cleft*. In the ends of synaptic knobs there are spherical *synaptic vesicles*, containing a chemical, the *neurotransmitter*, which is released into synaptic clefts. Neurotransmitters are synthesised by nerve cells, actively transported along the axons and stored in the synaptic vesicles. They are released by exocytosis in response to the action potential and diffuse across the synaptic cleft. They act on specific receptor sites on the postsynaptic membranes. Their action is short lived as immediately they have stimulated the postsynaptic neurone or effector organ, such as a muscle fibre, they are either inactivated by enzymes or taken back into the synaptic knob. A knowledge of the action of different neurotransmitters is important because some drugs neutralise or prolong their effect. Usually neurotransmitters have an excitatory effect at the synapse but they are sometimes inhibitory.

The neurotransmitters in the brain and spinal cord and their modes of action are not yet fully understood. It is believed however that *noradrenaline, gamma amino-*

Figure 7.7 Sensory nerve endings in the skin.

butyric acid (GABA) and *acetylcholine* act as neurotransmitters. Other substances, such as dopamine, serotonin (5-hydroxytryptamine), enkephalins, endorphins and substance P, have similar functions. Figure 7.9 summarises the neurotransmitters known to function in the peripheral nervous system. Somatic nerves carry impulses directly

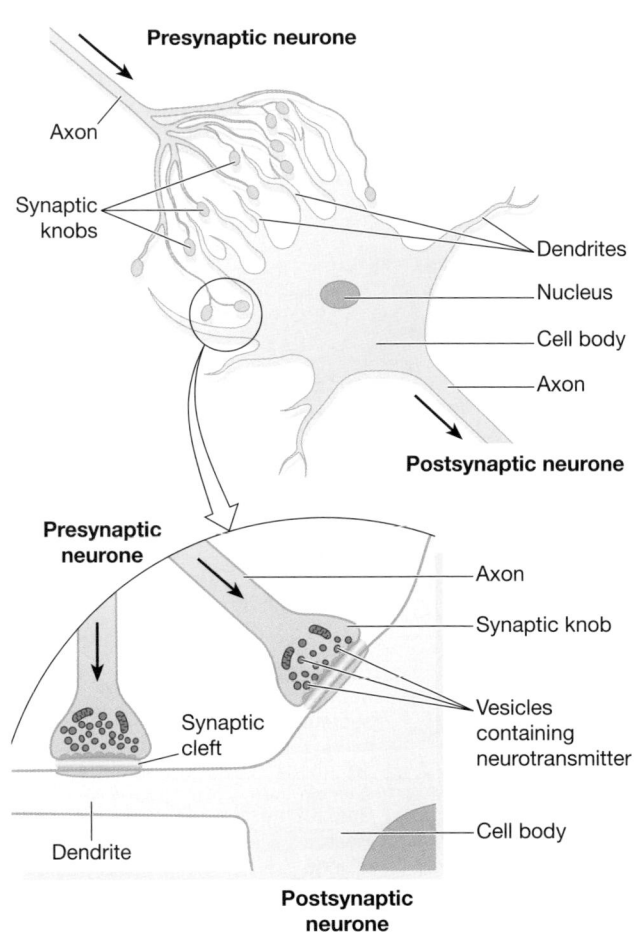

Presynaptic neurone

Axon

Synaptic knobs

Dendrites

Nucleus

Cell body

Axon

Postsynaptic neurone

Presynaptic neurone

Axon

Synaptic knob

Vesicles containing neurotransmitter

Synaptic cleft

Dendrite

Cell body

Postsynaptic neurone

Figure 7.8 Diagram of a synapse.

to the synapses at skeletal muscles: the neuromuscular junctions. In autonomic nerves, impulses travel along two nerves (preganglionic and postganglionic) and across two synapses to the effector organs in both the sympathetic and the parasympathetic divisions.

The neuromuscular junction

The axons of *motor neurones*, conveying impulses to skeletal muscle to produce contraction, divide into fine filaments terminating in minute pads called *motor end-plates* (Fig. 7.10). At the point where the nerve reaches the muscle, the myelin sheath is absent and the fine filament passes to a sensitive area on the surface of the muscle fibre. Each muscle fibre is stimulated through a single motor end-plate, and one motor nerve has many motor end-plates. The motor end-plate and the sensitive area of muscle fibre through which it is stimulated is analogous to the synapse between neurones and is known as the neuromuscular junction. The nerve impulse is passed across the gap between the motor end-plate and the

muscle fibre by the neurotransmitter, *acetylcholine*. The group of muscle fibres and the motor end-plates of the nerve fibre that supplies them constitute a *motor unit*. Nerve impulses cause serial contraction of motor units in a muscle and each unit contracts to its full capacity. The *strength* of the contraction depends on the *number* of motor units in action at a particular time.

The endings of *autonomic nerves* supplying smooth muscle and glands branch near their effector structure and release a neurotransmitter which stimulates or depresses the activity of the structure (Figs 7.9, 7.43 and 7.44).

CENTRAL NERVOUS SYSTEM

Learning outcomes

After studying this section you should be able to:

■ outline the functions of 4 types of neuroglial cells

■ describe the structure of the meninges

■ describe the flow of cerebrospinal fluid in the brain

■ list the functions of cerebrospinal fluid.

The central nervous system consists of the brain and the spinal cord.

Neuroglia

The neurones of the central nervous system are supported by four types of non-excitable *glial cells* that make up a quarter to a half of the volume of brain tissue. Unlike nerve cells these continue to replicate throughout life. They are *astrocytes, oligodendrocytes, microglia* and *ependymal cells*.

Astrocytes

These cells form the main supporting tissue of the central nervous system. They are star-shaped with fine branching processes and they lie in a mucopolysaccharide ground substance. At the free ends of some of the processes there are small swellings called *foot processes*. Astrocytes are found in large numbers adjacent to blood vessels with their foot processes forming a sleeve round them. This means that the blood is separated from the neurones by the capillary wall and a layer of astrocyte foot processes which together constitute the *blood–brain*

Type of nerve	Neurotransmitter at synapse in ganglion		Neurotransmitter at effector organ
Somatic Motor			Skeletal muscle — Acetylcholine
Autonomic Sympathetic (adrenergic)	Acetylcholine		Smooth muscle, Heart, Glands — Noradrenaline
Sympathetic (cholinergic)	Acetylcholine		Sweat glands, Blood vessels in skeletal muscles and skin — Acetylcholine
Sympathetic (splanchnic)	Acetylcholine	Adrenal medulla	Adrenaline and noradrenaline secreted into blood
Parasympathetic	Acetylcholine		Smooth muscle, Heart, Glands — Acetylcholine

Figure 7.9 Neurotransmitters at synapses in the peripheral nervous system.

barrier (Fig. 7.11). Their functions are analogous to those of fibroblasts elsewhere in the body.

The blood–brain barrier is a selective barrier that protects the brain from potentially toxic substances and chemical variations in the blood, e.g. after a meal. Oxygen, carbon dioxide, alcohol, barbiturates, glucose and lipophilic substances quickly cross the barrier into the brain. Some large molecules, drugs, inorganic ions and amino acids pass slowly from the blood to the brain.

Oligodendrocytes

These cells are smaller than astrocytes and are found:

- in clusters round nerve cell bodies, the grey matter where they are thought to have a supportive function
- adjacent to, and along the length of, myelinated nerve fibres.

The oligodendrocytes form and maintain myelin, having the same functions as Schwann cells in peripheral nerves.

Microglia

These cells are derived from monocytes that migrate from the blood into the nervous system before birth. They are found mainly in the area of blood vessels. They enlarge and become phagocytic in areas of inflammation and cell destruction.

Ependymal cells

These cells form the epithelial lining of the ventricles of the brain and the central canal of the spinal cord.

Membranes covering the brain and spinal cord (the meninges)

The brain and spinal cord are completely surrounded by three membranes, the *meninges*, lying between the skull and the brain and between the vertebrae and the spinal cord (Fig. 7.12). Named from outside inwards they are:

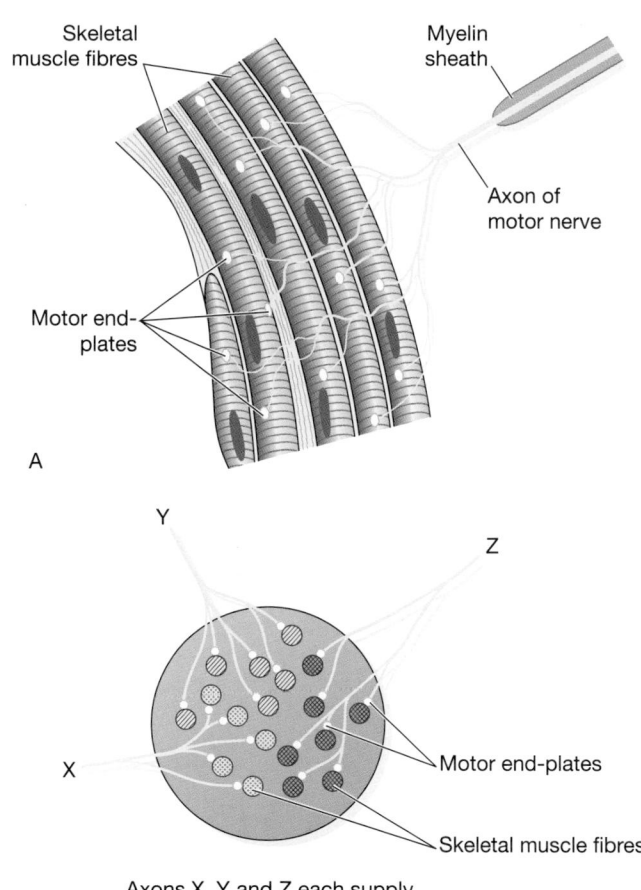

A

B

Axons X, Y and Z each supply
different bundles of muscle fibres

Figure 7.10 Motor unit: A. Longitudinal section. B. Cross-section.

Figure 7.11 Blood–brain barrier.

- dura mater
- arachnoid mater
- pia mater.

The dura and arachnoid maters are separated by a potential space, the *subdural space*. The arachnoid and pia maters are separated by the *subarachnoid space*, containing *cerebrospinal fluid*.

Dura mater

The cerebral dura mater consists of two layers of dense fibrous tissue. The outer layer takes the place of the periosteum on the inner surface of the skull bones and the inner layer provides a protective covering for the brain. There is only a potential space between the two layers except where the inner layer sweeps inwards between the cerebral hemispheres to form the *falx cerebri*; between the cerebellar hemispheres to form the *falx cerebelli*; and between the cerebrum and cerebellum to form the *tentorium cerebelli* (Fig. 7.12).

Venous blood from the brain drains into venous sinuses between the layers of dura mater. The *superior*

Figure 7.12 The meninges covering the brain and spinal cord.

sagittal sinus is formed by the falx cerebri, and the tentorium cerebelli forms the *straight* and *transverse sinuses* (see Figs 5.37 and 5.38, p. 101).

147

Spinal dura mater forms a loose sheath round the spinal cord, extending from the foramen magnum to the second sacral vertebra. Thereafter it encloses the *filum terminale* and fuses with the periosteum of the coccyx. It is an extension of the inner layer of cerebral dura mater and is separated from the periosteum of the vertebrae and ligaments within the neural canal by the *epidural* or *extradural* space, containing blood vessels and areolar tissue. It is attached to the foramen magnum and, by a number of fibrous slips, to the posterior longitudinal ligament at intervals along its length. Nerves entering and leaving the spinal cord pass through the epidural space. These attachments stabilise the spinal cord in the neural canal. Dyes, used for diagnostic purposes, and local anaesthetics or analgesics to relieve pain, may be injected into the epidural space.

Arachnoid mater

This delicate serous membrane lies between the dura and pia maters. It is separated from the dura mater by the *subdural space*, and from the pia mater by the *subarachnoid space*, containing *cerebrospinal fluid*. The arachnoid mater passes over the convolutions of the brain and accompanies the inner layer of dura mater in the formation of the falx cerebri, tentorium cerebelli and falx cerebelli. It continues downwards to envelop the spinal cord and ends by merging with the dura mater at the level of the 2nd sacral vertebra.

Pia mater

This is a fine connective tissue containing many minute blood vessels. It adheres to the brain, completely covering the convolutions and dipping into each fissure. It continues downwards surrounding the spinal cord. Beyond the end of the cord it continues as the *filum terminale*, pierces the arachnoid tube and goes on, with the dura mater, to fuse with the periosteum of the coccyx.

Ventricles of the brain and the cerebrospinal fluid

Within the brain there are four irregular-shaped cavities, or *ventricles*, containing *cerebrospinal fluid* (CSF) (Fig. 7.13). They are:

- right and left lateral ventricles
- third ventricle
- fourth ventricle.

The lateral ventricles

These cavities lie within the cerebral hemispheres, one on each side of the median plane just below the *corpus callosum*. They are separated from each other by a thin

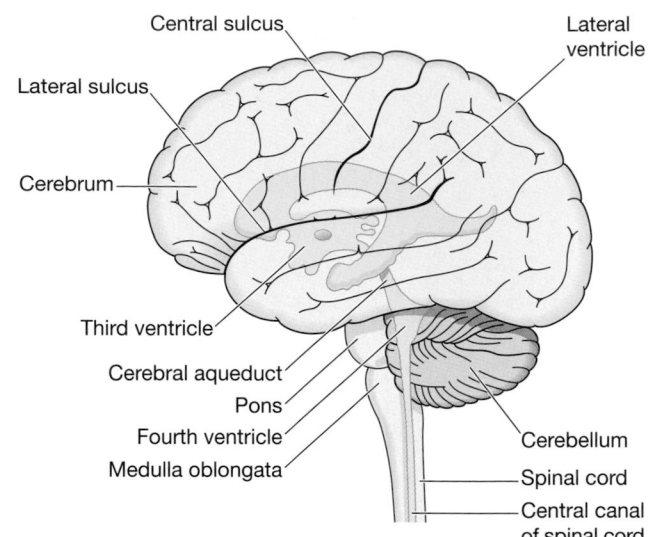

Figure 7.13 The positions of the ventricles of the brain (in yellow) superimposed on its surface. Viewed from the left side.

membrane, the *septum lucidum*, and are lined with ciliated epithelium. They communicate with the third ventricle by *interventricular foramina*.

The third ventricle

The third ventricle is a cavity situated below the lateral ventricles between the two parts of the *thalamus*. It communicates with the fourth ventricle by a canal, the *cerebral aqueduct* or *aqueduct of the midbrain*.

The fourth ventricle

The fourth ventricle is a diamond-shaped cavity situated below and behind the third ventricle, between the *cerebellum* and *pons*. It is continuous below with the *central canal* of the spinal cord and communicates with the subarachnoid space by foramina in its roof. Cerebrospinal fluid enters the subarachnoid space through these openings and through the open distal end of the central canal of the spinal cord.

Cerebrospinal fluid (CSF) (Fig. 7.14)

Cerebrospinal fluid is secreted into each ventricle of the brain by *choroid plexuses*. These are vascular areas where there is a proliferation of blood vessels surrounded by ependymal cells in the lining of ventricle walls. CSF passes back into the blood through tiny diverticula of arachnoid mater, called *arachnoid villi* (arachnoid granulations), that project into the venous sinuses. The movement of CSF from the subarachnoid space to venous sinuses depends upon the difference in pressure on each side of the walls of the arachnoid villi, which act as one-way valves. When

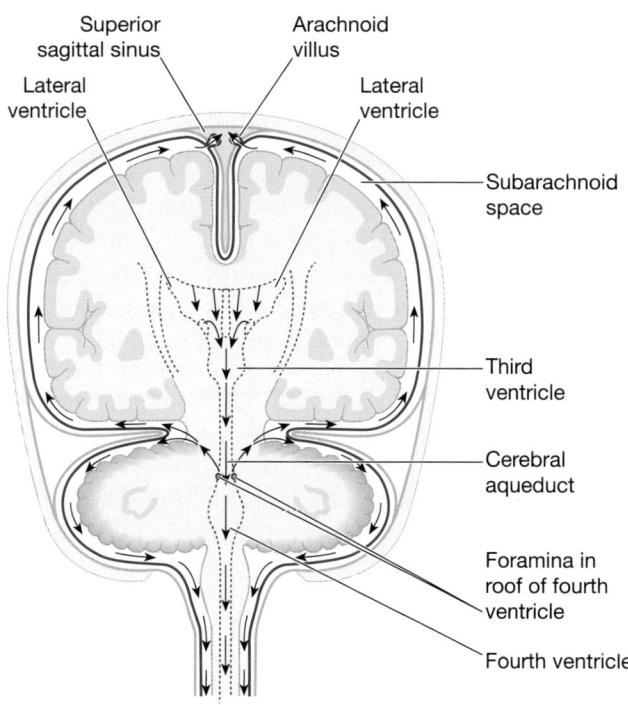

Figure 7.14 Arrows showing the flow of cerebrospinal fluid.

CSF pressure is higher than venous pressure CSF passes into the blood and when the venous pressure is higher the arachnoid villi collapse, preventing the passage of blood constituents into the CSF. There may also be some reabsorption of CSF by cells in the walls of the ventricles.

From the roof of the fourth ventricle CSF flows through foramina into the subarachnoid space and completely surrounds the brain and spinal cord. There is no intrinsic system of CSF circulation but its movement is aided by pulsating blood vessels, respiration and changes of posture.

CSF is secreted continuously at a rate of about 0.5 ml per minute, i.e. 720 ml per day. The amount around the brain and spinal cord remains fairly constant at about 120 ml, which means that absorption keeps pace with secretion. CSF pressure may be measured using a vertical tube attached to a lumbar puncture needle. It remains fairly constant at about 10 cmH$_2$O when the individual is lying on his side and about 30 cmH$_2$O when sitting up. If the brain is enlarged by, e.g. haemorrhage or tumour, some compensation is made by a reduction in the amount of CSF. When the volume of brain tissue is reduced, such as in degeneration or atrophy, the volume of CSF is increased. CSF is a clear, slightly alkaline fluid with a specific gravity of 1.005, consisting of:

- water
- mineral salts

- glucose
- plasma proteins: small amounts of albumin and globulin
- creatinine ⎫ small amounts
- urea ⎭
- a few leukocytes.

Functions of cerebrospinal fluid

- It supports and protects the brain and spinal cord.
- It maintains a uniform pressure around these delicate structures.
- It acts as a cushion and shock absorber between the brain and the cranial bones.
- It keeps the brain and spinal cord moist and there may be interchange of substances between CSF and nerve cells, such as nutrients and waste products.

BRAIN

Learning outcomes

After studying this section you should be able to:

- describe the blood supply to the brain
- name the lobes and sulci of the brain
- outline the functions of the cerebrum
- identify the main sensory and motor areas of the cerebrum
- describe the position and functions of the midbrain, pons, medulla oblongata and reticular activating system
- outline the position and functions of the basal nuclei, thalamus and hypothalamus
- describe the structure and functions of the cerebellum.

The brain constitutes about one-fiftieth of the body weight and lies within the cranial cavity. The parts are (Fig. 7.15):

- cerebrum
- midbrain ⎫
- pons ⎬ the brain stem
- medulla oblongata ⎭
- cerebellum.

149

Blood supply to the brain

The circulus arteriosus and its contributing arteries (see Fig. 5.34, p. 100) play a vital role in maintaining a constant supply of oxygen and glucose to the brain even when a contributing artery is narrowed or the head is moved. The brain receives about 15% of the cardiac output, approximately 750 ml of blood per minute. Autoregulation keeps blood flow to the brain constant by adjusting the diameter of the arterioles across a wide range of arterial blood pressure (about 65–140 mmHg) with changes occurring only outside these limits.

Cerebrum

This is the largest part of the brain and it occupies the anterior and middle cranial fossae (see Fig. 16.8, p. 393). It is divided by a deep cleft, the *longitudinal cerebral fissure*, into *right* and *left cerebral hemispheres*, each containing one of the lateral ventricles. Deep within the brain the hemispheres are connected by a mass of white matter (nerve fibres) called the *corpus callosum*. The falx cerebri is formed by the dura mater (Fig. 7.12). It separates the two hemispheres and penetrates to the depth of the corpus callosum. The superficial (peripheral) part of the cerebrum is composed of nerve cell bodies or grey matter, forming the *cerebral cortex*, and the deeper layers consist of nerve fibres or white matter.

The cerebral cortex shows many infoldings or furrows of varying depth. The exposed areas of the folds are the *gyri* or *convolutions* and these are separated by *sulci* or *fissures*. These convolutions greatly increase the surface area of the cerebrum.

For descriptive purposes each hemisphere of the cerebrum is divided into *lobes* which take the names of the bones of the cranium under which they lie:

- frontal
- parietal
- temporal
- occipital.

The boundaries of the lobes are marked by deep sulci (fissures). These are the *central, lateral* and *parieto-occipital sulci* (Fig. 7.16).

Interior of the cerebrum (Fig. 7.17)

The surface of the cerebral cortex is composed of grey matter (nerve cell bodies). Within the cerebrum the lobes are connected by masses of nerve fibres, or tracts, which make up the white matter of the brain. The afferent and

Figure 7.15 The parts of the central nervous system.

Figure 7.16 The lobes and sulci of the cerebrum.

Figure 7.17 labels: Longitudinal fissure between hemispheres · Cerebral cortex · Corpus callosum · Internal capsule · Thalamus · Basal nuclei · Hypothalamus

Figure 7.17 A section of the cerebrum showing some connecting nerve fibres.

Figure 7.18 labels: Premotor area · Motor area · Central sulcus · Sensory area · Sensory speech area · Frontal area · Motor speech area · Taste area · Auditory area · Visual area

Figure 7.18 The cerebrum showing the functional areas.

efferent fibres linking the different parts of the brain and spinal cord are as follows.

- *Association (arcuate) fibres* connect different parts of a cerebral hemisphere by extending from one gyrus to another, some of which are adjacent and some distant.
- *Commissural fibres* connect corresponding areas of the two cerebral hemispheres; the largest and most important commissure is the corpus callosum.
- *Projection fibres* connect the cerebral cortex with grey matter of lower parts of the brain and with the spinal cord, e.g. the internal capsule.

The *internal capsule* is an important area consisting of projection fibres. It lies deep within the brain between the basal nuclei (ganglia) and the thalamus. Many nerve impulses passing to and from the cerebral cortex are carried by fibres that form the internal capsule. Motor fibres within the internal capsule form the *pyramidal tracts* (corticospinal tracts) that cross over (decussate) at the medulla oblongata.

Functions of the cerebrum

There are three main varieties of activity associated with the cerebral cortex:

- mental activities involved in memory, intelligence, sense of responsibility, thinking, reasoning, moral sense and learning are attributed to the *higher centres*
- sensory perception, including the perception of pain, temperature, touch, sight, hearing, taste and smell
- initiation and control of skeletal (voluntary) muscle contraction.

Functional areas of the cerebrum (Fig. 7.18)

The main areas of the cerebrum associated with sensory perception and voluntary motor activity are known but it is unlikely that any area is associated exclusively with only one function. Except where specially mentioned, the different areas are active in both hemispheres.

Motor areas of the cerebrum

The precentral (motor) area. This lies in the frontal lobe immediately anterior to the *central sulcus*. The cell bodies are pyramid shaped (Betz's cells) and they initiate the contraction of skeletal muscles. A nerve fibre from a Betz's cell passes downwards through the internal capsule to the medulla oblongata where it crosses to the opposite side then descends in the spinal cord. At the appropriate level in the spinal cord the nerve impulse crosses a synapse to stimulate a second neurone which terminates at the motor end-plate of a muscle fibre. This means that the motor area of the *right hemisphere* of the cerebrum controls voluntary muscle movement on the left side of the body and vice versa. The neurone with its cell body in the cerebrum is the *upper motor neurone* and the other, with its cell body in the spinal cord, is the *lower motor neurone* (Fig. 7.19). Damage to either of these neurones may result in paralysis.

In the motor area of the cerebrum the body is represented upside down, i.e. the cells nearest the vertex control the feet and those in the lowest part control the head, neck, face and fingers (Fig. 7.20A). The sizes of the areas of cortex representing different parts of the body are proportional to the *complexity of movement* of the body part, not to its size. Figure 7.20A shows that, in comparison with the trunk, the hand, foot, tongue and lips are represented by large cortical areas.

151

The premotor area. This lies in the frontal lobe immediately anterior to the motor area. The cells are thought to exert a controlling influence over the motor area, ensuring an orderly series of movements. For example, in tying a shoe lace or writing, many muscles contract but the movements must be coordinated and carried out in a particular sequence. Such a pattern of movement, when established, is described as *manual dexterity*.

In the lower part of this area just above the lateral sulcus there is a group of nerve cells known as the *motor speech (Broca's) area* which controls the movements necessary for speech. It is dominant in the *left hemisphere* in *right-handed people* and vice versa.

The frontal area. This extends anteriorly from the premotor area to include the remainder of the frontal lobe. It is a large area and is more highly developed in humans than in other animals. It is thought that communications between this and the other regions in the cerebrum are responsible for the behaviour, character and emotional state of the individual. No particular behaviour, character or intellectual trait has, so far, been attributed to the activity of any one group of cells.

Sensory areas of the cerebrum

The postcentral (sensory) area. This is the area behind the central sulcus. Here sensations of pain, temperature, pressure and touch, knowledge of muscular movement and the position of joints are perceived. The sensory area of the *right hemisphere* receives impulses from the *left side of the body* and vice versa. The size of the areas representing different parts of the body (Fig. 7.20B) is proportional to the *extent of sensory innervation*, e.g. the large area for the face is consistent with the extensive sensory nerve supply by the three branches of the trigeminal nerves (5th cranial nerves).

The parietal area. This lies behind the postcentral area and includes the greater part of the parietal lobe of the cerebrum. Its functions are believed to be associated with obtaining and retaining accurate knowledge of objects. It has been suggested that objects can be recognised by touch alone because of the knowledge from past experience (memory) retained in this area.

The sensory speech area. This is situated in the lower part of the parietal lobe and extends into the temporal lobe. It is here that the spoken word is perceived. There is a dominant area in the *left hemisphere* in *right-handed* people and vice versa.

The auditory (hearing) area. This lies immediately below the lateral sulcus within the temporal lobe. The cells receive and interpret impulses transmitted from the inner ear by the cochlear (auditory) part of the vestibulocochlear nerves (8th cranial nerves).

Figure 7.19 The motor nerve pathways: upper and lower motor neurones.

The olfactory (smell) area. This lies deep within the temporal lobe where impulses from the nose via the olfactory nerves (1st cranial nerves) are received and interpreted.

The taste area. This is thought to lie just above the lateral sulcus in the deep layers of the sensory area. This is the area where impulses from special nerve endings in taste buds in the tongue and in the lining of the cheeks, palate and pharynx are perceived as taste.

The visual area. This lies behind the parieto-occipital sulcus and includes the greater part of the occipital lobe. The optic nerves (2nd cranial nerves) pass from the eye to this area which receives and interprets the impulses as visual impressions.

Other areas of the cerebrum

Deep within the cerebral hemispheres there are groups of cell bodies called *nuclei* (previously called ganglia) which act as relay stations where impulses are passed from one neurone to the next in a chain (Fig. 7.17). Important masses of grey matter include:

- basal nuclei
- thalamus
- hypothalamus.

152

Figure 7.20 A. The *motor homunculus* showing how the body is represented in the motor area of the cerebrum. B. The *sensory homunculus* showing how the body is represented in the sensory area of the cerebrum. (Both A and B are from Penfield W, Rasmussen T 1950 The cerebral cortex of man. Macmillan, New York. © 1950 Macmillan Publishing Co., renewed 1978 Theodore Rasmussen.)

153

Basal nuclei. These are areas of grey matter, lying deep within the cerebral hemispheres, with connections to the cerebral cortex and thalamus. The basal nuclei form part of the extrapyramidal tracts and are thought to be involved in initiating muscle tone in slow and coordinated activities. If control is inadequate or absent, movements are jerky, clumsy and uncoordinated.

Thalamus. The thalamus consists of two masses of nerve cells and fibres situated within the cerebral hemispheres just below the corpus callosum, one on each side of the third ventricle. Sensory input from the skin, viscera and special sense organs is transmitted to the thalamus before redistribution to the cerebrum.

Hypothalamus. The hypothalamus is composed of a number of groups of nerve cells. It is situated below and in front of the thalamus, immediately above the *pituitary gland*. The hypothalamus is linked to the posterior lobe of the pituitary gland by nerve fibres and to the anterior lobe by a complex system of blood vessels. Through these connections, the hypothalamus controls the output of hormones from both lobes of the gland (see p. 215).

Other functions with which the hypothalamus is concerned include control of:

- the autonomic nervous system (p. 170)
- appetite and satiety
- thirst and water balance
- body temperature (p. 365)
- emotional reactions, e.g. pleasure, fear, rage
- sexual behaviour including mating and child rearing
- biological clocks or circadian rhythms, e.g. sleeping and waking cycles, body temperature and secretion of some hormones.

Brain stem

Midbrain

The midbrain is the area of the brain situated around the cerebral aqueduct between the cerebrum above and the *pons* below. It consists of groups of cell bodies and nerve fibres (tracts) which connect the cerebrum with lower parts of the brain and with the spinal cord. The cell bodies act as relay stations for the ascending and descending nerve fibres.

Pons

The pons is situated in front of the cerebellum, below the midbrain and above the medulla oblongata. It consists mainly of nerve fibres which form a bridge between the two hemispheres of the cerebellum, and of fibres passing between the higher levels of the brain and the spinal cord. There are groups of cells within the pons which act as relay stations and some of these are associated with the cranial nerves.

The anatomical structure of the pons differs from that of the cerebrum in that the cell bodies (grey matter) lie deeply and the nerve fibres are on the surface.

Medulla oblongata

The medulla oblongata extends from the pons above and is continuous with the spinal cord below. It is about 2.5 cm long and it lies just within the cranium above the foramen magnum. Its anterior and posterior surfaces are marked by central fissures. The outer aspect is composed of *white matter* which passes between the brain and the spinal cord, and *grey matter* lies centrally. Some cells constitute relay stations for sensory nerves passing from the spinal cord to the cerebrum.

The vital centres, consisting of groups of cells associated with autonomic reflex activity, lie in its deeper structure. These are the:

- cardiac centre
- respiratory centre
- vasomotor centre
- reflex centres of vomiting, coughing, sneezing and swallowing.

The medulla oblongata has several special features:

- *Decussation (crossing) of the pyramids.* In the medulla *motor nerves* descending from the motor area in the cerebrum to the spinal cord in the pyramidal (corticospinal) tracts cross from one side to the other. This means that the left hemisphere of the cerebrum controls the right half of the body, and vice versa. These tracts are the main pathway for impulses to skeletal (voluntary) muscles.
- *Sensory decussation.* Some of the *sensory nerves* ascending to the cerebrum from the spinal cord cross from one side to the other in the medulla. Others decussate at lower levels, i.e. in the spinal cord.
- *The cardiovascular centre* controls the rate and force of cardiac contraction (p. 87). Sympathetic and parasympathetic nerve fibres originating in the medulla pass to the heart. Sympathetic stimulation increases the rate and force of the heartbeat and parasympathetic stimulation has the opposite effect.

- *The respiratory centre* controls the rate and depth of respiration. From this centre, nerve impulses pass to the phrenic and intercostal nerves which stimulate contraction of the diaphragm and intercostal muscles, thus initiating inspiration. The respiratory centre is stimulated by excess carbon dioxide and, to a lesser extent, by deficiency of oxygen in its blood supply and by nerve impulses from the chemoreceptors in the carotid bodies (p. 256).
- *The vasomotor centre* (p. 80) controls the diameter of the blood vessels, especially the small arteries and arterioles which have a large proportion of smooth muscle fibres in their walls. Vasomotor impulses reach the blood vessels through the autonomic nervous system. Stimulation may cause either constriction or dilatation of blood vessels depending on the site (see Figs 7.43 and 7.44, pp. 171 and 172).

  The sources of stimulation of the vasomotor centre are the arterial baroreceptors, body temperature and emotions such as sexual excitement and anger. Pain usually causes vasoconstriction although severe pain may cause vasodilatation, a fall in blood pressure and fainting.
- *Reflex centres.* When irritating substances are present in the stomach or respiratory tract, nerve impulses pass to the medulla oblongata, stimulating the reflex centres which initiate the reflex actions of vomiting, coughing and sneezing to expel the irritant.

Reticular formation

The reticular formation is a collection of neurones in the core of the brain stem, surrounded by neural pathways which conduct ascending and descending nerve impulses between the brain and the spinal cord. It has a vast number of synaptic links with other parts of the brain and is therefore constantly receiving 'information' being transmitted in ascending and descending tracts.

Functions
The reticular formation is involved in:

- coordination of skeletal muscle activity associated with voluntary motor movement and the maintenance of balance
- coordination of activity controlled by the autonomic nervous system, e.g. cardiovascular, respiratory and gastrointestinal activity
- selective awareness that functions through the *reticular activating system* (RAS) which selectively blocks or passes sensory information to the cerebral cortex, e.g. the slight sound made by a sick child moving in bed may arouse his mother but the noise of regularly passing trains may be suppressed.

Cerebellum

The cerebellum (Fig. 7.21) is situated behind the pons and immediately below the posterior portion of the cerebrum occupying the posterior cranial fossa. It is ovoid in shape and has two hemispheres, separated by a narrow median strip called the *vermis*. Grey matter forms the surface of the cerebellum, and the white matter lies deeply.

Functions

The cerebellum is concerned with the coordination of voluntary muscular movement, posture and balance. Cerebellar activities are not under voluntary control. The cerebellum controls and coordinates the movements of various groups of muscles ensuring smooth, even, precise actions. It coordinates activities associated with the *maintenance of the balance and equilibrium* of the body. The sensory input for these functions is derived from the muscles and joints, the eyes and the ears. *Proprioceptor impulses* from the muscles and joints indicate their position in relation to the body as a whole and those impulses from the eyes and the semicircular canals in the ears provide information about the position of the head in space. Impulses from the cerebellum influence the contraction of skeletal muscle so that balance and posture are maintained.

Damage to the cerebellum results in clumsy uncoordinated muscular movement, staggering gait and inability to carry out smooth, steady, precise movements.

SPINAL CORD

Learning outcomes

After studying this section you should be able to:

- describe the gross structure of the spinal cord
- state the functions of the sensory (afferent) nerve tracts in the spinal cord
- state the functions of the motor (efferent) nerve tracts in the spinal cord
- explain the events of a simple reflex arc.

The spinal cord is the elongated, almost cylindrical part of the central nervous system, which is suspended in the vertebral canal surrounded by the meninges and cerebrospinal fluid (Fig. 7.22). It is continuous above with the medulla oblongata and extends from the *upper border of the atlas* to the lower border of the *1st lumbar vertebra* (Fig. 7.23). It is approximately 45 cm long in an adult Caucasian male, and is about the thickness of the little finger. When a specimen of cerebrospinal fluid is required it is taken from a point below the end of the cord, i.e. below the level of the 2nd lumbar vertebra. This procedure is called *lumbar puncture*.

Except for the cranial nerves, the spinal cord is the nervous tissue link between the brain and the rest of the body (Fig. 7.24). Nerves conveying impulses from the

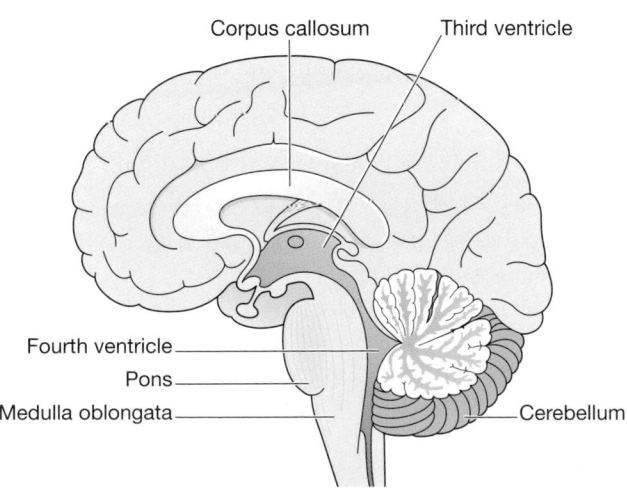

Figure 7.21 The cerebellum and associated structures.

Corpus callosum — Third ventricle — Fourth ventricle — Pons — Medulla oblongata — Cerebellum

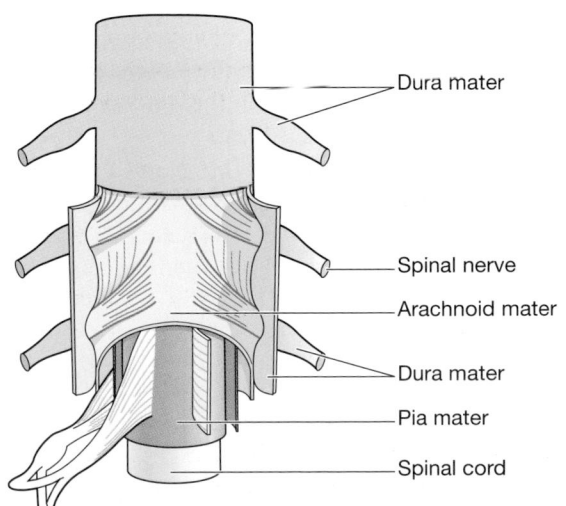

Figure 7.22 The meninges covering the spinal cord. Each cut away to show the underlying layers.

Dura mater — Spinal nerve — Arachnoid mater — Dura mater — Pia mater — Spinal cord

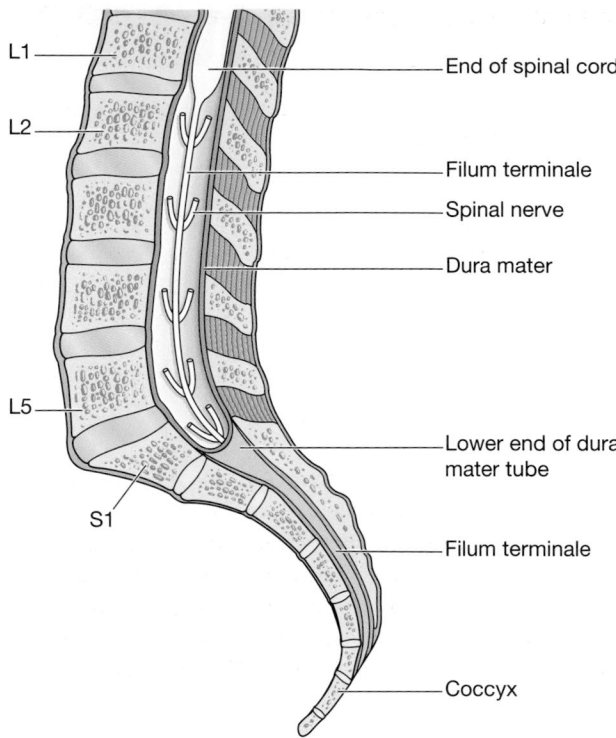

Figure 7.23 Section of the distal end of the vertebral canal.

brain to the various organs and tissues descend through the spinal cord. At the appropriate level they leave the cord and pass to the structure they supply. Similarly, sensory nerves from organs and tissues enter and pass upwards in the spinal cord to the brain.

Some activities of the spinal cord are independent of the brain, i.e. *spinal reflexes*. To facilitate these there are extensive neurone connections between sensory and motor neurones at the same or different levels in the cord.

The spinal cord is incompletely divided into two equal parts, anteriorly by a short, shallow *median fissure* and posteriorly by a deep narrow septum, the *posterior median septum*.

A cross-section of the spinal cord shows that it is composed of grey matter in the centre surrounded by white matter supported by neuroglia. Figure 7.25 shows the parts of the spinal cord and the nerve roots on one side. The other side is the same.

Grey matter

The arrangement of grey matter in the spinal cord resembles the shape of the letter H, having *two posterior, two anterior* and *two lateral columns*. The area of grey matter lying transversely is the *transverse commissure* and it is pierced by the central canal, an extension from the fourth

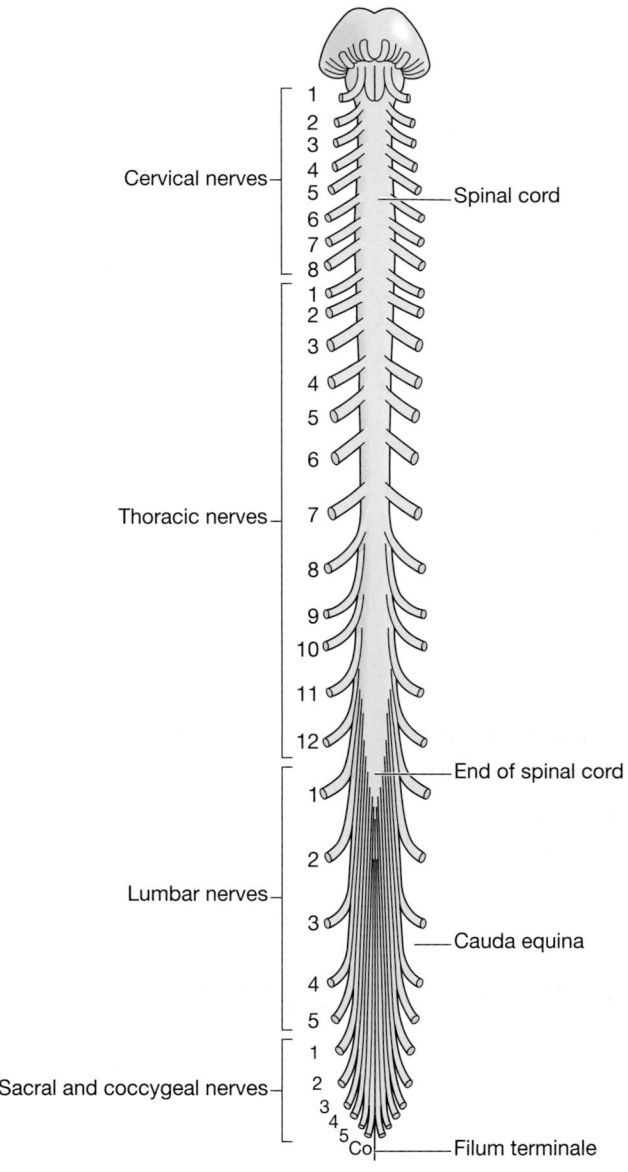

Figure 7.24 The spinal cord and spinal nerves.

ventricle, containing cerebrospinal fluid (Fig. 7.25). The cell bodies may be:

- *sensory cells*, which receive impulses from the periphery of the body
- *lower motor neurones*, which transmit impulses to the skeletal muscles
- *connector neurones*, linking sensory and motor neurones, at the same or different levels, which form spinal reflex arcs.

At each point where nerve impulses are passed from one neurone to another there is a synaptic cleft and a neurotransmitter (Fig. 7.8).

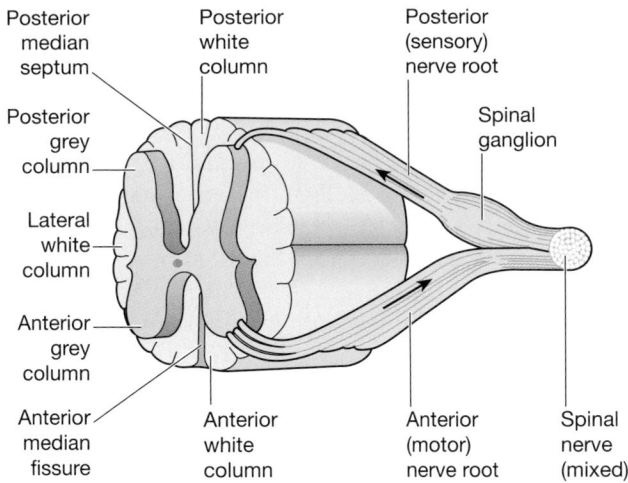

Figure 7.25 A section of the spinal cord showing nerve roots on one side.

Posterior columns of grey matter

These are composed of cell bodies which are stimulated by *sensory impulses* from the periphery of the body. The nerve fibres of these cells contribute to the formation of the white matter of the cord and transmit the sensory impulses upwards to the brain.

Anterior columns of grey matter

These are composed of the *cell bodies of the lower motor neurones* which are stimulated by the axons of the upper motor neurones or by the *cell bodies of connector neurones* linking the anterior and posterior columns to form reflex arcs.

    The posterior root (spinal) ganglia are composed of cell bodies which lie just outside the spinal cord on the pathway of the sensory nerves. All sensory nerve fibres pass through these ganglia. The only function of the cells is to promote the onward movement of nerve impulses.

White matter

The white matter of the spinal cord is arranged in three *columns* or *tracts*; anterior, posterior and lateral. These tracts are formed by *sensory nerve fibres* ascending to the brain, *motor nerve fibres* descending from the brain and fibres of *connector neurones*.

    Tracts are often named according to their points of origin and destination, e.g. spinothalamic, corticospinal.

Sensory nerve tracts (afferent or ascending) in the spinal cord

There are two main sources of sensation transmitted to the brain via the spinal cord.

1. *The skin.* Sensory receptors (nerve endings) in the skin, called *cutaneous receptors*, are stimulated by pain, heat, cold and touch, including pressure. Nerve impulses generated are conducted by three neurones to the sensory area in the *opposite hemisphere of the cerebrum* where the sensation and its location are perceived (Fig. 7.26). Crossing to the other side, or *decussation*, occurs either at the level of entry into the cord or in the medulla.

2. *The tendons, muscles and joints.* Sensory receptors are nerve endings in these structures, called *proprioceptors*, and they are stimulated by stretch. Together with impulses from the eyes and the ears they are associated with the maintenance of balance and posture and with perception of the position of the body in space. These nerve impulses have two destinations:

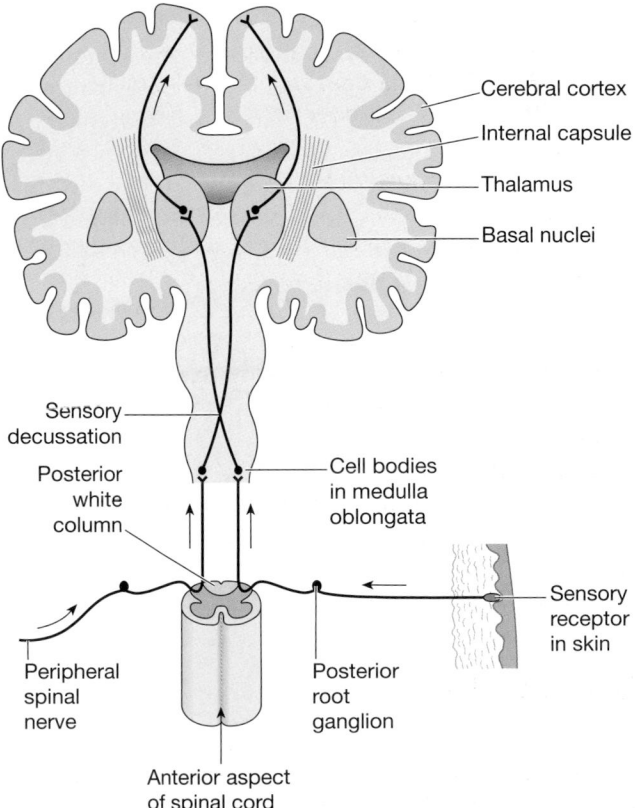

Figure 7.26 One of the sensory nerve pathways from the skin to the cerebrum.

- by a three-neurone system the impulses reach the sensory area of the *opposite hemisphere of the cerebrum*
- by a two-neurone system the nerve impulses reach the *cerebellar hemisphere on the same side*.

Table 7.1 provides further information about the origins, routes of transmission and the destinations of sensory nerve impulses.

Motor nerve tracts (efferent or descending) in the spinal cord

Neurones which transmit nerve impulses away from the brain are motor (efferent or descending) neurones. Motor neurone stimulation results in:

- contraction of skeletal (striated, voluntary) muscle
- contraction of smooth (involuntary) muscle, cardiac muscle and the secretion by glands controlled by nerves of the *autonomic nervous system* (p. 170).

Voluntary muscle movement

The contraction of the muscles which move the joints is, in the main, under conscious (voluntary) control, which means that the stimulus to contract originates at the level of consciousness in the cerebrum. However, some nerve impulses which affect skeletal muscle contraction are initiated in the midbrain, brain stem and cerebellum. This involuntary activity is associated with coordination of muscle activity, e.g. when very fine movement is required and in the maintenance of posture and balance.

Efferent nerve impulses are transmitted from the brain to the body via bundles of nerve fibres or *tracts* in the spinal cord. The *motor pathways* from the brain to the muscles are made up of two *neurones* (Fig. 7.19). These tracts are either:

- pyramidal (corticospinal)
- extrapyramidal.

The motor fibres that form the pyramidal tracts travel through the internal capsule and are the main pathway for impulses to voluntary (skeletal) muscles. Those motor fibres that do not pass through the internal capsule form the extrapyramidal tracts and have connections with many parts of the brain including the basal nuclei and the thalamus.

The upper motor neurone. This has its cell body (Betz's cell) in the *precentral sulcus area* of the cerebrum. The axons pass through the internal capsule, pons and medulla. In the spinal cord they form the *lateral corticospinal tracts* of white matter and the fibres terminate in close association with the cell bodies of the *lower motor neurones* in the anterior columns of grey matter. The axons of these upper motor neurones make up the pyramidal tracts and decussate in the medulla oblongata, forming the pyramids.

The lower motor neurone. This has its cell body in the *anterior horn of grey matter* in the spinal cord. Its axon emerges from the spinal cord by the *anterior root*, joins with the incoming sensory fibres and forms the *mixed spinal nerve* which passes through the *intervertebral foramen*. Near its termination in muscle the axon branches into a variable number of tiny fibres which form *motor end-plates*, each of which is in close association with a sensitive area on the wall of a muscle fibre. The motor

Table 7.1 Sensory nerve impulses: origins, routes, destinations		
Receptor	**Route**	**Destination**
Pain, touch, temperature	Neurone 1 – to spinal cord by posterior root Neurone 2 – decussation on entering spinal cord then in anterolateral spinothalamic tract to thalamus Neurone 3 –	 to parietal lobe of cerebrum
Touch, proprioceptors	Neurone 1 – to medulla in posterior spinothalamic tract Neurone 2 – decussation in medulla, transmission to thalamus Neurone 3 –	 to parietal lobe of cerebrum
Proprioceptors	Neurone 1 – to spinal cord Neurone 2 –	 no decussation, to cerebellum in posterior spinocerebellar tract

Table 7.2 Extrapyramidal upper motor neurones: origins and tracts

Origin	Name of tract	Site in spinal cord	Functions
Midbrain and pons	Rubrospinal tract decussates in brain stem	Lateral column	Control of skilled muscle movement
Reticular formation	Reticulospinal tract does not decussate	Lateral column	Coordination of muscle movement
Midbrain and pons	Tectospinal tract decussates in midbrain	Anterior column	Maintenance of posture and balance
Midbrain and pons	Vestibulospinal tract, some fibres decussate in the cord	Anterior column	

end-plates of each nerve and the muscle fibres they supply form a *motor unit* (Fig. 7.10). The neurotransmitter that conveys the nerve impulse across the synapse to stimulate the muscle fibre is *acetylcholine*. Motor units contract as a whole and the strength of contraction of a muscle depends on the number of motor units in action at a time.

The lower motor neurone has been described as the *final common pathway* for the transmission of nerve impulses to skeletal muscles. The cell body of this neurone is influenced by a number of upper motor neurones originating from various sites in the brain and by some neurones which begin and end in the spinal cord. Some of these neurones stimulate the cell bodies of the lower motor neurone while others have an inhibiting effect. The outcome of these influences is smooth, coordinated muscle movement, some of which is voluntary and some involuntary.

Involuntary muscle movement

Upper motor neurones. These have their cell bodies in the brain at a level *below* the cerebrum, i.e. in the midbrain, brain stem, cerebellum or spinal cord. They influence muscle activity in relation to the maintenance of posture and balance, the coordination of muscle movement and the control of muscle tone.

Table 7.2 shows details of the area of origin of these neurones and the tracts which their axons form before reaching the cell of the lower motor neurone in the spinal cord.

Spinal reflexes. These consist of three elements:

- sensory neurones
- connector neurones in the spinal cord
- lower motor neurones.

In the simplest *reflex arc* there is only one of each (Fig. 7.27). A *reflex action* is an immediate motor response to a sensory stimulus. Many connector and motor neurones may be stimulated by afferent impulses from a small area of skin, e.g. the pain impulses initiated by touching a very hot surface with the finger are transmitted to the spinal cord by sensory nerves. These stimulate many connector and lower motor neurones in the cord which results in the contraction of many skeletal muscles of the

159

Figure 7.27 A simple reflex arc involving one side only.

hand, arm and shoulder, and the removal of the finger. Reflex action takes place very quickly, in fact, the motor response may have occurred simultaneously with the perception of the pain in the cerebrum. Reflexes of this type are invariably protective but they can on occasion be inhibited. For example, if it is a precious plate that is very hot when lifted every effort will be made to overcome the pain to prevent dropping it!

Stretch reflexes. Only two neurones are involved. The cell body of the lower motor neurone is stimulated by the sensory neurone. There is no connector neurone involved. The *knee jerk* is one example, but this type of reflex can be demonstrated at any point where a stretched tendon crosses a joint. By tapping the tendon just below the knee when it is bent, the sensory nerve endings in the tendon and in the thigh muscles are stretched. This initiates a nerve impulse which passes into the spinal cord to the cell body of the lower motor neurone in the anterior column of grey matter on the same side. As a result the thigh muscles suddenly contract and the foot kicks forward. This is used as a test of the integrity of the reflex arc. This type of reflex has a protective function—it prevents excessive joint movement that may damage tendons, ligaments and muscles.

Autonomic reflexes. See page 172.

PERIPHERAL NERVOUS SYSTEM

Learning outcomes

After studying this section you should be able to:

- state the origins of the paired spinal nerves
- outline the function of a nerve plexus
- list the spinal nerves entering each plexus and the main nerves emerging from it
- describe the areas innervated by the thoracic nerves
- outline the functions of the 12 cranial nerves.

This part of the nervous system consists of:

- 31 pairs of spinal nerves
- 12 pairs of cranial nerves
- the autonomic part of the nervous system.

Most of the nerves of the peripheral nervous system are composed of *sensory nerve fibres* conveying afferent impulses from sensory end organs to the brain, and *motor nerve fibres* conveying efferent impulses from the brain through the spinal cord to the effector organs, e.g. skeletal muscles, smooth muscle and glands.

Each nerve consists of numerous nerve fibres collected into bundles. Each bundle has several coverings of protective connective tissue (Fig. 7.28).

- *Endoneurium* is a delicate tissue, surrounding each individual fibre, which is continuous with the septa that pass inwards from the perineurium.
- *Perineurium* is a smooth connective tissue, surrounding each *bundle* of fibres.
- *Epineurium* is the fibrous tissue which surrounds and encloses a number of bundles of nerve fibres. Most large nerves are covered by epineurium.

Spinal nerves

There are *31 pairs of spinal nerves* that leave the vertebral canal by passing through the intervertebral foramina formed by adjacent vertebrae. They are named and grouped according to the vertebrae with which they are associated (Fig. 7.24):

- 8 cervical
- 12 thoracic
- 5 lumbar
- 5 sacral
- 1 coccygeal.

Although there are only seven cervical vertebrae, there are eight nerves because the first pair leave the vertebral

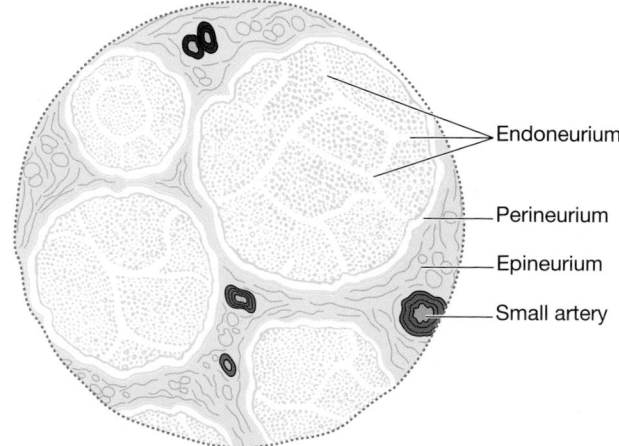

Figure 7.28 Transverse section of a peripheral nerve showing the protective coverings.

canal between the occipital bone and the atlas and the eighth pair leave below the last cervical vertebra. Thereafter the nerves are given the name and number of the vertebra immediately *above*.

The lumbar, sacral and coccygeal nerves leave the *spinal cord* near its termination at the level of the first lumbar vertebra, and extend downwards inside the vertebral canal in the subarachnoid space, forming a sheaf of nerves which resembles a horse's tail, the *cauda equina*. These nerves leave the vertebral canal at the appropriate lumbar, sacral or coccygeal level, depending on their destination.

The spinal nerves arise from both sides of the spinal cord and emerge through the intervertebral foramina. Each nerve is formed by the union of a *motor and a sensory nerve root* and is, therefore, a *mixed nerve*. Each spinal nerve has a contribution from the sympathetic part of the autonomic nervous system in the form of a *preganglionic fibre* (see Fig. 7.43, p. 171).

For details of the bones and muscles mentioned in the following section see Chapters 16 to 18. Bones and joints are supplied by adjacent nerves.

Nerve roots (Fig. 7.29)

The anterior nerve root consists of *motor nerve fibres* which are the axons of the nerve cells in the anterior column of grey matter in the spinal cord and, in the thoracic and lumbar regions, *sympathetic nerve fibres* which are the axons of cells in the lateral columns of grey matter.

The posterior nerve root consists of *sensory nerve fibres*. Just outside the spinal cord there is a *spinal ganglion* (posterior root ganglion), consisting of a little cluster of cell bodies. Sensory nerve fibres pass through these ganglia before entering the spinal cord. The area of skin supplied by each nerve is called a *dermatome* (Figs 7.34 and 7.38).

For a very short distance after leaving the spinal cord the nerve roots have a covering of *dura* and *arachnoid maters*. These terminate before the two roots join to form the mixed spinal nerve. The nerve roots have no covering of pia mater.

Immediately after emerging from the intervertebral foramen each spinal nerve divides into a ramus communicans, a posterior ramus and an anterior ramus.

The rami communicans are part of preganglionic sympathetic neurones of the autonomic nervous system (p. 170).

The posterior rami pass backwards and divide into medial and lateral branches to supply skin and muscles of relatively small areas of the posterior aspect of the head, neck and trunk.

The anterior rami supply the anterior and lateral aspects of the neck, trunk and the upper and lower limbs.

In the cervical, lumbar and sacral regions the anterior rami unite near their origins to form large masses of nerves, or *plexuses*, where nerve fibres are regrouped and rearranged before proceeding to supply skin, bones, muscles and joints of a particular area (Fig. 7.30). This

161

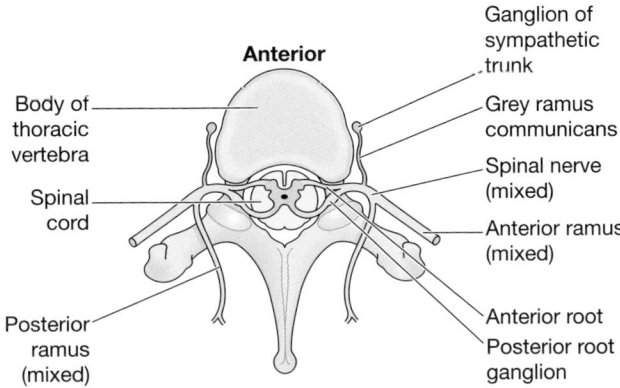

Figure 7.29 The relationship between sympathetic and mixed spinal nerves. Sympathetic part in green.

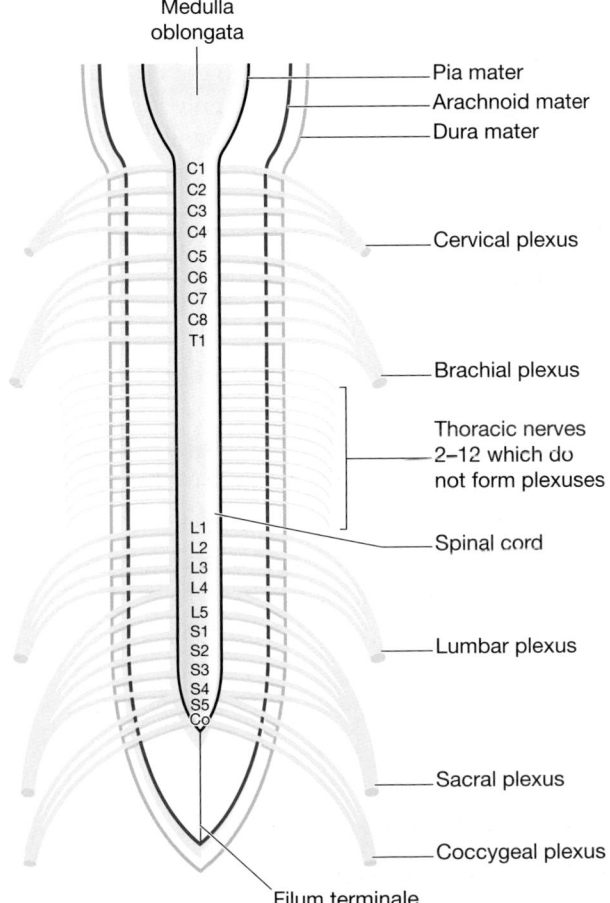

Figure 7.30 The meninges covering the spinal cord, spinal nerves and the plexuses they form.

means that these structures have a nerve supply from more than one spinal nerve and therefore damage to one spinal nerve does not cause loss of function of a region.

In the thoracic region the anterior rami do not form plexuses.

There are five large plexuses of mixed nerves formed on each side of the vertebral column. They are the:

- cervical plexuses
- brachial plexuses
- lumbar plexuses
- sacral plexuses
- coccygeal plexuses.

Cervical plexus (Fig. 7.31)

This is formed by the anterior rami of the first four cervical nerves. It lies opposite the 1st, 2nd, 3rd and 4th cervical vertebrae under the protection of the sterno-cleidomastoid muscle.

The superficial branches supply the structures at the back and side of the head and the skin of the front of the neck to the level of the sternum.

The deep branches supply muscles of the neck, e.g. the sternocleidomastoid and the trapezius.

The phrenic nerve originates from cervical roots 3, 4 and 5 and passes downwards through the thoracic cavity in front of the root of the lung to supply the muscle of the diaphragm with impulses which stimulate contraction.

Brachial plexus

The anterior rami of the lower four cervical nerves and a large part of the first thoracic nerve form the brachial plexus. Figure 7.32 shows its formation and the nerves which emerge from it. The plexus is situated in the neck and shoulder above and behind the subclavian vessels and in the axilla.

The branches of the brachial plexus supply the skin and muscles of the upper limbs and some of the chest muscles. Five large nerves and a number of smaller ones emerge from this plexus, each with a contribution from more than one nerve root, containing sensory, motor and autonomic fibres:

- axillary (circumflex) nerve: C5, 6
- radial nerve: C5, 6, 7, 8, T1
- musculocutaneous nerve: C5, 6, 7
- median nerve: C5, 6, 7, 8, T1
- ulnar nerve: C7, 8, T1
- medial cutaneous nerve: C8, T1.

The axillary (circumflex) nerve winds round the humerus at the level of the surgical neck. It then breaks up into minute branches to supply the deltoid muscle, shoulder joint and overlying skin.

The radial nerve is the largest branch of the brachial plexus. It supplies the triceps muscle behind the humerus, crosses in front of the elbow joint then winds round to the back of the forearm to supply extensors of the wrist and finger joints. It continues into the back of the hand to supply the skin of the thumb, the first two fingers and the lateral half of the third finger.

The musculocutaneous nerve passes downwards to the lateral aspect of the forearm. It supplies the muscles of the upper arm and the skin of the forearm.

The median nerve passes down the midline of the arm in close association with the brachial artery. It passes in front of the elbow joint then down to supply the muscles

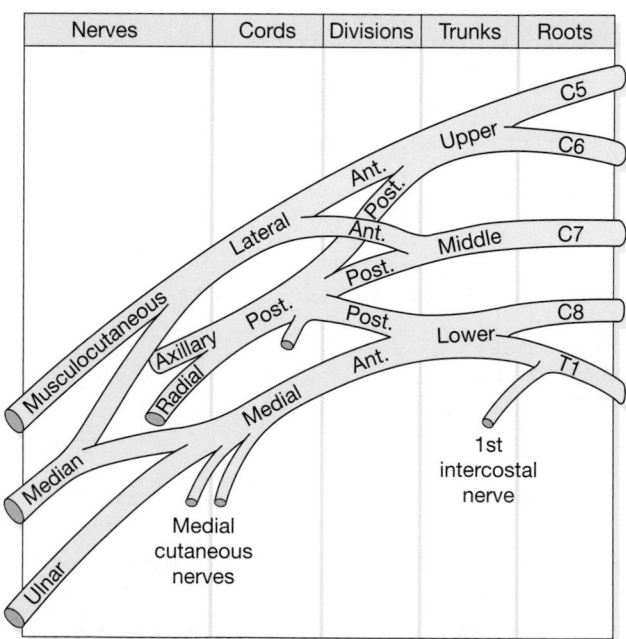

Figure 7.32 The brachial plexus.

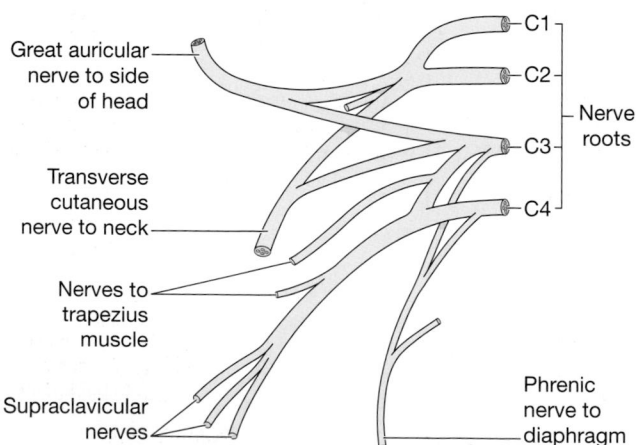

Figure 7.31 The cervical plexus.

162

of the front of the forearm. It continues into the hand where it supplies small muscles and the skin of the front of the thumb, the first two fingers and the lateral half of the third finger. It gives off no branches above the elbow.

The ulnar nerve descends through the upper arm lying medial to the brachial artery. It passes behind the medial epicondyle of the humerus to supply the muscles on the ulnar aspect of the forearm. It continues downwards to supply the muscles in the palm of the hand and the skin of the whole of the little finger and the medial half of the third finger. It gives off no branches above the elbow.

The main nerves of the arm are presented in Figure 7.33. The distribution and origins of the cutaneous sensory nerves of the arm are shown in Figure 7.34, i.e. the dermatomes.

Lumbar plexus (Figs 7.35, 7.37 and 7.38)

The lumbar plexus is formed by the anterior rami of the first three and part of the fourth lumbar nerves. The plexus is situated in front of the transverse processes of the lumbar vertebrae and behind the psoas muscle. The main branches, and their nerve roots are:

- iliohypogastric nerve: L1
- ilioinguinal nerve: L1
- genitofemoral: L1, 2
- lateral cutaneous nerve of thigh: L2, 3

- femoral nerve: L2, 3, 4
- obturator nerve: L2, 3, 4
- lumbosacral trunk: L4, (5).

The iliohypogastric, ilioinguinal and *genitofemoral nerves* supply muscles and the skin in the area of the lower abdomen, upper and medial aspects of the thigh and the inguinal region.

The lateral cutaneous nerve of the thigh supplies the skin of the lateral aspect of the thigh including part of the anterior and posterior surfaces.

The femoral nerve is one of the larger branches. It passes behind the inguinal ligament to enter the thigh in close association with the femoral artery. It divides into cutaneous and muscular branches to supply the skin and the muscles of the front of the thigh. One branch, the *saphenous nerve*, supplies the medial aspect of the leg, ankle and foot.

The obturator nerve supplies the adductor muscles of the thigh and skin of the medial aspect of the thigh. It ends just above the level of the knee joint.

The lumbosacral trunk descends into the pelvis and makes a contribution to the sacral plexus.

Sacral plexus (Figs 7.36, 7.37 and 7.38)

The sacral plexus is formed by the anterior rami of the lumbosacral trunk and the first, second and third sacral

163

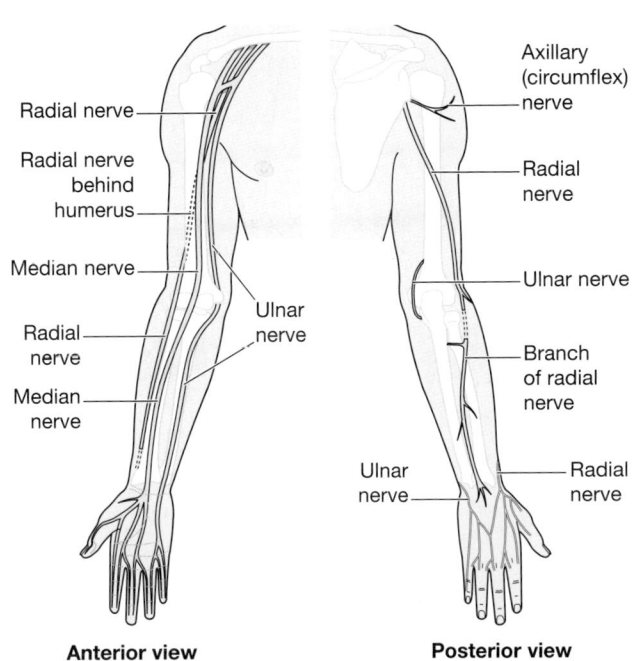

Figure 7.33 The main nerves of the arm.

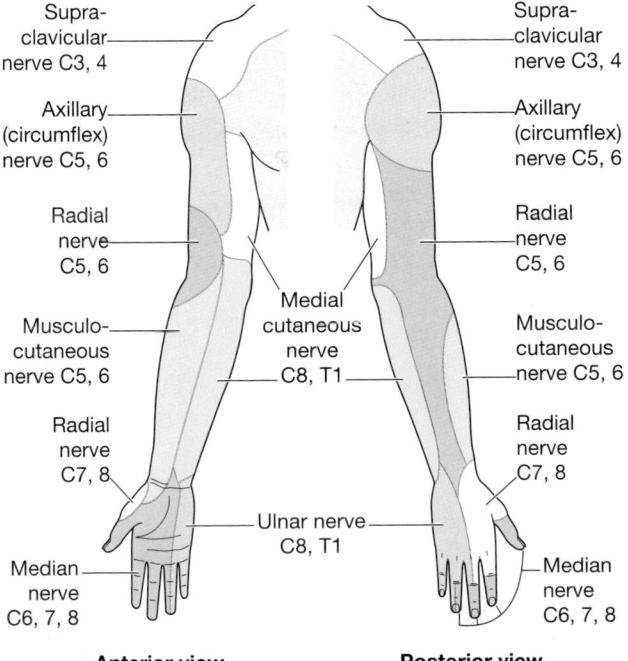

Figure 7.34 The distribution and origins of the cutaneous nerves of the arm.

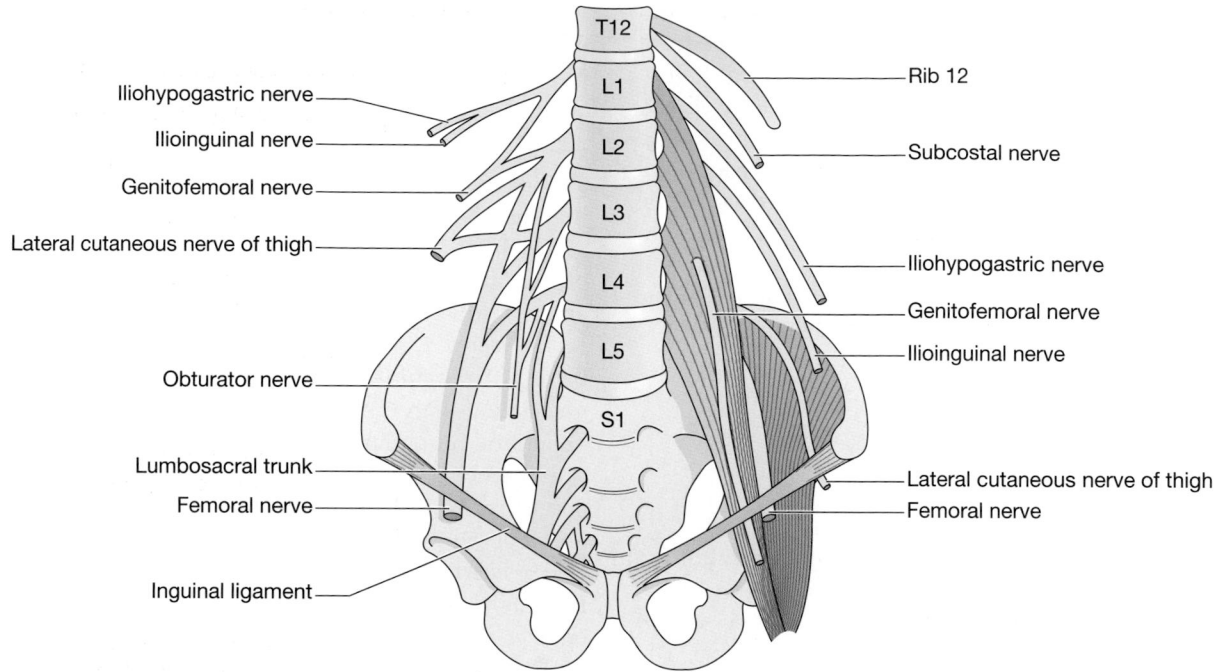

Figure 7.35 The lumbar plexus.

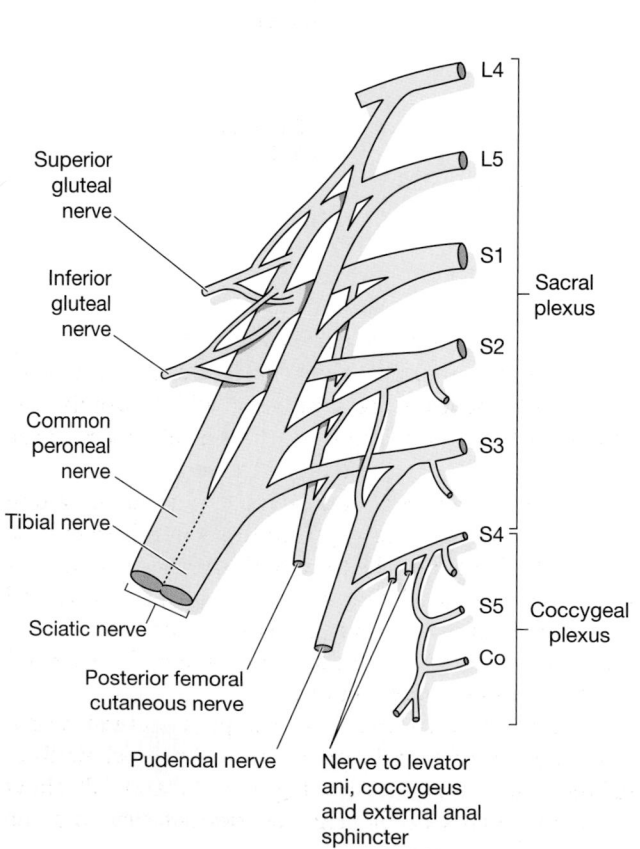

Figure 7.36 Sacral and coccygeal plexuses.

Figure 7.37 The main nerves of the leg.

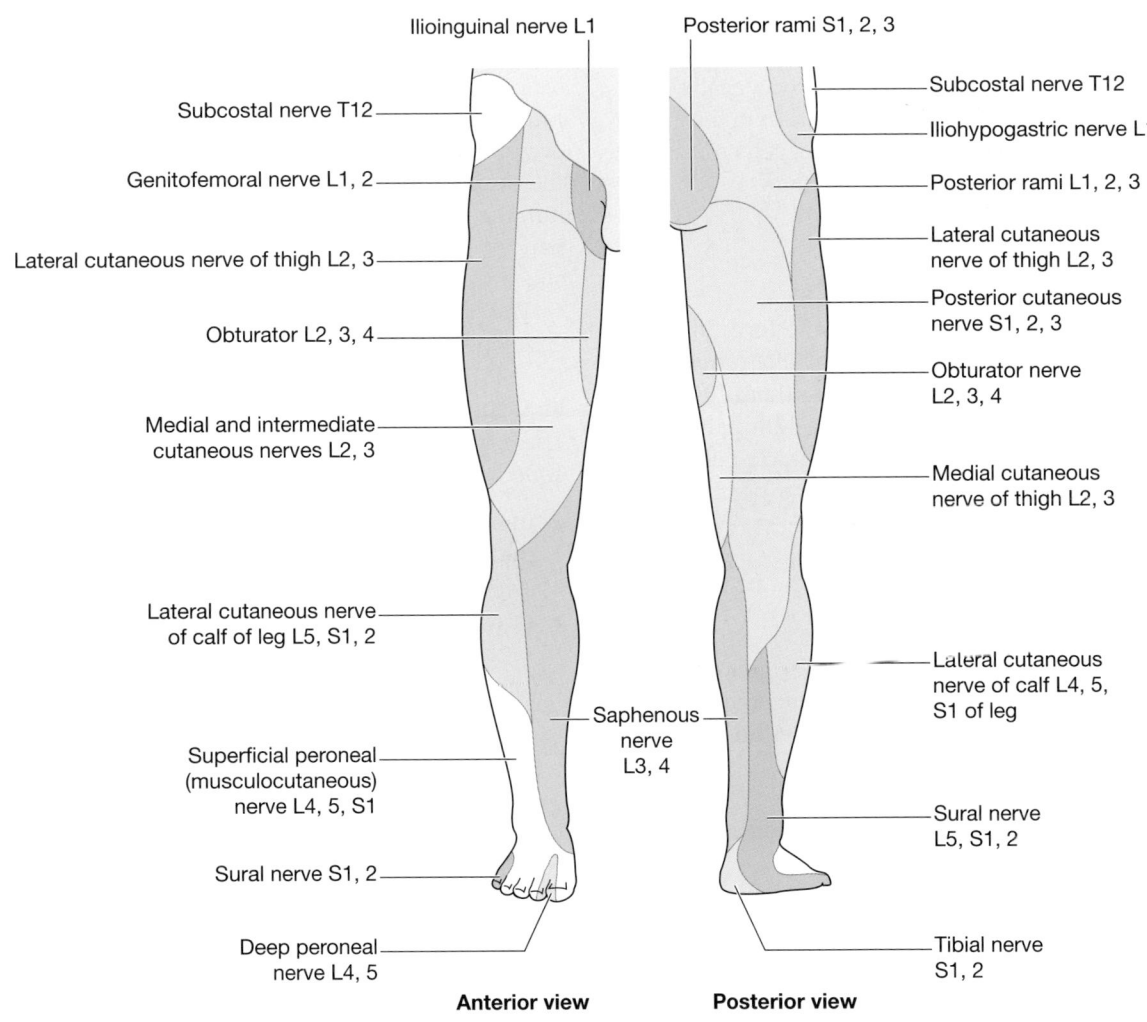

Ilioinguinal nerve L1

Posterior rami S1, 2, 3

Subcostal nerve T12

Genitofemoral nerve L1, 2

Lateral cutaneous nerve of thigh L2, 3

Obturator L2, 3, 4

Medial and intermediate cutaneous nerves L2, 3

Lateral cutaneous nerve of calf of leg L5, S1, 2

Superficial peroneal (musculocutaneous) nerve L4, 5, S1

Sural nerve S1, 2

Deep peroneal nerve L4, 5

Anterior view

Subcostal nerve T12

Iliohypogastric nerve L1

Posterior rami L1, 2, 3

Lateral cutaneous nerve of thigh L2, 3

Posterior cutaneous nerve S1, 2, 3

Obturator nerve L2, 3, 4

Medial cutaneous nerve of thigh L2, 3

Lateral cutaneous nerve of calf L4, 5, S1 of leg

Saphenous nerve L3, 4

Sural nerve L5, S1, 2

Tibial nerve S1, 2

Posterior view

Figure 7.38 Distribution and origins of the cutaneous nerves of the leg.

nerves. The lumbosacral trunk is formed by the fifth and part of the fourth lumbar nerves. It lies in the posterior wall of the pelvic cavity.

The sacral plexus divides into a number of branches, supplying the muscles and skin of the pelvic floor, muscles around the hip joint and the pelvic organs. In addition to these it provides the *sciatic nerve* which contains fibres from L4, 5, S1, 2, 3.

The sciatic nerve is the largest nerve in the body. It is about 2 cm wide at its origin. It passes through the greater sciatic foramen into the buttock then descends through the posterior aspect of the thigh supplying the hamstring muscles. At the level of the middle of the femur it divides to form the *tibial* and the *common peroneal nerves*.

The tibial nerve descends through the popliteal fossa to the posterior aspect of the leg where it supplies muscles

and skin. It passes under the medial malleolus to supply muscles and skin of the sole of the foot and toes. One of the main branches is the *sural nerve* which supplies the tissues in the area of the heel, the lateral aspect of the ankle and a part of the dorsum of the foot.

The common peroneal nerve descends obliquely along the lateral aspect of the popliteal fossa, winds round the neck of the fibula into the front of the leg where it divides into the *deep peroneal* (anterior tibial) and the *superficial peroneal* (musculocutaneous) nerves. These nerves supply the skin and muscles of the anterior aspect of the leg and the dorsum of the foot and toes.

The pudendal nerve (S2, 3, 4). The perineal branch supplies the external anal sphincter, the external urethral sphincter and adjacent skin. Figures 7.37 and 7.38 show the main nerves of the leg, the dermatomes and the origins of the main nerves.

Coccygeal plexus (Fig. 7.36)

The coccygeal plexus is a very small plexus formed by part of the fourth and fifth sacral and the coccygeal nerves. The nerves from this plexus supply the skin in the area of the coccyx and the levators ani and coccygeus muscles of the pelvic floor and the external anal sphincter.

Thoracic nerves

The thoracic nerves *do not* intermingle to form plexuses. There are 12 pairs and the first 11 are the *intercostal nerves*. They pass between the ribs supplying them, the intercostal muscles and overlying skin. The 12th pair are the *subcostal nerves*. The 7th to the 12th thoracic nerves also supply the muscles and the skin of the posterior and anterior abdominal walls (Fig. 7.39).

Cranial nerves (Fig. 7.40)

There are 12 pairs of cranial nerves originating from nuclei in the inferior surface of the brain, some sensory, some motor and some mixed. Their names and numbers are:

I.	Olfactory: sensory
II.	Optic: sensory
III.	Oculomotor: motor
IV.	Trochlear: motor
V.	Trigeminal: mixed
VI.	Abducent: motor
VII.	Facial: mixed
VIII.	Vestibulocochlear (auditory): sensory
IX.	Glossopharyngeal: mixed
X.	Vagus: mixed
XI.	Accessory: motor
XII.	Hypoglossal: motor.

I. Olfactory nerves (sensory)

These are the nerves of the *sense of smell*. Their nerve endings and fibres originate in the upper part of the mucous membrane of the nasal cavity, pass upwards through the cribriform plate of the ethmoid bone and then go to the *olfactory bulb* (see Fig. 8.23, p. 206). The nerves then proceed backwards as the olfactory tract, to the area for the perception of smell in the temporal lobe of the cerebrum.

II. Optic nerves (sensory)

These are the nerves of the *sense of sight*. The fibres originate in the retinae of the eyes and they combine to form the optic nerves (see Fig. 8.13, p. 200). They are directed backwards and medially through the posterior part of the orbital cavity. They then pass through the *optic foramina* of the sphenoid bone into the cranial cavity and join at the *optic chiasma*. The nerves proceed backwards as the *optic tracts* to the *lateral geniculate bodies* of the thalamus. Impulses pass from these to the centre for sight in the occipital lobes of the cerebrum and to the cerebellum. In the occipital lobe sight is perceived, and in the cerebellum the impulses from the eyes contribute to the maintenance of balance, posture and orientation of the head in space.

The central retinal artery and vein enter the eye enveloped by the fibres of the optic nerve.

III. Oculomotor nerves (motor)

These nerves arise from nerve cells near the cerebral aqueduct. They supply:

- four extraocular muscles, which move the eyeball, i.e. the *superior, medial* and *inferior recti* and the *inferior oblique muscle*
- intraocular muscles:
  - *ciliary muscles* which alter the shape of the lens, changing its refractive power
  - *circular muscles of the iris* which constrict the pupil
- the *levator palpebrae* muscle which raises the upper eyelid.

IV. Trochlear nerves (motor)

These nerves arise from nerve cells near the cerebral aqueduct. They supply the *superior oblique muscles* of the eyes.

V. Trigeminal nerves (mixed)

These nerves contain motor and sensory fibres and are among the largest of the cranial nerves. They are the chief sensory nerves for the face and head (including the oral and nasal cavities and teeth), receiving impulses of pain, temperature and touch. The motor fibres stimulate the muscles of mastication.

There are three main branches of the trigeminal nerves. The dermatomes supplied by the sensory fibres on the right side are shown in Figure 7.41.

The ophthalmic nerves are sensory only and supply the lacrimal glands, conjunctiva of the eyes, forehead, eyelids, anterior aspect of the scalp and mucous membrane of the nose.

The maxillary nerves are sensory only and supply the cheeks, upper gums, upper teeth and lower eyelids.

The mandibular nerves contain both sensory and motor fibres. These are the largest of the three divisions and they supply the teeth and gums of the lower jaw, pinnae of the ears, lower lip and tongue. The motor fibres supply the muscles of mastication.

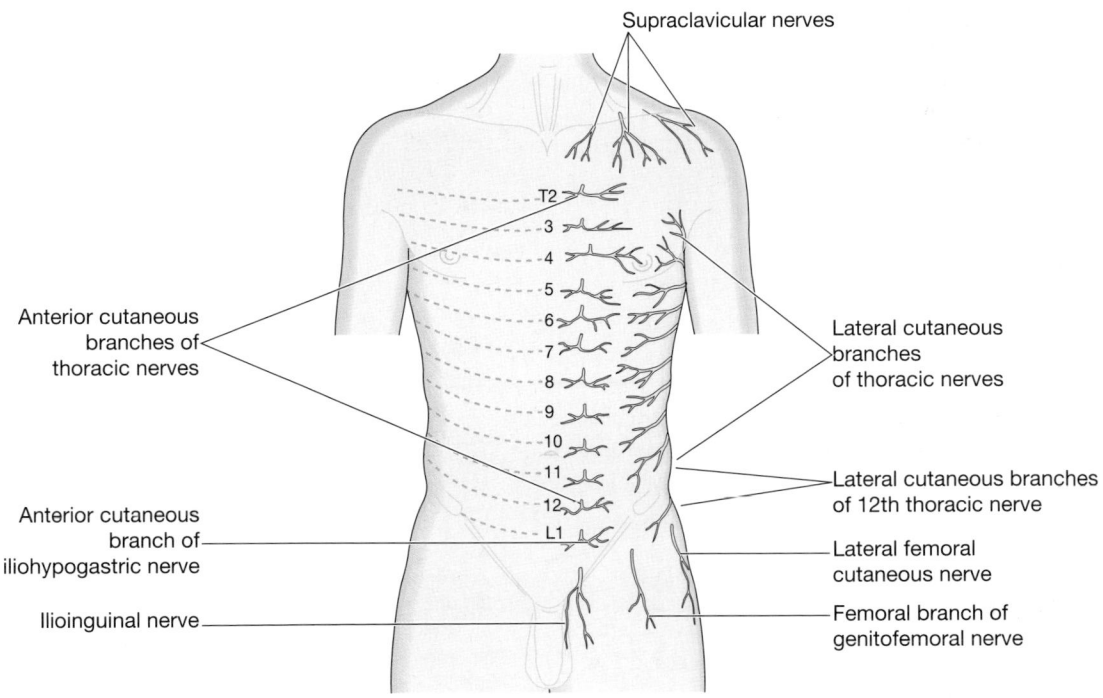

Figure 7.39 Segmental distribution of the thoracic cutaneous nerves.

Figure 7.40 The inferior surface of the brain showing the cranial nerves.

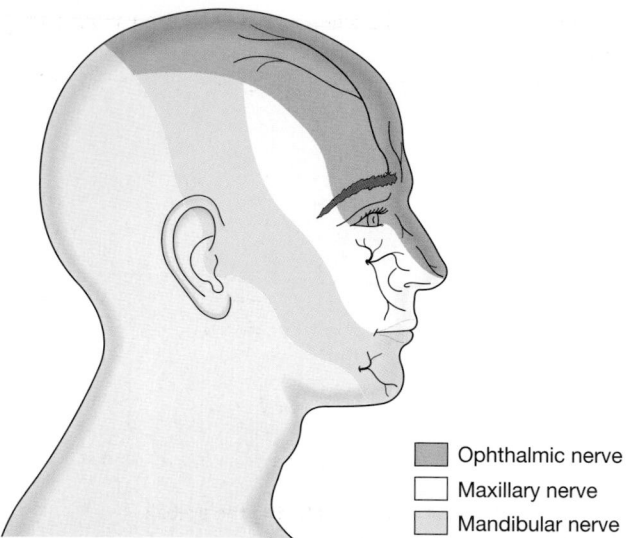

Figure 7.41 The cutaneous distribution of the main branches of the right trigeminal nerve.

Ophthalmic nerve
Maxillary nerve
Mandibular nerve

VI. Abducent nerves (motor)

These nerves arise from a group of nerve cells lying under the floor of the fourth ventricle. They supply the *lateral rectus muscles* of the eyeballs.

VII. Facial nerves (mixed)

These nerves are composed of both motor and sensory nerve fibres, arising from nerve cells in the lower part of the pons. The motor fibres supply the muscles of facial expression. The sensory fibres convey impulses from the taste buds in the anterior two-thirds of the tongue to the taste perception area in the cerebral cortex.

VIII. Vestibulocochlear (auditory) nerves (sensory)

These nerves are composed of two distinct sets of fibres, vestibular nerves and cochlear nerves.

The vestibular nerves arise from the semicircular canals of the inner ear and convey impulses to the cerebellum. They are associated with the maintenance of posture and balance.

The cochlear nerves originate in the organ of Corti in the inner ear and convey impulses to the hearing areas in the cerebral cortex where sound is perceived.

IX. Glossopharyngeal nerves (mixed)

These nerves arise from nuclei in the medulla oblongata. The motor fibres stimulate the muscles of the tongue and pharynx and the secretory cells of the parotid (salivary) glands.

The sensory fibres convey impulses to the cerebral cortex from the posterior third of the tongue, the tonsils

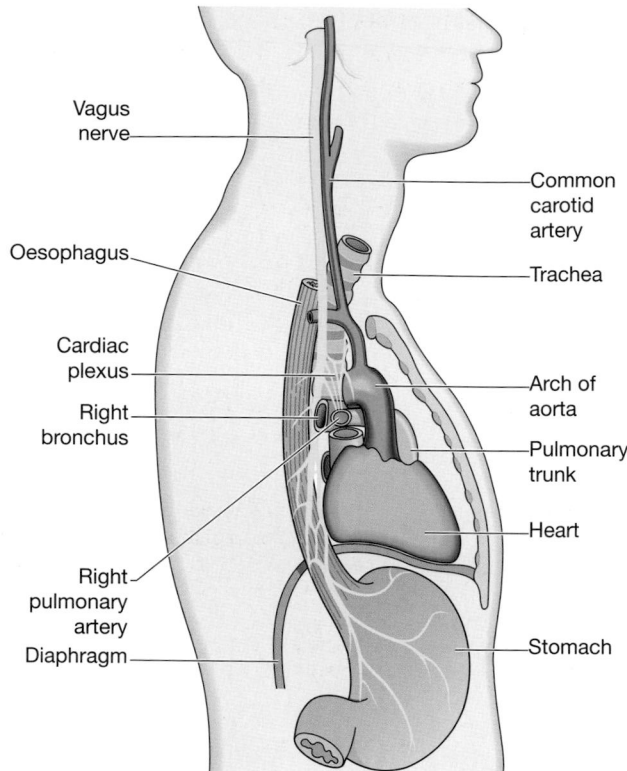

Vagus nerve
Oesophagus
Cardiac plexus
Right bronchus
Right pulmonary artery
Diaphragm
Common carotid artery
Trachea
Arch of aorta
Pulmonary trunk
Heart
Stomach

Figure 7.42 The position of the vagus nerve in the thorax viewed from the right side.

and pharynx and from taste buds in the tongue and pharynx. These nerves are essential for the swallowing and gag reflexes.

X. Vagus nerves (mixed) (Fig. 7.42)

These nerves have a more extensive distribution than any other cranial nerves. They arise from nerve cells in the medulla oblongata and other nuclei, and pass down through the neck into the thorax and the abdomen. These nerves form an important part of the parasympathetic nervous system (Fig. 7.44).

The motor fibres supply the smooth muscles and secretory glands of the pharynx, larynx, trachea, heart, oesophagus, stomach, intestines, pancreas, gall bladder, bile ducts, spleen, kidneys, ureter and blood vessels in the thoracic and abdominal cavities.

The sensory fibres convey impulses from the lining membranes of the same structures to the brain.

XI. Accessory nerves (motor)

These nerves arise from cell bodies in the medulla oblongata and in the spinal cord. The fibres supply the *sternocleidomastoid* and *trapezius muscles*. Branches join the vagus nerves and supply the *pharyngeal* and *laryngeal muscles*.

XII. Hypoglossal nerves (motor)

These nerves arise from cells in the medulla oblongata. They supply the muscles of the tongue and muscles surrounding the hyoid bone and contribute to swallowing and speech.

A summary of the cranial nerves is given in Table 7.3.

Table 7.3 Summary of the cranial nerves

Name and no.	Central connection	Peripheral connection	Function
I. Olfactory (sensory)	Smell area in temporal lobe of cerebrum through olfactory bulb	Mucous membrane in roof of nose	Sense of smell
II. Optic (sensory)	Sight area in occipital lobe of cerebrum Cerebellum	Retina of the eye	Sense of sight Balance
III. Oculomotor (motor)	Nerve cells near floor of aqueduct of midbrain	Superior, inferior and medial rectus muscles of the eye Ciliary muscles of the eye Circular muscle fibres of the iris	Moving the eyeball Focusing Regulating the size of the pupil
IV. Trochlear (motor)	Nerve cells near floor of aqueduct of midbrain	Superior oblique muscles of the eye	Movement of the eyeball
V. Trigeminal (mixed)	Motor fibres from the pons Sensory fibres from the trigeminal ganglion	Muscles of mastication Sensory to gums, cheek, lower jaw, iris, cornea	Chewing Sensation from the face
VI. Abducent (motor)	Floor of fourth ventricle	Lateral rectus muscle of the eye	Movement of the eye
VII. Facial (mixed)	Pons	Sensory fibres to the tongue Motor fibres to the muscles of the face	Sense of taste Movements of facial expression
VIII. Vestibulocochlear (sensory) (a) Vestibular (b) Cochlear	 Cerebellum Hearing area of cerebrum	 Semicircular canals in the inner ear Organ of Corti in cochlea	 Maintenance of balance Sense of hearing
IX. Glossopharyngeal (mixed)	Medulla oblongata	Parotid gland Back of tongue and pharynx	Secretion of saliva Sense of taste Movement of pharynx
X. Vagus (mixed)	Medulla oblongata	Pharynx, larynx; organs, glands ducts, blood vessels in the thorax and abdomen	Movement and secretion
XI. Accessory (motor)	Medulla oblongata	Sternocleidomastoid, trapezius, laryngeal and pharyngeal muscles	Movement of the head, shoulders, pharynx and larynx
XII. Hypoglossal (motor)	Medulla oblongata	Tongue	Movement of tongue

AUTONOMIC NERVOUS SYSTEM

Learning outcomes

After studying this section you should be able to:

- identify the two divisions of the autonomic nervous system

- compare and contrast the structures and neurotransmitters of the two divisions

- compare and contrast the effects of stimulation of the two divisions on body systems

- explain how referred pain occurs.

The autonomic or involuntary part of the nervous system (Fig. 7.6) controls the functions of the body carried out 'automatically', i.e. initiated in the brain below the level of the cerebrum. Although stimulation does not occur voluntarily the individual may be conscious of its effects, e.g. an increase in the heart rate.

The effects of autonomic control are rapid and essential for homeostasis.

The effector organs are:

- smooth muscle
- cardiac muscle
- glands (Fig. 7.6).

Effects of autonomic stimulation include:

- changes in rate and force of the heartbeat
- stimulation or depression of secretion of glands
- vasoconstriction or vasodilatation
- bronchoconstriction or bronchodilation
- changes in size of the pupils of the eyes.

The *efferent (motor) nerves* of the autonomic nervous system arise from nerve cells in the brain and emerge at various levels between the midbrain and the sacral region of the spinal cord. Many of them travel within the same nerve sheath as the peripheral nerves of the central nervous system to reach the organs which they innervate.

The autonomic nervous system is divided into two divisions:

- *sympathetic* (thoracolumbar outflow)
- *parasympathetic* (craniosacral outflow).

The two divisions have both structural and functional differences. They normally work in an opposing manner, enabling or restoring balance of involuntary functions, maintaining homeostasis. Sympathetic activity tends to predominate in stressful situations and parasympathetic activity during rest.

Each division has two efferent neurones in its peripheral pathways between the central nervous system and effector organs. These are:

- the preganglionic neurone
- the postganglionic neurone.

The cell body of the preganglionic neurone is in the brain or spinal cord. Its axon terminals synapse with the cell body of the postganglionic neurone in an *autonomic ganglion* outside the central nervous system. The postganglionic neurone conducts impulses to the effector organ (Fig. 7.9).

Sympathetic nervous system

Neurones convey impulses from their origin in the hypothalamus, reticular formation and medulla oblongata to effector organs and tissues (Fig. 7.43). The first neurone has its cell body in the brain and its fibre extends into the spinal cord.

The preganglionic neurone. This has its cell body in the *lateral column of grey matter* in the spinal cord between the levels of the 1st thoracic and 2nd or 3rd lumbar vertebrae. The nerve fibre of this cell leaves the cord by the anterior root and terminates in one of the ganglia either in the *lateral chain of sympathetic ganglia* or passes through it to one of the *prevertebral ganglia*. Acetylcholine is the neurotransmitter.

The postganglionic neurone. This has its cell body in a ganglion and terminates in the organ or tissue supplied. Noradrenaline is usually the neurotransmitter.

Sympathetic ganglia

The lateral chains of sympathetic ganglia. These are chains of ganglia which extend from the upper cervical level to the sacrum, one chain lying on each side of the bodies of the vertebrae. The ganglia are attached to each other by nerve fibres. Preganglionic neurones that emerge from the cord may synapse with the cell body of the postganglionic neurone at the same level or they may pass up or down the chain through one or more ganglia before synapsing. For example, the nerve which dilates the pupil of the eye leaves the cord at the level of the 1st thoracic vertebra and passes up the chain to the superior cervical ganglion before it synapses with the cell body of the postsynaptic neurone. The postganglionic neurones then pass to the eyes. The major exception is that there is no parasympathetic supply to the sweat glands, the skin

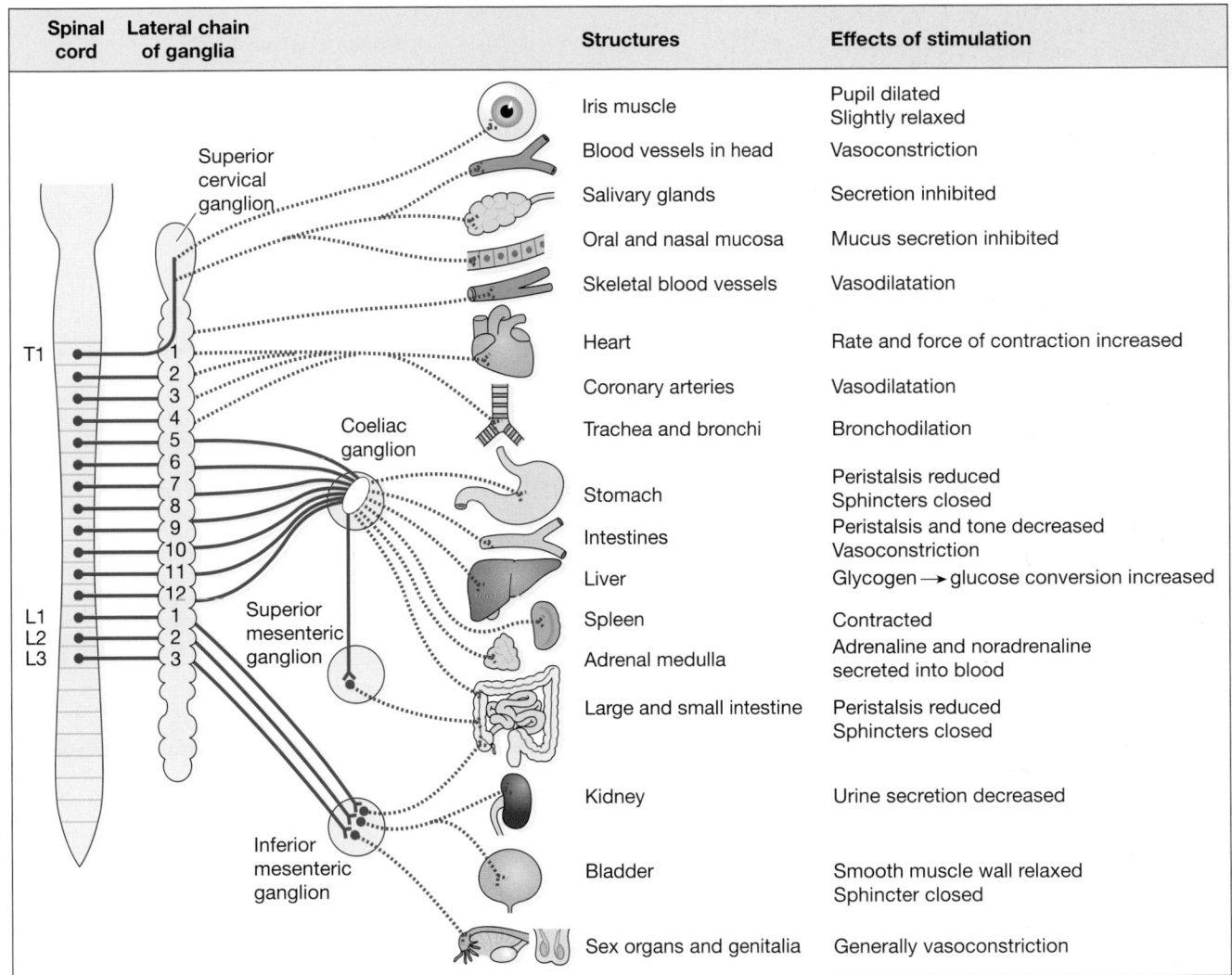

Spinal cord	Lateral chain of ganglia		Structures	Effects of stimulation
			Iris muscle	Pupil dilated Slightly relaxed
			Blood vessels in head	Vasoconstriction
			Salivary glands	Secretion inhibited
			Oral and nasal mucosa	Mucus secretion inhibited
			Skeletal blood vessels	Vasodilatation
			Heart	Rate and force of contraction increased
			Coronary arteries	Vasodilatation
			Trachea and bronchi	Bronchodilation
			Stomach	Peristalsis reduced Sphincters closed
			Intestines	Peristalsis and tone decreased Vasoconstriction
			Liver	Glycogen → glucose conversion increased
			Spleen	Contracted
			Adrenal medulla	Adrenaline and noradrenaline secreted into blood
			Large and small intestine	Peristalsis reduced Sphincters closed
			Kidney	Urine secretion decreased
			Bladder	Smooth muscle wall relaxed Sphincter closed
			Sex organs and genitalia	Generally vasoconstriction

Figure 7.43 The sympathetic outflow, the main structures supplied and the effects of stimulation. Solid red lines – preganglionic fibres; broken lines – postganglionic fibres. There is a right and left lateral chain of ganglia.

and blood vessels of skeletal muscles. These structures are supplied by only sympathetic fibres, some of which have acetylcholine and some adrenaline and noradrenaline as their neurotransmitter. They have, therefore, the effects of both sympathetic and parasympathetic nerve supply (Fig. 7.43).

Prevertebral ganglia. There are three prevertebral ganglia situated in the abdominal cavity close to the origins of arteries of the same names:

- coeliac ganglion
- superior mesenteric ganglion
- inferior mesenteric ganglion.

The ganglia consist of nerve cell bodies rather diffusely distributed among a network of nerve fibres which form plexuses. Preganglionic sympathetic fibres pass through the lateral chain to reach these ganglia.

Parasympathetic nervous system

Two neurones (preganglionic and postganglionic) are involved in the transmission of impulses from their source to the effector organ (Fig. 7.44). The neurotransmitter at both synapses is acetylcholine.

The preganglionic neurone. This has its cell body either in the brain or in the spinal cord. Those originating in the brain are the *cranial nerves* III, VII, IX and X, arising from nuclei in the midbrain and brain stem, and their nerve fibres terminate outside the brain. The cell bodies of the *sacral outflow* are in the lateral columns of grey

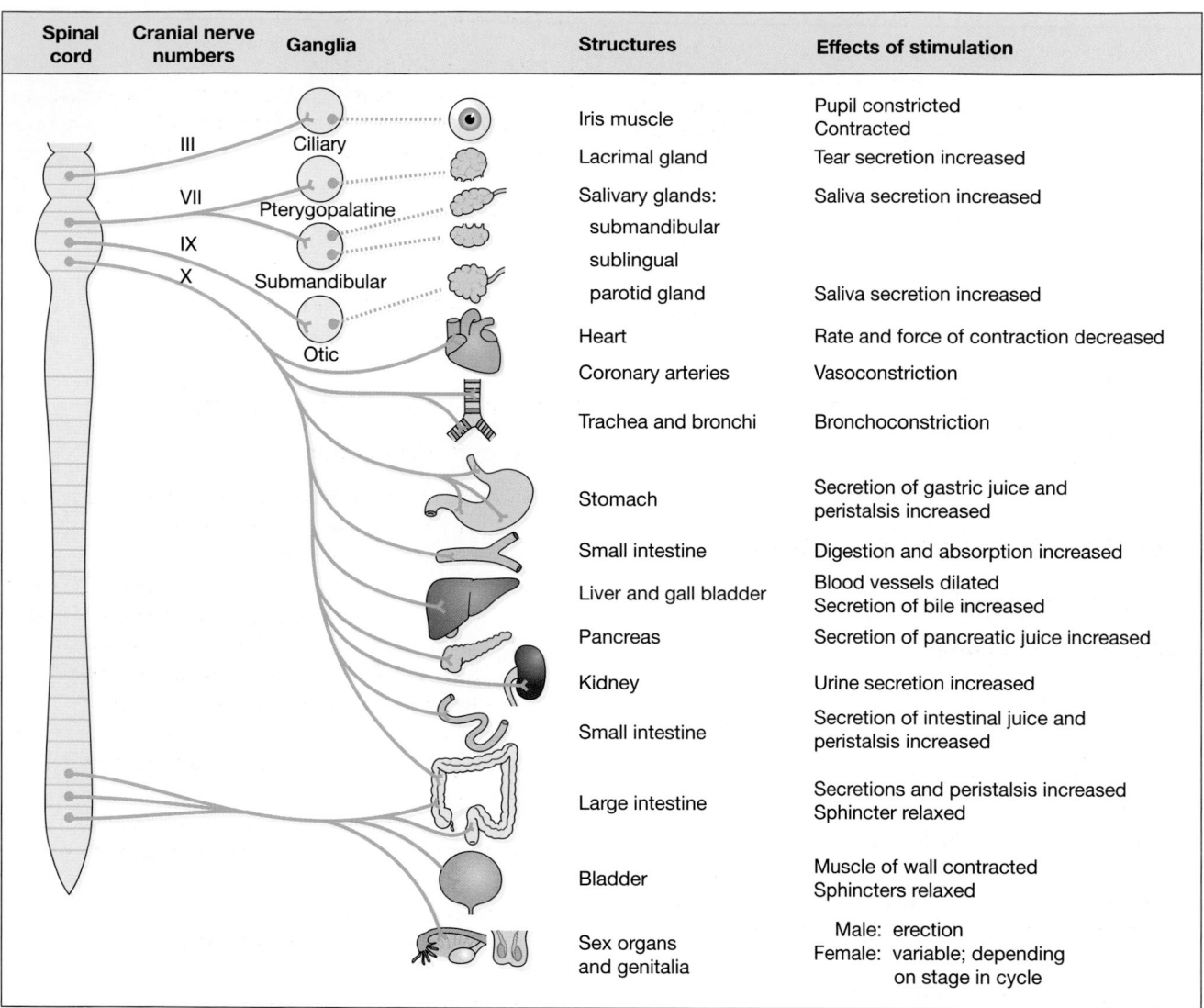

Spinal cord	Cranial nerve numbers	Ganglia	Structures	Effects of stimulation
	III	Ciliary	Iris muscle	Pupil constricted Contracted
	VII	Pterygopalatine	Lacrimal gland	Tear secretion increased
	IX		Salivary glands: submandibular sublingual	Saliva secretion increased
	X	Submandibular	parotid gland	Saliva secretion increased
		Otic	Heart	Rate and force of contraction decreased
			Coronary arteries	Vasoconstriction
			Trachea and bronchi	Bronchoconstriction
			Stomach	Secretion of gastric juice and peristalsis increased
			Small intestine	Digestion and absorption increased
			Liver and gall bladder	Blood vessels dilated Secretion of bile increased
			Pancreas	Secretion of pancreatic juice increased
			Kidney	Urine secretion increased
			Small intestine	Secretion of intestinal juice and peristalsis increased
			Large intestine	Secretions and peristalsis increased Sphincter relaxed
			Bladder	Muscle of wall contracted Sphincters relaxed
			Sex organs and genitalia	Male: erection Female: variable; depending on stage in cycle

Figure 7.44 The parasympathetic outflow, the main structures supplied and the effects of stimulation. Solid blue lines – preganglionic fibres; broken lines – postganglionic fibres. Where there are no broken lines, the postganglionic neurone is in the wall of the structure.

matter at the distal end of the spinal cord. Their fibres leave the cord in sacral segments 2, 3 and 4 and synapse with postganglionic neurones in the walls of pelvic organs.

The postganglionic neurone. This has its cell body either in a ganglion or in the wall of the organ supplied.

Functions of the autonomic nervous system

The autonomic nervous system is involved in a complex of reflex activities which, like the reflexes described

previously, depend on sensory input to the brain or spinal cord, and on motor output. In this case the reflex action is rapid contraction, or inhibition of contraction, of involuntary (smooth and cardiac) muscle or glandular secretion. These reflexes are coordinated subconsciously in the brain, i.e. below the level of the cerebrum. Some sensory input does reach consciousness and may result in temporary inhibition of the reflex action, e.g. reflex micturition can be inhibited temporarily.

The majority of the organs of the body are supplied by both sympathetic and parasympathetic nerves which have opposite effects that are finely balanced to ensure the optimum functioning of the organ.

Sympathetic stimulation prepares the body to deal with exciting and stressful situations, e.g. strengthening its defences in danger and in extremes of environmental temperature. The adrenal glands are stimulated to secrete the hormones adrenaline and noradrenaline into the bloodstream. These hormones potentiate and sustain the effects of sympathetic stimulation. It is sometimes said that sympathetic stimulation mobilises the body for 'fight or flight'.

Parasympathetic stimulation has a tendency to slow down body processes except digestion and absorption of food and the functions of the genitourinary systems. Its general effect is that of a 'peace maker' allowing restoration processes to occur quietly and peacefully.

Normally the two systems function together maintaining a regular heartbeat, normal temperature and an internal environment compatible with the immediate external surroundings.

Effects of autonomic stimulation

Cardiovascular system

Sympathetic stimulation

- Exerts an accelerating effect upon the sinoatrial node in the heart, increasing the rate and force of the heartbeat.
- Causes dilatation of the coronary arteries, increasing the blood supply to cardiac muscle.
- Causes dilatation of the blood vessels supplying skeletal muscle, increasing the supply of oxygen and nutritional materials and the removal of metabolic waste products, thus increasing the capacity of the muscle to work.
- Raises peripheral resistance and blood pressure by constricting the small arteries and arterioles in the skin. In this way an increased blood supply is available for highly active tissue, such as skeletal muscle, heart, brain.
- Constricts the blood vessels in the secretory glands of the digestive system, reducing the flow of digestive juices. This raises the volume of blood available for circulation in dilated blood vessels.
- Blood coagulation occurs more quickly because of vasoconstriction.

Parasympathetic stimulation

- Decreases the rate and force of the heartbeat.
- Causes constriction of the coronary arteries reducing the blood supply to cardiac muscle.

The parasympathetic nervous system exerts little or no effect on blood vessels except the coronary arteries.

Respiratory system

Sympathetic stimulation

This causes dilatation of the airways, especially the bronchioles, allowing a greater amount of air to enter the lungs at each inspiration and increases the respiratory rate. In conjunction with the increased heart rate, the oxygen intake and carbon dioxide output of the body are increased.

Parasympathetic stimulation

Produces constriction of the bronchi.

Digestive and urinary systems

Sympathetic stimulation

- *The liver* converts an increased amount of glycogen to glucose, making more carbohydrate immediately available to provide energy.
- *The adrenal (suprarenal) glands* are stimulated to secrete adrenaline and noradrenaline which potentiate and sustain the effects of sympathetic stimulation.
- *The stomach* and *small intestine*. Smooth muscle contraction and secretion of digestive juices are inhibited, delaying digestion, onward movement and absorption of food and the tone of sphincter muscles is increased.
- *Urethral* and *anal sphincters*. The muscle tone of the sphincters is increased, inhibiting micturition and defecation.
- *The bladder wall* relaxes.
- *The metabolic rate* is greatly increased.

Parasympathetic stimulation

- *The stomach* and *small intestine*. The rate of digestion and absorption of food is increased.
- *The pancreas*. There is an increase in the secretion of pancreatic juice and the hormone insulin.
- *Urethral* and *anal sphincters*. Relaxation of the internal urethral sphincter is accompanied by contraction of the muscle of the bladder wall and micturition occurs. Similar relaxation of the internal anal sphincter is accompanied by contraction of the muscle of the rectum and defecation occurs. In both cases there is voluntary relaxation of the external sphincters.

Eye

Sympathetic stimulation

This causes contraction of the radiating muscle fibres of the iris, *dilating* the pupil. Retraction of the levator palpebral muscles occurs, opening the eyes wide and giving the appearance of alertness and excitement. The ciliary muscle that adjusts the thickness of the lens is slightly relaxed.

Parasympathetic stimulation

This causes contraction of the circular muscle fibres of the iris, constricting the pupil. The eyelids tend to close, giving the appearance of sleepiness.

Skin

Sympathetic stimulation

- Causes increased secretion of sweat, leading to increased heat loss from the body.
- Produces contraction of the arrectores pilorum (the muscles in the hair follicles of the skin), giving the appearance of 'goose flesh'.
- Causes constriction of the blood vessels preventing heat loss.

There is no parasympathetic nerve supply to the skin. Some sympathetic fibres are adrenergic, causing vasoconstriction, and some are cholinergic, causing vasodilatation (Fig. 7.9).

Afferent impulses from viscera

Sensory fibres from the viscera travel with autonomic fibres and are sometimes called *autonomic afferents*. The impulses they transmit are associated with:

- visceral reflexes, usually at an unconscious level, e.g. cough, blood pressure
- sensation of, e.g., hunger, thirst, nausea, sexual sensation, rectal and bladder distension
- visceral pain.

Visceral pain

Normally the viscera are insensitive to cutting, burning and crushing. However, a sensation of dull, poorly located pain is experienced when:

- visceral nerves are stretched
- a large number of fibres are stimulated
- there is ischaemia and local accumulation of metabolites
- the sensitivity of nerve endings to painful stimuli is increased, e.g. during inflammation.

If the cause of the pain, e.g. inflammation, affects the parietal layer of a serous membrane (pleura, peritoneum)

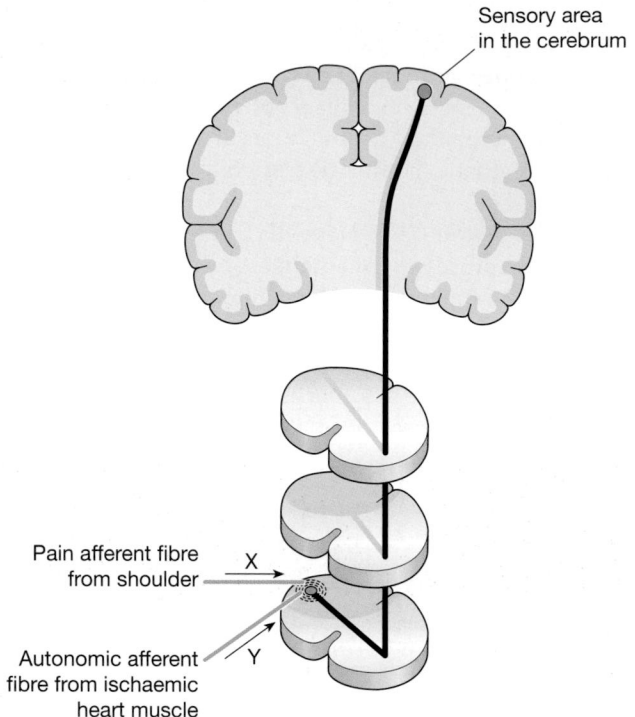

Figure 7.45 Referred pain. Pain perceived to originate from the tissues supplied by the damaged nerve. Y stimulates X and pain is perceived in the shoulder.

the pain is acute and easily located over the site of inflammation. This is because the peripheral spinal (somatic) nerves supplying the superficial tissues also supply the parietal layer of serous membrane. They transmit the impulses to the cerebral cortex where *somatic pain* is perceived and accurately located. Appendicitis is an example of this type of pain. Initially it is dull and vaguely located around the midline of the abdomen. As the condition progresses the parietal peritoneum becomes involved and acute pain is clearly located in the right iliac fossa, i.e. over the appendix.

Referred pain (Fig. 7.45)

In some cases of visceral disease pain may be perceived to occur in superficial tissues remote from the viscus, i.e. referred pain. This occurs when sensory fibres from the viscus enter the same segment of the spinal cord as somatic nerves, i.e. those from the superficial tissues. It is believed that the sensory nerve from the viscus stimulates the closely associated nerve in the spinal cord and it transmits the impulses to the sensory area in the cerebral cortex where the pain is perceived as originating in the area supplied by the somatic nerve. Examples of referred pain are given in Table 7.4.

Table 7.4 Referred pain	
Tissue of origin of pain	**Site of referred pain**
Heart	Left shoulder
Liver Biliary tract	Right shoulder
Kidney Ureter	Loin and groin
Uterus	Low back
Male genitalia	Low abdomen
Prolapsed intervertebral disc	Leg

RESPONSE OF NERVOUS TISSUE TO INJURY

Learning outcome

After studying this section you should be able to:

■ outline the response of nervous tissue to injury.

Neurone damage

Damage to the nerve cells or their processes can lead to rapid necrosis with sudden acute functional failure, or to slow atrophy with gradually increasing dysfunction. These changes are associated with:

■ hypoxia and anoxia
■ nutritional deficiencies
■ poisons, e.g. organic lead
■ trauma
■ infections
■ ageing
■ hypoglycaemia.

Neurone regeneration (Fig. 7.46)

Neurones of the brain, spinal cord and ganglia reach maturity a few weeks after birth and are not replaced when they are damaged or die.

The axons of *peripheral nerves* may regenerate if the cell body remains intact. Distal to the damage the axon and myelin sheath disintegrate and are removed by macrophages, but the Schwann cells survive and proliferate within the neurilemma. The live proximal part of the

175

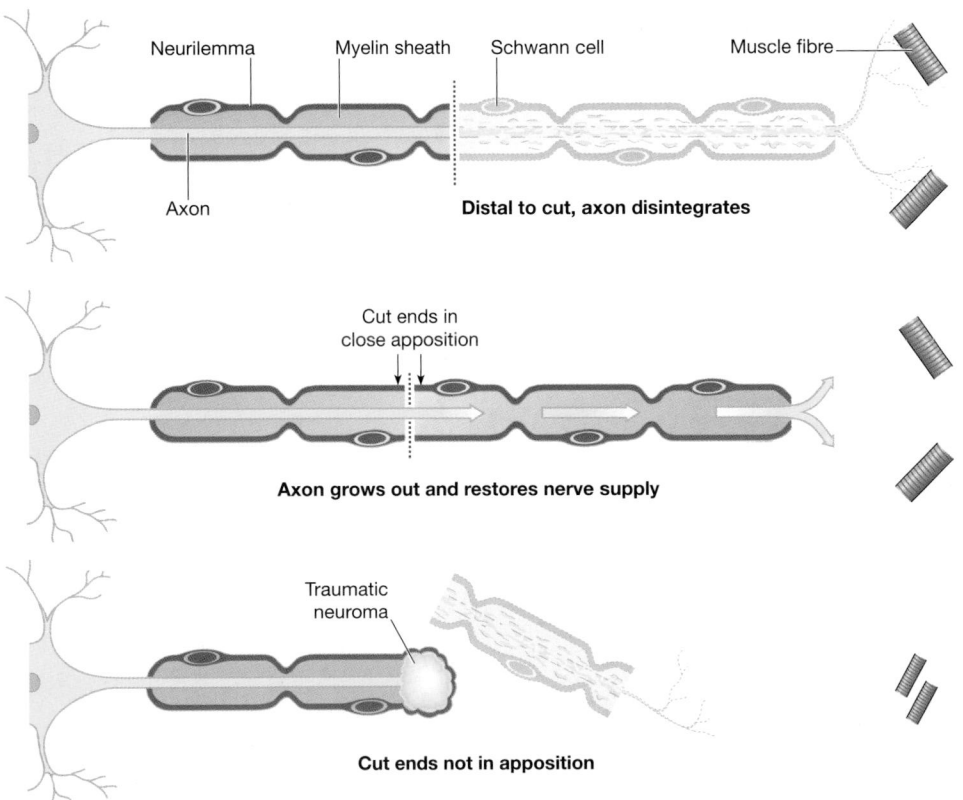

Distal to cut, axon disintegrates

Axon grows out and restores nerve supply

Cut ends not in apposition

Figure 7.46 Regrowth of peripheral nerves following injury.

axon grows along the original track (about 3 mm per day), provided the two parts of neurilemma are correctly positioned and in close apposition. Restoration of function depends on the re-establishment of satisfactory connections with the end organ. When the neurilemma is out of position or destroyed the sprouting axons and Schwann cells form a tumour-like cluster (*traumatic neuroma*) producing severe pain, e.g. following some fractures and amputation of limbs.

Neuroglia damage

Astrocytes

When severely damaged, astrocytes undergo necrosis and disintegrate. In less severe and chronic conditions there is proliferation of astrocyte processes and later cell atrophy (*gliosis*). This process occurs in many diseases and is analogous to fibrosis in other tissues.

Oligodendrocytes

These cells form and maintain myelin, having the same functions as Schwann cells in peripheral nerves. They increase in number around degenerating neurones and are destroyed in demyelinating diseases such as *multiple sclerosis* (p. 184).

Microglia

Microglia are derived from monocytes that migrate from the blood into the nervous system before birth, and are found mainly around blood vessels. Where there is inflammation and cell destruction the microglia increase in size and become phagocytic.

Effects of poisons on the central nervous system

Many chemical substances encountered either as drugs or in the environment may damage the nervous system. Neurone metabolism may be disturbed directly or result from damage to other organs, e.g. liver, kidneys. The outcome depends on the toxicity of the substance, the dose and the duration of exposure, ranging from short-term neurological disturbance to encephalopathy which may cause coma and death.

DISORDERS OF THE BRAIN

Learning outcomes

After studying this section you should be able to:

- list three causes of raised intracranial pressure (ICP)
- relate the effects of raised ICP to the functions of the brain and changes in vital signs
- outline how the brain is damaged during different types of head injury
- describe four complications of head injury
- explain the effects of cerebral hypoxia and stroke
- outline the causes and effects of dementia
- relate the pathology of Parkinson's disease to its effects on body function.

Increased intracranial pressure

This is a very serious complication of many conditions. The cranium forms a rigid cavity enclosing:

- the brain
- cerebral blood vessels and blood
- cerebrospinal fluid (CSF).

An increase in volume of any one of these will lead to raised intracranial pressure. Sometimes its effects are more serious than the condition causing it, e.g. by disrupting the blood supply or distorting the shape of the brain especially if the intracranial pressure (ICP) rises rapidly. A slow rise in ICP allows time for compensatory adjustment to be made, i.e. a slight reduction in the volume of circulating blood and of CSF. The slower the rise in ICP, the more effective the compensation. Rising ICP is accompanied by bradycardia and hypertension. As it reaches its limit a further small increase in pressure is followed by a sudden and usually serious reduction in the cerebral blood flow. The result is hypoxia and a rise in carbon dioxide levels, causing arteriolar dilatation which further increases the ICP. This leads to progressive loss of functioning neurones, which exacerbates bradycardia and hypertension. Further cerebral hypoxia causes *vasomotor paralysis* and death.

The causes of increased ICP are described on the following pages and include:

- cerebral oedema
- hydrocephalus, the accumulation of excess CSF
- expanding lesions inside the skull, also known as space-occupying lesions
  –haemorrhage, haematoma (traumatic or spontaneous)
  –tumours (primary or secondary).

Expanding lesions may occur in the brain or in the meninges and they may damage the brain in various ways (Fig. 7.47).

Effects of increased ICP

Displacement of the brain
Lesions causing displacement are usually one-sided but may affect both sides. Such lesions may cause:

- *herniation* (displacement of part of the brain from its usual compartment) of the cerebral hemisphere between the corpus callosum and the free border of the falx cerebri on the same side

A Subdural haematoma   B Subarachnoid haemorrhage   C Tumour or intracerebral haemorrhage

Figure 7.47 Effects of different types of expanding lesions inside the skull: A. Subdural haematoma. B. Subarachnoid haemorrhage. C. Tumour or intracerebral haemorrhage.

- herniation of the midbrain between the pons and the free border of the tentorium cerebelli on the same side
- compression of the subarachnoid space and flattening of the cerebral convolutions
- distortion of the shape of the ventricles and their ducts
- herniation of the cerebellum through the foramen magnum
- protrusion of the medulla oblongata through the foramen magnum ('*coning*').

Obstruction of the flow of cerebrospinal fluid

The ventricles or their ducts may be pushed out of position or a duct obstructed. The effects depend on the position of the lesion, e.g. compression of the aqueduct of the midbrain causes dilatation of the lateral ventricles and the third ventricle, further increasing the ICP.

Vascular damage

There may be stretching or compression of blood vessels, causing:

- haemorrhage when stretched blood vessels rupture
- ischaemia and infarction due to compression of blood vessels
- papilloedema (oedema round the optic disc) due to compression of the retinal vein in the optic nerve sheath where it crosses the subarachnoid space.

Neural damage

The vital centres in the medulla oblongata may be damaged when the increased ICP causes 'coning'. Stretching may damage cranial nerves, especially the oculomotor (III) and the abducent (VI), causing disturbances of eye movement and accommodation.

Bone changes

Prolonged increase of ICP causes bony changes, e.g.:

- erosion, especially of the sphenoid
- stretching and thinning before ossification is complete.

Cerebral oedema

There is movement of fluid from its normal compartment when oedema develops (p. 118). Cerebral oedema occurs when there is excess fluid in brain cells and/or in the interstitial spaces, causing increased intracranial pressure. It is associated with:

- traumatic injury
- haemorrhage
- infections, abscesses
- hypoxia

- local ischaemia, infarcts
- tumours
- inflammation of the brain or meninges
- hypoglycaemia.

Cytotoxic oedema

The neurones and neuroglial cells contain excess water due to disturbances of their osmotic pressure caused by retention of excess electrolytes. The permeability of the capillary walls is normal.

Vaosgenic oedema

Excess fluid collects in the interstitial spaces, especially round nerve fibres. The permeability of the capillary walls is increased and plasma proteins pass out of the capillaries, increasing the osmotic pressure in the interstitial spaces which causes oedema.

Hydrocephalus

In this condition the volume of CSF is abnormally high and is usually accompanied by increased ICP. An obstruction to CSF flow (Fig. 7.14) is the most common cause. It is described as *communicating* when there is free flow of CSF from the ventricular system to the subarachnoid space and *non-communicating* when there is not, i.e. there is obstruction in the system of ventricles, foramina or ducts.

Enlargement of the head occurs in children when ossification of the cranial bones is incomplete but, in spite of this, the ventricles dilate and cause stretching and thinning of the brain. After ossification is complete, hydrocephalus leads to a marked increase in ICP and destruction of neural tissue.

Primary hydrocephalus

This is usually caused by obstruction to the flow of CSF and may be communicating or non-communicating. Occasionally it is caused by malabsorption of CSF by the arachnoid villi.

Congenital primary hydrocephalus is due to malformation of the ventricles, foramina or ducts, usually at a narrow point.

Acquired primary hydrocephalus is caused by lesions that obstruct the circulation of the CSF, usually expanding lesions, e.g. tumours, haematomas or adhesions between arachnoid and pia maters, following meningitis.

Secondary hydrocephalus

Compensatory increases in the amount of CSF and ventricle capacity occur when there is atrophy of brain tissue, e.g. in dementia and following cerebral infarcts. There may not be a rise in ICP.

Head injuries

The brain may be injured by a blow to the head or movement of the brain during sudden acceleration or deceleration of the head. The damage to the brain may be serious even when there is no outward sign of injury.

Blow to the head

At the site of injury there may be:

- a scalp wound, with haemorrhage between scalp and skull bones
- damage to the underlying meninges and/or brain with local haemorrhage inside the skull
- depressed fracture of the skull, causing local damage to the underlying meninges and brain tissue
- temporal bone fracture, making an opening between the middle ear and the meninges
- fracture involving the air sinuses of the sphenoid, ethmoid or frontal bones, making an opening between the nose and the meninges.

Acceleration–deceleration injuries

Because the brain floats relatively freely in 'a cushion' of CSF, sudden acceleration or deceleration has an inertia effect, i.e. there is delay between the movement of the head and the corresponding movement of the brain. During this period the brain may be compressed and damaged at the site of impact. In '*contre coup*' injuries, brain damage is more severe on the side opposite to the site of impact. Other injuries include:

- nerve cell damage, usually to the frontal and parietal lobes, due to movement of the brain over the rough surface of bones of the base of the skull
- nerve fibre damage due to stretching, especially following rotational movement
- haemorrhage due to rupture of blood vessels in the subarachnoid space *on the side opposite* the impact or more diffuse small haemorrhages, following rotational movement.

Complications of head injury

If the individual survives the immediate effects, complications may develop hours or days later. Sometimes they are the first indication of serious damage caused by a seemingly trivial injury. Their effects may be to increase ICP, damage brain tissue or provide a route of entry for microbes.

Traumatic intracranial haemorrhage

Haemorrhage may occur causing secondary brain damage at the site of injury, on the opposite side of the brain or diffusely throughout the brain. If bleeding continues, the expanding haematoma damages the brain and increases the ICP.

Extradural haemorrhage

This may follow a direct blow that may or may not cause a fracture. The individual may recover quickly and indications of increased ICP only appear several hours later as the haematoma grows and the outer layer of dura mater (periosteum) is stripped off the bone. The haematoma grows rapidly when arterial blood vessels are damaged. In children there is rarely a fracture because the skull bones are still soft and the joints have not fused. The haematoma usually remains localised.

Acute subdural haemorrhage

This is due to haemorrhage from small veins in the dura mater or from larger veins between the layers of dura mater before they enter the venous sinuses. The blood may spread in the subdural space over one or both hemispheres (Fig. 7.47B). There may be concurrent subarachnoid haemorrhage, especially when there are extensive brain contusions and lacerations.

Chronic subdural haemorrhage

This may occur weeks or months after minor injuries and sometimes there is no history of injury. It occurs most commonly in people in whom there is some cerebral atrophy, e.g. the elderly and alcoholics. Evidence of increased ICP may be delayed when brain volume is reduced. The haematoma formed gradually increases in size due to repeated small haemorrhages and causes mild chronic inflammation and accumulation of inflammatory exudate. In time it is isolated by a wall of fibrous tissue.

Intracerebral haemorrhage and cerebral oedema

These occur following contusions, lacerations and shearing injuries associated with acceleration and deceleration, especially rotational movements.

Cerebral oedema is a common complication of contusions of the brain, leading to increased ICP, hypoxia and further brain damage.

Meningitis

Inflammation of the meninges may occur following a compound fracture of the skull that is accompanied by leakage of CSF and blood from the site, providing a route

179

of entry for microbes. The escape of CSF and blood may be through:

- skin, in compound fractures of the skull
- middle ear, in fractures of the temporal bone (CSF otorrhoea)
- nose, in fractures of sphenoid, ethmoid or frontal bones when the air sinuses are involved (CSF rhinorrhoea).

Post-traumatic epilepsy

This is usually characterised by seizures (fits) and may develop in the first week or several months after injury. Early development is most common after severe injuries, although in children the injury itself may have appeared trivial. After depressed fractures or large haematomas epilepsy tends to develop later.

Persistent vegetative state

In this condition there is severe brain damage that results in unconsciousness but the vital centres that control homeostasis remain intact, e.g. breathing, blood pressure.

Circulatory disturbances affecting the brain

A number of abnormalities of the circulation, not associated with head injuries, commonly affect the brain.

Cerebral hypoxia

Hypoxia may be due to:

- disturbances in the autoregulation of blood supply to the brain
- conditions affecting cerebral blood vessels.

When the mean blood pressure falls below about 60 mmHg there is failure of the autoregulating mechanisms that control the blood flow to the brain by adjusting the diameter of the arterioles. The consequent rapid decrease in the cerebral blood supply leads to hypoxia and lack of glucose. If severe hypoxia is sustained for more than a few minutes there is irreversible brain damage. The neurones are affected first, then the neuroglial cells and later the meninges and blood vessels. Conditions in which autoregulation breaks down include:

- cardiorespiratory arrest
- sudden severe hypotension

- carbon monoxide poisoning
- hypercapnia (excess blood carbon dioxide)
- drug overdosage with, e.g., narcotics, hypnotics, analgesics.

Conditions affecting cerebral blood vessels that may lead to hypoxia include:

- occlusion of a cerebral artery by, e.g., atheroma, thrombosis, rapidly expanding lesion, embolism
- arterial stenosis that occurs in arteritis, e.g. polyarteritis nodosa, syphilis, diabetes, degenerative changes in the elderly.

If the individual survives the initial episode of ischaemia, infarction, necrosis and loss of function of the affected area of brain occurs.

Stroke (cerebrovascular disease)

This condition is a common cause of death and disability, especially in the elderly. Predisposing factors include:

- hypertension
- atheroma
- cigarette smoking
- diabetes mellitus.

It occurs when a vascular disease suddenly interrupts flow of blood to the brain causing hypoxia. The effects include paralysis of a limb or one side of the body and disturbances of speech and vision. The nature and extent of cerebral impairment depends on the size and location of the affected blood vessels. The main causes are cerebral infarction (approx 85%) and spontaneous intracranial haemorrhage (15%).

Cerebral infarction

This is caused by atheroma complicated by thrombosis (p. 113) or blockage of an artery by an embolus from, e.g., infective endocarditis. When complete recovery occurs within 24 hours, the event is called a *transient ischaemic attack* (TIA). Recurrence or *completed stroke* associated with permanent damage may follow.

Spontaneous intracranial haemorrhage

The haemorrhage may be into the subarachnoid space or intracerebral (Fig. 7.48). It is commonly associated with an aneurysm or hypertension. In each case the escaped blood may cause arterial spasm, leading to ischaemia, infarction, fibrosis (gliosis) and hypoxic brain damage. A severe haemorrhage may be instantly fatal while repeated small haemorrhages have a cumulative effect in extending brain damage (multi-infarct dementia).

Figure 7.48 Types of haemorrhage causing stroke: A. Intracerebral. B. Subarachnoid.

Intracerebral haemorrhage

Prolonged hypertension leads to the formation of multiple microaneurysms in the walls of very small arteries in the brain. Rupture of one or more of these, due to continuing rise in blood pressure, is usually the cause of intracerebral haemorrhage. The most common sites are branches of the middle cerebral artery in the region of the internal capsule and the basal nuclei (ganglia).

Severe haemorrhage. This causes compression and destruction of tissue, a sudden increase in ICP and distortion and herniation of the brain. Death follows when the vital centres in the medulla oblongata are damaged by haemorrhage or if there is coning due to increased ICP.

Less severe haemorrhage. This causes paralysis and loss of sensation of varying severity, affecting the side of the body opposite the haemorrhage. If the bleeding stops and does not recur an *apoplectic cyst* develops, i.e. the haematoma is walled off by gliosis, the blood clot is gradually absorbed and the cavity filled with tissue exudate. When the ICP returns to normal some functions may be restored, e.g. speech and movement of limbs.

Subarachnoid haemorrhage

This is mostly due to rupture of a berry aneurysm on one of the major cerebral arteries or bleeding from a congenitally malformed blood vessel. The blood may remain localised but usually spreads in the subarachnoid space round the brain and spinal cord, causing a general increase in ICP without distortion of the brain (Fig. 7.47B). The irritant effect of the blood may cause arterial spasm, leading to ischaemia, infarction, gliosis and the effects of localised brain damage. It occurs most commonly in middle life, but occasionally in young people due to rapture of a malformed blood vessel. This condition is often fatal or results in permanent disability.

Dementia

Dementia is caused by progressive, irreversible degeneration and atrophy of the cerebral cortex and results in mental deterioration, usually over several years. There is gradual impairment of memory (especially short term), intellect and reasoning. Emotional lability and personality change may also occur.

Alzheimer's disease

This condition was previously called pre-senile dementia and is the commonest form of dementia. It is of unknown aetiology although genetic factors may be involved. Females are affected twice as often as males and it usually affects those over 60 years, the incidence increasing with age. There is progressive atrophy of the cerebral cortex accompanied by deteriorating mental functioning. Death usually occurs between 2 and 8 years after onset.

Huntington's disease (chorea)

This usually manifests itself between the ages of 30 and 50 years. It is caused by a genetic abnormality associated with deficient production of the neurotransmitter gamma aminobutyric acid (GABA). By the time of onset, the individual may have passed the genetic abnormality on to the next generation. Extrapyramidal changes cause *chorea*, rapid uncoordinated jerking movements of the limbs and involuntary twitching of the facial muscles. As the disease progresses, cortical atrophy causes personality changes and dementia.

Secondary dementias

Dementia may occur in association with other diseases:

- cerebrovascular disease—*multi-infarct dementia* is the cumulative result of several small cerebral infarcts leading to the gradually increasing impairment of mental function
- infections, e.g. encephalitis, neurosyphilis, human immunodeficiency virus (HIV), Creutzfeldt–Jakob disease

Figure 7.49 Shuffling gait of Parkinson's disease.

- cerebral trauma
- chronic abuse of alcohol and some drugs
- vitamin B deficiency
- effects of metabolic disorders, e.g. hypothyroidism, uraemia, liver failure.

182

Parkinson's disease

In this disease there is gradual degeneration of dopamine-releasing neurones in the extrapyramidal system. This leads to lack of control and coordination of muscle movement resulting in:

- fixed muscle tone causing expressionless facial features, rigidity of voluntary muscles causing the slow and characteristic stiff shuffling gait and stooping posture
- muscle tremor of extremities, e.g. 'pill rolling' movement of the fingers.

The cause is usually unknown but some cases are associated with repeated trauma as in, e.g., 'punch drunk' boxers; tumours, causing midbrain compression; drugs, e.g. phenothiazines; heavy metal poisoning. There is progressive physical disability but the intellect is not impaired (Fig. 7.49).

INFECTIONS OF THE CENTRAL NERVOUS SYSTEM

Learning outcome

After studying this section you should be able to:

- describe common infections of the nervous system and their effects on body function.

The brain and spinal cord are relatively well protected from microbial infection by the blood–brain barrier. When infection does occur microbes may be:

- blood-borne from infection elsewhere in the body, e.g. lung abscess
- introduced through a skull fracture (p. 179)
- spread through the skull bones from, e.g., middle ear infection, mastoiditis, skull bone infection
- introduced during a surgical procedure, e.g. lumbar puncture.

The microbes usually involved are bacteria and viruses, occasionally protozoa and fungi. The infection may originate in the meninges (*meningitis*) or in the brain (*encephalitis*), then spread from one site to the other.

Pyogenic infection

Pyogenic meningitis

Meningitis is most commonly transmitted through contact with an infected individual. Pyogenic (bacterial) infection of the meninges is usually preceded by a mild respiratory tract infection during which a few bacteria enter the bloodstream. They are carried to the meninges where they may remain localised in the extradural or subdural space. If an abscess forms it may rupture into the subarachnoid space and spread to the brain, causing encephalitis and further abscess formation. Infection of the arachnoid mater tends to spread diffusely in the subarachnoid space round the brain and spinal cord.

The onset is usually sudden with severe headache, neck stiffness, photophobia and fever. This may be accompanied by a petechial rash in some cases. Mortality and morbidity rates are considerable.

Pyogenic encephalitis

This may involve single or multiple sites, usually with abscess formation. The microbes are either bloodborne or spread from adjacent meningeal infection. The effects include the following.

- Inflammatory oedema and abscess formation lead to increased ICP, hypoxia and further brain damage.
- When meningitis follows encephalitis, healing takes place with the formation of fibrous adhesions which may interfere with CSF circulation and cause hydrocephalus, or compress blood vessels, causing hypoxia.
- Following encephalitis and brain abscess, healing is associated with gliosis and, as destroyed nerve cells are not replaced, loss of function depends on the site and extent of brain damage.

Viral infections

Viral infections of the nervous system are relatively rare even when caused by *neurotropic viruses*, i.e. those with an affinity for the nervous system. Viruses may cause meningitis, encephalitis or lesions of the neurones of spinal cord and peripheral nerves. Most viruses are bloodborne although a few travel along peripheral nerves, e.g. rabies virus and possibly polioviruses. They enter the body via:

- alimentary tract, e.g. poliomyelitis
- respiratory tract, e.g. shingles
- skin abrasions, e.g. rabies.

The effects of viral infections vary according to the site and the amount of tissue destroyed. Viruses are believed to damage nerve cells by:

- 'taking over' their metabolism
- stimulating an immune reaction which may explain why signs of some infections do not appear until there is a high antibody titre, 1 to 2 weeks after infection.

Viral meningitis

This is sometimes called 'aseptic' meningitis because cultures for bacteria are sterile. It is usually a relatively mild infection followed by complete recovery.

Viral encephalitis

Viral encephalitis may affect a wide variety of sites and, as nerve cells are not replaced, loss of function reflects the extent of damage. In severe infection neurones and neuroglia may be affected, followed by necrosis and gliosis. Early senility may develop or, if vital centres in the medulla oblongata are involved, death may ensue. In mild cases recovery is usually complete with little loss of function.

Herpes simplex encephalitis. This is an acute, often fatal, condition causing necrosis of areas of the cerebrum, usually the temporal lobes. If the patient survives the initial acute phase there may be residual dysfunction, e.g. behavioural disturbance and loss of memory.

Herpes zoster neuritis (shingles)

Herpes zoster viruses cause chickenpox (varicella) mainly in children and shingles (zoster) in adults. Susceptible children may contract chickenpox from a patient with shingles but not the reverse. Adults infected with the viruses may show no immediate signs of disease. The viruses may remain dormant in posterior root ganglia of the spinal nerves then become active years later, causing shingles. Reactivation may be either spontaneous or associated with the following factors:

- local trauma involving the dermatome, i.e. the area supplied by the affected peripheral nerve
- exposure of the dermatome to irradiation, e.g. sun, X-rays
- depression of the immunological system, e.g. by drugs, old age, AIDS.

The posterior root ganglion becomes acutely inflamed. From there the *viruses* pass along the sensory nerve to the surface tissues supplied, e.g. skin, cornea. The tissues become inflamed and vesicles, containing serous fluid and viruses, develop along the course of the nerve. This is accompanied by persistent pain and hypersensitivity to touch (*hyperaesthesia*). Recovery is usually slow and there may be some loss of sensation, depending on the severity of the disease. The infection is usually unilateral and the most common sites are:

- nerves supplying the trunk, sometimes two or three adjacent dermatomes (Fig. 7.39)
- the ophthalmic division of the trigeminal nerve (Fig. 7.41), causing *trigeminal neuralgia*, and, if vesicles form on the cornea, there may be ulceration, scarring and residual interference with vision.

Poliomyelitis

This disease is usually caused by *polioviruses* and, occasionally, by other *enteroviruses*. The infection is spread by food contaminated by infected faecal matter and the initial virus multiplication occurs in the alimentary tract. The viruses are then bloodborne to the nervous system and invade anterior horn cells in the spinal cord. Usually there is a mild febrile illness with no indication of nerve damage. In mild cases there is complete recovery but there is permanent disability in many others. Paralytic disease is believed to be precipitated by muscular exercise during the early febrile stage. Irreversible damage to lower motor neurones causes muscle paralysis which, in the limbs, may lead to deformity because of the unopposed tonal contraction of antagonistic muscles. Death may occur owing to respiratory paralysis. Vaccination programmes have now almost eradicated this disease in developed countries.

Rabies

All warm-blooded animals are susceptible to the rabies virus, which is endemic in many countries but not in Britain. The main reservoirs of virus are wild animals, some of which may be carriers. These may infect domestic pets which then become the main source of human infection. The viruses multiply in the salivary glands and are present in large numbers in saliva. They enter the body through skin abrasions and are believed to travel to the brain along the nerves. The incubation period varies from about 2 weeks to several months, possibly reflecting the distance viruses travel between the site of entry and the brain. Extensive damage to the basal nuclei, midbrain, medulla oblongata and the posterior root ganglia of the peripheral nerves causes meningeal irritation, extreme hyperaesthesia, muscle spasm and convulsions. *Hydrophobia* and overflow of saliva from the mouth are due to painful spasm of the throat muscles that inhibits swallowing. In the advanced stages muscle spasm may alternate with flaccid paralysis and death is usually due to respiratory muscle spasm or paralysis.

Not all people exposed to the virus contract rabies, but in those who do, the mortality rate is high.

Human immunodeficiency virus (HIV)

The brain is often affected in individuals with AIDS (p. 385) resulting in, e.g.:

- opportunistic infection
- dementia.

Creutzfeldt–Jakob disease

This infective condition may be caused by a 'slow' virus, the nature and transmission of which is poorly understood. It is thought to be via a heat-resistant transmissible particle known as a *prion protein*. It is a rapidly progressive form of dementia for which there is no known treatment so the condition is always fatal.

Myalgic encephalitis (ME)

This condition is also known as post-viral syndrome or chronic fatigue syndrome. It affects mostly teenagers and young adults and the aetiology is unknown. Sometimes the condition follows a viral illness. The effects include malaise, severe fatigue, poor concentration and myalgia. Recovery is usually spontaneous but sometimes results in chronic disability.

DEMYELINATING DISEASES

Learning outcome

After studying this section you should be able to:

- explain how the signs and symptoms of demyelinating disease are related to pathological changes in the nervous system.

These diseases are caused either by injury to axons or by disorders of cells that secrete myelin, i.e. oligodendrocytes and Schwann cells.

Multiple (disseminated) sclerosis (MS)

In this disease there are areas of demyelinated white matter, called *plaques*, irregularly distributed throughout the brain and spinal cord. Grey matter in the brain and spinal cord may also be affected because of the arrangement of satellite oligodendrocytes round cell bodies. In the early stages there may be little damage to axons. It usually develops between the ages of 20 and 40 years and there is an increased incidence of MS among siblings, especially twins, and parents of patients. It is not known whether this is due to genetic or environmental factors or a combination of both. The actual cause(s) of MS are not known but several factors have been suggested, more than one of which may be involved.

Environment before adolescence is suggested because the disease is most prevalent in people who spend their pre-adolescent years in temperate climates, and people who move to other climates after that age retain their susceptibility to MS. People moving into a temperate area during adolescence or later life appear not to be susceptible.

Genetically abnormal myelin is present in many patients and may be antigenic, causing the development of autoimmunity.

Viral infection by slow-growing viruses that attack myelin has been suggested but so far no virus has been identified.

Effects of multiple sclerosis

Neuronal damage leads to a variety of dysfunctions, depending on the sites and sizes of demyelinated plaques. Plaques damage white matter leading to upper motor neurone dysfunction causing:

- weakness of skeletal muscles and sometimes paralysis
- lack of coordination and movement
- disturbed sensation, e.g. burning or pins and needles
- incontinence of urine
- visual disturbances especially blurring and double vision. The optic nerves are commonly affected early in the disease.

The disease pattern is usually one of relapses and remissions of widely varying duration. Each relapse causes further loss of nervous tissue and progressive dysfunction. In some cases there may be chronic progression without remission, or acute disease rapidly leading to death.

Acute disseminating encephalomyelitis

This is a rare but serious condition that may occur:

- during or very soon after a virus infection, e.g. measles, chickenpox, mumps, respiratory infection
- following primary immunisation against viral diseases, mainly in older children and adults.

The cause of the acute diffuse demyelination is not known. It has been suggested that autoimmunity to myelin is triggered either by viruses during a viral infection, such as measles or rubella, or by viruses present in vaccines. The effects vary considerably, according to the distribution and degree of demyelination. The early febrile state may progress to paralysis and coma. Most patients survive the initial phase and recover with no residual dysfunction but some have severe impairment of a wide variety of neurological functions.

PHENYLKETONURIA

Learning outcome

After studying this section you should be able to:

- describe the causes and effects of phenylketonuria.

This is a genetic disorder in which the gene needed for synthesising the enzyme *phenylalanine hydroxylase* is absent. This enzyme normally converts phenylalanine to tyrosine in the liver (see Figs 2.8 and 3.4, pp. 24 and 32). Phenylalanine is the intermediate metabolite that accumulates in the liver cells and overflows into the blood (Fig. 7.50). In high quantities it is toxic to the nervous system and if untreated this condition results in brain damage and mental retardation within a few months. Tyrosine is a constituent of the skin pigment melanin and depigmentation occurs: affected children are fair skinned and blonde. The incidence of this disease is now low in developed countries because it is detected by screening all newborn infants and providing early treatment.

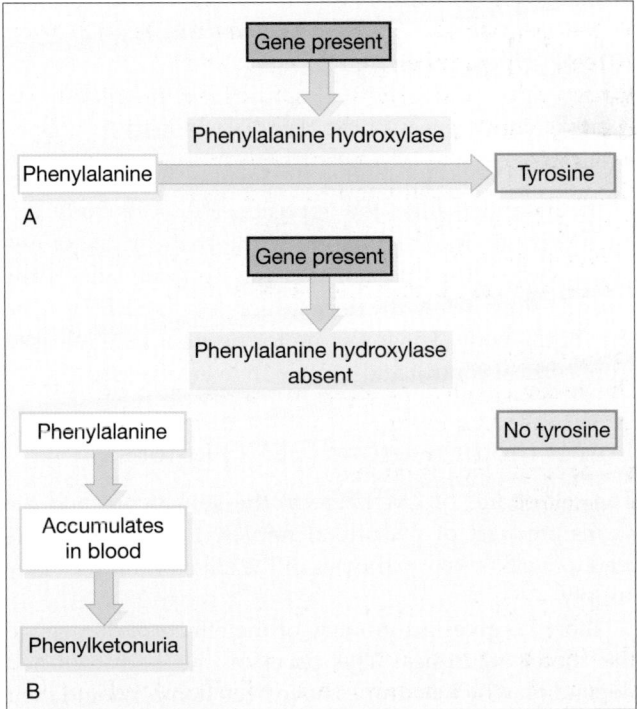

Figure 7.50 Phenylketonuria: A. Phenylalanine present. B. Phenylalanine absent.

DISEASES OF THE SPINAL CORD

Learning outcome

After studying this section you should be able to:

■ explain how disorders of the spinal cord cause abnormal body function.

Because space in the neural canal and intervertebral foramina is limited, any condition which distorts their shape or reduces the space may damage the spinal cord or peripheral nerve roots, or cause ischaemia by compressing blood vessels. Such conditions include:

■ fracture and/or dislocation of vertebrae
■ tumours of the meninges or vertebrae
■ prolapsed intervertebral disc.

The effects of disease or injury depend on the severity of the damage, the type and position of the neurones involved, i.e. motor, sensory, proprioceptor, autonomic, connector neurones in reflex arcs in the spinal cord or in peripheral nerves.

Motor neurones

Upper motor neurone (UMN) lesions

Lesions of the UMNs above the level of the decussation of the pyramids affect the opposite side of the body, e.g. haemorrhage or infarction in the internal capsule of one hemisphere causes paralysis of the opposite side of the body. Lesions below the decussation level affect the same side of the body. The lower motor neurones are released from cortical control and muscle tone is increased.

Lower motor neurone (LMN) lesions

The cell bodies of LMNs are in the spinal cord and the axons are part of peripheral nerves. Lesions of LMNs lead to weakness or paralysis of the effector muscles they supply.

Table 7.5 gives a summary of the effects of damage to the motor neurones. The parts of the body affected depend on which neurones have been damaged and their site in the brain, spinal cord or peripheral nerve.

Motor neurone disease

This is a chronic progressive degeneration of motor neurones, occurring mainly in men between 60 and 70 years

Table 7.5 Summary of effects of damage to motor neurones

Upper motor neurone	Lower motor neurone
Muscle weakness and spastic paralysis	Muscle weakness and flaccid paralysis
Exaggerated tendon reflexes	Absence of tendon reflexes
Muscle twitching	Muscle wasting Contracture of muscles Impaired circulation

of age. The cause is not known. Motor neurones in the cerebral cortex, brain stem and anterior horns of the spinal cord are destroyed and replaced by gliosis. Early effects are usually weakness and twitching of the small muscles of the hand, and muscles of the arm and shoulder girdle. The legs are affected later. Death is usually due to the involvement of the respiratory centre in the medulla oblongata.

Sensory neurones

The sensory functions lost as a result of disease or injury depend on which neurones have been damaged and their position in the brain or spinal cord, or the peripheral nerve involved. In the brain, neurones connecting the thalamus and the cerebrum pass through the internal capsule. Damage in this area by, e.g., haemorrhage, usually from a berry aneurysm, may lead to loss of sensation but does not affect cerebellar function unless upper motor neurones have also been damaged. Spinal cord damage leads to loss of sensation and cerebellar function. Peripheral nerve damage leads to loss of reflex activity, loss of sensation and of cerebellar function.

Mixed motor and sensory conditions

Subacute combined degeneration of the spinal cord

This condition most commonly occurs as a complication of pernicious anaemia. Vitamin B_{12} is associated with the formation and maintenance of myelin by Schwann cells and oligodendrocytes. Although degeneration of the spinal cord may be apparent before the anaemia it is arrested by treatment with vitamin B_{12}. This type of degeneration may occasionally complicate chronic conditions, such as diabetes mellitus, leukaemia and carcinoma.

The degeneration of nerve fibre myelin occurs in the posterior and lateral columns of white matter in the spinal cord, especially in the upper thoracic and lower cervical regions. Less frequently the changes occur in the posterior root ganglia and peripheral nerves. Demyelination of proprioceptor fibres (sensory) leads to ataxia and involvement of upper motor neurones leads to increased muscle tone and spastic paralysis.

Compression of the spinal cord and nerve roots

The causes include:

- prolapsed intervertebral disc
- syringomyelia
- tumours: metastatic, meningeal or nerve sheath
- fractures with displacement of bone fragments.

Prolapsed intervertebral disc (Fig. 7.51)

This is the most common cause of compression of the spinal cord and/or nerve roots. The bodies of the vertebrae are separated by the intervertebral discs, each consisting of an outer rim of cartilage, the *annulus fibrosus*, and a central core of soft gelatinous material, the *nucleus pulposus*.

Prolapse of a disc is herniation of the nucleus pulposus, causing the annulus fibrosus and the posterior longitudinal ligament to protrude into the neural canal. It is most common in the lumbar region usually below the level of the spinal cord, i.e. below L2, so the injury is to nerve roots only. If it occurs in the cervical region, the cord may also be compressed. Herniation may occur suddenly, typically in young adults during strenuous exercise or exertion, or progressively in older people when bone disease or degeneration of the disc leads to rupture during minimal exercise. The hernia may be:

- one-sided, causing pressure damage to a nerve root
- midline, compressing the spinal cord, the anterior spinal artery and possibly bilateral nerve roots.

The outcome depends upon the size of the hernia and the length of time the pressure is applied. Small herniations cause local pain due to pressure on the nerve endings in the posterior longitudinal ligament.

Large herniations may cause:

- unilateral or bilateral paralysis
- acute or chronic pain perceived to originate from the area supplied by the compressed sensory nerve, e.g. in the leg or foot
- compression of the anterior spinal artery, causing ischaemia and possibly necrosis of the spinal cord
- local muscle spasm due to pressure on motor nerves.

Syringomyelia

This dilatation (syrinx) of the central canal of the spinal cord occurs most commonly in the cervical region and is associated with congenital abnormality of the distal end of the fourth ventricle. As the central canal dilates, pressure causes progressive damage to sensory and motor neurones. Early effects include dissociated anaesthesia, i.e. insensibility to heat and pain, due to compression of the sensory fibres that cross the cord immediately they enter. In the long term there is destruction of motor and sensory tracts, leading to spastic paralysis and loss of sensation and reflexes.

Tumours and displaced fragments of fractured vertebrae

These may affect the spinal cord and nerve roots at any level. The pressure damage initially causes pain and later, if the pressure is not relieved, there may be loss of sensation and paralysis. The areas affected depend on the site of pressure.

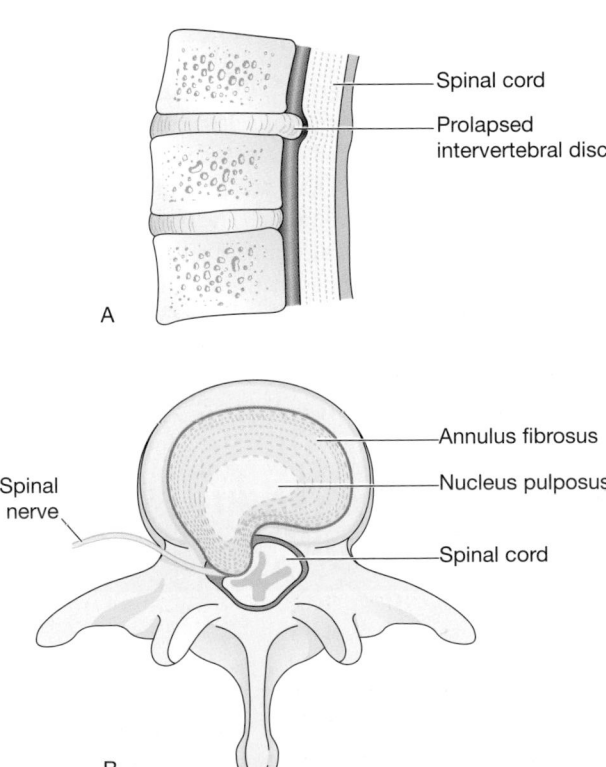

A

B

Figure 7.51 Prolapsed intervertebral disc. A. Viewed from the side. B. Viewed from above.

Labels:
- Spinal cord
- Prolapsed intervertebral disc
- Annulus fibrosus
- Nucleus pulposus
- Spinal cord
- Spinal nerve

187

DISEASES OF PERIPHERAL NERVES

Learning outcomes

After studying this section you should be able to:

- compare and contrast the causes and effects of parenchymal and interstitial neuropathies

- describe the effects of Guillain–Barré syndrome and Bell's palsy.

Neuropathies

This is a group of diseases of peripheral nerves not associated with inflammation. They are classified as:

- parenchymal (polyneuropathy): several neurones are affected
- interstitial (mononeuropathy): a single neurone is usually affected.

Parenchymal neuropathy

Polyneuropathy or damage to a number of neurones and their myelin sheaths occurs in metabolic or toxic disorders, e.g.:

- nutritional deficiencies, e.g. folic acid, vitamins B_1, B_2, B_6, B_{12}
- metabolic disorders, e.g. diabetes mellitus
- chronic diseases, e.g. renal failure, hepatic failure, carcinoma
- toxic reactions to, e.g., lead, arsenic, mercury, carbon tetrachloride, aniline dyes and some drugs, such as phenytoin, chloroquine
- infections, e.g. influenza, measles, typhoid fever, diphtheria, leprosy.

The long neurones are usually affected first, e.g. those supplying the feet and legs. The outcome depends upon the cause of the neuropathy and the extent of the damage.

Interstitial neuropathy

Usually only one neurone is damaged (*mononeuropathy*) and the most common cause is ischaemia due to pressure. Example include:

- pressure applied to cranial nerves in cranial bone foramina due to distortion of the brain by increased ICP
- compression of a nerve in a confined space caused by surrounding inflammation and oedema, e.g. the median nerve in the carpal tunnel (see p. 427)

- external pressure on a nerve, e.g. an unconscious person lying with an arm hanging over the side of a bed or trolley
- compression of the axillary (circumflex) nerve by ill-fitting crutches
- trapping a nerve between the broken ends of a bone
- ischaemia due to thrombosis of blood vessels supplying a nerve.

The resultant dysfunction depends on the site and extent of the injury.

Neuritis

Acute idiopathic inflammatory polyneuropathy (Guillain–Barré syndrome)

This is a sudden, acute, progressive, bilateral ascending paralysis, beginning in the lower limbs and spreading to the arms, trunk and cranial nerves. It usually occurs 1 to 3 weeks after an upper respiratory tract infection. There is widespread inflammation accompanied by some demyelination of spinal, peripheral and cranial nerves and the spinal ganglia. Paralysis may affect all the limbs and the respiratory muscles. Patients who survive the acute phase usually recover completely in weeks or months.

Bell's palsy

Compression of a facial nerve in the temporal bone foramen causes paralysis of facial muscles with drooping and loss of facial expression on the affected side. The immediate cause is inflammation and oedema of the nerve but the underlying cause is unknown. The onset may be sudden or develop over several hours. Distortion of the features is due to muscle tone on the unaffected side, the affected side being expressionless. Recovery is usually complete within a few months.

DEVELOPMENTAL ABNORMALITIES OF THE NERVOUS SYSTEM

Learning outcomes

After studying this section you should be able to:

- describe developmental abnormalities of the nervous system

- relate their effects to abnormal body function.

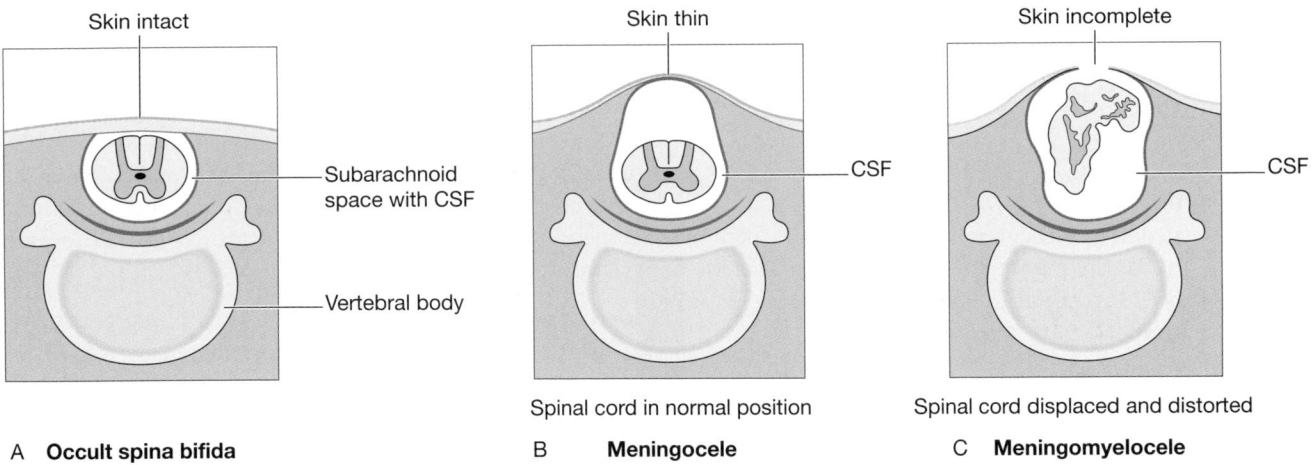

A **Occult spina bifida** Skin intact — Subarachnoid space with CSF — Vertebral body

B **Meningocele** Skin thin — CSF — Spinal cord in normal position

C **Meningomyelocele** Skin incomplete — CSF — Spinal cord displaced and distorted

Figure 7.52 Spina bifida.

Spina bifida

This is a congenital malformation of the neural canal and spinal cord (Fig. 7.52). The neural arches of the vertebrae are absent and the dura mater is abnormal, most commonly in the lumbosacral region. The causes are not known, although the condition is associated with dietary deficiency of folic acid at the time of conception. They may be of genetic origin or due to environmental factors, e.g. irradiation, or maternal infection (rubella) at a critical stage in development of the fetal vertebrae and spinal cord. The effects depend on the extent of the abnormality.

Occult spina bifida

The skin over the defect is intact and excessive growth of hair over the site may be the only sign of abnormality. This is sometimes associated with minor nerve defects that commonly affect the bladder.

Meningocele

The skin over the defect is very thin and there is dilatation of the subarachnoid space posteriorly. The spinal cord is correctly positioned.

Meningomyelocele

The subarachnoid space is dilated posteriorly, the spinal cord is displaced backwards and may be adherent to the posterior wall of the arachnoid dilatation. The skin is often deficient with leakage of CSF, and the meninges may become infected. Serious nerve defects result in paraplegia and lack of sphincter control causing incontinence of urine and faeces. There may also be mental retardation.

Hydrocephalus (see p. 178).

TUMOURS OF THE NERVOUS SYSTEM

Learning outcome

After studying this section you should be able to:

■ outline the effects of tumours of the nervous system.

Most tumours of the nervous system are of neuroglial origin. Neurones are rarely involved because they do not normally multiply. Metastases of nervous tissue tumours are rare. Because of this, the rate of growth of a tumour is more important than the likelihood of spread outside the nervous system. In this context, 'benign' means slow-growing and 'malignant' rapid-growing. Signs of raised ICP appear after the limits of compensation have been reached.

Within the confined space of the skull, haemorrhage in a tumour exacerbates the increased ICP caused by the tumour.

Slow-growing tumours

These allow time for adjustment to compensate for increasing intracranial pressure, so the tumour may be quite large before its effects are evident. Compensation involves gradual reduction in the volume of cerebrospinal fluid and circulating blood.

Rapidly growing tumours

These do not allow time for adjustment to compensate for the rapidly increasing ICP, so the effects quickly become apparent (Fig. 7.47C). Complications include:

- neurological impairment, depending on tumour site and size
- effects of increased ICP (p. 177)
- necrosis of the tumour, causing haemorrhage and oedema.

Specific tumours

Gliomas are usually astrocytomas, ranging from benign tumours to the highly malignant *glioblastoma multiforme*.

Meningiomas are usually benign, originating from arachnoid granulations.

Medulloblastomas are highly malignant neurone-cell tumours, occurring mainly in the cerebellum in children.

They are believed to originate from primitive cells prior to differentiation into neurones and neuroglia.

Metastases in the brain

The most common primary sites that metastasise to the brain are the breast, lungs and bone marrow (leukaemias). The prognosis of this condition is poor and the effects depend on the site(s) and rate of growth of metastases. There are two forms:

- discrete multiple tumours, mainly in the cerebrum
- diffuse tumours in the arachnoid mater.

8

The special senses

The special senses of hearing, sight, smell and taste all have specialised sensory receptors (nerve endings) outside the brain. These are found in the ears, eyes, nose and mouth. The ear is also involved in the maintenance of balance. In the brain the incoming nerve impulses undergo complex processes of integration and coordination that result in perception of sensory information and a variety of responses inside and outside the body.

HEARING AND THE EAR

Learning outcomes

After studying this section you should be able to:

- describe the structure of the outer, middle and inner parts of the ear

- explain the physiology of hearing.

The ear is the organ of hearing. It is supplied by the 8th *cranial nerve*, i.e. the *cochlear part* of the *vestibulocochlear* nerve which is stimulated by vibrations caused by sound waves.

With the exception of the auricle (pinna), the structures that form the ear are encased within the petrous portion of the temporal bone.

Structure

The ear is divided into three distinct parts (Figs 8.1 and 8.6):

- outer ear
- middle ear (tympanic cavity)
- inner ear.

Outer ear

The outer ear consists of the auricle (pinna) and the external acoustic meatus.

The auricle (pinna)

The auricle is the expanded portion projecting from the side of the head. It is composed of *fibroelastic cartilage* covered with skin. It is deeply grooved and ridged and the most prominent outer ridge is the *helix*.

The lobule (earlobe) is the soft pliable part at the lower extremity, composed of fibrous and adipose tissue richly supplied with blood.

External acoustic meatus (auditory canal)

This is a slightly 'S'-shaped tube about 2.5 cm long extending from the auricle to the *tympanic membrane* (eardrum). The lateral third is cartilaginous and the remainder is a canal in the temporal bone. The meatus is lined with skin containing hairs continuous with that of the auricle. There are numerous *sebaceous* and *ceruminous glands* in the skin of the lateral third. Ceruminous glands

Temporal bone   Malleus   Incus   Stapes   Semicircular canal

Vestibulocochlear nerve

Auricle

Cochlea

Pharyngotympanic (auditory) tube

To nasopharynx

Helix   Lobule   External acoustic meatus   Tympanic membrane

☐ Outer ear   ■ Middle ear   ▢ Inner ear

Figure 8.1 The parts of the ear.

are modified sweat glands that secrete *cerumen* (wax), a sticky material containing lysozyme and immunoglobulins. Foreign materials, e.g. dust, insects and microbes, are prevented from reaching the tympanic membrane by wax, hairs and the curvature of the meatus. Movements of the temporomandibular joint during chewing and speaking 'massage' the cartilaginous meatus, moving the wax towards the exterior.

The tympanic membrane (eardrum) (Fig. 8.2) completely separates the external acoustic meatus from the middle ear. It is oval-shaped with the slightly broader edge upwards and is formed by three types of tissue: the outer covering of *hairless skin*, the middle layer of *fibrous tissue* and the inner lining of *mucous membrane* continuous with that of the middle ear.

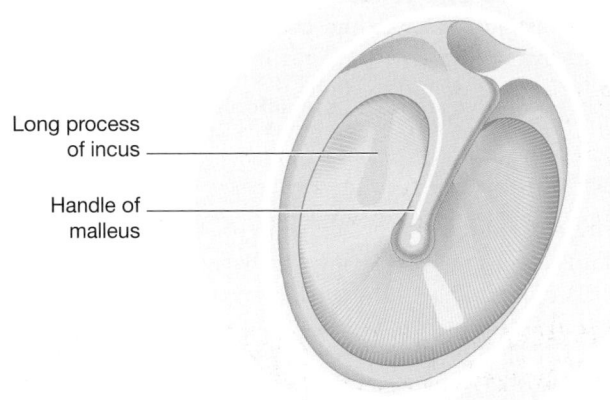

Figure 8.2 The tympanic membrane viewed through an auriscope showing the shadows cast by the malleus and the incus.

Middle ear (tympanic cavity)

This is an irregular-shaped air-filled cavity within the petrous portion of the temporal bone. The cavity, its contents and the air sacs which open out of it are lined with either simple squamous or cuboidal epithelium.

The lateral wall of the middle ear is formed by the tympanic membrane.

The roof and floor are formed by the temporal bone.

The posterior wall is formed by the temporal bone with openings leading to the *mastoid antrum* through which air passes to the air cells within the mastoid process.

The medial wall is a thin layer of temporal bone in which there are two openings:

- oval window
- round window (see Fig. 8.6).

The oval window is occluded by part of a small bone called the *stapes* and the round window, by a fine sheet of *fibrous tissue*.

Air reaches the cavity through the *pharyngotympanic (auditory or Eustachian)* tube which extends from the nasopharynx. It is about 4 cm long and is lined with ciliated epithelium. The presence of air at atmospheric pressure on both sides of the tympanic membrane is maintained by the pharyngotympanic tube and enables the membrane to vibrate when sound waves strike it. The pharyngotympanic tube is normally closed but when there is unequal pressure across the tympanic membrane, e.g. at high altitude, it is opened by swallowing or yawning and the ears 'pop', equalising the pressure again.

Auditory ossicles (Fig. 8.3)
These are three very small bones that extend across the middle ear from the tympanic membrane to the oval window (Fig. 8.1). They form a series of movable joints with each other and with the medial wall of the cavity at the oval window. They are named according to their shapes.

The malleus. This is the lateral hammer-shaped bone. The handle is in contact with the tympanic membrane and the head forms a movable joint with the incus.

The incus. This is the middle anvil-shaped bone. Its body articulates with the malleus, the long process with the stapes, and it is stabilised by the short process, fixed by fibrous tissue to the posterior wall of the tympanic cavity.

193

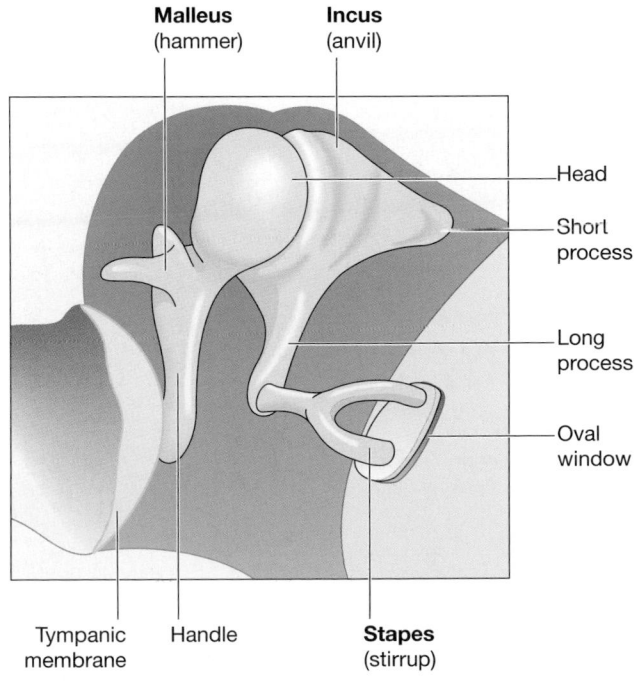

Figure 8.3 The auditory ossicles.

The stapes. This is the medial stirrup-shaped bone. Its head articulates with the incus and its footplate fits into the oval window.

The three ossicles are held in position by fine ligaments.

Inner ear (Fig. 8.4)

The inner (internal) ear or labyrinth (meaning 'maze') ear contains the organs of hearing and balance. It is generally described in two parts, the *bony labyrinth* and the *membranous labyrinth*.

Bony labyrinth

This is a cavity within the temporal bone lined with periosteum. It is larger than, and encloses, the membranous labyrinth of the same shape which fits into it, like a tube within a tube. Between the bony and membranous labyrinth there is a layer of watery fluid called *perilymph* and within the membranous labyrinth there is a similarly watery fluid, *endolymph*.

The bony labyrinth consists of:

- 1 vestibule
- 1 cochlea
- 3 semicircular canals.

The vestibule. This is the expanded part nearest the middle ear. It contains the oval and round windows in its lateral wall.

The cochlea. This resembles a snail's shell. It has a broad base where it is continuous with the vestibule and a narrow apex, and it spirals round a central bony column.

The semicircular canals. These are three tubes arranged so that one is situated in each of the three planes of space. They are continuous with the vestibule.

Membranous labyrinth

This contains endolymph and lies within its bony counterpart. It comprises:

- the vestibule, which contains the *utricle* and *saccule*
- the cochlea
- three semicircular canals.

The cochlea

A cross-section of the cochlea (Fig. 8.5) contains three compartments:

- the scala vestibuli
- the scala media, or *cochlear duct*
- the scala tympani.

In cross-section the bony cochlea has two compartments containing perilymph: the scala vestibuli, which originates at the oval window, and the scala tympani, which ends at the round window. The two compartments are continuous with each other and Figure 8.6 shows the relationship between these structures. The cochlear duct

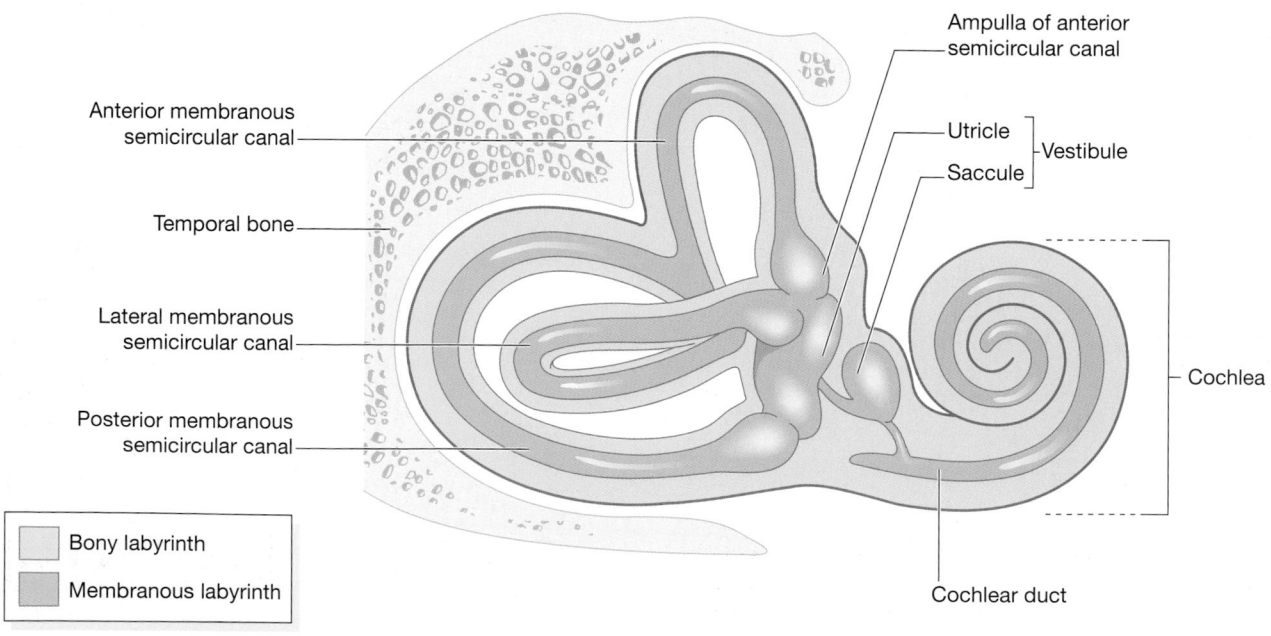

Figure 8.4 The inner ear. The membranous labyrinth within the bony labyrinth.

is part of the membranous labyrinth and is triangular in shape. On the *basilar membrane*, or base of the triangle, there are *supporting cells* and specialised *cochlear hair cells* containing auditory receptors. These cells form the *spiral organ* (of Corti), the sensory organ that responds to vibration by initiating nerve impulses that are then perceived as hearing by the brain. The *auditory receptors* are dendrites of efferent nerves that combine forming the cochlear (auditory) part of the vestibulocochlear nerve (8th cranial nerve), which passes through a foramen in the temporal bone to reach the hearing area in the temporal lobe of the cerebrum (see Fig. 7.18, p. 151).

Physiology of hearing

Every sound produces *sound waves* or vibrations in the air, which travel at about 332 metres (1088 feet) per second. The auricle, because of its shape, concentrates the waves and directs them along the auditory meatus causing the tympanic membrane to vibrate. Tympanic membrane vibrations are transmitted and amplified through the middle ear by movement of the ossicles (Fig. 8.6). At their medial end the footplate of the stapes rocks to and fro in the oval window, setting up fluid waves in the perilymph of the scala vestibuli. Some of the force of these waves is transmitted along the length of the scala vestibuli and scala tympani, but most of the pressure is transmitted into the cochlear duct. This causes a corresponding wave motion in the endolymph, resulting in vibration of the basilar membrane and stimulation of the auditory receptors in the hair cells of the spiral organ. The nerve impulses generated pass to the brain in the cochlear (auditory) portion of the *vestibulocochlear nerve* (8th cranial nerve). The fluid wave is finally expended into the middle ear by vibration of the membrane of the round window. The vestibulocochlear nerve transmits the impulses to the hearing area in the cerebrum where sound is perceived and to various nuclei in the pons and the midbrain.

Sound waves have properties of *pitch* and *volume*, or intensity (Fig. 8.7). Pitch is determined by the frequency of the sound waves and is measured in hertz (Hz). The volume depends on the amplitude of the sound waves and is measured in decibels (dB). Very loud noise is damaging to the ear, particularly when prolonged because it damages the sensitive hair cells of the spiral organ.

Because of the structure of the inner ear, sounds of different frequencies stimulate the basilar membrane at different places along its length allowing discrimination of pitch. Additionally, the greater the amplitude of the wave created in the endolymph, the greater the stimulation of the auditory receptors in the hair cells in the spiral organ, enabling perception of volume.

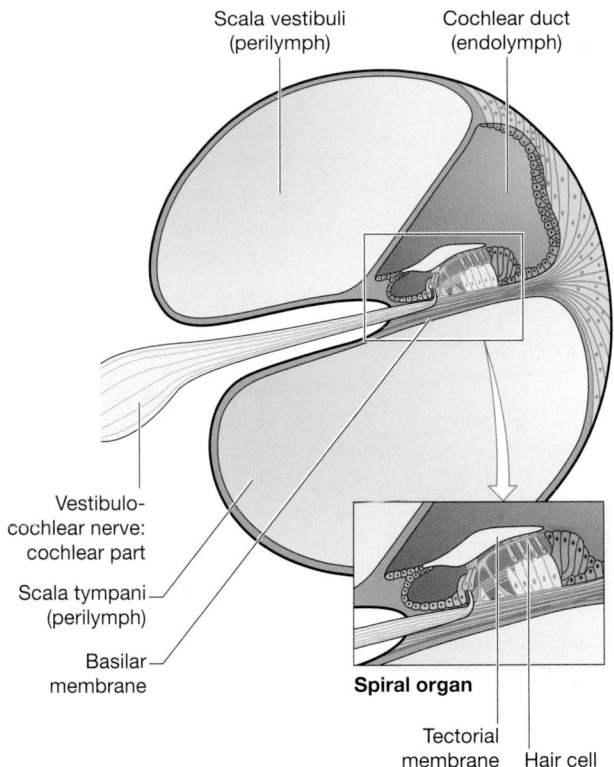

Figure 8.5 A cross-section of the cochlea showing the spiral organ (of Corti).

195

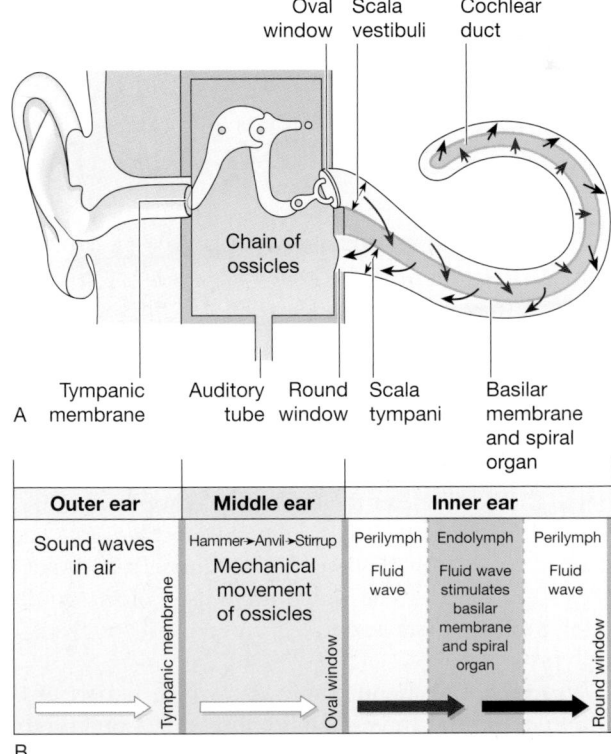

Figure 8.6 Passage of sound waves: A. The ear with cochlea uncoiled. B. Summary of transmission.

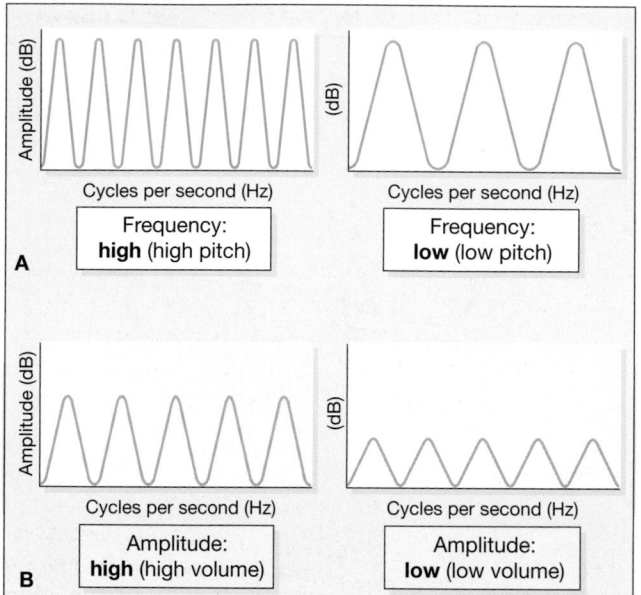

A

B

Figure 8.7 Behaviour of sound waves. A. Difference in frequency but of the same amplitude. B. Difference in amplitude but of the same frequency.

BALANCE AND THE EAR

> **Learning outcome**
>
> After studying this section you should be able to:
>
> ■ describe the physiology of balance.

The semicircular canals and vestibule (Fig. 8.4)

The semicircular canals have no auditory function although they are closely associated with the cochlea. They provide information about the position of the head in space, contributing to maintenance of posture and balance.

There are three semicircular canals, one lying in each of the three planes of space. They are situated above and behind the vestibule of the inner ear and open into it.

The semicircular canals, like the cochlea, are composed of an outer bony wall and inner membranous tubes or *ducts*. The membranous ducts contain endolymph and are separated from the bony wall by perilymph.

The utricle is a membranous sac which is part of the vestibule and the three membranous ducts open into it at their dilated ends, the *ampullae*. The *saccule* is a part of the vestibule and communicates with the utricle and the cochlea.

In the walls of the utricle, saccule and ampullae there are fine specialised epithelial cells with minute projections, called *hair cells*. Amongst the hair cells there are sensory nerve endings which combine forming the *vestibular part* of the vestibulocochlear nerve.

Physiology of balance

The semicircular canals and the vestibule (utricle and saccule) are concerned with balance. Any change of position of the head causes movement in the perilymph and endolymph, which bends the hair cells and stimulates the sensory nerve endings in the utricle, saccule and ampullae. The resultant nerve impulses are transmitted by the vestibular nerve which joins the cochlear nerve to form the vestibulocochlear nerve. The vestibular branch passes first to the *vestibular nucleus*, then to the *cerebellum*.

The cerebellum also receives nerve impulses from the eyes and proprioceptors (sensory receptors) in the skeletal muscles and joints. Impulses from these three sources are coordinated and efferent nerve impulses pass to the cerebrum and to skeletal muscles. This results in awareness of body position, maintenance of upright posture and fixing of the eyes on the same point, independently of head movements.

SIGHT AND THE EYE

> **Learning outcomes**
>
> After studying this section you should be able to:
>
> ■ describe the gross structure of the eye
>
> ■ describe the route taken by a nerve impulse from the retina to the cerebrum
>
> ■ describe how light entering the eye is focused on the retina
>
> ■ state the functions of the extraocular muscles of the eye
>
> ■ describe the functions of the accessory organs of the eye.

The eye is the organ of the sense of sight situated in the orbital cavity and it is supplied by the *optic nerve* (2nd cranial nerve).

It is almost spherical in shape and is about 2.5 cm in diameter. The space between the eye and the orbital cavity is occupied by adipose tissue. The bony walls of the orbit and the fat help to protect the eye from injury.

Structurally the two eyes are separate but, unlike the ear, some of their activities are coordinated so that they function as a pair. It is possible to see with only one eye but three-dimensional vision is impaired when only one eye is used, especially in relation to the judgement of distance.

Structure (Fig. 8.8)

There are three layers of tissue in the walls of the eye. They are:

- the outer fibrous layer: sclera and cornea
- the middle vascular layer or *uveal tract*: choroid, ciliary body and iris
- the inner nervous tissue layer: retina.

Structures inside the eyeball are the lens, aqueous fluid (humour) and vitreous body (humour).

Sclera and cornea

The sclera, or white of the eye, forms the outermost layer of tissue of the posterior and lateral aspects of the eyeball and is continuous anteriorly with the transparent *cornea*. It consists of a firm fibrous membrane that maintains the shape of the eye and gives attachment to the *extraocular* or *extrinsic muscles* of the eye (p. 203).

Anteriorly the sclera continues as a clear transparent epithelial membrane, the *cornea*. Light rays pass through the cornea to reach the retina. The cornea is convex anteriorly and is involved in *refracting* or bending light rays to focus them on the retina.

Choroid (Figs 8.8 and 8.9)

The choroid lines the posterior five-sixths of the inner surface of the sclera. It is very rich in blood vessels and is deep chocolate brown in colour. Light enters the eye through the pupil, stimulates the nerve endings in the retina and is then absorbed by the choroid.

Ciliary body

The ciliary body is the anterior continuation of the choroid consisting of *ciliary muscle* (smooth muscle fibres) and secretory epithelial cells. It gives attachment to the *suspensory ligament* which, at its other end, is attached to the capsule enclosing the lens. Contraction and relaxation of the ciliary muscle changes the thickness of the lens which *bends*, or *refracts* light rays entering the eye to focus them on the retina. The epithelial cells secrete *aqueous fluid* into the anterior segment of the eye, i.e. the space between the lens and the cornea (anterior and posterior chambers). The ciliary body is supplied by parasympathetic branches of the oculomotor nerve (3rd cranial nerve). Stimulation causes contraction of the smooth muscle and accommodation of the eye (p. 202).

197

Figure 8.8 Section of the eye.

Iris

The iris is the visible coloured part of the eye and extends anteriorly from the ciliary body, lying behind the cornea in front of the lens. It divides the anterior segment of the eye into *anterior* and *posterior chambers* which contain *aqueous fluid* secreted by the ciliary body. It is a circular body composed of pigment cells and two layers of smooth muscle fibres, one circular and the other radiating (Fig. 8.9). In the centre there is an aperture called the *pupil*.

The iris is supplied by parasympathetic and sympathetic nerves. Parasympathetic stimulation constricts the pupil and sympathetic stimulation dilates it (see Figs 7.43 and 7.44, pp. 171 and 172).

The colour of the iris is genetically determined and depends on the number of pigment cells present. Albinos have no pigment cells and people with blue eyes have fewer than those with brown eyes.

Lens (Fig. 8.10)

The lens is a *highly elastic* circular biconvex body, lying immediately behind the pupil. It consists of fibres enclosed within a capsule and it is suspended from the ciliary body by the *suspensory ligament*. Its thickness is controlled by the ciliary muscle through the suspensory ligament. The lens bends (refracts) light rays reflected by objects in front of the eye. It is the only structure in the eye that can vary its refractory power, achieved by changing its thickness. When the ciliary muscle contracts, it moves forward, releasing its pull on the lens, increasing its thickness. The nearer is the object being viewed the thicker the lens becomes to allow focusing.

Retina

The retina is the innermost layer of the wall of the eye (Fig. 8.8). It is an extremely delicate structure and is especially adapted for stimulation by light rays. It is composed of several layers of nerve cell bodies and their axons, lying on a pigmented layer of epithelial cells which attach it to the choroid. The layer highly sensitive to light is the layer of sensory receptor cells: rods and cones.

The retina lines about three-quarters of the eyeball and is thickest at the back and thins out anteriorly to end just behind the ciliary body. Near the centre of the posterior part is the *macula lutea*, or yellow spot (Figs 8.11 and 8.12). In the centre of the area there is a little depression called the *fovea centralis*, consisting of only cone-shaped cells. Towards the anterior part of the retina there are fewer cone- than rod-shaped cells (Fig. 8.11).

The rods and cones contain photosensitive pigments that convert light rays into nerve impulses and this is explained on page 202.

About 0.5 cm to the nasal side of the macula lutea all the nerve fibres of the retina converge to form the *optic*

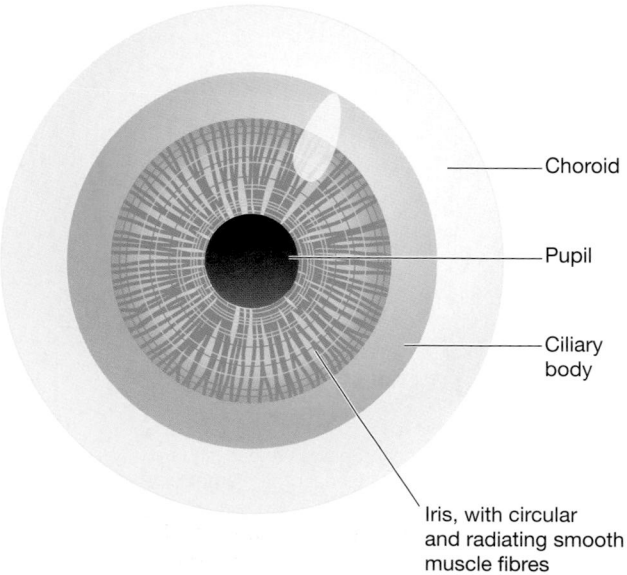

Choroid

Pupil

Ciliary body

Iris, with circular and radiating smooth muscle fibres

Figure 8.9 The choroid, ciliary body and iris. Viewed from the front.

Sclera

Ciliary body

Lens

Suspensory ligament

Figure 8.10 The lens and suspensory ligament viewed from the front. The iris has been removed.

nerve. The small area of retina where the optic nerve leaves the eye is the *optic disc* or *blind spot*. It has no light-sensitive cells.

Blood supply to the eye

The eye is supplied with arterial blood by the *ciliary arteries* and the *central retinal artery*. These are branches of the ophthalmic artery, one of the branches of the internal carotid artery.

Venous drainage is by a number of veins, including the *central retinal vein*, which eventually empty into a deep venous sinus.

The central retinal artery and vein are encased in the optic nerve, entering the eye at the optic disc.

Interior of the eye

The anterior segment of the eye, i.e. the space between the cornea and the lens, is incompletely divided into *anterior* and *posterior chambers* by the iris (Fig. 8.8). Both chambers contain a clear *aqueous fluid (humour)* secreted into the posterior chamber by ciliary glands. It circulates in front of the lens, through the pupil into the anterior chamber and returns to the venous circulation through the *scleral venous sinus* (canal of Schlemm) in the angle between the iris and cornea (Fig. 8.8). There is continuous production and drainage but the intraocular pressure remains fairly constant between 1.3 and 2.6 kPa (10 to 20 mmHg). An increase in this pressure causes *glaucoma* (p. 210). Aqueous fluid supplies nutrients and removes waste from the transparent structures in the front of the eye that have no blood supply, i.e. the cornea, lens and lens capsule.

Behind the lens and filling the posterior segment (cavity) of the eyeball is the *vitreous body (humour)*. This is a soft, colourless, transparent, jelly-like substance composed of 99% water, some salts and mucoprotein. It maintains sufficient intraocular pressure to support the retina against the choroid and prevent the walls of the eyeball from collapsing.

The eye keeps its shape because of the intraocular pressure exerted by the vitreous body and the aqueous fluid. It remains fairly constant throughout life.

Optic nerves (second cranial nerves) (Fig. 8.13)

The fibres of the optic nerve originate in the retina of the eye. All the fibres converge to form the optic nerve about 0.5 cm to the nasal side of the macula lutea. The nerve pierces the choroid and sclera to pass backwards and medially through the orbital cavity. It then passes through the optic foramen of the sphenoid bone, backwards and medially to meet the nerve from the other eye at the *optic chiasma*.

Optic chiasma

This is situated immediately in front of and above the pituitary gland which is in the hypophyseal fossa of the sphenoid bone (see Fig. 9.2, p. 215). In the optic chiasma the nerve fibres of the optic nerve from the nasal side of each retina cross over to the opposite side. The fibres from the temporal side do not cross but continue backwards on the same side. This crossing over provides both cerebral hemispheres with sensory input from each eye.

199

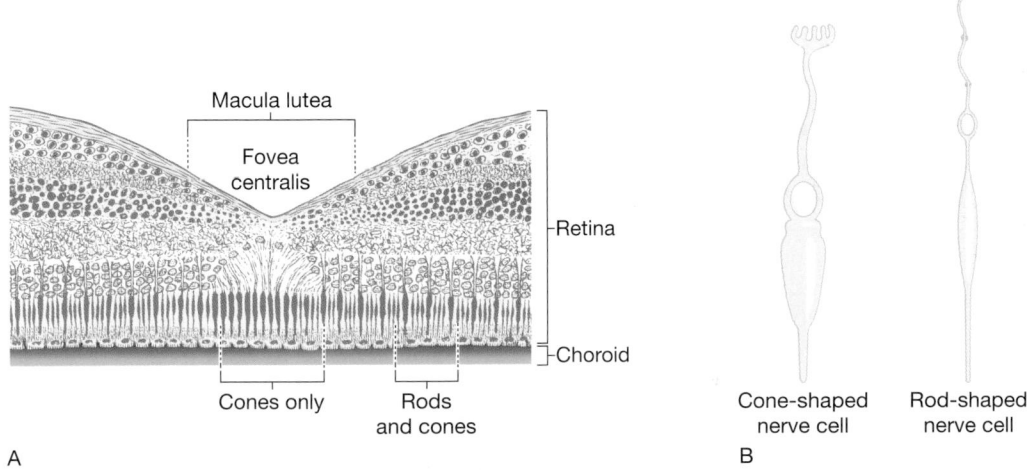

Figure 8.11 The retina: A. Magnified section. B. Light-sensitive nerve cells: rods and cones.

Optic tracts

These are the pathways of the optic nerves, posterior to the optic chiasma. Each tract consists of the nasal fibres from the retina of one eye and the temporal fibres from the retina of the other. The optic tracts pass backwards through the cerebrum to synapse with nerve cells of the *lateral geniculate bodies* of the thalamus. From there the nerve fibres proceed backwards and medially as the *optic radiations* to terminate in the *visual area* of the cerebral cortex in the occipital lobes of the cerebrum. Other neurones originating in the lateral geniculate bodies convey impulses from the eyes to the *cerebellum* where, together with impulses from the semicircular canals of the ears and from the skeletal muscles and joints, they contribute to the maintenance of posture and balance.

Figure 8.12 The retina as seen through the pupil with an ophthalmoscope.

Physiology of sight

Light waves travel at a speed of 186 000 miles (300 000 kilometres) per second. Light is reflected into the eyes by objects within the field of vision. White light is a combination of all the colours of the visual spectrum (rainbow), i.e. red, orange, yellow, green, blue, indigo and violet. This is demonstrated by passing white light through a glass prism which *refracts* or bends the rays of the different colours to a greater or lesser extent, depending on their wavelengths (Fig. 8.14). Red light has the longest wavelength and violet the shortest.

This range of colour is the *spectrum of visible light*. In a rainbow, white light from the sun is broken up by raindrops which act as prisms and reflectors.

The electromagnetic spectrum

The electromagnetic spectrum is broad but only a small part is visible to the human eye (Fig. 8.15). Beyond the long end there are infrared waves (heat), microwaves and radio waves. Beyond the short end there are ultraviolet (UV), X-rays and gamma rays. UV light is not normally visible because it is absorbed by a yellow pigment in the lens. Following removal of the lens (cataract extraction), UV light is visible and it has been suggested that long-term exposure may damage the retina.

A specific colour is perceived when only one wavelength is *reflected* by the object and all the others are *absorbed*, e.g. an object appears red when only the red wavelength is reflected. Objects appear white when all wavelengths are reflected, and black when they are all absorbed.

In order to achieve clear vision, light reflected from objects within the visual field is focused on to the retina of each eye. The processes involved in producing a clear image are *refraction of the light rays*, changing the *size of the pupils* and *accommodation of the eyes*.

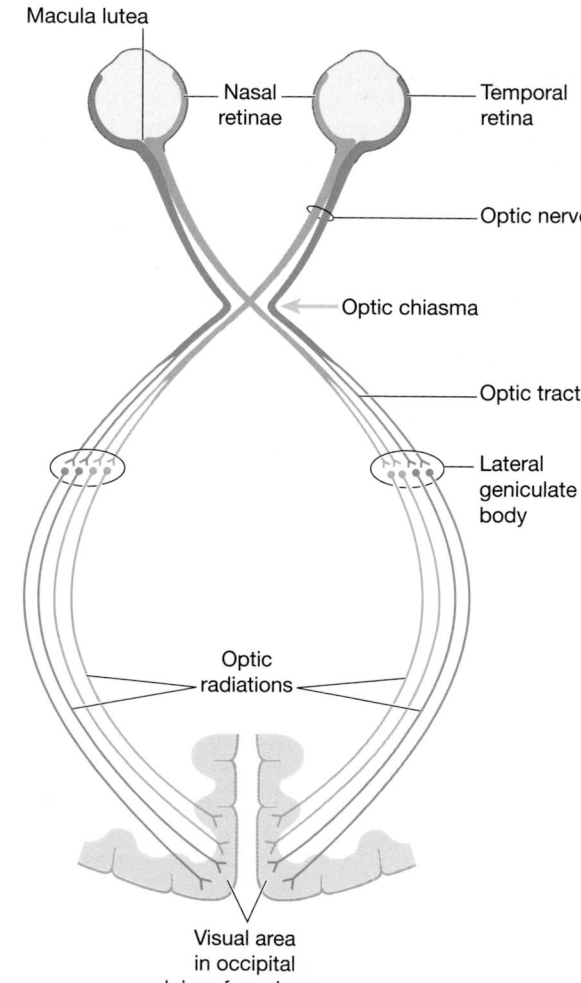

Figure 8.13 The optic nerves and their pathways.

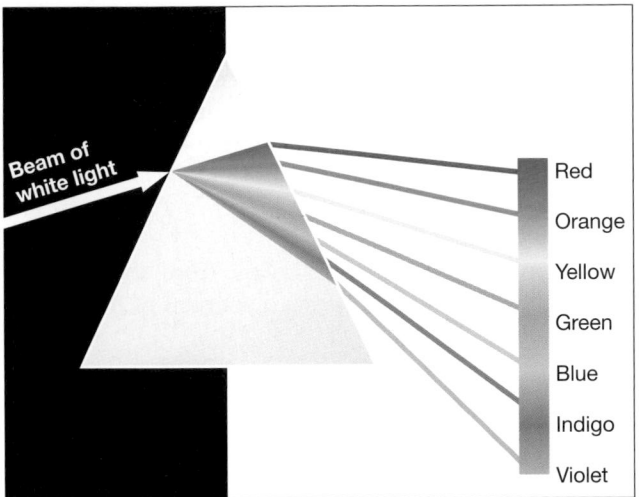

Figure 8.14 Refraction: white light broken into the colours of the visible spectrum when passed through a prism.

Although these may be considered as separate processes, effective vision is dependent upon their coordination.

Refraction of the light rays

When light rays pass from a medium of one density to a medium of a different density they are refracted or bent; for example in the eye the biconvex lens bends and focuses light rays (Fig. 8.16). This principle is used to focus light on the retina. Before reaching the retina light rays pass successively through the conjunctiva, cornea, aqueous fluid, lens and vitreous body. They are all more dense than air and, with the exception of the lens, they have a constant refractory power, similar to that of water.

Abnormal refraction within the eye is corrected using biconvex or biconcave lenses, which are shown on page 212.

Lens

The lens is a biconvex elastic transparent body suspended behind the iris from the ciliary body by the suspensory ligament. It is the only structure in the eye that changes its refractive power. Light rays entering the eye need to be bent (refracted) to focus them on the retina. Light from distant objects needs least refraction and, as the object comes closer, the amount of refraction needed is increased. To increase the refractive power the ciliary muscle contracts, releasing its pull on the suspensory ligament and the anterior surface of the lens bulges forward, increasing its convexity. This focuses light rays from near objects on the retina. When the ciliary muscle relaxes it slips backwards, increasing its pull on the suspensory ligament, making the lens thinner (Fig. 8.17). This focuses light rays from distant objects on the retina.

Size of the pupils

Pupil size influences accommodation by controlling the amount of light entering the eye. In a bright light the pupils are constricted. In a dim light they are dilated.

If the pupils were dilated in a bright light, too much light would enter the eye and damage the sensitive retina. In a dim light, if the pupils were constricted, insufficient light would enter the eye to activate the photosensitive pigments in the rods and cones which stimulate the nerve endings in the retina.

The iris consists of one layer of circular and one of radiating smooth muscle fibres. Contraction of the circular fibres constricts the pupil, and contraction of the radiating fibres dilates it. The size of the pupil is controlled by the autonomic nervous system. Sympathetic stimulation dilates the pupils and parasympathetic stimulation causes constriction.

201

Figure 8.15 The electromagnetic spectrum.

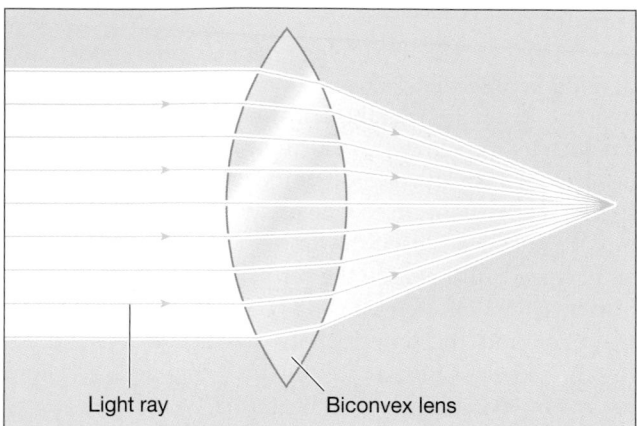

Figure 8.16 Refraction of light rays passing through a biconvex lens.

Accommodation of the eyes to light
(Figs 8.17 and 8.18)

Close vision

In order to focus on near objects, i.e. within about 6 metres, the eye must make the following adjustments:

- constriction of the pupils
- convergence of the eyeballs
- changing the power of the lens.

Constriction of the pupils. This assists accommodation by reducing the width of the beam of light entering the eye so that it passes through the central curved part of the lens.

Convergence (movement) of the eyeballs. Light rays from nearby objects enter the two eyes at different angles and for clear vision they must stimulate *corresponding areas* of the two retinae. Extraocular muscles move the eyes and to obtain a clear image they rotate the eyes so that they *converge* on the object viewed. This coordinated muscle activity is under autonomic control. When there is voluntary movement of the eyes both eyes move and convergence is maintained. The nearer an object is to the eyes the greater the eye rotation needed to achieve convergence, e.g. an individual focusing near the tip of his nose appears to be 'cross-eyed'. If convergence is not complete the eyes are focused on different objects or on different points of the same object. There are then two images sent to the brain and this leads to double vision, *diplopia*. After a period of time during which convergence is not possible the brain tends to ignore the impulses received from the divergent eye (see squint, p. 211).

Changing the power of the lens. Changes in the thickness of the lens are made to focus light on the retina. The amount of adjustment depends on the distance of the object from the eyes, i.e. the lens is thicker for near vision and at its thinnest when focusing on objects at more than 6 metres' distance (Fig. 8.17). Looking at near objects 'tires' the eyes more quickly, owing to the continuous use of the ciliary muscle.

Distant vision

Objects more than 6 metres away from the eyes are focused on the retina without adjustment of the lens or convergence of the eyes.

Functions of the retina

The retina is the *photosensitive* part of the eye. The light-sensitive nerve cells are the *rods* and *cones* and their distribution in the retina is shown in Figure 8.11A. Light rays cause chemical changes in photosensitive pigments in these cells and they generate nerve impulses which are conducted to the occipital lobes of the cerebrum via the optic nerves.

The rods are more sensitive than the cones. They are stimulated by low-intensity or dim light, e.g. by the dim light in the interior of a darkened room.

The cones are sensitive to bright light and colour. The different wavelengths of visible light stimulate photosensitive pigments in the cones, resulting in the perception of different colours. In bright light the light rays are focused on the macula lutea.

The rods are more numerous towards the periphery of the retina. *Visual purple (rhodopsin)* is a photosensitive pigment present only in the rods. It is bleached (degraded)

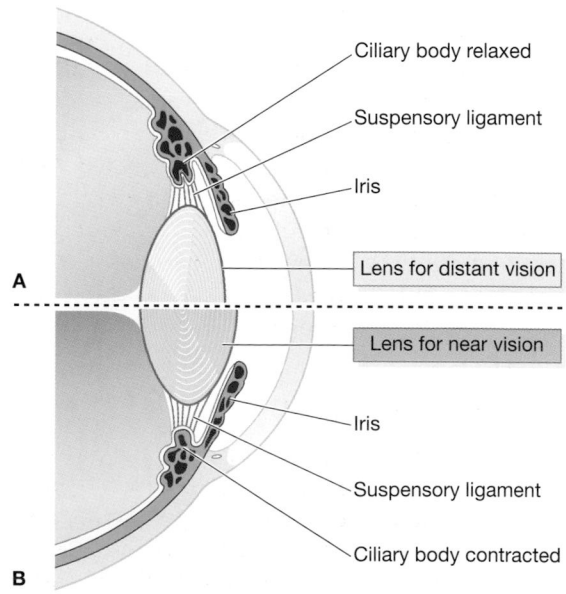

Figure 8.17 The shape of the lens: A. Distant vision. B. Near vision.

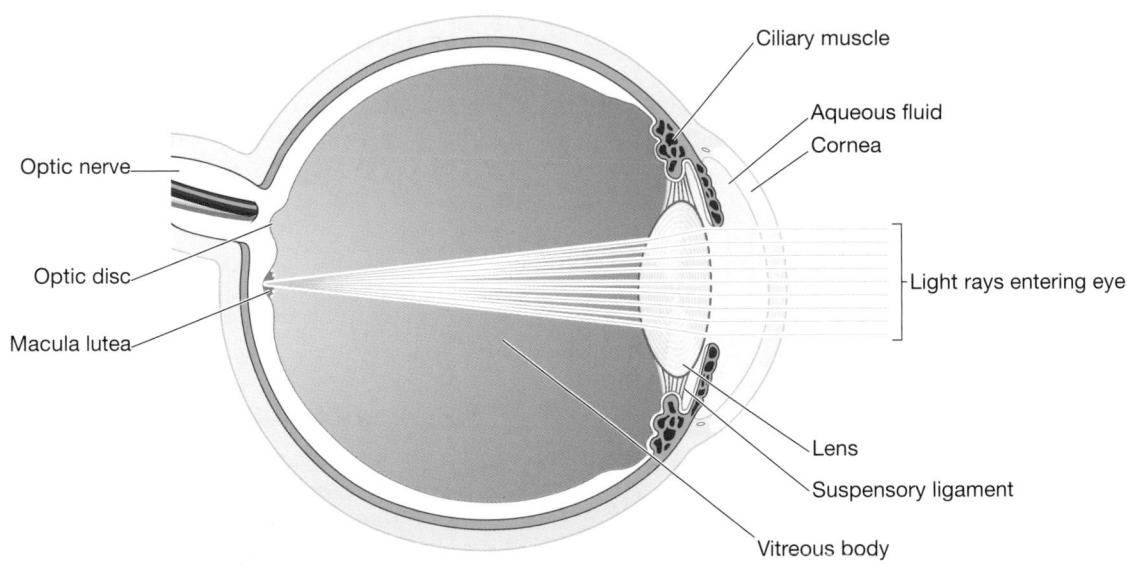

Figure 8.18 Section of the eye showing the focusing of light rays on the retina.

by bright light and is quickly regenerated when an adequate supply of vitamin A is available (p. 274).

Dark adaptation. When exposed to bright light, the rhodopsin within the sensitive rods is completely degraded. This is not significant until the individual moves into a darkened area where the light intensity is insufficient to stimulate the cones, and temporary visual impairment results whilst the rhodopsin is being regenerated within the rods, 'dark adaptation'. When regeneration of rhodopsin occurs, normal sight returns.

It is easier to see a dim star in the sky at night if the head is turned slightly away from it because light of low intensity is then focused on an area of the retina where there is a greater concentration of rods. If looked at directly the light intensity of a dim star is not sufficient to stimulate the less sensitive cones in the area of the macula lutea. In dim evening light different colours cannot be distinguished because the light intensity is insufficient to stimulate colour-sensitive pigments in cones.

Breakdown and regeneration of the visual pigments in cones is similar to that of rods.

Binocular vision (Fig. 8.19)

Binocular or stereoscopic vision has certain advantages. Each eye 'sees' a scene slightly differently. There is an overlap in the middle but the left eye sees more on the left than can be seen by the other eye and vice versa. The images from the two eyes are fused in the cerebrum so that only one image is perceived.

Binocular vision provides a much more accurate assessment of one object relative to another, e.g. its distance, depth, height and width. People with monocular vision may find it difficult, for example, to judge the speed and distance of an approaching vehicle.

203

Extraocular muscles of the eye

The eyeballs are moved by six *extrinsic muscles*, attached at one end to the eyeball and at the other to the walls of the orbital cavity. There are four *straight* (rectus) muscles and two *oblique* muscles (Fig. 8.20). They are:

- medial rectus
- lateral rectus
- superior rectus
- inferior rectus
- superior oblique
- inferior oblique.

Movement of the eyes to look in a particular direction is under voluntary control, but coordination of movement, needed for convergence and accommodation to near or distant vision, is under autonomic (involuntary) control. Movements of the eyes made by the action of these muscles are shown in Table 8.1.

Nerve supply to the muscles of the eye

Nerves shown in Table 8.1 supply the extrinsic muscles. The *oculomotor nerves* supply the *intrinsic muscles* of the iris and ciliary body.

Table 8.1 Extrinsic muscles of the eye: their actions and cranial nerve supply

Name	Action	Cranial nerve supply
Medial rectus	Rotates eyeball inwards	Oculomotor nerve (3rd cranial nerve)
Lateral rectus	Rotates eyeball outwards	Abducent nerve (6th cranial nerve)
Superior rectus	Rotates eyeball upwards	Oculomotor nerve (3rd cranial nerve)
Inferior rectus	Rotates eyeball downwards	Oculomotor nerve (3rd cranial nerve)
Superior oblique	Rotates eyeball downwards and outwards	Trochlear nerve (4th cranial nerve)
Inferior oblique	Rotates eyeball upwards and outwards	Oculomotor nerve (3rd cranial nerve)

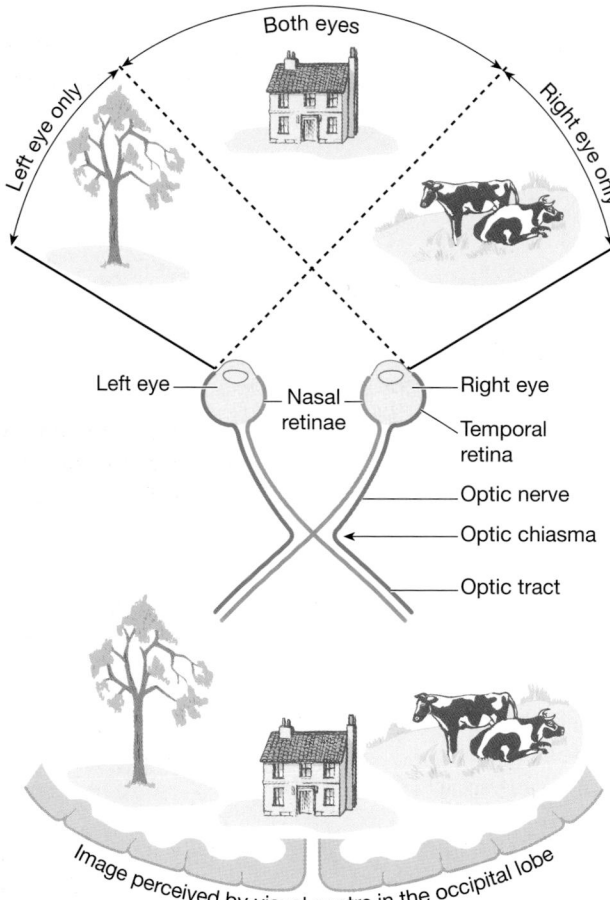

Figure 8.19 Parts of the visual field – monocular and binocular.

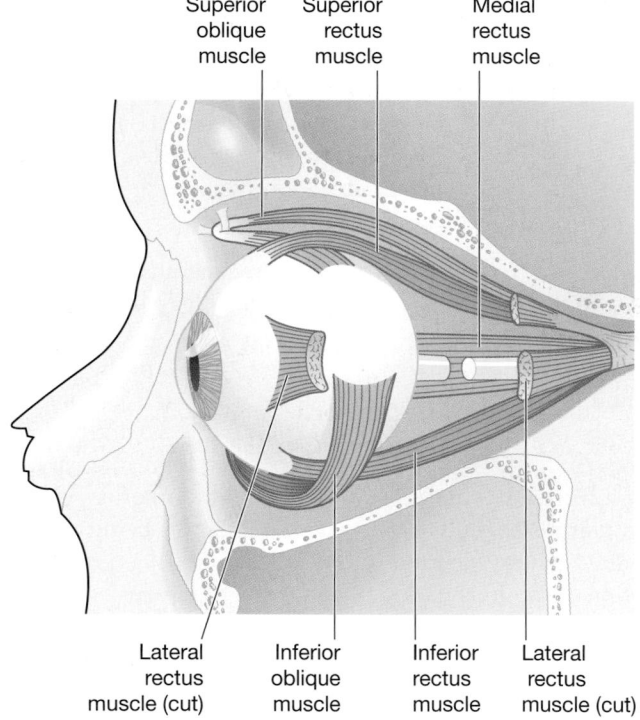

Figure 8.20 The extrinsic muscles of the eye.

Accessory organs of the eye

The eye is a delicate organ which is protected by several structures (Fig. 8.21):

- eyebrows
- eyelids and eyelashes
- lacrimal apparatus.

Eyebrows

These are two arched ridges of the supraorbital margins of the frontal bone. Numerous hairs (eyebrows) project obliquely from the surface of the skin. They protect the anterior aspect of the eyeball from sweat, dust and other foreign bodies.

Eyelids (palpebrae)

The eyelids are two movable folds of tissue situated above and below the front of each eye. On their free edges there are short curved hairs, the *eyelashes*. The layers of tissue which form the eyelids are:

- a thin covering of skin
- a thin sheet of loose (areolar) tissue
- two muscles — the *orbicularis oculi* and *levator palpebrae superioris*
- a thin sheet of dense connective tissue, the *tarsal plate*, larger in the upper than in the lower eyelid, which supports the other structures
- a lining of *conjunctiva*.

Conjunctiva

This is a fine transparent membrane which lines the eyelids and the front of the eyeball (Fig. 8.21). Where it lines the eyelids it consists of highly vascular columnar epithelium. Corneal conjunctiva consists of less-vascular stratified epithelium. When the eyelids are closed the conjunctiva becomes a closed sac. It protects the delicate cornea and the front of the eye. When eyedrops are administered they are placed in the lower conjunctival sac. The medial and lateral angles of the eye where the upper and lower lids come together are called respectively the *medial canthus* and the *lateral canthus*.

Eyelid margins

Along the edges of the lids there are numerous *sebaceous glands*, some with ducts opening into the hair follicles of the *eyelashes* and some on to the eyelid margins between the hairs. *Tarsal glands* (meibomian glands) are modified sebaceous glands embedded in the tarsal plates with ducts that open on to the inside of the free margins of the eyelids. They secrete an oily material, spread over the conjunctiva by blinking, which delays evaporation of tears.

Functions

The *eyelids* and *eyelashes* protect the eye from injury.

- Reflex closure of the lids occurs when the conjunctiva or eyelashes are touched, when an object comes close to the eye or when a bright light shines into the eye — this is called the *conjunctival* or *corneal reflex*.
- Blinking at about 3- to 7-second intervals spreads tears and oily secretions over the cornea, preventing drying.

When the *orbicularis oculi* contracts, the eyes close. When the *levator palpebrae* contract the eyelids open (see Fig. 18.1, p. 430).

Lacrimal apparatus (Fig. 8.22)

For each eye this consists of:

- 1 lacrimal gland and its ducts
- 2 lacrimal canaliculi
- 1 lacrimal sac
- 1 nasolacrimal duct.

The lacrimal glands are exocrine glands situated in recesses in the frontal bones on the lateral aspect of each eye just behind the supraorbital margin. Each gland is

205

Figure 8.21 Section of the eye and its accessory structures.

Frontal bone
Eyebrow
Lacrimal gland
Upper eyelid
Conjunctiva
Lower eyelid
Maxilla
Optic nerve

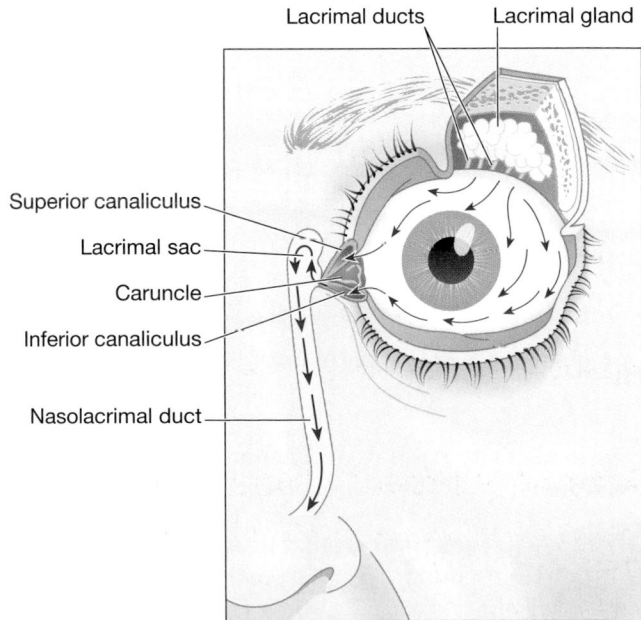

Figure 8.22 The lacrimal apparatus. Arrows show the direction of the flow of tears.

Lacrimal ducts
Lacrimal gland
Superior canaliculus
Lacrimal sac
Caruncle
Inferior canaliculus
Nasolacrimal duct

approximately the size and shape of an almond, and is composed of secretory epithelial cells. The glands secrete *tears* composed of water, mineral salts, antibodies, and *lysozyme*, a bactericidal enzyme.

The tears leave the lacrimal gland by several small ducts and pass over the front of the eye under the lids towards the medial canthus where they drain into the *two lacrimal canaliculi*; the opening of each is called the *punctum*. The two canaliculi lie one above the other, separated by a small red body, the *caruncle*. The tears then drain into the *lacrimal sac* which is the upper expanded end of the *nasolacrimal duct*. This is a membranous canal approximately 2 cm long, extending from the lower part of the lacrimal sac to the nasal cavity, opening at the level of the inferior concha. Normally the rate of secretion of tears keeps pace with the rate of drainage. When a foreign body or other irritant enters the eye the secretion of tears is greatly increased and the conjunctival blood vessels dilate. Secretion of tears is also increased in emotional states, e.g. crying.

Functions

The fluid that fills the conjunctival sac consists of tears and the oily secretion of tarsal glands and is spread over the cornea by blinking. The functions of this mixture of fluids include:

- washing away irritating materials, e.g. dust, grit
- the bacteriocidal enzyme lysozyme prevents microbial infection
- its oiliness delays evaporation and prevents drying of the conjunctiva
- nourishment of the cornea.

SENSE OF SMELL

Learning outcome

After studying this section you should be able to:

- describe the physiology of smell.

The nasal cavity has a dual function: a passageway for respiration (Ch. 10) and sense of smell.

Olfactory nerves (first cranial nerves)

These are the sensory nerves of smell. They originate as specialised olfactory nerve endings (*chemoreceptors*) in the mucous membrane of the roof of the nasal cavity above the superior nasal conchae (Fig. 8.23). On each side of the

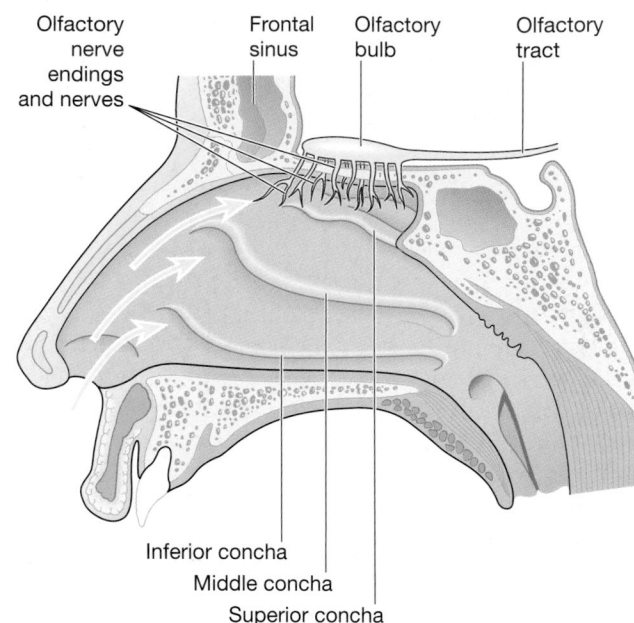

Figure 8.23 The olfactory structures.

Figure 8.24 An enlarged section of the olfactory apparatus in the nose and on the inferior surface of the cerebrum.

nasal septum nerve fibres pass through the cribriform plate of the ethmoid bone to the *olfactory bulb* where interconnections and synapses occur (Fig. 8.24). From the bulb, bundles of nerve fibres form the *olfactory tract* which passes backwards to the olfactory area in the *temporal lobe* of the cerebral cortex in each hemisphere where the impulses are interpreted and odour perceived.

Physiology of smell

The sense of smell in human beings is generally less acute than in other animals. Many animals are known to secrete odorous chemicals called *pheromones* that play an important part in chemical communication in, for example, territorial behaviour, mating and the bonding of mothers and their newborn offspring. The role of pheromones in human communication is unknown.

All odorous materials give off volatile molecules, which are carried into the nose with the inhaled air and stimulate the olfactory chemoreceptors when dissolved in mucus.

The air entering the nose is warmed and convection currents carry eddies of inspired air to the roof of the nasal cavity. 'Sniffing' concentrates volatile molecules in the roof of the nose. This increases the number of olfactory receptors stimulated and thus the perception of the smell. The sense of smell may affect the appetite. If the odours are pleasant the appetite may improve and vice versa. When accompanied by the sight of food, an appetising smell increases salivation and stimulates the digestive system (Ch. 12). The sense of smell may create long-lasting memories, especially to distinctive odours, e.g. hospital smells, favourite or least-liked foods.

Inflammation of the nasal mucosa prevents odorous substances from reaching the olfactory area of the nose, causing loss of the sense of smell (*anosmia*). The usual cause is the common cold.

Adaptation. When an individual is continuously exposed to an odour, perception of the odour decreases and ceases within a few minutes. This loss of perception only affects that specific odour and adaptation probably occurs both in the cerebrum and in the sensory receptors in the nasal cavity.

SENSE OF TASTE

Learning outcome

After studying this section you should be able to:

■ describe the physiology of taste.

Taste buds contain sensory receptors (chemoreceptors) that are found in the papillae of the tongue and widely distributed in the epithelia of the tongue, soft palate, pharynx and epiglottis. They consist of small sensory nerve endings of the glossopharyngeal, facial and vagus nerves (cranial nerves VII, IX and X). Some of the cells have hair-like microvilli on their free border, projecting towards tiny pores in the epithelium (Fig. 8.25). The sensory receptors are stimulated by chemicals that enter the pores dissolved in saliva. Nerve impulses are generated and conducted along the glossopharyngeal, facial and

vagus nerves before synapsing in the medulla and thalamus. Their final destination is the *taste area* in the parietal lobe of the cerebral cortex where taste is perceived (see Fig. 7.18, p. 151).

Physiology of taste

Four fundamental sensations of taste have been described—sweet, sour, bitter and salt. This is probably an oversimplification because perception varies widely and many 'tastes' cannot be easily classified. However, some tastes consistently stimulate taste buds in specific parts of the tongue (see Fig. 12.12, p. 290):

■ sweet and salty, mainly at the tip
■ sour, at the sides
■ bitter, at the back.

The sense of taste triggers salivation and the secretion of gastric juice (Ch. 12). It also has a protective function, e.g. when foul-tasting food is eaten then reflex gagging or vomiting may be induced.

The sense of taste is impaired when the mouth is dry because substances can be 'tasted' only if they are in solution.

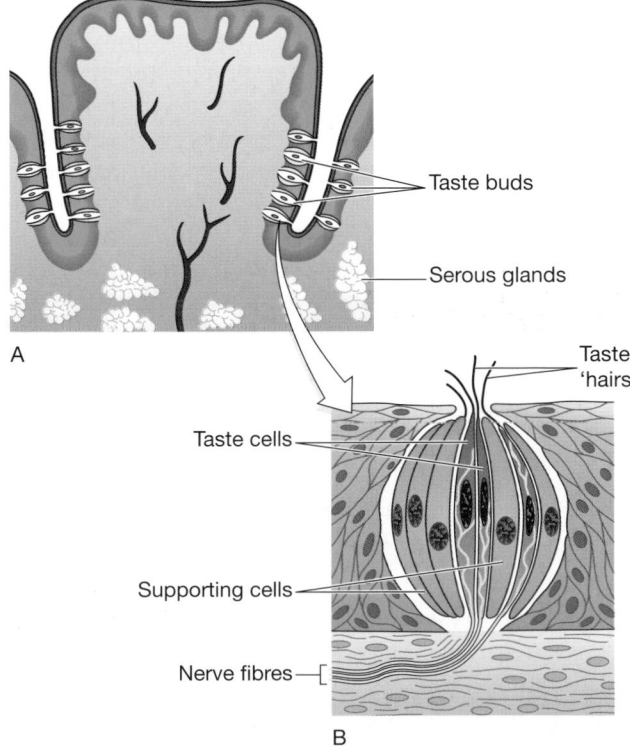

Figure 8.25 Structure of taste buds: A. A section of a papilla. B. A taste bud – greatly magnified.

DISEASES OF THE EAR

Learning outcomes

After studying this section you should be able to:

- describe the causes and effects of diseases of the ear

- compare and contrast the features of conductive and sensorineural deafness.

External otitis

Infection by *Staphylococcus aureus* is the usual cause of localised inflammation (boils) in the external auditory meatus. When more generalised, the inflammation may be caused by bacteria or fungi or by an allergic reaction to, e.g., dandruff, soaps, hair sprays, hair dyes.

Acute otitis media

This is inflammation of the middle ear cavity usually caused by upward spread of microbes from an upper respiratory tract infection via the auditory tube. It is very common in children and is accompanied by severe ear-ache on the affected side. Occasionally it spreads from the outer ear through a perforation in the tympanic membrane.

Microbial infection leads to the accumulation of pus and the outward bulging of the tympanic membrane. Sometimes there is rupture of the tympanic membrane and purulent discharge from the ear (*otorrhoea*). The spread of infection may cause *mastoiditis* and *labyrinthitis*. As the petrous portion of the temporal bone is very thin the infection may spread through the bone and cause meningitis and brain abscess.

Serous otitis media

Also known as '*glue ear*', or secretory otitis media, this is a collection of fluid (*effusion*) in the middle ear cavity. Causes include:

- obstruction of the auditory tube by, for example, pharyngeal swelling, enlarged adenoids or tumour
- barotrauma (usually caused by descent in an aeroplane when suffering from a cold)
- untreated acute otitis media.

In adults the individual suffers from deafness and (usually painless) blockage of the ear, whereas young children show delay in speech development and behavioural disorders owing to deafness. Air already present in the middle ear is absorbed and a negative pressure develops. At first there is retraction of the tympanic membrane, then fluid is drawn into the low-pressure cavity from surrounding blood vessels. Conductive hearing loss occurs and there may or may not be secondary infection. This is a common cause of hearing impairment in children.

Chronic otitis media

In this condition there is permanent perforation of the tympanic membrane following acute otitis media (especially when recurrent, persistent or untreated) and mechanical or blast injuries. During the healing process stratified epithelium from the outer ear sometimes grows into the middle ear, forming a *cholesteatoma*. This is a collection of desquamated epithelial cells and purulent material. Continued development of cholesteatoma may lead to:

- destruction of the ossicles and conduction deafness
- erosion of the roof of the middle ear and meningitis
- spread of infection to the inner ear that may cause labyrinthitis.

Otosclerosis

This is a common cause of progressive conductive hearing loss in young adults that may affect one ear but is more commonly bilateral. It is usually hereditary, more common in females than males and often worsens during pregnancy. Abnormal bone develops around the footplate of the stapes fusing it to the oval window, reducing the ability to transmit sound waves across the tympanic cavity.

Presbycusis

This form of hearing impairment commonly accompanies the ageing process. Degenerative changes in the sensory cells of the spiral organ (of Corti) result in sensorineural (perceptive) deafness. Perception of high-frequency sound is impaired first and later low-frequency sound may also be affected. The individual develops difficulty in discrimination, e.g. following a conversation, especially in the presence of background noise.

Ménière's disease

In this condition there is accumulation of endolymph causing distension and increased pressure within the membranous labyrinth with destruction of the sensory cells in the ampulla and cochlea. It is usually unilateral at first but both ears may be affected later. The cause is not known. Ménière's disease is associated with recurrent episodes of incapacitating dizziness (vertigo), nausea and vomiting, lasting for several hours. Periods of remission vary from days to months. During and between attacks there may be continuous ringing in the affected ear (tinnitus). Loss of hearing is experienced during episodes, and permanent hearing impairment may gradually develop over a period of years as the spiral organ (of Corti) is destroyed.

Labyrinthitis

This may be caused by development of a fistula from a cholesteatoma (see above) or rarely by spread of infection from the middle ear. In some cases the spiral organ is destroyed, causing sudden total nerve deafness in the affected ear.

Motion sickness

Repetitive motion causes excessive stimulation of the semicircular canals and vestibular apparatus and results in nausea and vomiting in some people.

Deafness

Hearing impairment can be classified in two main categories: *conductive* and *sensorineural*. Common causes are shown in Box 8.1. Hearing impairment can also be

---

Box 8.1 Common causes of deafness

Conductive	Sensorineural
Wax or foreign body	Presbycusis
Acute otitis media	Noise pollution
Serous otitis media	Congenital
Chronic otitis media	Ménière's disease
Barotrauma	Ototoxic drugs, e.g. aminoglycosides, diuretics, chemotherapy
Otosclerosis	
External otitis	Infections, e.g. mumps, herpes zoster, meningitis, syphilis
Injury of the tympanic membrane	

---

mixed when there is a combination of conductive and sensorineural deafness in one ear.

Conductive deafness

This is due to impaired transmission of sound waves from the outside to the oval window, i.e. an abnormality of the outer or middle ear.

Sensorineural (perceptive) deafness

This is the result of disease of the cochlea, the cochlear branch of the vestibular nerve or the hearing area of the brain. The individual usually perceives noise but cannot discriminate between sounds, i.e. hears but cannot understand.

Risk factors for *congenital deafness* include:

- family history of hereditary deafness
- viruses, e.g. maternal rubella during the first 3 months of pregnancy
- acute hypoxia at birth.

DISEASES OF THE EYE

Learning outcome

After studying this section you should be able to:

- describe the pathological changes and effects of diseases of the eye.

Inflammation

Stye (hordeolum)

This is an acute and painful bacterial infection of sebaceous or tarsal glands of the eyelid margin. A 'crop' of styes may occur due to localised spread to adjacent glands. Infection of tarsal glands may block their ducts, leading to cyst formation (*chalazion*) which may damage the cornea. The most common infecting organism is *Staphylococcus aureus*.

Blepharitis

This is chronic inflammation of the eyelid margins, which is usually caused by microbes or allergy, e.g. staphylococcal infection or seborrhoea (excessive sebaceous gland secretion). If ulceration occurs, healing by fibrosis may distort the eyelid margins, preventing complete closure of the eye. This may lead to drying of the eye, conjunctivitis and possibly corneal ulceration.

Conjunctivitis

Inflammation of the conjunctiva may be caused by irritants, such as smoke, dust, wind, cold or dry air, microbes or antigens. Corneal ulceration (see below) is a rare complication.

Microbial infection. In adults this is usually caused by strains of staphylococci, streptococci, pneumococci and haemophilus.

Neonatal conjunctivitis. This occurs within 28 days of birth and is commonly caused by *Neisseria gonorrhoea*, *Chlamydia trachomatis* or herpes simplex virus. It is usually acquired when microbes contaminate the baby's eyes during delivery. Infection may cause corneal ulceration (see below).

Allergic conjunctivitis. This may be a complication of hay fever or be caused by a wide variety of airborne antigens, e.g. dust, pollen, fungus spores, animal dander, cosmetics, hair sprays, soaps. The condition sometimes becomes chronic.

Trachoma. This is a chronic inflammatory condition caused by *Chlamydia trachomatis* in which fibrous tissue forms in the conjunctiva and cornea, leading to eyelid deformity, and is a common cause of blindness in tropical countries. The microbes are spread by flies, communal use of contaminated washing water, cross-infection between mother and child, contaminated towels and clothing.

Corneal ulcer

This is local necrosis of corneal tissue, usually associated with corneal infection (*keratitis*) following trauma (e.g. abrasion), or infection spread from the conjunctiva or eyelids. Common infecting microbes include staphylococci, pneumococci and herpes simplex viruses. Acute pain, injection (redness of the cornea), photophobia and lacrimation interfere with sight during the acute phase. In severe cases extensive ulceration or perforation and healing by fibrosis can cause opacity of the cornea and irreversible loss of sight.

Inflammation of the uveal tract (iris, ciliary body, choroid)

Anterior uveitis (iritis, iridocyclitis). Iridocyclitis (inflammation of iris and ciliary body) is the more common and it may be acute or chronic. The infection may have spread from the outer eye but in most cases the cause is unknown. There is usually moderate to severe pain, redness, blurring of vision, lacrimation and photophobia. In severe cases adhesions form between the iris and lens capsule, preventing the circulation of aqueous fluid in the posterior and anterior chambers. This may cause the lens to bulge and

occlude the scleral venous sinus (canal of Schlemm), raising intraocular pressure causing *chronic closed-angle glaucoma* (see below). Acute infection usually resolves in several days or weeks while the chronic form may last for months or years.

Posterior uveitis (choroiditis, chorioretinitis). This affects the posterior segment of the eye and chorioretinitis is the more common condition. It may be caused by spread of infection from the anterior segment (front) of the eye or be secondary to a wide variety of systemic conditions, including rheumatoid arthritis, Reiter's syndrome, inflammatory bowel disease and brucellosis. Complications of uveitis include retinal detachment due to accumulation of inflammatory exudate, secondary glaucoma, cataract.

Glaucoma

This is a group of conditions in which there is increased intraocular pressure due to impaired drainage of aqueous fluid through the scleral venous sinus (canal of Schlemm) in the angle between the iris and cornea in the anterior chamber. Persistently raised intraocular pressure may damage the optic nerve by:

- mechanical compression of the axons
- compression of the blood supply causing ischaemia of the axons.

Damage to the optic nerve impairs vision and the extent varies from some visual impairment to complete blindness.

Primary glaucomas

Chronic open-angle glaucoma. There is a gradual painless rise in intraocular pressure with progressive loss of vision. Peripheral vision is lost first but may not be noticed until only central (*tunnel*) vision remains. As the condition progresses, atrophy of the optic disc occurs leading to irreversible blindness. It is commonly bilateral and occurs mostly in people over 40 years of age. The cause is not known but there is a familial tendency.

Acute closed-angle glaucoma. This is most common in people over 40 years of age and usually affects one eye. During life the lens gradually increases in size, pushing the iris forward. In dim light when the pupil dilates the lax iris bulges still further forward, and may come into contact with the cornea blocking the scleral venous sinus (canal of Schlemm) suddenly raising the intraocular pressure. Sudden severe pain, photophobia, lacrimation and loss of vision accompany an acute attack. It may resolve spontaneously if the iris responds to bright light, constricting the pupil and releasing the pressure on the scleral venous sinus. After repeated attacks spontaneous recovery may be incomplete and vision is progressively impaired.

Chronic closed-angle glaucoma. The intraocular pressure rises gradually without symptoms. Peripheral vision deteriorates first followed by atrophy of the optic disc and blindness.

Congenital glaucoma. This abnormal development of the anterior chamber is often familial or due to maternal infection with rubella in early pregnancy.

Secondary glaucoma

The most common primary disorder is anterior uveitis with the formation of adhesions (see above). Other predisposing primary conditions include intraocular tumours, enlarged cataracts, central retinal vein occlusion, intraocular haemorrhage, trauma to the eye.

Strabismus (squint, cross-eye)

This is the inability of the eyes to move together so that the same image falls on the corresponding parts of the retina in both eyes. The result is that two images are sent to the brain, one from each eye, instead of one integrated image. It is caused by extraocular muscle weakness or defective nerve supply to the muscle, i.e. defective cranial nerves III, IV or VI. In most cases the image falling on the squinting eye is suppressed by the brain, otherwise there is double vision (diplopia).

Cataract

This is opacity of the lens which may be age-related or congenital, bilateral or unilateral.

In *age-related cataract* there is gradual development of lens opacity that usually develops during older age as the result of exposure to a variety of predisposing factors including: UV light, X-rays, cigarette smoke, diabetes mellitus, ocular trauma, uveitis, systemic drug therapy, e.g. corticosteroids, chlorpromazine.

Congenital cataract may be due to genetic abnormality, e.g. Down's syndrome, or maternal infection in early pregnancy, e.g. rubella. Early treatment is required to prevent permanent blindness.

The extent of visual impairment depends on the location and extent of the opacity.

Retinopathies

Vascular retinopathies

Occlusion of the central retinal artery or vein causes sudden painless unilateral loss of vision. *Arterial occlusion* is usually due to embolism from, e.g. atheromatous plaques, endocarditis, retinal artery sclerosis. *Venous occlusion* is usually associated with arteriosclerosis in the elderly or with venous thrombosis elsewhere in the body. The retinal veins become distended and retinal haemorrhages occur. Predisposing factors include glaucoma, diabetes mellitus, hypertension, increased blood viscosity.

Diabetic retinopathy

This occurs in Type I and Type II diabetes mellitus (p. 234) and changes in retinal blood vessels are associated more with the duration of diabetes than with its severity. Capillary microaneurysms develop and later there may be proliferation of blood vessels. Haemorrhages, fibrosis and secondary retinal detachment may occur, leading to retinal degeneration and loss of vision.

Retinopathy of prematurity

Previously known as retrolental fibroplasia this condition affects premature babies. Known risk factors include: birth before 32 weeks' gestation, birth weight less than 1500 g, requirement for oxygen therapy, apnoea and sepsis. There is abnormal development of retinal blood vessels and formation of fibrovascular tissue in the vitreous body causing varying degrees of interference with light transmission. In severe cases there may also be haemorrhage in the vitreous body, retinal detachment and blindness.

211

Retinal detachment

This painless condition occurs when a tear or hole in the retina allows fluid to accumulate between the layers of retinal cells or between the retina and choroid. It is usually localised at first but as fluid collects the detachment spreads. There are spots before the eyes, flashing lights due to abnormal stimulation of sensory cells, and progressive loss of vision, sometimes described as a 'shadow' or 'curtain'. In many cases the cause is unknown but it may be associated with trauma to the eye or head, tumours, haemorrhage, cataract surgery when the pressure in the eye is reduced or diabetic retinopathy.

Retinitis pigmentosa

This is an hereditary disease in which there is degeneration of the retina, mainly affecting the rods. Defective vision in dim light usually becomes apparent in early childhood, leading to tunnel vision and eventually, blindness.

Keratomalacia

In this condition there is corneal ulceration, usually with secondary infection. The lacrimal glands and conjunctiva may be involved. It is caused by chronic vitamin A and protein deficiency in the diet. There may be softening or even perforation of the cornea. Night blindness (defective adaptation to dim light) is usually an early sign of deficiency of vitamin A which is required for the regeneration of rhodopsin (visual purple) after it has been exposed to light.

Tumours

Choroidal malignant melanoma

This is the most common ocular malignancy and it occurs between 40 and 70 years of age. Vision is not normally affected until the tumour causes retinal detachment or secondary glaucoma, usually when well advanced. The tumour spreads locally in the choroid, and bloodborne metastases develop mainly in the liver.

Retinoblastoma

This is a malignant tumour derived from embryonic retinal cells. A small number of cases are familial. It is usually evident before the age of 4 years and may be bilateral. The condition presents with a squint and enlargement of the eye. As the tumour grows visual impairment develops and the pupil looks pale. It spreads locally to the vitreous body and may grow along the optic nerve, invading the brain.

Disorders of the lacrimal apparatus

Acute dacryoadenitis

This is inflammation of the lacrimal gland, usually unilateral. It may be due to spread of infection from the eyelids or surrounding structures, or be associated with measles, mumps or influenza. This rare infection usually resolves but occasionally an abscess forms.

Dacryocystitis

This inflammation of the lacrimal sac is usually associated with partial or complete obstruction of the lacrimal duct. In infants there may be congenital stenosis of the duct. In adults the blockage may be due to nasal trauma, deviated nasal septum, nasal polyp or acute inflammatory nasal congestion.

REFRACTIVE ERRORS OF THE EYE

Learning outcome

After studying this section you should be able to:

- describe the corrective lenses used to treat refractive errors of the eye.

In the *emetropic* or normal eye, light from near and distant objects is focused on the retina (Fig. 8.26A).

In *hypermetropia*, or farsightedness, a near image is focused behind the retina because the eyeball is too short (Fig. 8.26B). A *biconvex lens* corrects this (Fig. 8.26C). Distant objects are focused normally.

In *myopia*, or nearsightedness, the eyeball is too long and distant objects are focused in front of the retina (Fig. 8.26D). Correction is achieved using a *biconcave lens* (Fig. 8.26E). Near objects are seen in focus as the eye can accommodate normally.

Astigmatism results in blurred vision when there is abnormal curvature of part of the cornea or lens that prevents focusing on the retina. Correction requires cylindrical lenses.

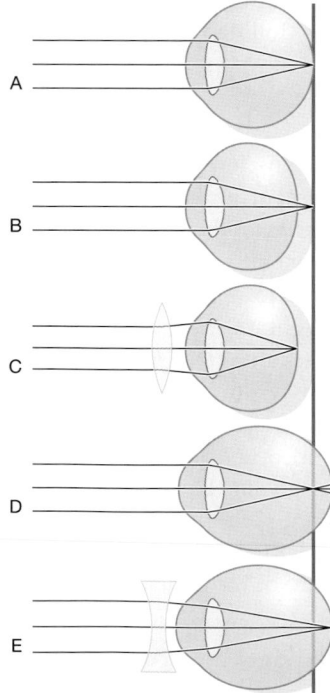

Figure 8.26 Common refractive errors of the eye and corrective lenses. A. Normal eye. B and C. Farsightedness. D and E. Nearsightedness.

9 The endocrine system

The endocrine system consists of glands widely separated from each other with no direct anatomical links (Fig. 9.1). Endocrine glands consist of groups of secretory cells surrounded by an extensive network of capillaries which facilitates diffusion of *hormones* (chemical messengers) from the secretory cells into the bloodstream. They are commonly referred to as the *ductless glands* because the hormones are secreted and diffuse directly into the bloodstream.

A hormone is formed in one organ or gland and carried in the blood to another organ (*target organ* or *tissue*), probably quite distant, where it influences cellular activity, especially growth and metabolism. Most hormones are synthesised from amino acids (amines, polypeptides and proteins; see p. 23) or are cholesterol-based lipids (steroids).

Homeostasis of the internal environment is maintained partly by the autonomic nervous system and partly by the endocrine system. The autonomic nervous system is concerned with rapid changes, while hormones of the endocrine system are mainly involved in slower and more precise adjustments.

The endocrine system consists of a number of distinct glands and some tissues in other organs. Although the hypothalamus is classified as a part of the brain and not as an endocrine gland it controls the pituitary gland and has an indirect effect on many others. The endocrine glands are:

- 1 pituitary gland
- 1 thyroid gland
- 4 parathyroid glands
- 2 adrenal (suprarenal) glands
- the pancreatic islets (islets of Langerhans)
- 1 pineal gland or body
- 1 thymus gland
- 2 ovaries in the female
- 2 testes in the male.

The ovaries and the testes secrete hormones associated with the reproductive system after puberty. Their functions are described in Chapter 19.

When a hormone arrives at its target cell, it binds to a specific area, the *receptor*, where it acts as a switch influencing chemical or metabolic reactions inside the cell. The receptors for water-soluble hormones are situated on the cell membrane and those for lipid-soluble hormones are inside the cell. Examples are shown in Box 9.1.

The level of a hormone in the blood is variable and self-regulating within its normal range. A hormone is released in response to a specific stimulus and usually its action reverses or negates the stimulus through a *negative feedback mechanism* (see p. 6). This may be controlled

Box 9.1 Examples of lipid-soluble and water-soluble hormones

Lipid-soluble hormones	Water-soluble hormones
Steroids e.g. glucocorticoids, mineralocorticoids	Adrenaline, noradrenaline
Thyroid hormones	Insulin
	Glucagon

either indirectly through the release of hormones by the hypothalamus and the anterior pituitary gland, e.g. steroid and thyroid hormones, or directly by blood levels of the stimulus, e.g. insulin and glucagon.

The effect of a *positive feedback mechanism* is amplification of the stimulus and increasing release of the hormone until a particular process is complete and the stimulus ceases, e.g. release of oxytocin during labour (pp. 7 and 218).

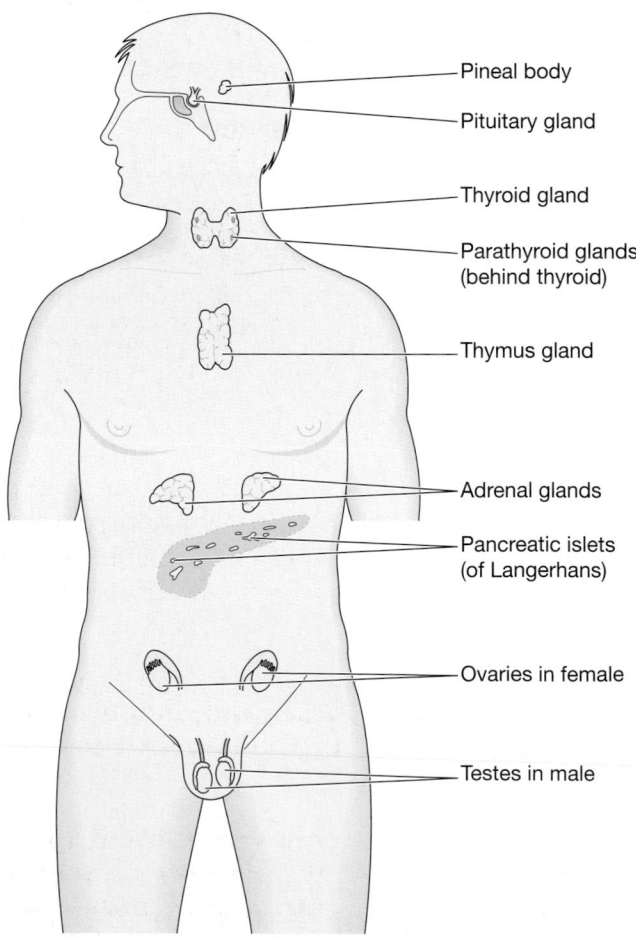

Figure 9.1 Positions of the endocrine glands.

PITUITARY GLAND AND HYPOTHALAMUS

Learning outcomes

After studying this section you should be able to:

- describe the structure of the hypothalamus and the pituitary gland

- explain the influence of the hypothalamus on the lobes of the pituitary gland

- outline the actions of the hormones secreted by the anterior and posterior lobes of the pituitary gland.

The pituitary gland (hypophysis) and the hypothalamus act as a unit, regulating the activity of most of the other endocrine glands. The pituitary gland lies in the hypophyseal fossa of the sphenoid bone below the hypothalamus, to which it is attached by a *stalk* (Fig. 9.2). It is the size of a pea, weighs about 500 mg and consists of three distinct parts that originate from different types of cells. The *anterior pituitary* (adenohypophysis) is an upgrowth of glandular epithelium from the pharynx and the *posterior pituitary* (neurohypophysis) is a downgrowth of nervous tissue from the brain. There is a network of nerve fibres between the hypothalamus and the posterior pituitary. Between these lobes there is a thin strip of tissue called the *intermediate lobe* and its function in humans is not known.

Blood supply

Arterial blood. This is supplied by branches from the internal carotid artery. The anterior lobe is supplied indirectly by blood that has already passed through a capillary bed in the hypothalamus but the posterior lobe is supplied directly.

Venous blood. This comes from both lobes, containing hormones, and leaves the gland in short veins that enter the venous sinuses between the layers of dura mater.

The influence of the hypothalamus on the pituitary gland

The influence of the hypothalamus on the release of hormones is different in the anterior and posterior lobes of the pituitary gland.

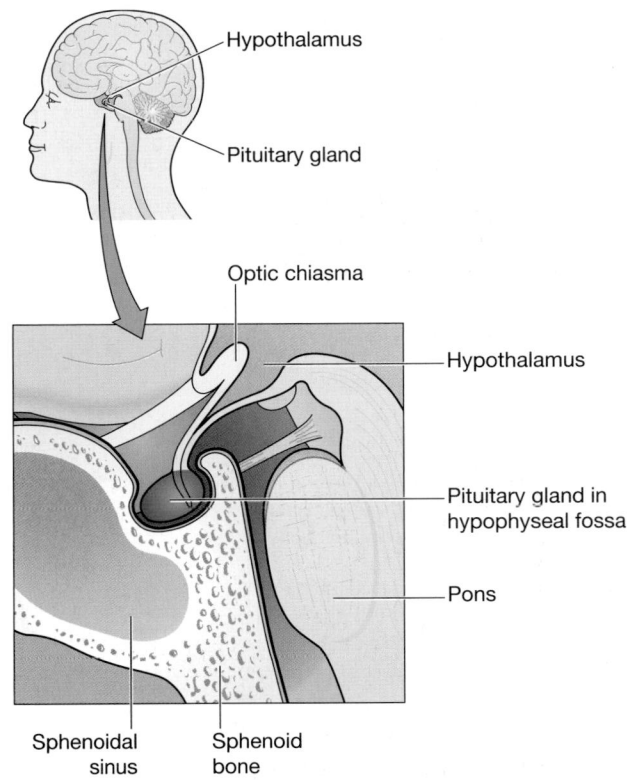

Figure 9.2 The position of the pituitary gland and its associated structures.

The anterior pituitary. This is supplied indirectly with arterial blood that has already passed through a capillary bed in the hypothalamus (Fig. 9.3A). This network of blood vessels forms part of the *pituitary portal system*, which transports blood from the hypothalamus to the anterior pituitary where it enters thin-walled vascular sinusoids and is in very close contact with the secretory cells. As well as providing oxygen and nutrients, this blood transports *releasing* and *inhibiting hormones* secreted by the *hypothalamus*. These hormones influence secretion and release of other hormones formed in the anterior pituitary. The releasing and inhibiting hormones that stimulate and inhibit secretion of specific anterior pituitary hormones are shown in Table 9.1.

The posterior pituitary. This is formed from nervous tissue and consists of nerve cells surrounded by supporting cells called *pituicytes*. These neurones have their cell bodies in the supraoptic and paraventricular nuclei of the hypothalamus and their axons form a bundle known as the *hypothalamohypophyseal tract* (Fig. 9.3A). Posterior pituitary hormones are synthesised in the nerve cell bodies, transported along the axons and then stored in vesicles within the axon terminals (Fig. 9.3B). Their release by exocytosis is triggered by nerve impulses from the hypothalamus.

Table 9.1 Hormones of the hypothalamus, anterior pituitary and their target tissues

Hypothalamus	Anterior pituitary	Target gland or tissue
GHRH	GH	Most tissues
		Many organs
GHRIH	GH inhibition	Thyroid gland
	TSH inhibition	Pancreatic islets
		Most tissues
TRH	TSH	Thyroid gland
CRH	ACTH	Adrenal cortex
PRH	PRL	Breast
PIH	PRL inhibition	Breast
LHRH or	FSH	Ovaries and testes
GnRH	LH	Ovaries and testes

GHRH	=	growth hormone releasing hormone
GH	=	growth hormone (somatotrophin)
GHRIH	=	growth hormone release inhibiting hormone (somatostatin)
TRH	=	thyroid releasing hormone
TSH	=	thyroid stimulating hormone
CRH	=	corticotrophin releasing hormone
ACTH	=	adrenocorticotrophic hormone
PRH	=	prolactin releasing hormone
PRL	=	prolactin (lactogenic hormone)
PIH	=	prolactin inhibiting hormone (dopamine)
LHRH	=	luteinising hormone releasing hormone
GnRH	=	gonadotrophin releasing hormone
FSH	=	follicle stimulating hormone
LH	=	luteinising hormone

Anterior pituitary

Some of the hormones secreted by the anterior lobe (adenohypophysis) stimulate or inhibit secretion by other endocrine glands (target glands) while others have a direct effect on target tissues. Table 9.1 summarises the main relationships between the hormones of the hypothalamus, the anterior pituitary and target glands or tissues.

The release of an anterior pituitary hormone follows stimulation of the gland by a specific *releasing hormone* produced by the hypothalamus and conveyed to the gland through the pituitary portal system of blood vessels. The whole system is controlled by a *negative feedback mechanism*. That is, when there is a low level of a hormone in the blood supplying the hypothalamus it produces the appropriate releasing hormone which stimulates release of a *trophic hormone* by the anterior pituitary. This in turn stimulates the target gland to produce and release its hormone. As a result the blood level of that hormone rises and inhibits the secretion of releasing factor by the hypothalamus (Fig. 9.4).

Figure 9.3 The pituitary gland: A. The lobes of the pituitary gland and their relationship with the hypothalamus. B. Synthesis and storage of antidiuretic hormone and oxytocin.

Figure 9.4 Negative feedback regulation of secretion of hormones by the anterior lobe of the pituitary gland.

Growth hormone (GH)

This is the most abundant hormone synthesised by the anterior pituitary. It stimulates growth and division of most body cells but especially those in the bones and skeletal muscles. It also regulates aspects of metabolism in many organs, e.g. liver, intestines and pancreas; stimulates protein synthesis; promotes breakdown of fats; and increases blood glucose levels (see Ch. 12).

Its release is stimulated by *growth hormone releasing hormone* (GHRH) and suppressed by *growth hormone release inhibiting hormone* (GHRIH) both of which are secreted by the hypothalamus. Secretion of GH is greater at night during sleep although hypoglycaemia, exercise and anxiety also stimulate release. The daily amount secreted peaks in adolescence and then declines with age. Inhibition of GH secretion occurs by a negative feedback mechanism when the blood level rises and also when GHRIH (*somatostatin*) is released by the hypothalamus. GHRIH also suppresses secretion of TSH and gastrointestinal secretions, e.g. gastric juice, gastrin and cholecystokinin (see Ch. 12).

Thyroid stimulating hormone (TSH)

This hormone is synthesised by the anterior pituitary and its release is stimulated by TRH from the hypothalamus. It stimulates growth and activity of the thyroid gland, which secretes the hormones *thyroxine* (T_4) and *triiodothyronine* (T_3). Release is lowest in the early evening and highest during the night. Secretion is regulated by a negative feedback mechanism (Fig. 9.4). When the blood level of thyroid hormones is high, secretion of TSH is reduced, and vice versa.

Adrenocorticotrophic hormone (corticotrophin, ACTH)

Corticotrophin releasing hormone (CRH) from the hypothalamus promotes the synthesis and release of ACTH by the anterior pituitary. This increases the concentration of cholesterol and steroids within the adrenal context and the output of steroid hormones, especially *cortisol.*

ACTH levels are highest at about 8 a.m. and fall to their lowest about midnight, although high levels sometimes occur at midday and 6 p.m. This circadian rhythm is maintained throughout life. It is associated with the sleep pattern and adjustment to changes takes several days, following, e.g., shift work changes, travel to a different time zone (jet lag).

Secretion is also regulated by a negative feedback mechanism, being suppressed when the blood level of ACTH rises (Fig. 9.4). Other factors that stimulate secretion include hypoglycaemia, exercise and other stressors, e.g. emotional states and fever.

Prolactin

This hormone stimulates *lactation* (milk production) and has a direct effect on the breasts immediately after parturition (childbirth). The blood level of prolactin is stimulated by prolactin releasing hormone (PRH) released from the hypothalamus and it is lowered by prolactin inhibiting hormone (PIH, *dopamine*) and by an increased blood level of prolactin. After birth, suckling stimulates prolactin secretion and lactation. The resultant high blood level is a factor in reducing the incidence of conception during lactation.

Prolactin together with oestrogens, corticosteroids, insulin and thyroxine is involved in initiating and maintaining lactation. Prolactin secretion is related to sleep, i.e. it is raised during any period of sleep, night or day. Emotional stress increases production.

Gonadotrophins

After puberty two gonadotrophins (sex hormones) are secreted by the anterior pituitary in response to *luteinising hormone releasing hormone* (LHRH), also known as

217

gonadotrophin releasing hormone (GnRH). In both males and females these are:

- follicle stimulating hormone (FSH)
- luteinising hormone (LH).

In both sexes. FSH stimulates production of gametes (ova or spermatozoa).

In females. LH and FSH are involved in secretion of the hormones *oestrogen* and *progesterone* during the menstrual cycle (see Figs 19.8 and 19.9, pp. 444 and 445). As the levels of oestrogen and progesterone rise secretion of LH and FSH is suppressed.

In males. LH, also called interstitial cell stimulating hormone (ICSH) stimulates the interstitial cells of the testes to secrete the hormone *testosterone* (see Ch. 19).

Table 9.2 summarises the hormonal secretions of the anterior pituitary.

Posterior pituitary

The structure of the posterior pituitary gland and its relationship with the hypothalamus is explained on page 215. *Oxytocin* and *antidiuretic hormone* (ADH or vasopressin) are the hormones synthesised in the hypothalamus and then released from the axon terminals within the posterior pituitary gland (Fig. 9.3B). These hormones act directly on non-endocrine tissue and their release by exocytosis is stimulated by nerve impulses from the hypothalamus.

Oxytocin

Oxytocin stimulates two target tissues during and after parturition (childbirth): uterine smooth muscle and the muscle cells of the lactating breast.

During parturition increasing amounts of oxytocin are released by the posterior pituitary into the bloodstream in response to increasing distension of sensory stretch receptors in the uterine cervix by the baby's head. Sensory impulses are generated and travel to the control centre in the hypothalamus, stimulating the posterior pituitary to release more oxytocin. In turn this stimulates more forceful uterine contractions and greater stretching of the uterine cervix as the baby's head is forced further downwards. This is an example of a *positive feedback mechanism* which stops soon after the baby is delivered when distension of the uterine cervix is greatly reduced (Fig. 9.5).

The process of milk ejection also involves a positive feedback mechanism. Suckling generates sensory impulses that are transmitted from the breast to the hypothalamus. The impulses trigger the release of oxytocin from the posterior pituitary and oxytocin stimulates contraction of the myoepithelial cells around the glandular cells and ducts of the lactating breast to contract, ejecting milk. Suckling also inhibits the release of *prolactin inhibiting hormone* (PIH), prolonging prolactin secretion and lactation. The role of this hormone in males and non-lactating females remains unclear.

Antidiuretic hormone (ADH) or vasopressin

The main effect of antidiuretic hormone is to reduce urine output (diuresis is the production of a large volume of urine). ADH increases the permeability to water of the distal convoluted and collecting tubules of the nephrons of the kidneys (Ch. 13). As a result the reabsorption of water from the glomerular filtrate is increased. The amount of ADH secreted is influenced by the osmotic pressure of the blood circulating to the *osmoreceptors* in the hypothalamus.

As the osmotic pressure rises, the secretion of ADH increases as in, for example, dehydration and following

Table 9.2 Summary of the hormones secreted by the anterior pituitary gland and their functions

Hormone	Function
Growth hormone (GH)	Regulates metabolism, promotes tissue growth especially of bones and muscles
Thyroid stimulating hormone (TSH)	Stimulates growth and activity of thyroid gland and secretion of T_3 and T_4
Adrenocorticotrophic hormone (ACTH)	Stimulates the adrenal cortex to secrete glucocorticoids
Prolactin (PRL)	Stimulates milk production in the breasts
Follicle stimulating hormone (FSH)	Stimulates production of sperm in the testes, stimulates secretion of oestrogen by the ovaries, maturation of ovarian follicles, ovulation
Luteinising hormone (LH)	Stimulates secretion of testosterone by the testes, stimulates secretion of progesterone by the corpus luteum

Figure 9.5 Regulation of secretion of oxytocin through a positive feedback mechanism.

haemorrhage. More water is therefore reabsorbed and the urine output is reduced. This means that the body retains more water and the rise in osmotic pressure is reversed. Conversely, when the osmotic pressure of the blood is low, for example after a large fluid intake, secretion of ADH is reduced, less water is reabsorbed and more urine is produced (Fig. 9.11).

At high concentrations, for example after severe blood loss, ADH causes smooth muscle contraction, especially vasoconstriction in the blood vessels of the skin and abdominal organs. This has a *pressor effect*, raising systemic blood pressure; the alternative name of this hormone, vasopressin, reflects this effect.

THYROID GLAND (Fig. 9.6)

Learning outcomes

After studying this section you should be able to:

- describe the position of the thyroid gland and its related structures

- describe the microscopic structure of the thyroid gland

- outline the actions of the thyroid hormones

- explain how blood levels of the thyroid hormones T_3 and T_4 are regulated.

The thyroid gland is situated in the neck in front of the larynx and trachea at the level of the 5th, 6th and 7th cervical and 1st thoracic vertebrae. It is a highly vascular gland that weighs about 25 g and is surrounded by a fibrous capsule. It resembles a butterfly in shape, consisting of *two lobes*, one on either side of the thyroid

219

Table 9.3 Common effects of abnormal secretion of thyroid hormones

Hyperthyroidism: increased T_3 and T_4 secretion	Hypothyroidism: decreased T_3 and T_4 secretion
Increased basal metabolic rate	Decreased basal metabolic rate
Anxiety, physical restlessness, mental excitability	Depression, psychosis, mental slowness, lethargy
Hair loss	Dry skin, brittle hair
Tachycardia, palpitations, atrial fibrillation	Bradycardia
Warm sweaty skin, heat intolerance	Dry cold skin, prone to hypothermia
Diarrhoea	Constipation
Weight loss, good appetite	Weight gain, anorexia
Exophthalmos in Graves' disease	

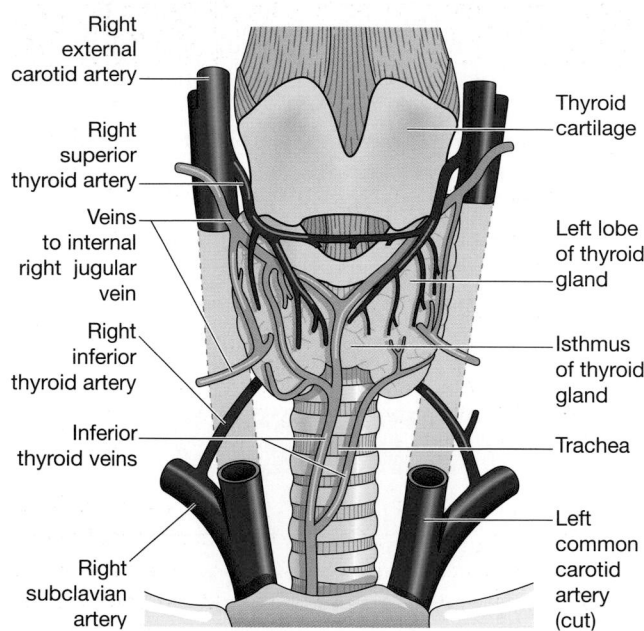

Figure 9.6 The position of the thyroid gland and its associated structures.

cartilage and upper cartilaginous rings of the trachea. The lobes are joined by a narrow *isthmus*, lying in front of the trachea.

The lobes are roughly cone-shaped, about 5 cm long and 3 cm wide.

The *arterial blood supply* to the gland is through the superior and inferior thyroid arteries. The superior thyroid artery is a branch of the external carotid artery and the inferior thyroid artery is a branch of the subclavian artery.

The *venous return* is by the thyroid veins which drain into the internal jugular veins.

Two parathyroid glands lie against the posterior surface of each lobe and are sometimes embedded in thyroid tissue. The recurrent laryngeal nerve passes upwards close to the lobes of the gland and on the right side it lies near the inferior thyroid artery (Fig. 9.9).

The gland is composed of cuboidal epithelium that forms spherical follicles. These secrete and store *colloid*, a thick sticky protein material (Fig. 9.7). Between the follicles there are other cells found singly or in small groups: *parafollicular cells*, also called C-cells, which secrete the hormone *calcitonin*.

Thyroxine and triiodothyronine

Iodine is essential for the formation of the thyroid gland hormones, thyroxine (T_4) and triiodothyronine (T_3). The body's main sources of iodine are seafood, vegetables grown in iodine-rich soil and iodinated table salt in the diet. The thyroid gland selectively takes up iodine from the blood, a process called *iodine trapping*.

Figure 9.7 The microscopic structure of the thyroid gland.

The thyroid hormones are synthesised as large precursor molecules called *thyroglobulin*, the major constituent of colloid. The release of T_3 and T_4 into the blood is regulated by *thyroid stimulating hormone* (TSH) from the anterior pituitary.

Secretion of TSH is stimulated by the *thyroid releasing hormone* (TRH) from the hypothalamus and secretion of TRH is stimulated by exercise, stress, malnutrition, low plasma glucose and sleep. The level of secretion of TSH depends on the plasma levels of T_3 and T_4 because these hormones affect the sensitivity of the anterior pituitary to TRH. Increased levels of T_3 and T_4 decrease TSH secretion and vice versa (Fig. 9.8). When the supply of iodine is deficient, excess TSH is secreted and there is proliferation of thyroid gland cells and enlargement of the gland (see Goitre, p. 230). Secretion of T_3 and T_4 begins about the third month of fetal life and is increased at puberty and in women during the reproductive years, especially during pregnancy. Otherwise, it remains fairly constant throughout life.

Thyroid hormones enter the target cells and regulate the expression of genes in the nucleus, i.e. they increase or decrease the synthesis of some proteins including enzymes. They combine with specific receptor sites and enhance the effects of other hormones, e.g. adrenaline and noradrenaline.

T_3 and T_4 affect most cells of the body by:

- increasing the basal metabolic rate and heat production
- regulating metabolism of carbohydrates, proteins and fats.

T_3 and T_4 are essential for normal growth and development, especially of the skeleton and nervous system. Most other organs and systems are also influenced by thyroid hormones—physiological effects of T_3 and T_4 on the heart, skeletal muscles, skin, digestive and reproductive systems are more evident when there is underactivity or overactivity of the thyroid gland. These changes are listed in Table 9.3.

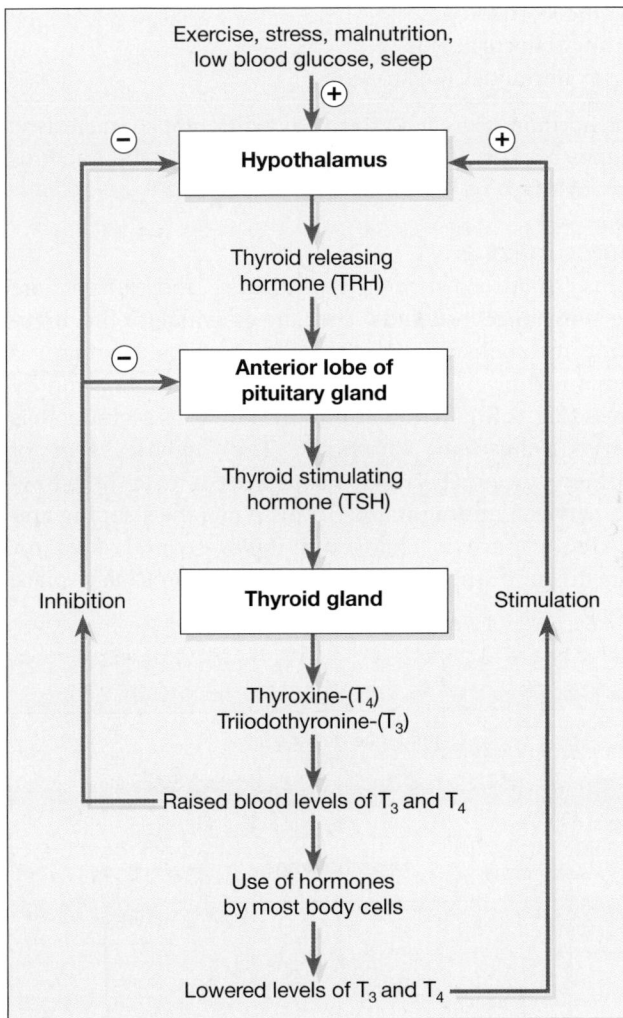

Figure 9.8 Regulation of the secretion of thyroxine (T_4) and triiodothyronine (T_3).

PARATHYROID GLANDS

Learning outcomes

After studying this section you should be able to:

- describe the position and gross structure of the parathyroid glands

- outline the functions of parathyroid hormone and calcitonin

- explain how blood levels of parathyroid hormone and calcitonin are regulated.

There are four small parathyroid glands, two embedded in the posterior surface of each lobe of the thyroid gland (Fig. 9.9). They are surrounded by fine connective tissue capsules. The cells forming the glands are spherical in shape and are arranged in columns with channels containing blood between them.

Function

The parathyroid glands secrete *parathyroid hormone* (PTH, parathormone). Secretion is regulated by the blood level of calcium. When this falls, secretion of PTH is increased and vice versa.

The main function of PTH is to increase the blood calcium level when it is low. This is achieved by indirectly increasing the amount of calcium absorbed from the small

221

Calcitonin

This hormone is secreted by the parafollicular or C-cells in the thyroid gland. It acts on bone and the kidneys to reduce the blood calcium (Ca^{2+}) level when it is raised. It reduces the reabsorption of calcium from bones and inhibits reabsorption of calcium by the renal tubules. Its effect is opposite to that of parathyroid hormone (PTH, parathormone), the hormone secreted by the parathyroid glands. Release of calcitonin is stimulated by an increase in the blood calcium level.

This hormone is important during childhood when bones undergo considerable changes in size and shape.

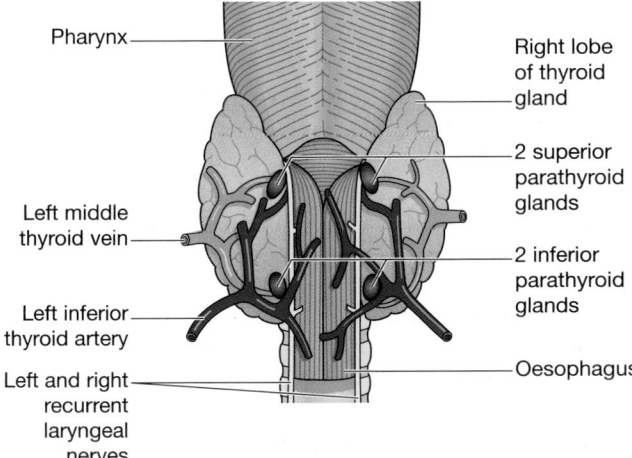

Figure 9.9 The positions of the parathyroid glands and their related structures, viewed from behind.

intestine and reabsorbed from the renal tubules. If these sources provide inadequate supplies then PTH stimulates osteoclasts (bone-destroying cells) and resorption of calcium from bones.

Parathormone and calcitonin from the thyroid gland act in a complementary manner to maintain blood calcium levels within the normal range. This is needed for:

- muscle contraction
- blood clotting
- nerve impulse transmission.

ADRENAL (SUPRARENAL) GLANDS

Learning outcomes

After studying this section you should be able to:

- describe the structure of the adrenal glands
- describe the actions of each of the three groups of adrenocorticoid hormones
- explain how blood levels of glucocorticoids are regulated
- describe the actions of adrenaline and noradrenaline
- outline how the adrenal glands respond to stress.

There are two adrenal glands, one situated on the upper pole of each kidney enclosed within the renal fascia (see Fig. 13.2, p. 340). They are about 4 cm long and 3 cm thick.

The *arterial blood supply* to the glands is by branches from the abdominal aorta and renal arteries.

The *venous return* is by suprarenal veins. The right gland drains into the inferior vena cava and the left into the left renal vein.

The glands are composed of two parts which have different structures and functions. The outer part is the *cortex* and the inner part the *medulla*. The adrenal cortex is essential to life but the medulla is not.

Adrenal cortex

The adrenal cortex produces three groups of steroid hormones from cholesterol. They are collectively called *adrenocorticocoids* (corticosteroids, corticoids). They are:

- glucocorticoids
- mineralocorticoids
- sex hormones (androgens).

The hormones in each group have different characteristic actions but due to their structural similarity their actions may overlap.

Glucocorticoids

Cortisol (hydrocortisone), *corticosterone* and *cortisone* are the main glucocorticoids. They are essential for life, regulating metabolism and responses to stress. Secretion is stimulated by ACTH from the anterior pituitary and by stress (Fig. 9.10). In non-stressful conditions secretion has marked circadian variations. The highest level of hormones occurs between 4 a.m. and 8 a.m. and the lowest, between midnight and 3 a.m. When the sleeping and waking pattern is changed it takes several days for adjustment of the ACTH/cortisol secretion to take place (see p. 217).

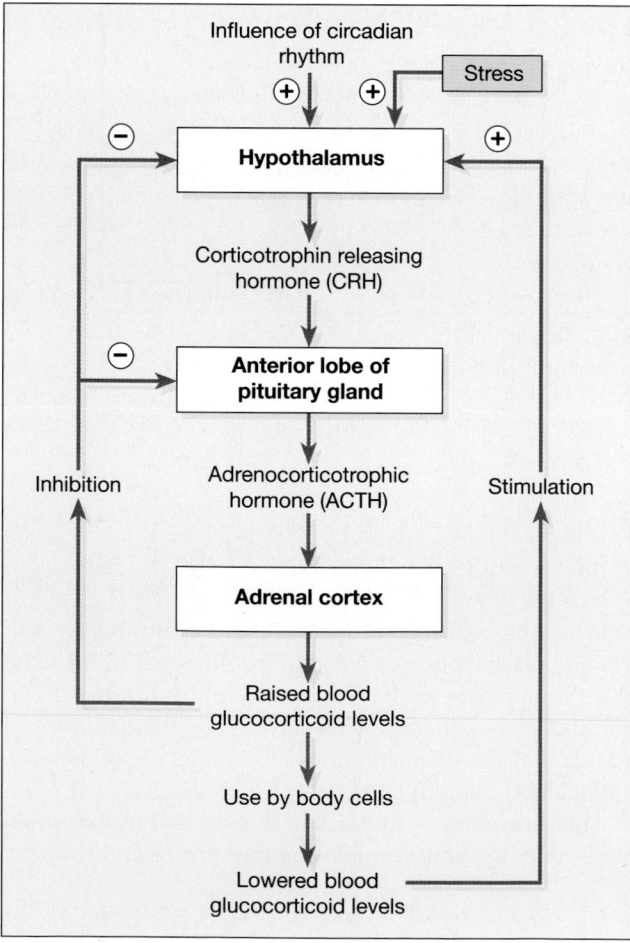

Figure 9.10 Regulation of glucocorticoid secretion.

Glucocorticoids have widespread effects and these include:

- *gluconeogenesis* (formation of new sugar from, for example, protein) and hyperglycaemia (raised blood glucose level)
- *lipolysis* (breakdown of triglycerides into fatty acids and glycerol for energy production)
- stimulating breakdown of protein, releasing amino acids, which can be used for synthesis of other proteins, e.g. enzymes, or for energy (ATP) production (p. 316)
- promoting absorption of sodium and water from renal tubules (a weak mineralocorticoid effect).

In pathological and pharmacological quantities glucocorticoids:

- have an anti-inflammatory action
- suppress the immune response
- suppress the response of tissues to injury
- delay wound healing.

Mineralocorticoids (aldosterone)

Aldosterone is the main mineralocorticoid. Its functions are associated with the maintenance of water and electrolyte balance in the body. It stimulates the reabsorption of sodium (Na^+) by the renal tubules and excretion of potassium (K^+) in the urine. Sodium reabsorption is also accompanied by retention of water and therefore aldosterone is involved in the regulation of blood volume and blood pressure too.

The blood potassium level regulates the amount of aldosterone produced by the adrenal cortex. When the blood potassium level rises, more aldosterone is secreted (Fig. 9.11). Low blood potassium has the opposite effect. *Angiotensin* (see below) also stimulates the release of aldosterone.

Renin–angiotensin–aldosterone system. When renal blood flow is reduced or blood sodium levels fall the enzyme *renin* is secreted by kidney cells. Renin converts the plasma protein *angiotensinogen*, produced by the liver, to *angiotensin 1*. Angiotensin converting enzyme (ACE), formed in small quantities in the lungs, proximal kidney tubules and other tissues converts angiotensin 1 to *angiotensin 2*, which stimulates secretion of aldosterone (Fig. 9.11). It also causes vasoconstriction and increases blood pressure.

Sex hormones

Sex hormones secreted by the adrenal cortex are mainly *androgens* (male sex hormones) and the amounts produced are insignificant compared with those secreted by the

testes and ovaries in late puberty and adulthood. Their role is unclear but it is thought that they contribute to the onset of puberty (see Ch. 19). An elevated level in females causes masculinisation. Control of secretion is poorly understood.

Adrenal medulla

The medulla is completely surrounded by the cortex. It develops from nervous tissue in the embryo and is part of the sympathetic division of the autonomic nervous system. It is stimulated by its extensive sympathetic nerve supply to produce the hormones *adrenaline* and *noradrenaline*.

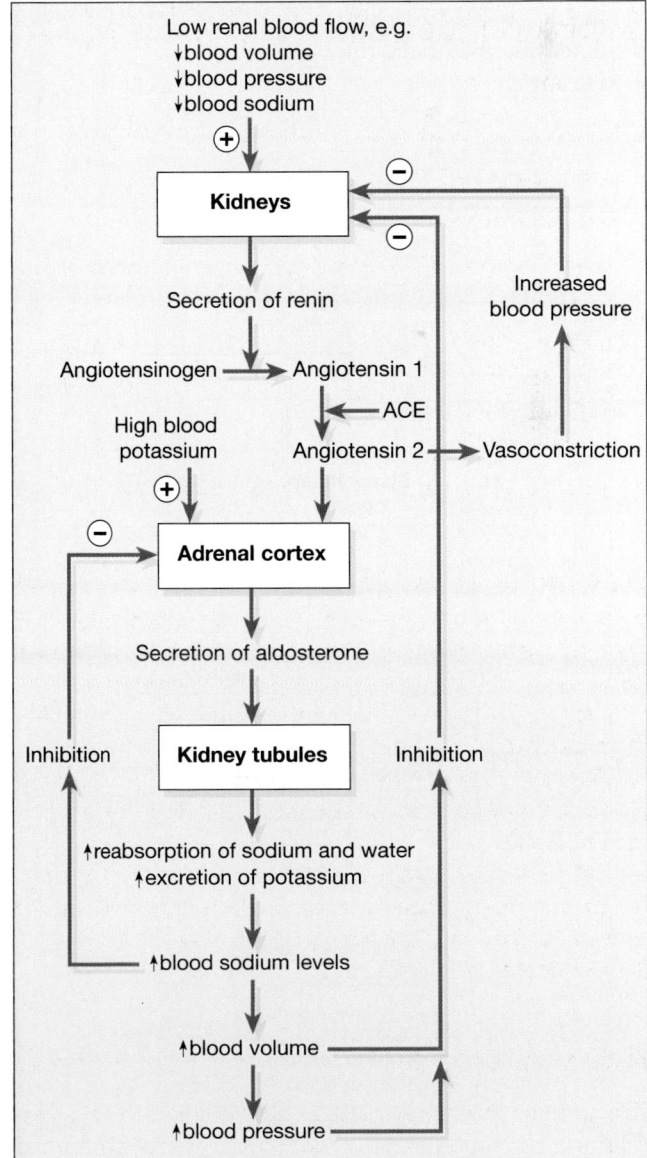

Figure 9.11 Regulation of aldosterone secretion.

223

Adrenaline and noradrenaline

Noradrenaline is the postganglionic neurotransmitter of the sympathetic division of the autonomic nervous system (see Fig. 7.9, p. 146). Adrenaline and some noradrenaline are released into the blood from the adrenal medulla during stimulation of the sympathetic nervous system (see Fig. 7.43, p. 171). They are structurally very similar and this explains their similar effects. Together they potentiate the fight or flight response after initial sympathetic stimulation by:

- increasing heart rate
- increasing blood pressure
- diverting blood to essential organs including the heart, brain and skeletal muscles by dilating their blood vessels and constricting those of less essential organs, such as the skin
- increasing metabolic rate
- dilating the pupils.

Adrenaline has a greater effect on the heart and metabolic processes whereas noradrenaline has more influence on blood vessels.

Response to stress

When the body is under stress homeostasis is disturbed. To restore it and, in some cases, to maintain life there are immediate and, if necessary, longer-term responses. Stressors include exercise, fasting, fright, temperature changes, infection, disease and emotional disturbances/situations.

The *immediate response* is sometimes described as preparing for 'fight or flight'. This is mediated by the sympathetic part of the autonomic nervous system and the principal effects are shown in Figure 9.12.

In the *longer term*, ACTH from the anterior pituitary stimulates the release of glucocorticoids and mineralocorticoids from the adrenal cortex and a more prolonged response to stress occurs.

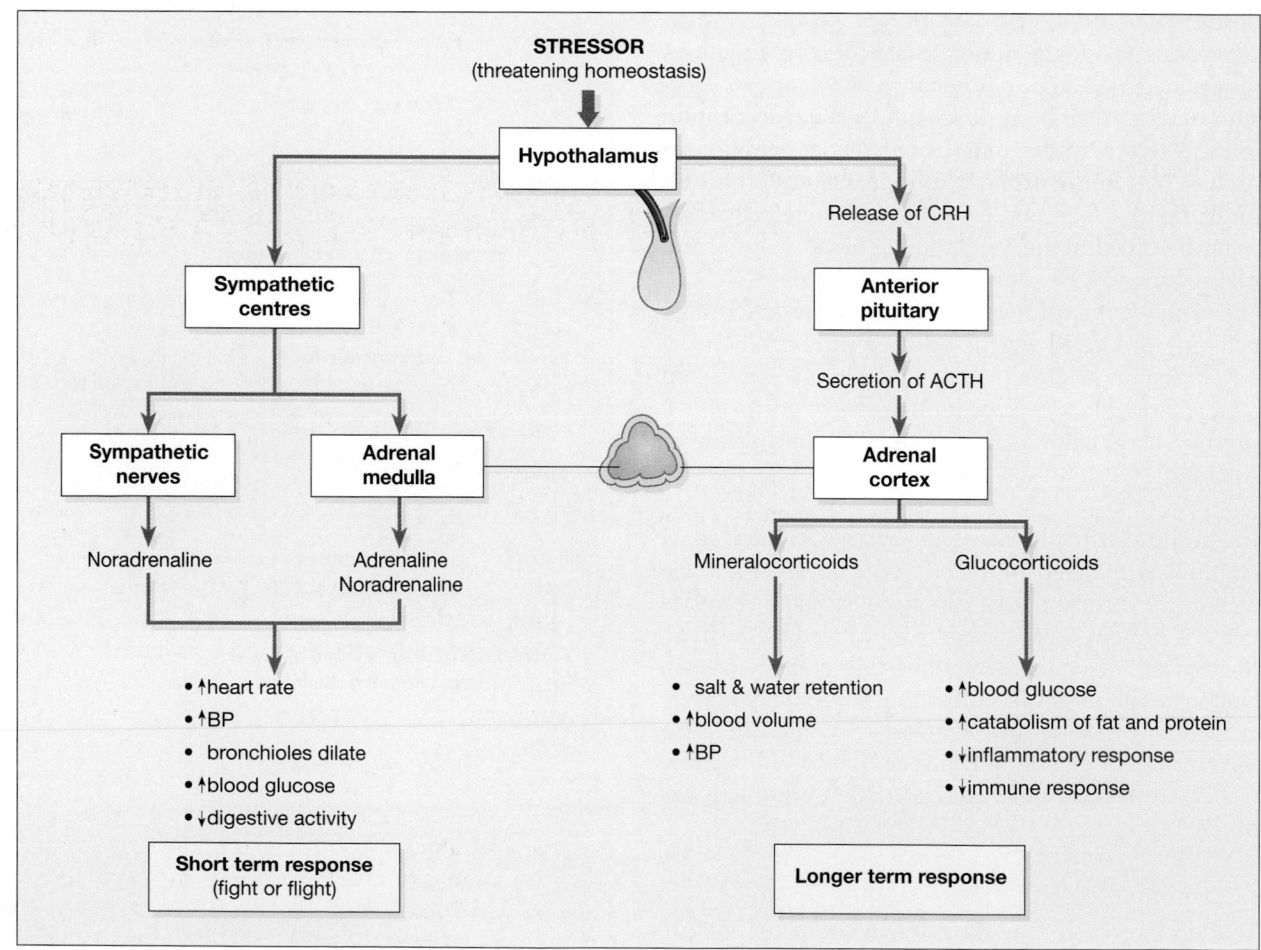

Figure 9.12 Responses to stressors that threaten homeostasis. CRH = corticotrophin releasing hormone. ACTH = adrenocorticotrophic hormone.

PANCREATIC ISLETS

Learning outcomes

After studying this section you should be able to:

■ list the hormones secreted by the endocrine pancreas

■ describe the actions of insulin and glucagon

■ explain how blood glucose levels are regulated.

The cells which make up the pancreatic islets (islets of Langerhans) are found in clusters irregularly distributed throughout the substance of the pancreas. Unlike the exocrine pancreas, which produces pancreatic juice, there are no ducts leading from the clusters of islet cells. Pancreatic hormones are secreted directly into the bloodstream and circulate throughout the body.

There are three main types of cells in the pancreatic islets:

■ α (alpha) cells that secrete *glucagon*
■ β (beta) cells that secrete *insulin*
■ δ (delta) cells that secrete *somatostatin* (GHRIH, p. 217).

The normal blood glucose level is between 2.5 and 5.3 mmol/litre (45 to 95 mg/100 ml). Blood glucose levels are controlled mainly by the opposing actions of insulin and glucagon:

■ glucagon increases blood glucose levels
■ insulin reduces blood glucose levels.

Insulin

The main function of insulin is to lower blood levels of absorbed nutrients when they rise above normal. When these nutrients, especially glucose, are in excess of immediate needs insulin promotes storage by:

■ acting on cell membranes and stimulating uptake and use of glucose by muscle and connective tissue cells
■ increasing conversion of glucose to glycogen (glycogenesis), especially in the liver and skeletal muscles
■ accelerating uptake of amino acids by cells, and the synthesis of protein
■ promoting synthesis of fatty acids and storage of fat in adipose tissue (lipogenesis)
■ decreasing glycogenolysis
■ preventing the breakdown of protein and fat, and *gluconeogenesis* (formation of new sugar from, e.g. protein).

Secretion of insulin is stimulated by increased blood glucose and amino acid levels, and gastrointestinal hormones, e.g. gastrin, secretin and cholecystokinin. Secretion is decreased by sympathetic stimulation, glucagon, adrenaline, cortisol and somatostatin (GHRIH) secreted by cells of the pancreatic islets.

Insulin is a polypeptide consisting of about 50 amino acids. Amounts are expressed in international units (IU).

Glucagon

The effects of glucagon increase blood glucose levels by stimulating, e.g.:

■ conversion of glycogen to glucose in the liver and skeletal muscles (glycogenolysis)
■ gluconeogenesis.

Secretion of glucagon is stimulated by a low blood glucose level and exercise and decreased by somatostatin and insulin.

Somatostatin (GHRIH)

The effect of this hormone, also produced by the hypothalamus, is to inhibit the secretion of both insulin and glucagon.

PINEAL GLAND OR BODY

Learning outcomes

After studying this section you should be able to:

■ state the position of the pineal gland

■ outline the actions of melatonin.

The pineal gland is a small body attached to the roof of the third ventricle and is connected to it by a short stalk containing nerves, many of which terminate in the hypothalamus. The pineal gland is about 10 mm long, is reddish brown in colour and is surrounded by a capsule.

Melatonin

This is the hormone secreted by the pineal gland. Secretion is influenced by the amount of light entering the eye stimulating the optic pathways and levels fluctuate during each 24-hour period, being highest at night and lowest around midday. Although its functions are not fully understood, it is believed to be associated with:

- coordination of the circadian and diurnal rhythms of many tissues, possibly by influencing the hypothalamus
- inhibition of growth and development of the sex organs before puberty, possibly by preventing synthesis or release of gonadotrophins.

The gland tends to atrophy after puberty and may become calcified in later life.

THYMUS GLAND

Learning outcomes

After studying this section you should be able to:

- state the position of the thymus gland
- outline the actions of thymosin.

The location and structure of the thymus gland are described on page 134.

Thymosin

This is the hormone secreted by the thymus gland and is required for the development of T-lymphocytes for cell-mediated immunity (Ch. 15).

LOCAL HORMONES

Learning outcome

After studying this section you should be able to:

- name substances that act as local hormones.

A number of body tissues not normally described as endocrine glands secrete substances that act locally. Some of these are described below.

Histamine

This hormone is synthesised by mast cells in the tissues and basophils in blood. It is released as part of the inflammatory process, increasing capillary permeability and dilatation. It also causes contraction of smooth muscle of the bronchi and alimentary tract and stimulates the secretion of gastric juice.

Serotonin (5-hydroxytryptamine, 5-HT)

This is present in platelets, in the brain and in the intestinal wall. It causes intestinal secretion and contraction of smooth muscle and its role in haemostasis (blood clotting) is outlined in Chapter 4.

Prostaglandins (PGs)

These are lipid substances that act as local hormones and have wide-ranging physiological effects in:

- the inflammatory response
- potentiating pain
- fever
- regulating blood pressure
- blood clotting
- uterine contractions during labour.

Other chemically similar compounds include *leukotrienes* and *thromboxanes*. They are active substances found in only small amounts, as they are rapidly degraded.

Erythropoietin

This hormone is synthesised by the kidneys and increases erythropoiesis (the rate of red blood cell formation, see Fig. 4.4, p. 63).

Gastrointestinal hormones

Several local hormones, including gastrin, secretin and cholecystokinin (CCK), influence the secretion of digestive juices and their functions are explained in Chapter 12.

DISORDERS OF THE ANTERIOR PITUITARY

Learning outcomes

After studying this section you should be able to:

- list the causes of diseases in this section

- relate the features of the diseases in this section to abnormal growth and development.

Endocrine disorders are commonly caused by *tumours* or *autoimmune diseases* and their effects are usually the result of:

- hypersecretion (overproduction) of hormones
- hyposecretion (underproduction) of hormones.

The abnormalities described in this section are those in which there is a general effect but no specific target gland. Abnormal secretion of *stimulating hormones* are included with the disorders of their target glands.

Hypersecretion of anterior pituitary hormones

Gigantism and acromegaly

The most common cause is prolonged hypersecretion of growth hormone (GH), usually by a hormone-secreting pituitary tumour. The conditions are only occasionally due to excess growth hormone releasing hormone (GHRH) secreted by the hypothalamus. As the tumour increases in size compression of nearby structures may lead to:

- hyposecretion of other pituitary hormones of both the anterior and posterior lobes
- hyposecretion of hormone-releasing factors by the hypothalamus
- damage to the optic nerves, causing visual disturbances.

Effects of excess GH
These include:

- excessive growth of bones
- enlargement of internal organs
- growth of excess connective tissue

- enlargement of the heart and a rise in blood pressure
- reduced glucose tolerance and a predisposition to diabetes mellitus.

Gigantism. This occurs when there is excess GH while epiphyseal cartilages of long bones are still growing, i.e. during childhood before ossification of bones is complete. It is evident mainly in the bones of the limbs and affected individuals may grow to heights of 2.1 to 2.4 m, although body proportions remain normal (Fig. 9.13).

Acromegaly (meaning 'large extremities'). This occurs when there is excess GH after ossification is complete. The bones become abnormally thick due to ossification of periosteum and there is thickening of the soft tissues. These changes are most noticeable as coarse facial features, an enlarged tongue and excessively large hands and feet (Fig. 9.14).

Figure 9.13 Effects of normal and abnormal growth hormone secretion.

227

Figure 9.14 Facial features in acromegaly.

Hyperprolactinaemia

This is caused by a hormone-secreting tumour. It causes galactorrhoea, amenorrhoea and sterility in women and impotence in men.

Hyposecretion of anterior pituitary hormones

The number of hormones and the extent of hyposecretion varies. *Panhypopituitarism* is absence of all hormones. Causes of hyposecretion include:

- tumours of the hypothalamus or pituitary
- trauma, usually caused by fractured base of skull or surgery
- pressure caused by a tumour adjacent to the pituitary gland, e.g. glioma, meningioma
- infection, e.g. meningitis, encephalitis, syphilis
- ischaemic necrosis
- ionising radiation or cytotoxic drugs.

Ischaemic necrosis

Simmond's disease is hypofunction of the anterior pituitary gland that only rarely affects the posterior lobe. The arrangement of the blood supply makes the gland unusually susceptible to a fall in systemic BP. Ischaemic necrosis of the gland may follow severe hypotensive shock causing deficient stimulation of target glands and hypofunction of all or some of the thyroid, adrenal cortex and gonads. The outcome depends on the extent of pituitary necrosis and hormone deficiency. In severe cases, glucocorticoid deficiency may be life threatening or fatal. When this condition is associated with severe haemorrhage during or after childbirth it is known as *Sheehan's syndrome* and in this situation the other effects are preceded by failure of lactation.

Pituitary dwarfism (Lorain–Lévi syndrome)

This is caused by severe deficiency of GH, and possibly of other hormones, in childhood. The individual is of small stature but is well proportioned and mental development is not affected. Puberty is delayed and there may be episodes of hypoglycaemia. The condition may be due to genetic abnormality or a tumour.

Fröhlich's syndrome

In this condition there is panhypopituitarism but the main features are associated with deficiency of GH, FSH and LH. In children the effects are diminished growth, lack of sexual development, obesity with female distribution of fat and retarded mental development. In a similar condition in adults, obesity and sterility are the main features. It may be the result of a tumour of the anterior pituitary and/or the hypothalamus but in most cases the cause is unknown.

DISORDERS OF THE POSTERIOR PITUITARY

Learning outcomes

After studying this section you should be able to:

- list the causes of diabetes insipidus
- relate the features of diabetes insipidus to abnormal secretion of antidiuretic hormone.

Diabetes insipidus

This is a relatively rare condition usually caused by hyposecretion of ADH due to damage to the hypothalamus by, e.g., trauma, tumour, encephalitis. Occasionally it occurs when the renal tubules do not respond to ADH. Water reabsorption by the renal tubules is deficient, leading to excretion of excessive amounts of dilute urine, often more than 10 litres daily, causing dehydration, extreme thirst and polydipsia. Water balance is disturbed unless fluid intake is greatly increased to compensate for excess losses.

DISORDERS OF THE THYROID GLAND

Learning outcome

After studying this section you should be able to:

- compare and contrast the effects of hyperthyroidism and hypothyroidism, relating them to the actions of T_3 and T_4.

These fall into three main categories:

- abnormal secretion of thyroid hormones (T_3 and T_4)
  - hyperthyroidism
  - hypothyroidism
- *goitre*—enlargements of the thyroid gland
- *tumours*.

Abnormal thyroid function may arise not only from thyroid disease but also from disorders of the pituitary or hypothalamus; in addition, insufficient dietary iodine causes deficiency in thyroid hormone production. The main effects are caused by an abnormally high or low basal metabolic rate.

Abnormal secretion of thyroid hormones

Hyperthyroidism

This syndrome, also known as *thyrotoxicosis*, arises as the body tissues are exposed to excessive levels of T_3 and T_4. The main effects are due to increased basal metabolic rate (Table 9.3).

In the elderly, cardiac failure is another common consequence as the ageing heart works harder to deliver more blood and nutrients to the hyperactive body cells. The main causes are:

- Graves' disease
- toxic nodular goitre
- toxic adenoma (a benign tumour, p. 231).

Graves' disease (Fig. 9.15)

Sometimes called *exophthalmic goitre*, this accounts for 90% of cases of thyrotoxicosis. More women are affected than

Figure 9.15 Features of Graves' disease.

men and this disorder usually occurs between the ages of 30 and 50 years. There is diffuse swelling (hyperplasia) of the gland with secretion of excess T_3 and T_4. In addition to the effects of hyperthyroidism, there may also be exophthalmos. This is an 'organ-specific' autoimmune condition where autoantibodies that mimic the action of TSH are produced and stimulate high levels of T_3 and T_4 secretion.

Exophthalmos (protrusion of the eyeballs). This is due to the deposition of excess fat and fibrous tissue behind the eyes; it is often present in Graves' disease. It may be caused by autoimmunity different from that associated with hyperplasia of the gland. Effective treatment of thyrotoxicosis does not reduce the exophthalmos. In severe cases the eyelids may not completely cover the eyes during blinking and sleep, leading to drying of the conjunctiva and predisposing to infection. It does not occur in other forms of thyrotoxicosis.

Toxic nodular goitre

In this condition one or two nodules of a gland that is already affected by goitre (see Simple goitre, p. 230) become active and secrete excess T_3 and T_4 causing the effects of hyperthyroidism (Table 9.3). It is more common in women than men and after middle age. As this condition affects an older age group than Graves' disease, arrhythmias and cardiac failure are more common. Exophthalmos does not occur in this type of hyperthyroidism.

Hypothyroidism

This occurs when there is insufficient T_3 and T_4 secretion causing:

- cretinism in children
- myxoedema in adults.

229

Cretinism

This condition is *endemic* in areas remote from the sea where the soil and diet are severely deficient in iodine and there is therefore insufficient iodine for synthesis of T_3 and T_4. In *sporadic* cases there is congenital absence of the thyroid gland. In both situations retarded physical growth and mental development become evident within a few weeks or months of birth. Unless treatment begins early in life the individual remains severely mentally retarded, has disproportionately short limbs, a large protruding tongue, coarse dry skin, poor abdominal muscle tone and an umbilical hernia (Fig. 9.16).

Myxoedema

This condition is prevalent in the elderly and is five times more common in females than males. Deficiency of T_3 and T_4 in adults results in an abnormally low metabolic rate and other effects shown in Table 9.3. There may be accumulation of polysaccharide substances in the subcutaneous tissues especially of the face (Fig. 9.17). The commonest causes are:

- autoimmune thyroiditis
- severe iodine deficiency (see goitre)
- iatrogenic, e.g. antithyroid drugs, surgical removal of thyroid tissue, ionising radiation.

Autoimmune thyroiditis

The most common cause of acquired hypothyroidism is *Hashimoto's disease*. It is more common in women than men. Similar conditions that are less common include *primary myxoedema* and *focal thyroiditis* and like Graves'

disease it is also an organ-specific autoimmune condition. Autoantibodies that react with thyroglobulin and thyroid gland cells develop and prevent synthesis and release of thyroid hormones causing hypothyroidism.

Simple goitre

This is enlargement of the thyroid gland without signs of hyperthyroidism. Secretion of T_3 and T_4 is reduced and the low levels stimulate secretion of TSH resulting in hyperplasia of the thyroid gland (Fig. 9.18). Sometimes the extra thyroid tissue is able to maintain normal hormone levels but if not, hypothyroidism develops. Causes are:

- persistent iodine deficiency
- genetic abnormality
- iatrogenic, e.g. antithyroid drugs, surgical removal of excess thyroid tissue.

Figure 9.17 Facial features of myxoedema.

Figure 9.16 Features of cretinism.

Figure 9.18 Enlarged thyroid gland in simple goitre.

The enlarged gland may cause pressure damage to adjacent tissues, especially if it lies in an abnormally low position, i.e. behind the sternum. The structures most commonly affected are the oesophagus, causing dysphagia; the trachea, causing dyspnoea; and the recurrent laryngeal nerve, causing hoarseness of voice.

Tumours of the thyroid gland

Benign tumours

Single adenomas are fairly common and may become cystic. Sometimes the adenoma secretes hormones and thyrotoxicosis may develop. The tumours have a tendency to become malignant especially in the elderly.

Malignant tumours

These are rare and are usually well differentiated but are sometimes anaplastic.

DISORDERS OF THE PARATHYROID GLANDS

Learning outcome

After studying this section you should be able to:

- explain how the diseases in this section are related to abnormal secretion of parathyroid hormone.

Hyperparathyroidism

Excess secretion of parathyroid hormone (PTH), usually by benign tumours of a gland, causes reabsorption of calcium from bones, raising the blood calcium level (hypercalcaemia). The effects may be:

- formation of renal calculi complicated by pyelonephritis and renal failure
- polyuria and polydipsia
- anorexia
- muscle weakness
- general fatigue
- calcification of soft tissue.

Figure 9.19 Characteristic positions adopted during tetanic spasms.

Hypoparathyroidism

Parathyroid hormone (PTH) deficiency causes hypocalcaemia, i.e. an abnormally low level of calcium in the blood. This reduces absorption of calcium from the small intestine and reabsorption from bones and glomerular filtrate. Low blood calcium causes:

- *tetany* (Fig. 9.19)
- psychiatric disturbances
- paraesthesia
- grand mal epilepsy
- development of cataract (opacity of the lens) and brittle nails.

The causes of hypoparathyroidism include:

- damage to or removal of the glands during thyroidectomy
- ionising radiation, usually from radioactive iodine used to treat hyperthyroidism
- development of autoantibodies to PTH and parathyroid cells
- congenital abnormality of the glands.

Tetany

This is caused by hypocalcaemia. There are very strong painful spasms of skeletal muscles, causing characteristic bending inwards of the hands, forearms and feet (Fig. 9.19). In children there may be laryngeal spasm and convulsions. Hypocalcaemia is associated with:

- hypoparathyroidism
- deficiency of vitamin D or dietary deficiency of calcium

- chronic renal failure when there is excretion of excess calcium in the urine
- alkalosis; metabolic due to persistent vomiting, ingestion of excess alkali to alleviate gastric disturbances or respiratory due to hyperventilation.

DISORDERS OF THE ADRENAL CORTEX

Learning outcomes

After studying this section you should be able to:

- relate the features of Cushing's syndrome to the actions of adrenocorticoids
- relate the features of Addison's disease to the actions of adrenocorticoids.

Hypersecretion of glucocorticoids (Cushing's syndrome)

Cortisol is the main glucocorticoid hormone secreted by the adrenal cortex. Causes of hypersecretion include:

- hormone-secreting adrenal tumours, benign or malignant
- hypersecretion of adrenocorticotrophic hormone (ACTH) by the anterior pituitary
- abnormal secretion of ACTH by a non-pituitary tumour, e.g. bronchial carcinoma, pancreatic tumour, carcinoid tumours
- prolonged therapeutic use of ACTH or glucocorticoids, e.g. prednisolone, in high doses.

Hypersecretion of cortisol has a wide variety of effects but they may not all be present (Fig. 9.20). They include:

- painful adiposity of the face (*moon face*), neck and abdomen
- excess protein catabolism, causing thinning of subcutaneous tissue and muscle wasting, especially of the limbs

232

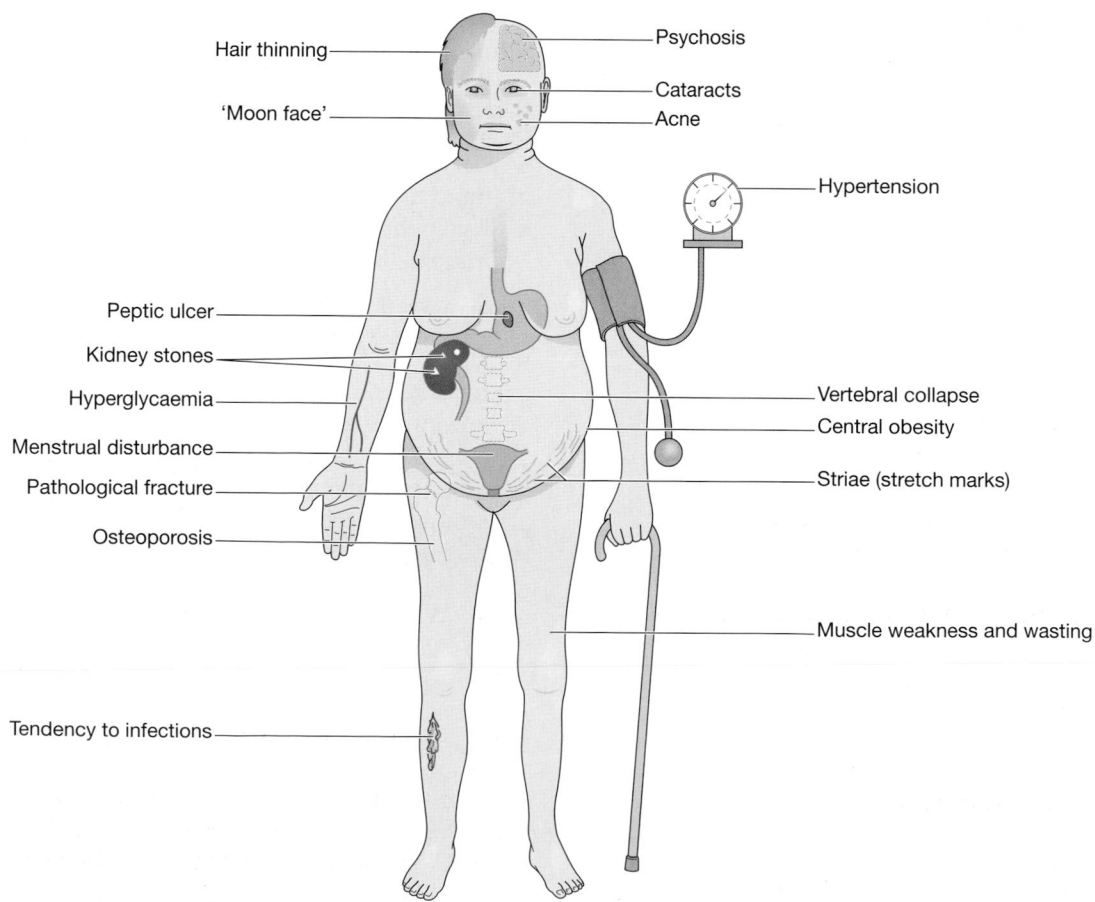

Figure 9.20 The systemic features of Cushing's syndrome.

- diminished protein synthesis
- suppression of growth hormone, causing arrest of growth in children
- osteoporosis and kyphosis if vertebral bodies are involved
- pathological fractures
- excessive gluconeogenesis with hyperglycaemia and glycosuria
- atrophy of lymphoid tissue and depressed immune response
- susceptibility to infection due to reduced febrile response, depressed immune response and phagocytosis, impaired migration of phagocytes
- insomnia, excitability, euphoria, psychosis, depression
- hypertension
- menstrual disturbances
- formation of renal calculi
- peptic ulceration.

Hyposecretion of glucocorticoids

Inadequate secretion of cortisol causes diminished gluconeogenesis, low blood glucose, muscle weakness and pallor. It may be primary, i.e. due to adrenal cortex disease, or secondary due to deficiency of ACTH from the anterior pituitary. In primary deficiency there is also hyposecretion of aldosterone (see below) but in secondary deficiency, aldosterone secretion is not usually affected.

Hypersecretion of mineralocorticoids

Excess aldosterone affects kidney function, causing:

- excessive reabsorption of sodium chloride and water, causing increased blood volume and hypertension
- excessive excretion of potassium, causing *hypokalaemia*, which leads to cardiac arrhythmia, alkalosis, syncope and muscle weakness.

Primary aldosteronism (Conn's syndrome)

This is due to an excessive secretion of mineralocorticoids, independent of the renin–angiotensin–aldosterone system. It is usually caused by a tumour affecting only one adrenal gland.

Secondary aldosteronism

This is caused by overstimulation of normal glands by the excessively high blood levels of renin and angiotensin that result from low renal perfusion or low blood sodium.

Hyposecretion of mineralocorticoids

Hypoaldosteronism results in failure of the kidneys to regulate sodium, potassium and water excretion, leading to:

- blood sodium deficiency (hyponatraemia) and potassium excess (hyperkalaemia)
- dehydration, low blood volume and low blood pressure, especially if arteriolar constriction is defective due to deficiency of noradrenaline.

There is usually hyposecretion of other cortical hormones, as in Addison's disease.

Chronic adrenal cortex insufficiency (Addison's disease)

This is due to hyposecretion of glucocorticoid and mineralocorticoid hormones. The most common causes are development of autoantibodies to cortical cells, metastatic tumours and infections. Autoimmune disease of some other glands is associated with Addison's disease, e.g. thyrotoxicosis and hypoparathyroidism. The most important effects are:

- muscle weakness and wasting
- gastrointestinal disturbances, e.g. vomiting, diarrhoea, anorexia
- increased pigmentation of the skin, especially of exposed areas, due to excess ACTH and the related melanin-stimulating hormone secreted by the anterior pituitary
- listlessness and tiredness
- hypoglycaemia
- mental confusion
- menstrual disturbances and loss of body hair in women
- electrolyte imbalance, including hyponatraemia, low blood chloride levels and hyperkalaemia
- chronic dehydration, low blood volume and hypotension.

The adrenal glands have a considerable reserve of tissue and Addison's disease is not usually severely debilitating unless more than 90% of cortical tissue is destroyed.

Acute adrenal cortical insufficiency (Addisonian crisis)

This is characterised by sudden severe nausea, vomiting, diarrhoea, hypotension, electrolyte imbalance and, in severe cases, circulatory collapse. It is precipitated when an individual with chronic adrenal cortex insufficiency is subjected to stress, e.g. an acute infection.

DISORDERS OF THE ADRENAL MEDULLA

Learning outcome

After studying this section you should be able to:

- explain how the features of the diseases in this section are related to excessive secretion of adrenaline and noradrenaline.

Tumours

Hormone-secreting tumours are the main abnormality. The effects of excess adrenaline and noradrenaline include:

- hypertension, often associated with arteriosclerosis and cerebral haemorrhage
- hyperglycaemia and glycosuria
- excessive sweating and alternate flushing and blanching
- raised metabolic rate
- nervousness
- headache.

Phaeochromocytoma

This is a *benign tumour*, occurring in one or both glands. The secretion of hormones may be at a steady high level or in intermittent bursts.

Neuroblastoma

This is a *malignant tumour*, occurring in infants and children under 15 years of age. Tumours that develop early tend to be highly malignant but in this condition there may be spontaneous regression.

DISORDERS OF THE PANCREATIC ISLETS

Learning outcomes

After studying this section you should be able to:

- compare and contrast the onset and features of types I and II diabetes mellitus
- state the common causes of secondary diabetes
- relate the signs and symptoms of diabetes mellitus to deficient secretion of insulin
- explain how the causes and effects of the following conditions occur: diabetic ketoacidosis and hypoglycaemic coma
- describe the long term complications of diabetes mellitus

Diabetes mellitus

This is due to deficiency or absence of insulin or rarely to impairment of insulin activity (insulin resistance) causing varying degrees of disruption of carbohydrate and fat metabolism.

Type I, insulin-dependent diabetes mellitus (IDDM)

This occurs mainly in children and young adults and the onset is usually sudden. The deficiency or absence of insulin is due to the destruction of β-islet cells. The causes are unknown but there is a familial tendency, suggesting genetic involvement. In many cases an auto-immune reaction has occurred in which autoantibodies to β-islet cells are present. Antibodies to viruses are present in some cases and these may destroy the β-islet cells directly or by an autoimmune mechanism.

Type II, non-insulin-dependent diabetes mellitus (NIDDM)

This is the most common form of diabetes, accounting for about 90% of cases. Most patients are obese and it tends to develop in women over 75 years and men over 65 years. The cause is unknown. Insulin secretion may be below or above normal. Deficiency of glucose inside body cells may occur when there is hyperglycaemia and a high insulin level. This may be due to changes in cell membranes which block the insulin-assisted movement of glucose into cells (insulin resistance).

Secondary diabetes

This may develop as a complication of:

- acute and chronic pancreatitis
- some drugs, e.g. corticosteroids, phenytoin, thiazide diuretics
- secondary to other hormonal disturbances involving hypersecretion of e.g. growth hormone, thyroid hormones, cortisol, adrenaline
- pregnancy (gestational diabetes).

Gestational diabetes

This develops during pregnancy and usually disappears after delivery; however, diabetes often recurs in later life. Raised blood glucose levels during pregnancy predispose to the birth of excessively large babies and also to stillbirths and deaths shortly after birth.

Effects of diabetes mellitus

Raised blood glucose level

After the intake of a carbohydrate meal the blood glucose level remains high because:

- glucose uptake and use by body cells is defective
- conversion of glucose to glycogen in the liver and muscles is diminished
- there is gluconeogenesis from protein in response to deficiency of intracellular glucose.

Glycosuria and polyuria

The concentration of glucose in the glomerular filtrate is the same as in the blood and, although diabetes raises the renal threshold for glucose, it is not all reabsorbed by the tubules (p. 344). The remaining glucose in the filtrate raises the osmotic pressure, water reabsorption is reduced and the volume of urine produced is increased.

This causes electrolyte imbalance and excretion of urine of high specific gravity. Polyuria leads to hypovolaemia, extreme thirst and polydipsia.

Weight loss

In diabetes, cells fail to metabolise glucose in the normal manner, resulting in weight loss due to:

- gluconeogenesis from amino acids and body protein, causing tissue wasting, tissue breakdown and further increase in blood glucose
- catabolism of body fat, releasing some of its energy and excess production of ketoacids.

Ketoacidosis

This is due to the accumulation of the intermediate metabolite, acetyl coenzyme A, which cannot enter the citric acid cycle without oxaloacetic acid (see Fig. 12.48, p. 318). In diabetes the amount of available oxaloacetic acid is reduced because glucose metabolism is reduced. As a result excess acetyl coenzyme A is converted to ketones, which are acidic. When these accumulate in the blood, the pH drops, causing ketoacidosis. Ketones are excreted in the urine (ketonuria) and by the lungs. The consequences are:

- hyperventilation and the excretion of excess bicarbonate
- acidification of urine and high filtrate osmotic pressure which leads to excessive loss of water (polyuria), ammonia, sodium and potassium
- coma due to a combination of low blood pH (acidosis), high plasma osmotic pressure and electrolyte imbalance.

Acute complications of diabetes mellitus

Diabetic ketoacidosis (diabetic coma, hyperglycaemic coma)

This mainly affects insulin-dependent diabetics. Keto-acidosis develops owing to increased insulin requirement or increased resistance to insulin due to some added stress, such as pregnancy, microbial infection, infarction, cerebrovascular accident. The inadequate supply of insulin may also be due to failure by the patient to administer the prescribed dose or inadequate adjustment of the prescribed dose to meet the patient's increased needs. In some cases severe and dangerous ketoacidosis may occur without loss of consciousness.

The factors that predispose to the development of hyperglycaemic coma in either type of diabetes include:

- hypovolaemia with severe dehydration due to persistent polyuria
- high blood osmotic pressure due to excess blood glucose, leading to electrolyte imbalance
- acidosis due to accumulation of ketoacids.

Hypoglycaemic coma

This occurs in insulin-dependent diabetics when the insulin administered is in excess of that needed to balance the food intake and expenditure of energy. Because neurones are more dependent on glucose for their energy needs than are other cells, glucose deprivation causes disturbed neural function, leading to coma and, if prolonged, irreversible damage. Hypoglycaemia may be the result of:

- accidental overdose of insulin
- delay in eating after insulin administration
- gastrointestinal disturbances in which carbohydrate absorption is diminished, e.g., vomiting, diarrhoea
- increased metabolic rate in, e.g. unexpected exercise, acute febrile illness
- an insulin-secreting tumour, especially if it produces irregular bursts of secretion.

Common signs and symptoms of hypoglycaemia include drowsiness, confusion, speech difficulty, sweating, trembling and anxiety.

Long-term complications of diabetes mellitus

Cardiovascular disturbances

Changes in blood vessels occur even when the disease is well controlled by insulin and/or diet.

Diabetic macroangiopathy

The most common lesions are atheroma and calcification of the tunica media of the large muscular arteries. In insulin-dependent diabetics these changes may occur at a relatively early age. The most common sequelae are serious and often fatal: peripheral vascular disease, myocardial infarction, cerebral ischaemia and infarction.

Diabetic microangiopathy

There is thickening of the epithelial basement membrane of arterioles, capillaries and sometimes of venules. These changes may lead to:

- peripheral vascular disease, progressing to gangrene
- retinopathy, in which microaneurysms and small haemorrhages cause numerous small necrotic points in the retina, leading to loss of sight
- glomerulosclerosis, leading to nephrotic syndrome and renal failure
- peripheral neuropathy, especially when myelination is defective.

Infection

Diabetics are highly susceptible to infection, especially by bacteria and fungi, possibly because phagocyte activity is depressed by insufficient intracellular glucose. Infection may cause:

- complications in areas affected by *peripheral neuropathy* and changes in blood vessels, e.g. in the feet when sensation and blood supply are impaired
- boils and carbuncles
- vaginal candidiasis (thrush)
- pyelonephritis.

Renal failure

This is due to changes affecting the walls of small blood vessels and infection, and is a common cause of death in diabetics (see Diabetic kidney, p. 352).

Intake of raw materials and elimination of waste

3

The cells of the body need energy for their chemical activity that maintains homeostasis. Most of this energy is derived from chemical reactions which can only take place in the presence of oxygen (O_2). The main waste product of these reactions is carbon dioxide (CO_2). The respiratory system provides the route by which the supply of oxygen present in the atmospheric air gains entry to the body and it provides the route of excretion of carbon dioxide.

The condition of the atmospheric air entering the body varies considerably according to the external environment, e.g. it may be dry, cold and contain dust particles or it may be moist and hot. As the air breathed in moves through the air passages to reach the lungs, it is warmed or cooled to body temperature, moistened to become saturated with water vapour and 'cleaned' as particles of dust stick to the mucus which coats the lining membrane. Blood provides the transport system for these gases between the lungs and the cells of the body. Exchange of gases between the blood and the lungs is called *external respiration* and that between the blood and the cells *internal respiration*. The organs of the respiratory system are:

- nose
- pharynx
- larynx
- trachea
- two bronchi (one bronchus to each lung)
- bronchioles and smaller air passages
- two lungs and their coverings, the pleura

- muscles of respiration—the intercostal muscles and the diaphragm.

A general view of the organs of the respiratory system is given in Figure 10.1.

NOSE AND NASAL CAVITY

Learning outcomes

After studying this section, you should be able to:

- describe the location of the nasal cavities
- relate the structure of the nasal cavities to their function in respiration
- outline the physiology of smell.

Position and structure

The nasal cavity is the first of the respiratory organs and consists of a large irregular cavity divided into two equal passages by a *septum*. The posterior bony part of the septum is formed by the perpendicular plate of the ethmoid bone and the vomer. Anteriorly it consists of hyaline cartilage (Fig. 10.2).

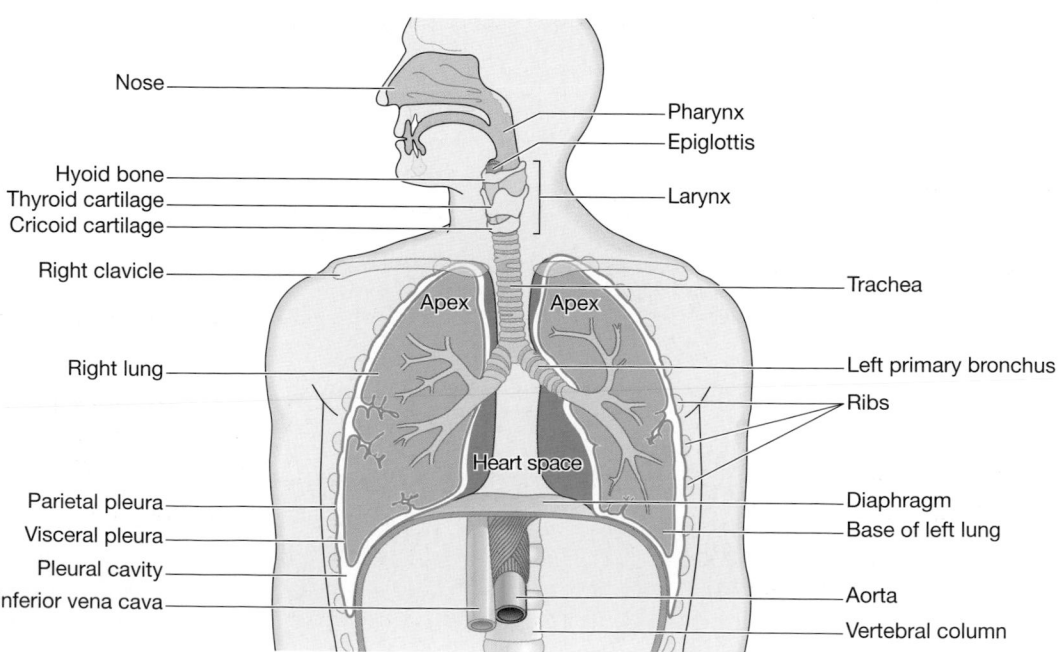

Figure 10.1 The organs of respiration.

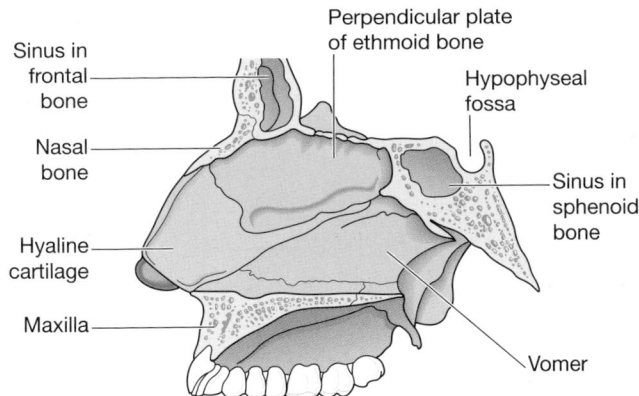

Figure 10.2 Structures forming the nasal septum.

The *roof* is formed by the cribriform plate of the ethmoid bone, and the sphenoid bone, frontal bone and nasal bones.

The *floor* is formed by the roof of the mouth and consists of the hard palate in front and the soft palate behind. The hard palate is composed of the maxilla and palatine bones and the soft palate consists of involuntary muscle.

The *medial wall* is formed by the *septum*.

The *lateral walls* are formed by the maxilla, the ethmoid bone and the inferior conchae (Fig. 10.3).

The *posterior wall* is formed by the posterior wall of the pharynx.

Lining of the nose

The nose is lined with very vascular *ciliated columnar epithelium* (ciliated mucous membrane) which contains mucus-secreting goblet cells (p. 43). At the anterior nares

this blends with the skin and posteriorly it extends into the nasal part of the pharynx.

Openings into the nasal cavity

The anterior nares, or nostrils, are the openings from the exterior into the nasal cavity. Hairs are present in this area.

The posterior nares are the openings from the nasal cavity into the pharynx.

The paranasal sinuses are cavities in the bones of the face and the cranium which contain air. There are tiny openings between the paranasal sinuses and the nasal cavity. They are lined with mucous membrane, continuous with that of the nasal cavity. The main sinuses are:

- maxillary sinuses in the lateral walls
- frontal and sphenoidal sinuses in the roof (Fig. 10.3)
- ethmoidal sinuses in the upper part of the lateral walls (Fig. 10.3).

The sinuses function in speech and also serve to lighten the skull. *The nasolacrimal ducts* extend from the lateral walls of the nose to the conjunctival sacs of the eye (p. 205). They drain tears from the eyes.

Respiratory function of the nose

The nose is the first of the respiratory passages through which the inspired air passes. The function of the nose is to begin the process by which the air is *warmed, moistened and 'filtered'*.

The projecting *conchae* (Figs 10.3 and 10.4) increase the surface area and cause turbulence, spreading inspired air

241

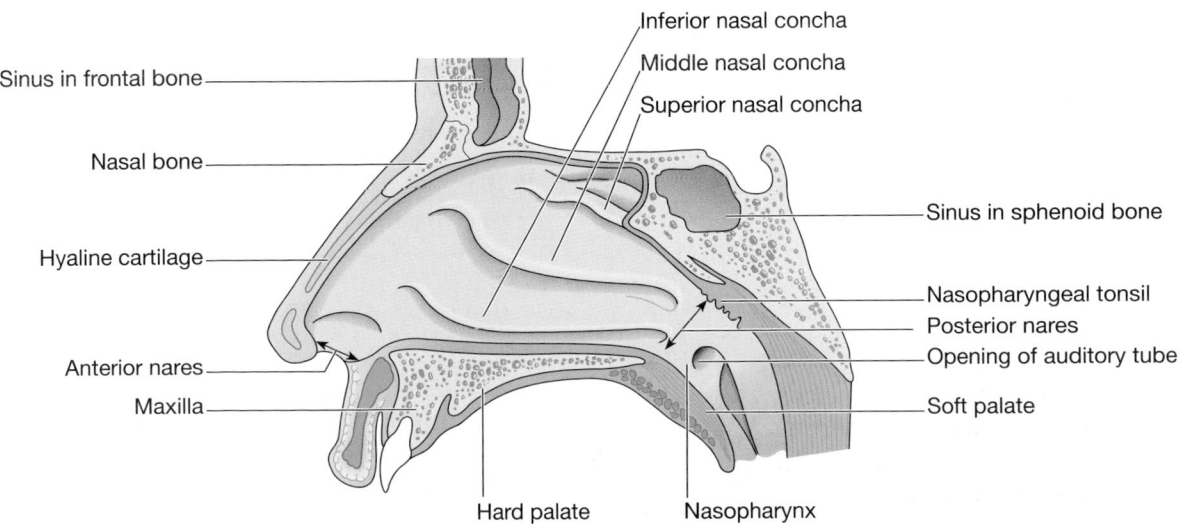

Figure 10.3 Lateral wall of right nasal cavity.

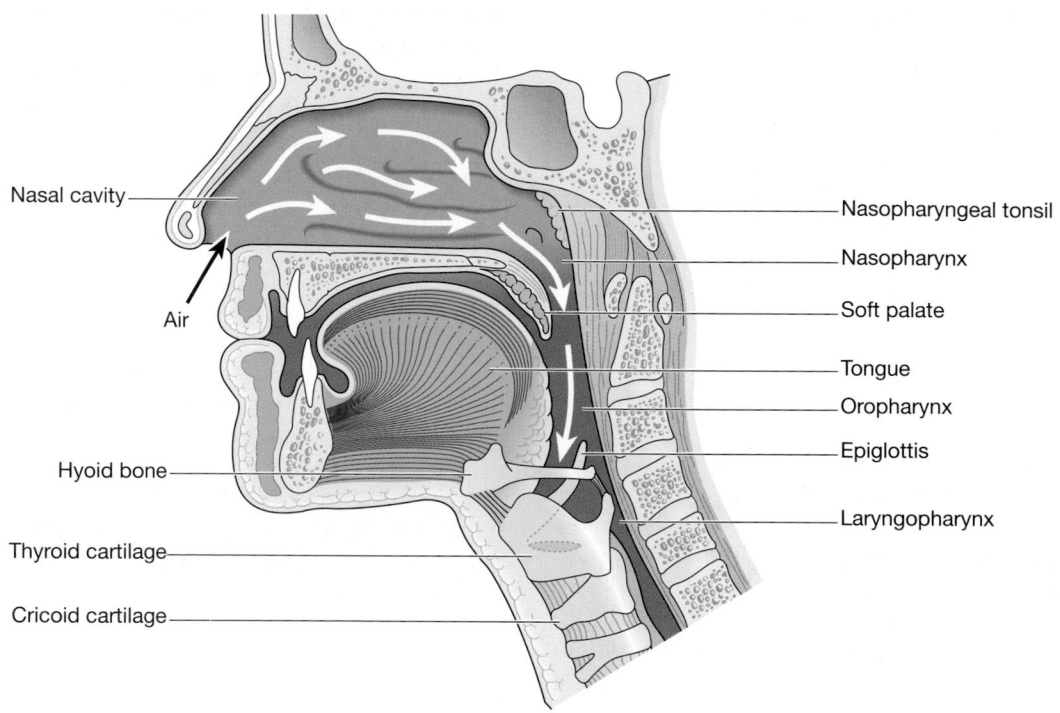

Figure 10.4 The pathway of air from the nose to the larynx.

Labels on figure: Nasal cavity, Air, Hyoid bone, Thyroid cartilage, Cricoid cartilage, Nasopharyngeal tonsil, Nasopharynx, Soft palate, Tongue, Oropharynx, Epiglottis, Laryngopharynx

242

over the whole nasal surface. The large surface area maximises warming, humidification and filtering.

Warming. This is due to the immense vascularity of the mucosa. This explains the large blood loss when a nose-bleed (epistaxis) occurs.

Filtering and cleaning of air. This occurs as hairs at the anterior nares trap larger particles. Smaller particles such as dust and microbes settle and adhere to the mucus. Mucus protects the underlying epithelium from irritation and prevents drying. Synchronous beating of the cilia wafts the mucus towards the throat where it is swallowed or expectorated.

Humidification. This occurs as air travels over the moist mucosa and becomes saturated with water vapour. Irritation of the nasal mucosa results in *sneezing*, a reflex action that forcibly expels an irritant.

Olfactory function of the nose

The nose is the organ of the sense of smell. There are nerve endings that detect smell, located in the roof of the nose in the area of the cribriform plate of the ethmoid bones and the superior conchae. These nerve endings are stimulated by chemical substances given off by odorous materials. The resultant nerve impulses are conveyed by the *olfactory nerves* to the brain where the sensation of smell is perceived (p. 206).

PHARYNX

Learning outcomes

After studying this section, you should be able to:

- describe the location of the pharynx
- relate the structure of the pharynx to its function.

Position

The pharynx is a tube 12 to 14 cm long that extends from the base of the skull to the level of the 6th cervical vertebra. It lies behind the nose, mouth and larynx and is wider at its upper end.

Structures associated with the pharynx

Superiorly — the inferior surface of the base of the skull

Inferiorly — it is continuous with the oesophagus

Anteriorly — the wall is incomplete because of the openings into the nose, mouth and larynx

Posteriorly — areolar tissue, involuntary muscle and the bodies of the first six cervical vertebrae

For descriptive purposes the pharynx is divided into three parts: *nasopharynx, oropharynx* and *laryngopharynx*.

The nasopharynx. The nasal part of the pharynx lies behind the nose above the level of the soft palate. On its lateral walls are the two openings of the *auditory tubes*, one leading to each middle ear. On the posterior wall there are the *pharyngeal tonsils* (adenoids), consisting of lymphoid tissue. They are most prominent in children up to approximately 7 years of age. Thereafter they gradually atrophy.

The oropharynx. The oral part of the pharynx lies behind the mouth, extending from below the level of the soft palate to the level of the upper part of the body of the 3rd cervical vertebra. The lateral walls of the pharynx blend with the soft palate to form two folds on each side. Between each pair of folds there is a collection of lymphoid tissue called the *palatine tonsil*.

During swallowing, the nasal and oral parts are separated by the soft palate and the *uvula*.

The laryngopharynx. The laryngeal part of the pharynx extends from the oropharynx above and continues as the oesophagus below, i.e. from the level of the 3rd to the 6th cervical vertebrae.

Structure

The pharynx is composed of three layers of tissue:

1. *Mucous membrane lining.* The mucosa varies slightly in the different parts. In the nasopharynx it is continuous with the lining of the nose and consists of ciliated columnar epithelium; in the oropharynx and laryngopharynx it is formed by tougher stratified squamous epithelium which is continuous with the lining of the mouth and oesophagus.
2. *Fibrous tissue.* This forms the intermediate layer. It is thicker in the nasopharynx, where there is little muscle, and becomes thinner towards the lower end, where the muscle layer is thicker.
3. *Muscle tissue.* This consists of several involuntary *constrictor muscles* that play an important part in the mechanism of swallowing (deglutition) which, in the pharynx, is not under voluntary control. The upper end of the oesophagus is closed by the lower constrictor muscle, except during swallowing.

Blood and nerve supply

Blood is supplied to the pharynx by several branches of the facial artery. The venous return is into the facial and internal jugular veins.

The nerve supply is from the pharyngeal plexus, formed by parasympathetic and sympathetic nerves. Parasympathetic supply is by the *vagus* and *glossopharyngeal* nerves. Sympathetic supply is by nerves from the *superior cervical ganglia* (p. 170).

Functions

Passageway for air and food. The pharynx is an organ involved in both the respiratory and the digestive systems: air passes through the nasal and oral parts, and food through the oral and laryngeal parts.

Warming and humidifying. By the same methods as in the nose, the air is further warmed and moistened as it passes through the pharynx.

Taste. There are olfactory nerve endings of the sense of taste in the epithelium of the oral and pharyngeal parts.

Hearing. The auditory tube, extending from the nasal part to each middle ear, allows air to enter the middle ear. Satisfactory hearing depends on the presence of air at atmospheric pressure on each side of the *tympanic membrane* (ear drum) (p. 193).

Protection. The lymphatic tissue of the pharyngeal and laryngeal tonsils produces antibodies in response to antigens, e.g. microbes (Ch. 15). The tonsils are larger in children and tend to atrophy in adults.

Speech. The pharynx functions in speech; by acting as a resonating chamber for the sound ascending from the larynx, it helps (together with the sinuses) to give the voice its individual characteristics.

LARYNX

Learning outcomes

After studying this section, you should be able to:

■ describe the structure and function of the larynx

■ outline the physiology of speech generation.

Position

The larynx or 'voice box' extends from the root of the tongue and the hyoid bone to the trachea. It lies in front of the laryngopharynx at the level of the 3rd, 4th, 5th and 6th cervical vertebrae. Until puberty there is little difference in the size of the larynx between the sexes. Thereafter it grows larger in the male, which explains the prominence of the 'Adam's apple' and the generally deeper voice.

Structures associated with the larynx

Superiorly	—	the hyoid bone and the root of the tongue
Inferiorly	—	it is continuous with the trachea
Anteriorly	—	the muscles attached to the hyoid bone and the muscles of the neck
Posteriorly	—	the laryngopharynx and 3rd to 6th cervical vertebrae
Laterally	—	the lobes of the thyroid gland

Structure

Cartilages

The larynx is composed of several irregularly shaped cartilages attached to each other by ligaments and membranes. The main cartilages are:

■ 1 thyroid cartilage ⎫
■ 1 cricoid cartilage ⎬ hyaline cartilage
■ 2 arytenoid cartilages ⎭
■ 1 epiglottis — elastic fibrocartilage.

The thyroid cartilage (Figs 10.6 and 10.7). This is the most prominent and consists of two flat pieces of hyaline cartilage, or *laminae*, fused anteriorly, forming the *laryngeal prominence* (Adam's apple). Immediately above the laryngeal prominence the laminae are separated, forming a V-shaped notch known as the *thyroid notch*. The thyroid cartilage is incomplete posteriorly and the posterior border of each lamina is extended to form two processes called the *superior* and *inferior cornu*.

The upper part of the thyroid cartilage is lined with stratified squamous epithelium like the larynx, and the lower part with ciliated columnar epithelium like the trachea. There are many muscles attached to its outer surface.

The cricoid cartilage (Fig. 10.5). This lies below the thyroid cartilage and is also composed of hyaline cartilage. It is shaped like a signet ring, completely encircling the larynx with the narrow part anteriorly and the broad part posteriorly. The broad posterior part articulates with the arytenoid cartilages above and with the inferior cornu of the thyroid cartilage below. It is lined with ciliated columnar epithelium and there are muscles and ligaments attached to its outer surface (Fig. 10.7). The lower border of the cricoid cartilage marks the end of the upper respiratory tract.

The arytenoid cartilages. These are two roughly pyramid-shaped hyaline cartilages situated on top of the broad part of the cricoid cartilage forming part of the posterior wall of the larynx. They give attachment to the vocal cords and to muscles and are lined with ciliated columnar epithelium.

The epiglottis. This is a leaf-shaped fibroelastic cartilage attached to the inner surface of the anterior wall of the thyroid cartilage immediately below the thyroid notch. It rises obliquely upwards behind the tongue and the body of the hyoid bone. It is covered with stratified squamous epithelium. If the larynx is likened to a box then the epiglottis acts as the lid; it closes off the larynx during swallowing, protecting the lungs from accidental inhalation of foreign objects.

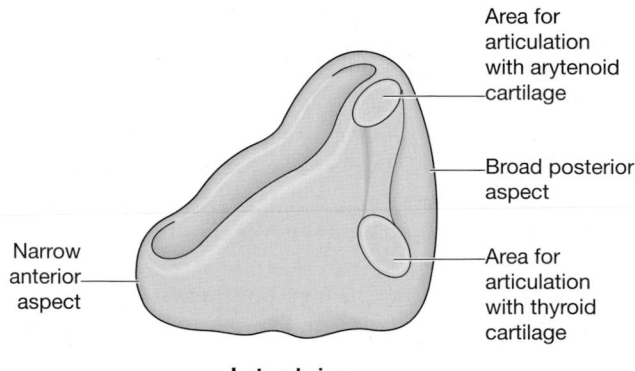

Area for articulation with arytenoid cartilage

Broad posterior aspect

Narrow anterior aspect

Area for articulation with thyroid cartilage

Lateral view

Figure 10.5 Cricoid cartilage.

Ligaments and membranes

There are several ligaments that attach the cartilages to each other and to the hyoid bone (Figs 10.6, 10.7 and 10.8).

Blood and nerve supply

Blood is supplied to the larynx by the superior and inferior laryngeal arteries and drained by the thyroid veins, which join the internal jugular vein.

The parasympathetic nerve supply is from the superior laryngeal and recurrent laryngeal nerves, which are branches of the vagus nerves, and the sympathetic nerves are from the superior cervical ganglia, one on each side. These provide the motor nerve supply to the muscles of the larynx and sensory fibres to the lining membrane.

Interior of the larynx

The *vocal cords* are two pale folds of mucous membrane with cord-like free edges which extend from the inner wall of the thyroid prominence anteriorly to the arytenoid cartilages posteriorly (Fig. 10.8).

When the muscles controlling the vocal cords are relaxed, the vocal cords open and the passageway for air coming up through the larynx is clear; the vocal cords are said to be *abducted* (Fig. 10.9A). The pitch of the sound produced by vibrating the vocal cords in this position is low. When the muscles controlling the vocal cords contract, the vocal cords are stretched out tightly across the larynx (Fig. 10.9B)—they are said to be *adducted*. When the vocal cords are stretched to this extent, and are vibrated by air passing through from the lungs, the sound produced is high pitched. The pitch of the voice is therefore determined by the tension applied to the vocal cords by the appropriate sets of muscles. When not in use, the vocal cords are adducted.

Functions

Production of sound. Sound has the properties of *pitch, volume* and *resonance*.

- Pitch of the voice depends upon the *length* and *tightness* of the cords. At puberty, the male vocal cords begin to grow longer, hence the lower pitch of the adult male voice.
- Volume of the voice depends upon the *force* with which the cords vibrate. The greater the force of expired air the more the cords vibrate and the louder the sound emitted.
- Resonance, or tone, is dependent upon the shape of the mouth, the position of the tongue and the lips, the facial muscles and the air in the paranasal sinuses.

Speech. This occurs during expiration when the sounds produced by the vocal cords are manipulated by the tongue, cheeks and lips.

Protection of the lower respiratory tract. During swallowing (deglutition) the larynx moves upwards, occluding the opening into it from the pharynx and the

245

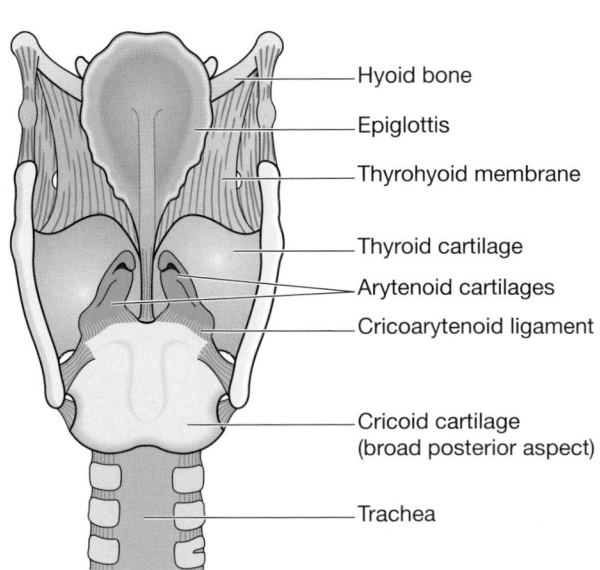

Figure 10.6 Larynx – viewed from behind.

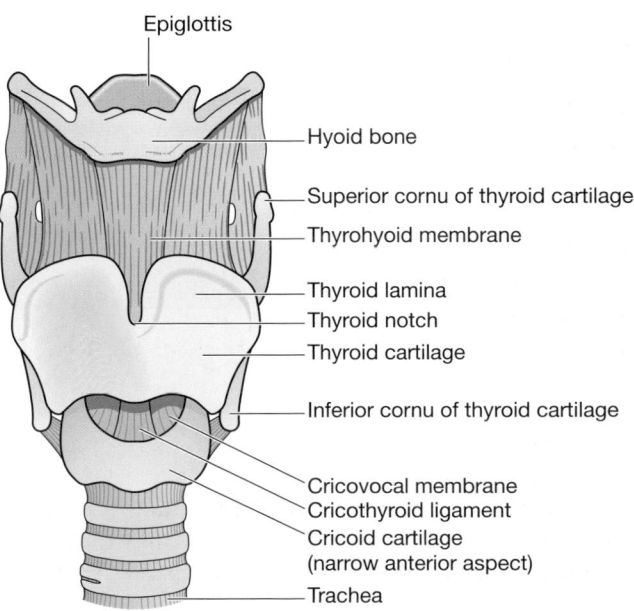

Figure 10.7 Larynx – viewed from the front.

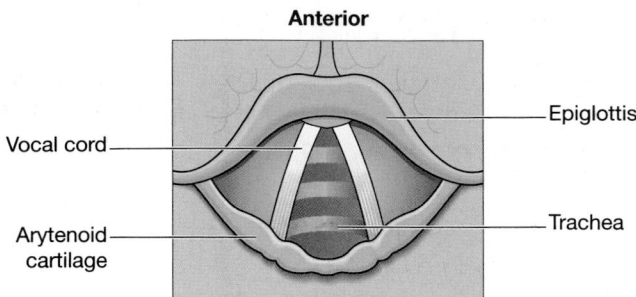

Figure 10.8 Interior of the larynx viewed from above.

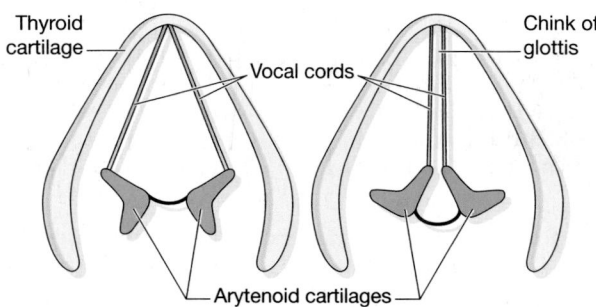

A   Vocal cords abducted   B   Vocal cords adducted

Figure 10.9 The extreme positions of the vocal cords.

hinged epiglottis closes over the larynx. This ensures that food passes into the oesophagus and not into the lower respiratory passages (p. 295).

Passageway for air. This is between the pharynx and trachea.

Humidifying, filtering and warming. These continue as inspired air travels through the larynx.

TRACHEA

Learning outcomes

After studying this section, you should be able to:

■ describe the location of the trachea

■ outline the structure of the trachea

■ explain the functions of the trachea in respiration.

Position

The trachea or windpipe is a continuation of the larynx and extends downwards to about the level of the 5th thoracic vertebra where it divides (bifurcates) at the *carina* into the right and left bronchi, one bronchus going to each lung. It is approximately 10 to 11 cm long and lies mainly in the median plane in front of the oesophagus (Fig. 10.10).

Structures associated with the trachea (Fig. 10.11)

Superiorly	—	the larynx
Inferiorly	—	the right and left bronchi
Anteriorly	—	upper part: the isthmus of the thyroid gland
		lower part: the arch of the aorta and the sternum
Posteriorly	—	the oesophagus separates the trachea from the vertebral column
Laterally	—	the lungs and the lobes of the thyroid gland.

Structure

The trachea is composed of from 16 to 20 incomplete (C-shaped) rings of hyaline cartilages lying one above the other. The cartilages are incomplete posteriorly. Connective tissue and involuntary muscle join the cartilages and form the posterior wall where they are incomplete. The soft tissue posterior wall is in contact with the oesophagus (Fig. 10.10).

There are three layers of tissue which 'clothe' the cartilages of the trachea.

The outer layer. This consists of fibrous and elastic tissue and encloses the cartilages.

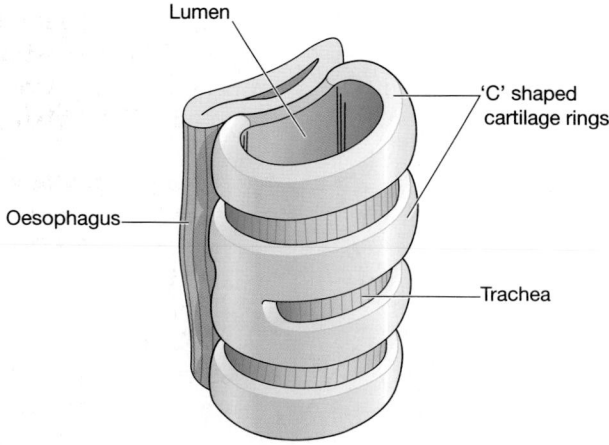

Figure 10.10 The relationship of the trachea to the oesophagus.

The middle layer. This consists of cartilages and bands of smooth muscle that wind round the trachea in a helical arrangement. There is some areolar tissue, containing blood and lymph vessels and autonomic nerves.

The inner lining. This consists of ciliated columnar epithelium, containing mucus-secreting goblet cells.

Blood and nerve supply, lymph drainage

The arterial blood supply. This is mainly by the inferior thyroid and bronchial arteries and the *venous return* is by the inferior thyroid veins into the brachiocephalic veins.

The *nerve supply.* This is by parasympathetic and sympathetic fibres. Parasympathetic supply is by the recurrent laryngeal nerves and other branches of the vagi. Sympathetic supply is by nerves from the sympathetic ganglia.

Lymph. Lymph from the respiratory passages passes through lymph nodes situated round the trachea and in the *carina*, the area where it divides into two bronchi.

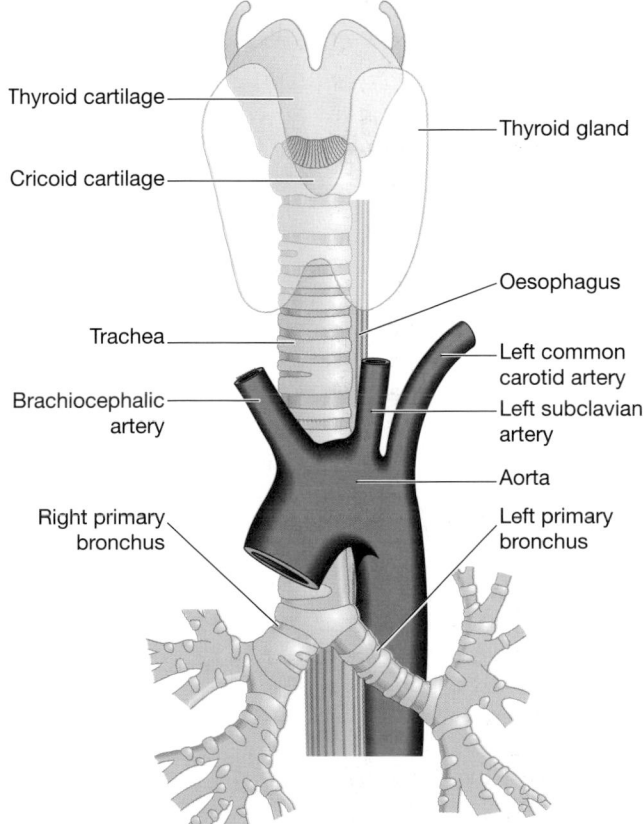

Figure 10.11 The trachea and some of its associated structures.

Functions

Support and patency. The arrangement of cartilage and elastic tissue prevents kinking and obstruction of the airway as the head and neck move. The absence of cartilage posteriorly allows the trachea to dilate and constrict in response to nerve stimulation, and for indentation as the oesophagus distends during swallowing. The cartilages prevent collapse of the tube when the internal pressure is less than intrathoracic pressure, i.e. at the end of forced expiration.

Mucociliary escalator. This is the synchronous and regular beating of the cilia of the mucous membrane lining that wafts mucus with adherent particles upwards towards the larynx where it is swallowed or expectorated (Fig. 10.12).

Cough reflex. Nerve endings in the larynx, trachea and bronchi are sensitive to irritation that generates nerve impulses which are conducted by the vagus nerves to the respiratory centre in the brain stem (p. 256). The reflex motor response is deep inspiration followed by closure of the glottis. The abdominal and respiratory muscles then contract and suddenly the air is released under pressure expelling mucus and/or foreign material from the mouth.

247

Warming, humidifying and filtering of air. These continue as in the nose, although air is normally saturated and at body temperature when it reaches the trachea.

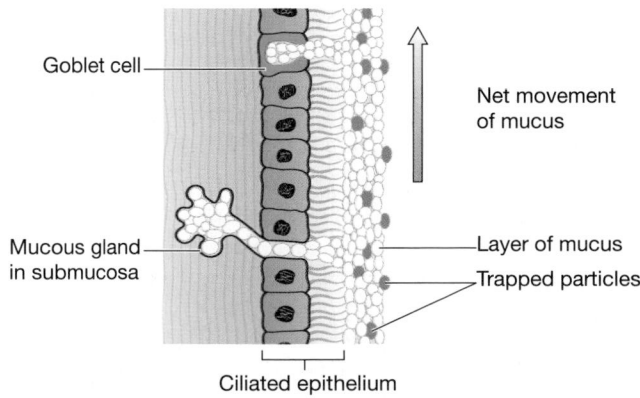

Figure 10.12 Microscopic view of ciliated mucous membrane.

BRONCHI AND SMALLER AIR PASSAGES

Learning outcomes

After studying this section, you should be able to:

- name the air passage of the bronchial tree in descending order of size

- describe the structure and changing functions of the different levels of airway.

The two primary bronchi are formed when the trachea divides, i.e. about the level of the 5th thoracic vertebra (Fig. 10.13).

The right bronchus. This is wider, shorter and more vertical than the left bronchus and is therefore the more likely of the two to become obstructed by an inhaled foreign body. It is approximately 2.5 cm long. After entering the right lung at the hilum it divides into three branches, one to each lobe. Each branch then subdivides into numerous smaller branches.

The left bronchus. This is about 5 cm long and is narrower than the right. After entering the lung at the hilum it divides into two branches, one to each lobe. Each branch then subdivides into progressively smaller tubes within the lung substance.

Bronchi and bronchioles

Structure

The bronchi are composed of the same tissues as the trachea. They are lined with ciliated columnar epithelium. The bronchi progressively subdivide into *bronchioles* (Fig. 10.13), *terminal bronchioles, respiratory bronchioles, alveolar ducts* and finally, *alveoli*. Towards the distal end of the bronchi the cartilages become irregular in shape and are absent at bronchiolar level. In the absence of cartilage the smooth muscle in the walls of the bronchioles becomes thicker and is responsive to autonomic nerve stimulation and irritation. Ciliated columnar mucous membrane changes gradually to non-ciliated cuboidal-shaped cells in the distal bronchioles.

Blood and nerve supply, lymph drainage

The arterial blood supply. The supply to the walls of the bronchi and smaller air passages is through branches of the *right and left bronchial arteries* and the *venous return* is mainly through the bronchial veins. On the right side they empty into the azygos vein and on the left into the superior intercostal vein (see Figs 5.42 and 5.43, p. 103)

The nerve supply. This is by parasympathetic and sympathetic nerves. The vagus nerves (parasympathetic) stimulate contraction of smooth muscle in the bronchial tree, causing bronchoconstriction, and sympathetic stimulation causes bronchodilatation (Ch. 7).

The lymphatic vessels and lymph nodes. Lymph is drained from the walls of the air passages in a network of lymph vessels. It passes through lymph nodes situated around the trachea and bronchial tree then into the thoracic duct on the left side and right lymphatic duct on the other.

Functions of air passages not involved in gaseous exchange

Control of air entry. The diameter of the respiratory passages may be altered by contraction or relaxation of

248

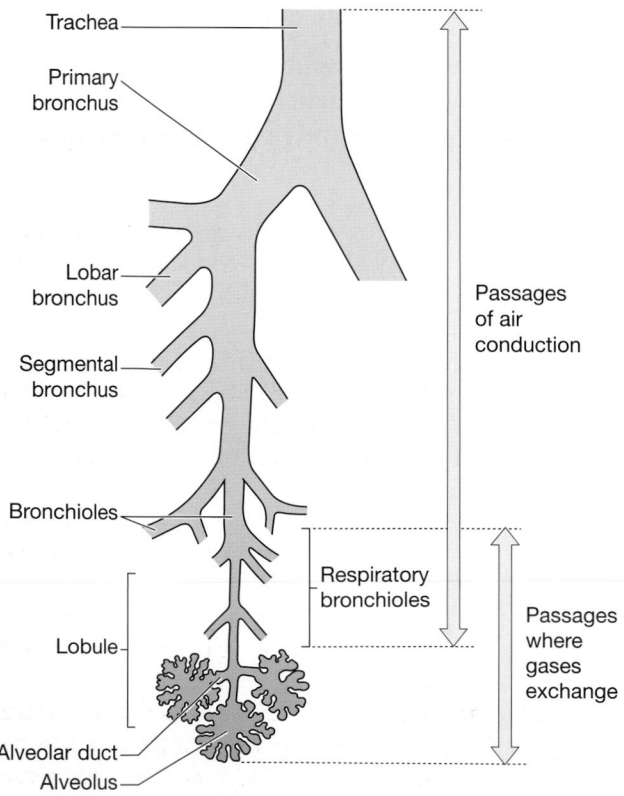

Figure 10.13 Lower respiratory tract.

the involuntary muscles in their walls, thus regulating the volume of air entering the lungs. These changes are controlled by the autonomic nerve supply: parasympathetic stimulation causes constriction and sympathetic stimulation causes dilatation (p. 173).

The following functions continue as in the upper airways:

- warming and humidifying
- support and patency
- removal of particulate matter
- cough reflex.

Respiratory bronchioles and alveoli

Structure

Lobules are the blind ends of the respiratory tract distal to the terminal bronchioles, consisting of: *respiratory bronchioles, alveolar ducts* and *alveoli* (tiny air sacs) (Fig. 10.13). It is in these structures that the process of gas exchange occurs. The walls gradually become thinner until muscle and connective tissue fade out leaving a single layer of simple squamous epithelial cells in the alveolar ducts and alveoli. These distal respiratory passages are supported by a loose network of elastic connective tissue in which macrophages, fibroblasts, nerves and blood and lymph vessels are embedded. The alveoli are surrounded by a network of capillaries. The exchange of gases during respiration takes place across two membranes, the alveolar and capillary membranes.

Interspersed between the squamous cells are other cells that secrete *surfactant*, a phospholipid fluid which prevents the alveoli from drying out. In addition, surfactant reduces surface tension and prevents alveolar walls collapsing during expiration. Secretion of surfactant into the distal air passages and alveoli begins about the 35th week of fetal life. Its presence in newborn babies facilitates expansion of the lungs and the establishment of respiration. It may not be present in sufficient amounts in the immature lungs of premature babies, causing difficulty in establishing respiration.

Functions of respiratory bronchioles and alveoli

External respiration. (See p. 255.)

Defence against microbes. At this level, ciliated epithelium, goblet cells and mucus are no longer present. Defence relies on protective cells present within the lung tissue. These include lymphocytes and plasma cells, which produce antibodies in the presence of antigens, and macrophages and polymorphonuclear lymphocytes, which are phagocytic. These cells are most active in the distal air passages where ciliated epithelium has been replaced by flattened cells.

Warming and humidifying. These continue as in the upper airways. Inhalation of dry or inadequately humidified air over a period of time causes irritation of the mucosa and facilitates the establishment of pathogenic microbes.

LUNGS

Learning outcomes

After studying this section, you should be able to:

- describe the location and gross anatomy of the lungs
- identify the functions of the pleura
- describe the pulmonary blood supply.

Position and associated structures

(Fig. 10.14)

There are two lungs, one lying on each side of the midline in the thoracic cavity. They are cone-shaped and are described as having an *apex*, a *base, costal surface* and *medial surface.*

The apex. This is rounded and rises into the root of the neck, about 25 mm (1 inch) above the level of the middle third of the clavicle. The structures associated with it are the first rib and the blood vessels and nerves in the root of the neck.

The base. This is concave and semilunar in shape and is closely associated with the thoracic surface of the diaphragm.

The costal surface. This surface is convex and is closely associated with the costal cartilages, the ribs and the intercostal muscles.

The medial surface. This surface is concave and has a roughly triangular-shaped area, called the *hilum*, at the level of the 5th, 6th and 7th thoracic vertebrae. Structures which form the *root of the lung* enter and leave at the hilum. These include the primary bronchus, the

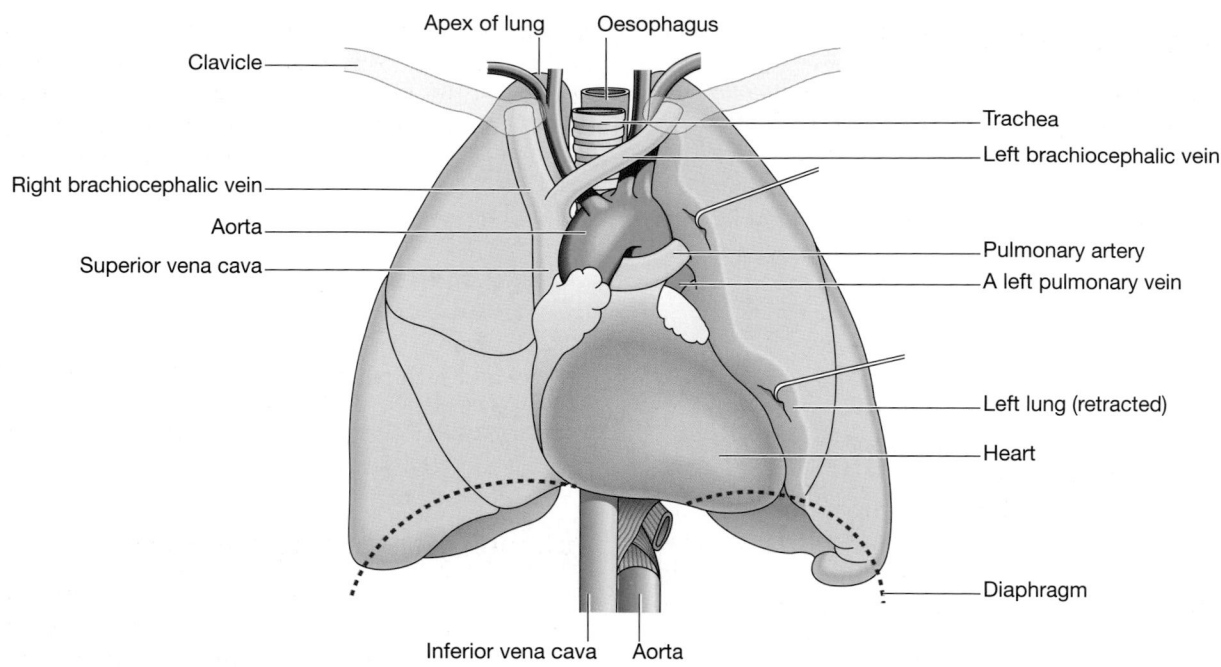

Figure 10.14 Organs associated with the lungs.

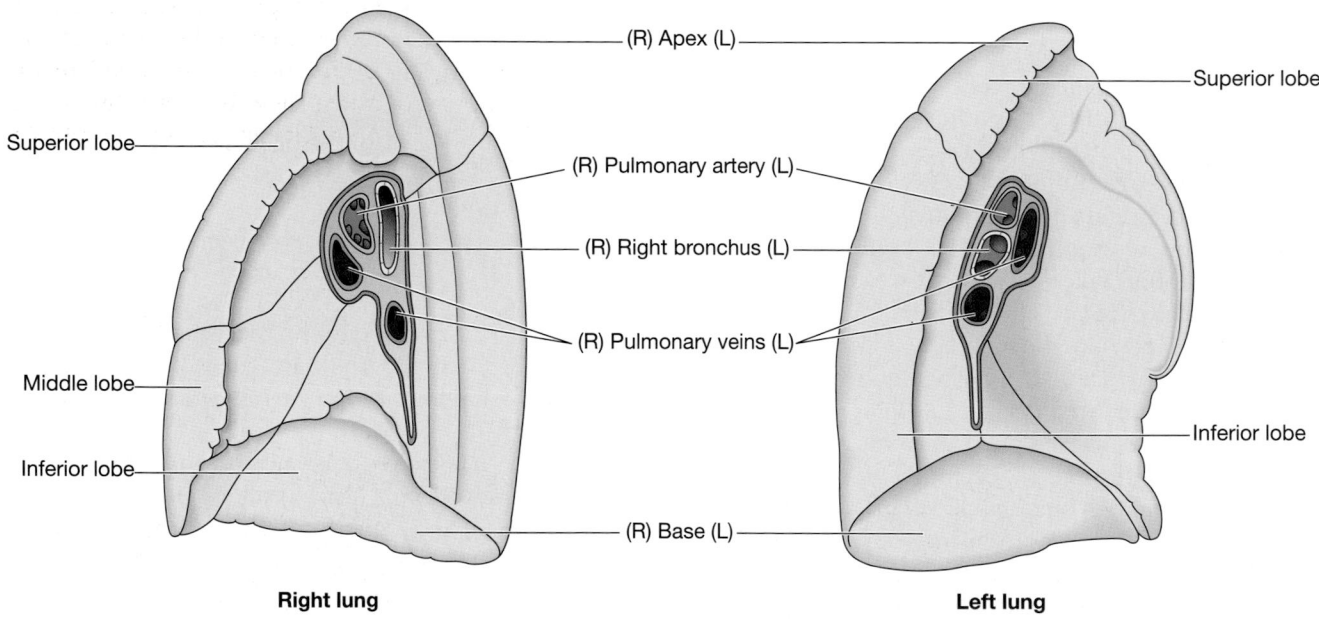

Right lung

Left lung

Figure 10.15 The lobes of the lungs and vessels/airways of each hilum – medial views.

pulmonary artery supplying the lung and the two pulmonary veins draining it, the bronchial artery and veins, and the lymphatic and nerve supply (Fig. 10.15).

The area between the lungs is the *mediastinum*. It is occupied by the heart, great vessels, trachea, right and left bronchi, oesophagus, lymph nodes, lymph vessels and nerves.

Organisation of the lungs

The *right lung* is divided into three distinct lobes: superior, middle and inferior.

The *left lung* is smaller as the heart is situated left of the midline. It is divided into only two lobes: superior and inferior.

Pleura and pleural cavity

The pleura consists of a closed sac of serous membrane (one for each lung) which contains a small amount of serous fluid. The lung is invaginated into this sac so that it forms two layers: one adheres to the lung and the other to the wall of the thoracic cavity (Figs 10.1 and 10.16).

The visceral pleura. This is adherent to the lung, covering each lobe and passing into the fissures which separate them.

The parietal pleura. This is adherent to the inside of the chest wall and the thoracic surface of the diaphragm. It remains detached from the adjacent structures in the mediastinum and is continuous with the visceral pleura round the edges of the hilum.

The *pleural cavity.* This is only a potential space. In health, the two layers of pleura are separated by only a thin film of serous fluid which allows them to glide over each other, preventing friction between them during breathing. The scrous fluid is secreted by the epithelial cells of the membrane.

The two layers of pleura, with serous fluid between them, behave in the same way as two pieces of glass separated by a thin film of water. They glide over each other easily but can be pulled apart only with difficulty, because of the surface tension between the membranes and the fluid. If either layer of pleura is punctured, the underlying lung collapses due to its inherent property of elastic recoil.

Interior of the lungs

The lungs are composed of the bronchi and smaller air passages, alveoli, connective tissue, blood vessels, lymph vessels and nerves. The left lung is divided into two lobes and the right, into three (Fig. 10.15). Each lobe is made up of a large number of lobules.

Pulmonary blood supply (Fig. 10.17)

The *pulmonary artery* divides into two, one branch conveying *deoxygenated blood* to each lung. Within the lungs each pulmonary artery divides into many branches which eventually end in a dense capillary network around the walls of the alveoli (Fig. 10.18). The walls of the alveoli and those of the capillaries each consist of only one layer of flattened epithelial cells. The exchange of gases between air in the alveoli and blood in the capillaries takes place across these two very fine membranes. The pulmonary capillaries join up, eventually

251

Fluid filled balloon

Pleural cavity with serous fluid

Visceral pleura

Parietal pleura

Ribs

Lung

Heart

Diaphragm

Figure 10.16 The relationship of the pleura to the lungs.

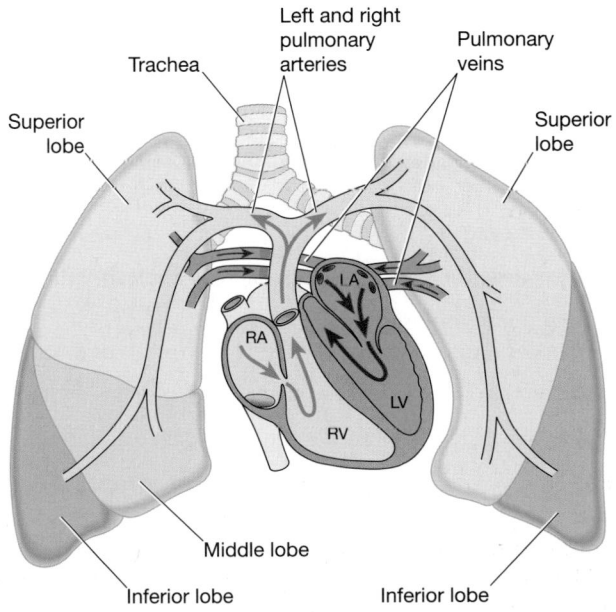

Left and right pulmonary arteries

Trachea

Pulmonary veins

Superior lobe

Superior lobe

LA

RA

LV

RV

Middle lobe

Inferior lobe

Inferior lobe

Figure 10.17 The flow of blood between heart and lungs.

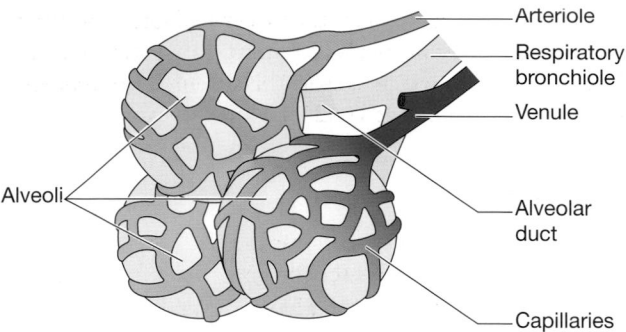

Figure 10.18 The capillary network surrounding the alveoli.

becoming *two pulmonary veins* in each lung. They leave the lungs at the hilum and convey *oxygenated blood* to the left atrium of the heart. The innumerable blood capillaries and blood vessels in the lungs are supported by connective tissue.

The blood supply to the respiratory passages, lymphatic drainage and nerve supply has already been described (p. 248).

RESPIRATION

Learning outcomes

After studying this section, you should be able to:

- describe the actions of the main muscles of respiration during ventilation

- compare and contrast the mechanical events occurring in inspiration and expiration

- define the terms compliance, elasticity and airflow resistance

- describe the principal lung volumes and capacities

- compare the processes of internal and external respiration, using the concept of diffusion of gases

- describe O_2 and CO_2 transport in the blood

- explain the main mechanisms by which respiration is controlled.

Inflation and deflation of the lungs occurring with each breath ensures that regular exchange of gases takes place between the alveoli and the external air.

Muscles of respiration

The expansion of the chest during inspiration occurs as a result of muscular activity, partly voluntary and partly involuntary. The main muscles of respiration in normal quiet breathing are the *intercostal muscles* and the *diaphragm*. During difficult or deep breathing they are assisted by the muscles of the neck, shoulders and abdomen.

Intercostal muscles

There are 11 pairs of intercostal muscles that occupy the spaces between the 12 pairs of ribs. They are arranged in two layers, the external and internal intercostal muscles (Fig. 10.19).

The external intercostal muscle fibres. These extend in a downwards and forwards direction from the lower border of the rib above to the upper border of the rib below.

The internal intercostal muscle fibres. These extend in a downwards and backwards direction from the lower border of the rib above to the upper border of the rib below, crossing the external intercostal muscle fibres at right angles.

The first rib is fixed. Therefore, when the intercostal muscles contract they pull all the other ribs towards the first rib. Because of the shape of the ribs they move outwards when pulled upwards. In this way the thoracic cavity is enlarged anteroposteriorly and laterally. The intercostal muscles are stimulated to contract by the *intercostal nerves.*

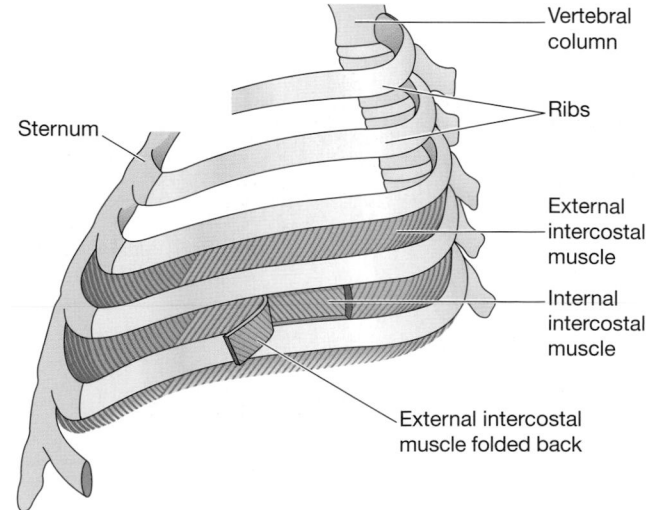

Figure 10.19 The intercostal muscles and the bones of the thorax.

Diaphragm

The diaphragm is a dome-shaped structure separating the thoracic and abdominal cavities. It forms the floor of the thoracic cavity and the roof of the abdominal cavity and consists of a central tendon from which muscle fibres radiate to be attached to the lower ribs and sternum and to the vertebral column by two crura. When the muscle of the diaphragm is relaxed, the central tendon is at the level of the 8th thoracic vertebra (Fig. 10.20). When it contracts, its muscle fibres shorten and the central tendon is pulled downwards to the level of the 9th thoracic vertebra, enlarging the thoracic cavity in length. This decreases pressure in the thoracic cavity and increases it in the abdominal and pelvic cavities. The diaphragm is supplied by the *phrenic nerves*.

The intercostal muscles and the diaphragm contract *simultaneously* ensuring the enlargement of the thoracic cavity in all directions, that is from back to front, side to side and top to bottom (Fig. 10.21).

Cycle of respiration

This occurs 12 to 15 times per minute and consists of three phases:

- inspiration
- expiration
- pause.

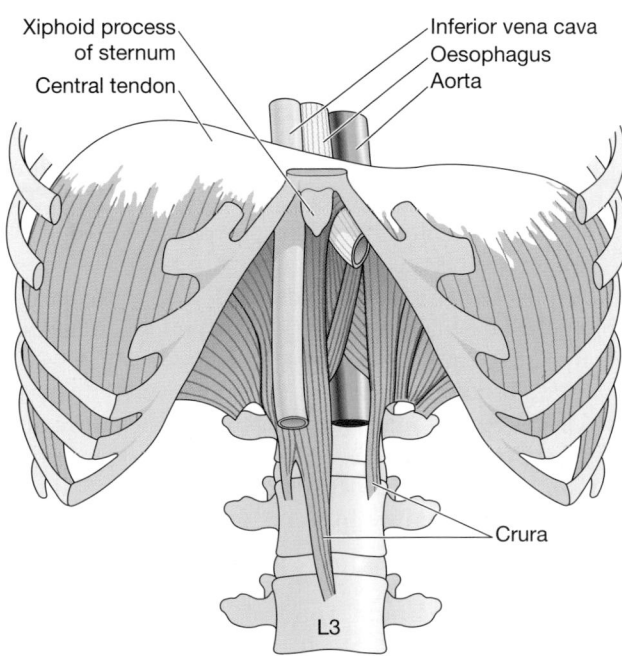

Xiphoid process of sternum
Central tendon
Inferior vena cava
Oesophagus
Aorta
Crura
L3

Figure 10.20 The diaphragm.

As described previously, the visceral pleura is adherent to the lungs and the parietal pleura to the inner wall of the thorax and to the diaphragm. Between them there is a thin film of serous fluid (p. 251).

Inspiration

When the capacity of the thoracic cavity is increased by simultaneous contraction of the intercostal muscles and the diaphragm, the parietal pleura moves with the walls of the thorax and the diaphragm. This reduces the pressure in the pleural cavity to a level considerably lower than atmospheric pressure. The visceral pleura follows the parietal pleura pulling the lung with it. This stretches the lungs and the pressure within the alveoli and in the air passages falls, drawing air into the lungs in an attempt to equalise the atmospheric and alveolar air pressures.

The process of inspiration is *active*, as it requires expenditure of energy for muscle contraction. The negative pressure created in the thoracic cavity aids venous return to the heart and is known as the *respiratory pump*.

Expiration

Relaxation of the intercostal muscles and the diaphragm results in downward and inward movement of the rib cage (Fig. 10.21) and elastic recoil of the lungs. As this occurs, pressure inside the lungs exceeds that in the atmosphere and therefore air is expelled from the respiratory tract. The lungs still contain some air and are prevented from complete collapse by the intact pleura. This process is *passive* as it does not require the expenditure of energy.

After expiration, there is a *pause* before the next cycle begins.

Physiological variables affecting respiration

Elasticity. Elasticity is the term used to describe the ability of the lung to return to its normal shape after each breath. Loss of elasticity of the connective tissue in the lungs necessitates forced expiration and increased effort on inspiration.

Compliance. This is a measure of the distensibility of the lungs, i.e. the effort required to inflate the alveoli. When compliance is low the effort needed to inflate the lungs is greater than normal, e.g. in some diseases where elasticity is reduced or when insufficient surfactant is present. It should be noted that compliance and elasticity are opposing forces.

Figure 10.21 The changes in capacity of the thoracic cavity and the lungs during breathing.

Airflow resistance. When this is increased, e.g. in bronchoconstriction, more respiratory effort is required to inflate the lungs.

Lung volumes and capacities (Fig. 10.22)

In normal quiet breathing there are about 15 complete respiratory cycles per minute. The lungs and the air passages are never empty and, as the exchange of gases takes place only across the walls of the alveolar ducts and alveoli, the remaining capacity of the respiratory passages is called the *anatomical dead space* (about 150 ml).

Figure 10.22 Lung volumes and capacities: IRV = inspiratory reserve volume; IC = inspiratory capacity; FRC = functional residual capacity; ERV = expiratory reserve volume; RV = residual volume; VC = vital capacity.

Tidal volume (TV). This is the amount of air which passes into and out of the lungs during each cycle of quiet breathing (about 500 ml).

Inspiratory reserve volume (IRV). This is the extra volume of air that can be inhaled into the lungs during maximal inspiration.

Inspiratory capacity (IC). This is the amount of air that can be inspired with maximum effort. It consists of the tidal volume (500 ml) plus the inspiratory reserve volume.

Functional residual capacity (FRC). This is the amount of air remaining in the air passages and alveoli at the end of quiet expiration. Tidal air mixes with this air, causing relatively small changes in the composition of alveolar air. As blood flows continuously through the pulmonary capillaries this means that the interchange of gases is not interrupted between breaths, preventing marked changes in the concentration of blood gases. The functional residual volume also prevents collapse of the alveoli on expiration.

Expiratory reserve volume (ERV). This is the largest volume of air which can be expelled from the lungs during maximal expiration.

Residual volume (RV). This cannot be directly measured but is the volume of air remaining in the lungs after forced expiration.

Vital capacity (VC). This is the maximum volume of air which can be moved into and out of the lungs:

VC = Tidal volume + IRV + ERV

Alveolar ventilation. This is the volume of air that moves into and out of the alveoli per minute. It is equal to the tidal volume minus the anatomical dead space, multiplied by the respiratory rate:

Alveolar ventilation = (TV − anatomical dead space)
$\times$ respiratory rate
= (500 − 150) ml $\times$ 15 per
minute
= 5.25 litres per minute

Lung function tests are carried out to determine respiratory function and are based on the parameters outlined above. Results of these tests can help in diagnosis and monitoring of respiratory disorders.

Composition of air

Atmospheric pressure at sea level is 101.3 kilopascals (kPa)* or 760 mmHg. With the increase in height above sea level, atmospheric pressure is progressively reduced and at 5500 m, about two-thirds the height of Mount Everest (8850 m), it is about half that at sea level. Under water, pressure increases by approximately 1 atmosphere per 10 m below sea level.

Air is a mixture of gases: nitrogen, oxygen, carbon dioxide, water vapour and small quantities of inert gases. The percentage of each is listed in Table 10.1. Each gas in the mixture exerts a part of the total pressure proportional to its concentration, i.e. the *partial pressure* (Table 10.2). This is denoted as, e.g. PO_2, PCO_2.

Alveolar air

The composition of alveolar air remains fairly constant and is different from atmospheric air. It is saturated with water vapour and contains more carbon dioxide, and less oxygen. Saturation with water vapour provides 6.3 kPa (47 mmHg) thus reducing the partial pressure of all the other gases present. Gaseous exchange between the alveoli and the bloodstream (*external respiration*) is a continuous process, as the alveoli are never empty, so it is independent of the respiratory cycle. During each inspiration only some of the alveolar gases are exchanged.

Expired air

This is a mixture of alveolar air and atmospheric air in the dead space. Its composition is shown in Table 10.1.

Diffusion of gases

Exchange of gases occurs when a difference in partial pressure exists across semipermeable membranes. Gases move by diffusion from the higher concentration to the lower until equilibrium is established (p. 26). Atmospheric nitrogen is not used by the body so its partial pressure remains unchanged and is the same in inspired and expired air, alveolar air and in the blood.

External respiration

This is exchange of gases by diffusion between the alveoli and the blood. Each alveolar wall is one cell thick and is surrounded by a network of tiny capillaries (the walls of which are also only one cell thick). The total area for gas exchange in the lungs is 70 to 80 square metres. Venous blood arriving at the lungs has travelled from all the active tissues of the body, and contains high levels of CO_2 and low levels of O_2. Carbon dioxide diffuses from venous blood down its concentration gradient into the alveoli until equilibrium with alveolar air is reached. By the same process, oxygen diffuses from the alveoli into the blood. The slow flow of blood through the capillaries increases the time available for diffusion to occur. When blood leaves the alveolar capillaries, the oxygen and carbon dioxide concentrations are in equilibrium with those of alveolar air (Fig. 10.23).

Internal respiration

This is exchange of gases by diffusion between blood in the capillaries and the body cells. Gaseous exchange does

255

Table 10.1 The composition of inspired and expired air

	Inspired air %	Expired air %
Oxygen	21	16
Carbon dioxide	0.04	4
Nitrogen and rare gases	78	78
Water vapour	Variable	Saturated

Table 10.2 Partial pressures of gases

Gas	Alveolar air kPa	Alveolar air mmHg	Deoxygenated blood kPa	Deoxygenated blood mmHg	Oxygenated blood kPa	Oxygenated blood mmHg
Oxygen	13.3	100	5.3	40	13.3	100
Carbon dioxide	5.3	40	5.8	44	5.3	40
Nitrogen and other inert gases	76.4	573	76.4	573	76.4	573
Water vapour	6.3	47				
	101.3	760				

*1 mmHg = 133.3 Pa = 0.133 kPa
1 kPa = 7.5 mmHg

Figure 10.23 External respiration: exchange of gases between alveolar air and capillary blood.

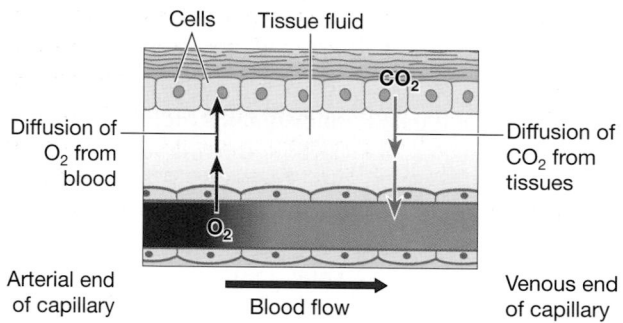

Figure 10.24 Internal respiration: exchange of gases between capillary blood and tissue cells.

not occur across the walls of the arteries carrying blood from the heart to the tissues, because their walls are too thick. PO_2 of blood arriving at the capillary bed is therefore the same as blood leaving the lungs. Blood arriving at the tissues has been cleansed of its CO_2 and saturated with O_2 during its passage through the lungs, and therefore has a higher PO_2 and a lower PCO_2 than the tissues. This creates concentration gradients between the blood and the tissues, and gaseous exchange therefore occurs (Fig. 10.24). O_2 diffuses from the bloodstream through the capillary wall into the tissues. CO_2 diffuses from the cells into the extracellular fluid then into the bloodstream towards the venous end of the capillary.

Transport of gases in the bloodstream

Transport of blood oxygen and carbon dioxide is essential for internal respiration to occur.

Oxygen
Oxygen is carried in the blood:

- in chemical combination with haemoglobin as *oxyhaemoglobin* (98.5% of blood O_2)
- in solution in plasma water (1.5% of blood O_2).

Oxyhaemoglobin is an unstable compound that under certain conditions readily dissociates releasing oxygen. Factors that increase dissociation include raised carbon dioxide content of tissue fluid, raised temperature and 2,3-diphosphoglycerate (2,3-DPG is a substance present in red blood cells). In active tissues there is increased production of carbon dioxide and heat which leads to increased release of oxygen. In this way oxygen is available to tissues in greatest need. When oxygen leaves the erythrocyte, the deoxygenated haemoglobin turns purplish in colour.

Carbon dioxide
Carbon dioxide is one of the waste products of metabolism. It is excreted by the lungs and is transported by three mechanisms:

- most of it is in the form of bicarbonate ions (HCO_3^-) in the plasma (70% of blood CO_2)
- some is dissolved in the plasma (7% of blood CO_2)
- some is carried in erythrocytes, loosely combined with haemoglobin as *carbaminohaemoglobin* (23% of blood CO_2).

Control of respiration

Control of respiration is normally involuntary. Voluntary control is exerted during activities such as speaking and singing but is overridden if blood CO_2 rises (hypercapnia).

The respiratory centre
This is formed by groups of nerve cells that control the rate and depth of respiration (Fig. 10.25). They are situated in the brain stem, in the *medulla oblongata* and the *pons*. The interrelationship between these groups of cells is complex. In the medulla there are *inspiratory neurones* and *expiratory neurones*. Neurones in the *pneumotaxic* and *apneustic centres*, situated in the pons, influence the inspiratory and expiratory neurones of the medulla.

Motor impulses leaving the respiratory centre pass in the *phrenic* and *intercostal nerves* to the diaphragm and intercostal muscles respectively.

Chemoreceptors
These are receptors that respond to changes in the partial pressures of oxygen and carbon dioxide in the blood and cerebrospinal fluid. They are located centrally and peripherally.

Central chemoreceptors. These are on the surface of the medulla oblongata and are bathed in cerebrospinal fluid. When the arterial PCO_2 rises (hypercapnia), even slightly, the central chemoreceptors respond by stimulating the respiratory centre, increasing ventilation of the lungs and reducing arterial PCO_2. The sensitivity of the central chemoreceptors to raised arterial PCO_2 is the most important factor in maintaining homeostasis of blood gases in health. A small reduction in PO_2 (hypoxaemia) has the same, but less pronounced effect, but a substantial reduction has a depressing effect.

Peripheral chemoreceptors. These are situated in the arch of the aorta and in the carotid bodies (Fig. 10.25). They are more sensitive to small rises in arterial PCO_2 than to similarly low arterial PO_2 levels. Nerve impulses, generated in the peripheral chemoreceptors, are conveyed by the *glossopharyngeal* and *vagus nerves* to the medulla and stimulate the respiratory centre. The rate and depth of breathing are then increased. An increase in blood acidity (decreased pH or raised [H^+]) stimulates the peripheral chemoreceptors, resulting in increased ventilation, increased CO_2 excretion and increased blood pH.

Other factors that influence respiration

Breathing may be modified by the higher centres in the brain by:

- speech, singing
- emotional displays, e.g. crying, laughing, fear
- drugs, e.g. sedatives, alcohol
- sleep.

Temperature influences breathing. In fever respiration is increased due to increased metabolic rate while in hypothermia it is depressed, as is metabolism. Temporary changes in respiration occur in swallowing, sneezing and coughing.

The *Hering–Breuer reflex* prevents overinflation of the lungs. Stretch receptors situated in the thoracic wall generate nerve inhibitory impulses when the lungs have inflated. They travel via the vagus nerves to the respiratory centre.

Normally, quiet breathing is adequate to maintain arterial PO_2 and PCO_2 levels; however, on strenous exercise, both the rate and depth of breathing increase, increasing oxygen uptake and carbon dioxide excretion in order to meet increased needs and so maintain homeostasis. When intense respiratory effort is required, the *accessory muscles of respiration* are used. The most important is the *sternocleidomastoid* (Fig. 18.1). Contraction of these muscles in addition to the diaphragm and intercostal muscles ensures the maximum increase in the capacity of the thoracic cavity.

Effective control of respiration enables the body to maintain homeostasis of blood gases over a wide range of physiological, environmental and pathological conditions.

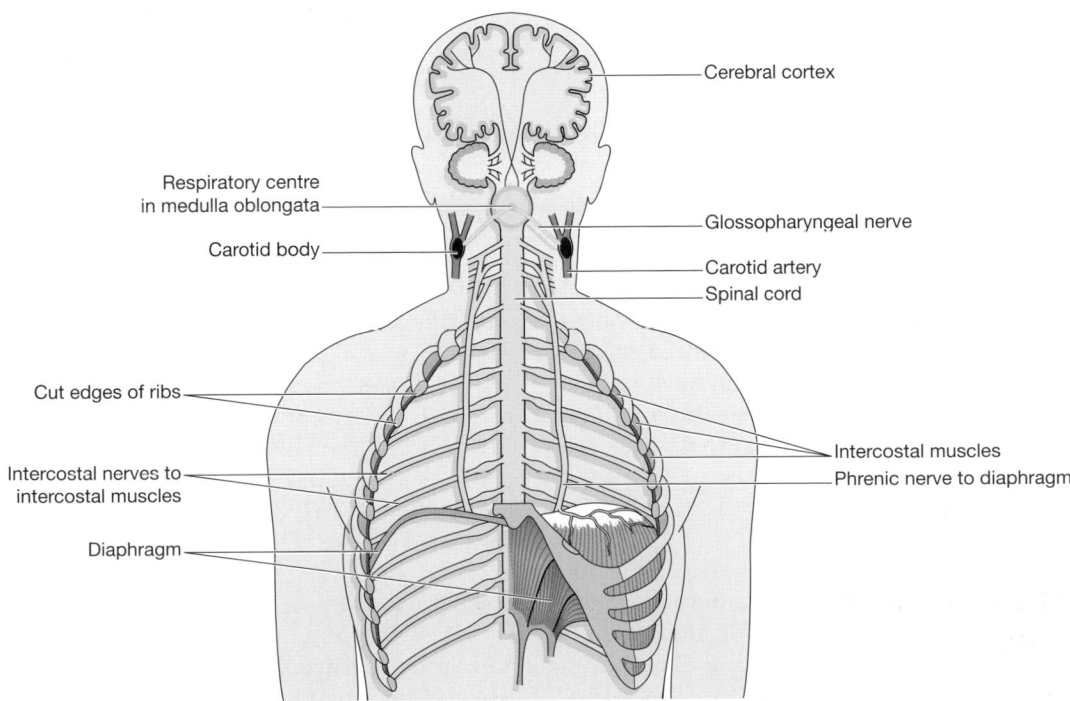

Cerebral cortex

Respiratory centre in medulla oblongata

Glossopharyngeal nerve

Carotid body

Carotid artery

Spinal cord

Cut edges of ribs

Intercostal muscles

Phrenic nerve to diaphragm

Intercostal nerves to intercostal muscles

Diaphragm

Figure 10.25 Some of the nerves involved in control of respiration.

DISORDERS OF THE UPPER RESPIRATORY TRACT

Learning outcomes

After studying this section, you should be able to:

- describe the main inflammatory and infectious disorders of the upper respiratory tract

- outline the main tumours of the upper respiratory tract.

Infectious and inflammatory disorders

Inflammation of the upper respiratory tract can be caused by inhaling irritants, but is commonly due to infection. Such infections are usually caused by viruses that lower the resistance of the respiratory tract to other infections. This allows bacteria dormant in the tract to invade the tissues. Such infections are a threat to life only if:

- they spread to the lungs or other organs
- inflammatory swelling and exudate block the airway.

Microbes are usually spread by droplet infection, in dust or by contaminated equipment and dressings. If not completely resolved, acute infection may become chronic.

Viruses enter host cells and replicate inside them, where they are protected both from the body's own defences and from many drug treatments. Interferons secreted by lymphocytes provide some degree of protection against viruses by limiting their ability to replicate (p. 374).

Viral infections cause acute inflammation of mucous membrane, leading to tissue congestion and profuse exudate of watery fluid. Secondary infection by bacteria usually results in purulent discharge.

Viral infections commonly cause severe illness and sometimes death in infants, young children and the elderly. In adults influenza is an incapacitating condition but is rarely fatal unless infection spreads to the lungs.

Common cold and influenza

The common cold (coryza) is usually caused by the rhinoviruses and is a highly infectious, normally mild illness characterised mainly by a runny nose (rhinorrhoea), sneezing, sore throat and sometimes slight fever. Normally a cold runs its course over a few days. Influenza is caused by a different group of viruses and produces far more severe symptoms than a cold, including very high temperatures and muscle pains; complete recovery can take weeks and secondary bacterial infections are more common than with a simple cold.

Sinusitis

This is usually caused by spread of microbes from the nose and pharynx to the mucous membrane lining the paranasal sinuses in maxillary, sphenoidal, ethmoidal and frontal bones. The primary viral infection is usually followed by bacterial infection, e.g. *Streptococcus pyogenes, Streptococcus pneumoniae, Staphylococcus aureus*. The congested mucosa may block the openings between the nose and the sinuses, preventing drainage of mucopurulent discharge. If there are repeated attacks or if recovery is not complete, the infection may become chronic.

Tonsillitis

Viruses and *Streptococcus pyogenes* are common causes of inflammation of the palatine tonsils, palatine arches and walls of the pharynx. Severe infection may lead to suppuration and abscess formation (*quinsy*). Occasionally the infection spreads into the neck causing cellulitis. Following acute tonsillitis, swelling subsides and the tonsil returns to normal but repeated infection may lead to chronic inflammation, fibrosis and permanent enlargement. Endotoxins from tonsillitis caused by *Streptococcus pyogenes* are associated with the development of rheumatic fever and glomerulonephritis.

The nasopharyngeal tonsils lie on the upper wall of the nasopharynx (Fig. 10.3) and, when inflamed, are better known as the *adenoids*. Temporary enlargement is a protective reaction to infection of nasal and pharyngeal mucosa, and the tissue returns to normal after the infection has subsided, but repeated infections can leave them enlarged and fibrotic. This can cause airway obstruction and can be a problem especially in children.

Pharyngitis

This usually accompanies common colds and tonsillitis. Viruses, with superimposed bacterial infection, cause acute inflammation of the mucous membrane of the pharynx, nose and sinuses.

Laryngitis and tracheitis

The larynx and trachea are subject to the same viral and bacterial infections as the nose and pharynx. The infection may become chronic, expecially in tobacco smokers and people who live or work in a polluted atmosphere. Acute inflammation may follow damage caused by an endotracheal tube, especially if it is used for long periods or has an inflated cuff.

Laryngotracheobronchitis (*croup* in children) is a rare but serious complication of upper respiratory tract infections. The airway is obstructed by marked swelling around the larynx and epiglottis, accompanied by wheeze and breathlessness (dyspnoea).

Diphtheria

This is an infection of the pharynx, caused by *Corynebacterium diphtheriae*, that may extend to the nasopharynx and trachea. A thick fibrous membrane forms over the area and may obstruct the airway. Powerful exotoxins may severely damage cardiac and skeletal muscle, the liver, kidneys and adrenal glands. Where immunisation is widespread diphtheria is comparatively rare.

Hay fever (allergic rhinitis)

In this condition, *atopic* ('immediate') hypersensitivity develops to foreign proteins (antigens), e.g. pollen, mites in pillow feathers, animal dander. The acute non-microbial inflammation of nasal mucosa and conjunctiva causes *rhinorrhoea* (excessive watery exudate from the nose), redness of the eyes and excessive secretion of tears. The first time the antigen is encountered and absorbed, IgE antibodies are produced by B-lymphocytes which adhere to the surface of mast cells and basophils in the mucosa. Subsequent contact with the same antigen causes an immediate antigen/antibody reaction, stimulating the release of histamine and related substances from the granules of mast cells and basophils. These substances cause vasodilatation, increased permeability of capillary walls, hypersecretion by glands and swelling of tissues (see Fig. 15.1, p. 375). Atopic hypersensitivity tends to run in families, but no genetic factor has yet been identified. Other forms of atopic hypersensitivity include:

- childhood onset asthma (see below)
- eczema in infants and young children
- food allergies.

Tumours

Benign (haemangiomata)

These occur in the nasal septum. They consist of abnormal proliferations of blood vessels interspersed with collagen fibres of irregular size and arrangement. The blood vessels tend to rupture and cause persistent bleeding (epistaxis).

Malignant

Carcinoma of the nose, sinuses, nasopharynx and larynx is relatively rare.

DISEASES OF THE BRONCHI

Learning outcomes

After studying this section, you should be able to:

- compare the causes and pathology of chronic and acute bronchitis
- discuss the causes and disordered physiology of asthma
- explain the main physiological abnormality in bronchiectasis.

Acute bronchitis

This is usually a secondary bacterial infection of the bronchi. It is usually preceded by a common cold or influenza and it may also complicate measles and whooping cough in children. The viruses depress normal defence mechanisms, allowing bacteria already present in the respiratory tract to multiply, e.g. *Streptococcus pneumoniae*, *Haemophilus influenzae*, *Streptococcus pyogenes*, *Staphylococcus aureus*. Downward spread of infection may lead to bronchiolitis, and bronchopneumonia may develop, especially in children and in debilitated, often elderly, adults.

Chronic bronchitis

Chronic bronchitis is defined clinically when an individual has had a cough with sputum for 3 months in 2 successive years. It is a progressive inflammatory disease resulting from prolonged irritation of the bronchial epithelium. One or more of the following predisposing factors are usually present:

- acute bronchitis commonly caused by *Haemophilus influenzae* or *Streptococcus pneumoniae*
- cigarette smoking
- atmospheric pollutants, e.g. motor vehicle exhaust fumes, industrial chemicals, sulphur dioxide, urban fog
- previous episodes of acute bronchitis.

It develops mostly in middle-aged men who are chronic heavy smokers and may have a familial predisposition.

259

The changes occurring in the mucous membrane of the bronchi include:

- thickening
- increase in the number and size of mucous glands
- oedema
- reduction in the number of ciliated cells
- narrowing of bronchioles due to fibrosis following repeated inflammatory episodes.

Reduced ciliary activity causes stagnation in the bronchi of the excessive amount of mucus secreted. If the mucus and bronchial lining are colonised by bacteria, pus is formed. Stagnant mucus may partially or completely obstruct small bronchioles. The severe difficulty in breathing (*dyspnoea*) with active expiratory effort raises the air pressure in the alveoli and may rupture the alveolar walls, causing *emphysema* (p. 261). Damp cold conditions tend to exacerbate the disease, and spread of infected mucus to the alveoli may cause pneumonia. As the disease progresses inflamed tissue of the bronchi is progressively replaced by fibrous tissue. Ventilation of the lungs is severely impaired, causing breathlessness, leading to hypoxia, pulmonary hypertension and right-sided heart failure. As respiratory failure develops, arterial blood PO_2 is reduced (*hypoxaemia*) and is accompanied by a rise in arterial blood PCO_2 (*hypercapnia*). When the condition becomes more severe, the respiratory centre in the medulla responds to hypoxaemia rather than to hypercapnia.

Asthma

Asthma is an inflammatory disease of the airways in which the mucous membrane and muscle layers of the bronchi become thickened and the mucous glands enlarge, reducing airflow in the lower respiratory tract. During an asthmatic attack spasmodic contraction of bronchial muscle (*bronchospasm*) constricts the airway and there is excessive secretion of thick sticky mucus which further reduces the airway. Inspiration is normal but only partial expiration is achieved, so the lungs become hyperinflated and there is severe dyspnoea and wheezing. The duration of attacks usually varies from a few minutes to hours, and very occasionally, days (*status asthmaticus*). In severe acute attacks the bronchi may be obstructed by mucus plugs, leading to acute respiratory failure, hypoxia and possibly death.

Non-specific factors that may precipitate asthma attacks include:

- cold air
- cigarette smoking
- air pollution

- upper respiratory tract infection
- emotional stress
- strenuous exercise.

There are two types of asthma which, generally, give rise to identical symptoms and are treated in the same way. Important differences include typical age of onset and the contribution of an element of allergy.

Childhood onset (extrinsic, allergic, atopic) asthma

This type occurs in children and young adults who have atopic (Type 1) hypersensitivity to foreign protein, e.g. pollen, dust containing mites from carpets, feather pillows, animal dander, fungi. A history of infantile eczema or food allergies is common and there are often close family members with a history of allergy.

The same disease process occurs as in hay fever. Antigens (allergens) are inhaled and absorbed by the bronchial mucosa. This stimulates the production of IgE antibodies that bind to the surface of mast cells and basophils round the bronchial blood vessels. When the allergen is encountered again, the antigen/antibody reaction results in the release of histamine and other related substances that stimulate mucus secretion and muscle contraction. Attacks tend to become less frequent and less severe with age.

Adult onset (intrinsic) asthma

This type occurs later in adult life and there is no history of childhood allergic reactions. It is associated with chronic inflammation of the upper respiratory tract, e.g. chronic bronchitis, nasal polyps. Antigens are rarely identified but drug hypersensitivity may develop later, especially to aspirin and penicillin. Attacks tend to increase in severity and there may be irreversible damage to the lungs. Eventually, impaired lung ventilation leads to hypoxia, pulmonary hypertension and right-sided heart failure.

Most asthmatics, whatever the aetiology, can usually have their disease well controlled with inhaled anti-inflammatory and bronchodilator agents, and live a normal life.

Bronchiectasis

This is permanent abnormal dilatation of bronchi and bronchioles. It is associated with chronic bacterial infection and in some cases there is a history of childhood bronchiolitis and bronchopneumonia, cystic fibrosis, or bronchial tumour. The bronchi become obstructed by mucus, pus and inflammatory exudate and the alveoli *distal* to the blockage collapse as trapped air is absorbed. Interstitial elastic tissue degenerates and is replaced by fibrous adhesions that attach the bronchi to the parietal pleura. The pressure of inspired air in these damaged bronchi leads to dilatation *proximal* to the blockage. The persistent severe coughing to remove copious purulent sputum causes intermittent increases in pressure in the blocked bronchi, leading to further dilatation.

The lower lobe of the lung is usually affected. Suppuration is common. If a blood vessel is eroded, haemoptysis may occur or pyaemia, leading to abscess formation elsewhere in the body, commonly the brain. Progressive fibrosis of the lung leads to hypoxia, pulmonary hypertension and right-sided heart failure.

DISORDERS OF THE LUNGS

Learning outcomes

After studying this section, you should be able to:

- discuss the pathologies of the main forms of emphysema

- describe the causes and effects of lung infection, including pneumonia, abscess and tuberculosis

- describe the main pneumoconioses

- outline the main causes and consequences of chemically-induced lung disease

- describe the main causes and consequences of lung cancer

- discuss the causes and effects of collapse of all or part of a lung

Emphysema (Fig. 10.26)

Pulmonary emphysema

In this form of the disease there is irreversible distension of the respiratory bronchioles, alveolar ducts and alveoli reducing the surface area for the exchange of gases. There are two main types and both are usually present.

Panacinar emphysema

The walls between *adjacent alveoli* break down, the *alveolar ducts* dilate and there is loss of interstitial elastic tissue. The lungs become distended and their capacity is

increased. Because the volume of air in each breath remains unchanged it constitutes a smaller proportion of the total volume of air in the distended alveoli, reducing the partial pressure of oxygen. The consequence of this is to reduce the concentration gradient of O_2 across the alveolar membrane, therefore decreasing diffusion of O_2 into the blood. The merging of alveoli reduces the surface area for diffusion of gases. Homeostasis of arterial blood O_2 and CO_2 levels is maintained at rest by hyperventilation. As the disease progresses the combined effect of these changes may lead to hypoxia, pulmonary hypertension and eventually right-sided heart failure. Predisposing factors include:

- cigarette smoking, believed to promote the release of proteolytic enzymes from mast cells and basophils in the lungs
- acute inflammation of bronchi and lungs
- increased pressure caused by coughing which stretches the already damaged structures
- congenital deficiency of an antiproteolytic enzyme, α_1-antitrypsin, which causes deficiency of supporting elastic tissue in the lungs.

Centrilobular emphysema

In this form there is irreversible dilatation of the *respiratory bronchioles* in the centre of lobules. When inspired air reaches the dilated area the pressure falls, leading to a reduction in alveolar air pressure, reduced ventilation efficiency and reduced partial pressure of oxygen. As the disease progresses the resultant hypoxia leads to pulmonary hypertension and right-sided heart failure. Predisposing conditions, exacerbated by persistent severe coughing, include recurrent bronchiolitis, pneumoconiosis, chronic bronchitis and cigarette smoking.

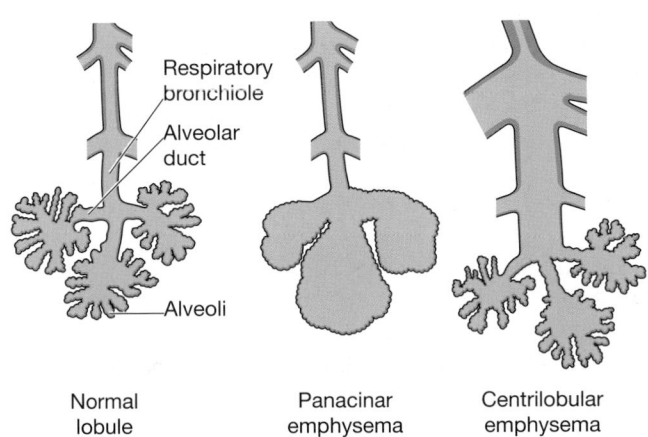

Figure 10.26 Emphysema.

Interstitial emphysema

Interstitial emphysema means the presence of air in the thoracic interstitial tissues, and this may happen in one of the following ways:

- from the outside by injury, e.g. fractured rib, stab wound
- from the inside when an alveolus ruptures through the pleura, e.g. during an asthmatic attack, in bronchiolitis, coughing as in whooping cough.

The air in the tissues usually tracks upwards to the soft tissues of the neck where it is gradually absorbed, causing no damage. A large quantity in the mediastinum may limit heart movement.

Pneumonia (Fig. 10.27)

This occurs when protective processes fail to prevent inhaled or blood-borne microbes reaching and *colonising* the lungs. The following are some predisposing factors.

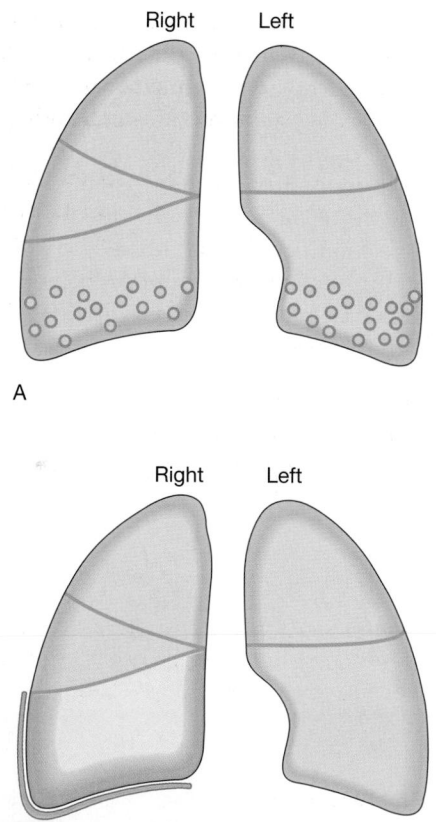

A

B

Figure 10.27 Distribution of infected tissue in: A. Bronchopneumonia. B. Lobar pneumonia.

Impaired coughing. The effectiveness of coughing as an aid to the removal of infected mucus may be reduced when the individual is unconscious or by damage to:

- sensory nerve endings in the walls of the respiratory passages
- the cough reflex centre in the medulla oblongata
- nerves to the respiratory passages, lungs and muscles of respiration
- the diaphragm and intercostal muscles.

Voluntary inhibition may occur if coughing causes pain, e.g. following abdominal surgery.

Damage to the epithelial lining of the tract. Ciliary action may be impaired or the epithelium destroyed by, e.g., tobacco smoking, inhaling noxious gases, infection.

Defective alveolar phagocytosis. Depressed macrophage activity may be caused by tobacco smoking, alcohol, anoxia, oxygen toxicity.

Pulmonary oedema and congestion. Bronchopneumonia frequently occurs in patients with hypostatic pulmonary oedema and congestive heart failure. The relationship is not clear.

General lowering of resistance to infection. Factors involved include:

- leukopenia
- chronic diseases
- impaired immune response caused by, e.g., ionising radiation, corticosteroid drugs
- unusually virulent infections
- hypothermia.

Lobar pneumonia

This is infection of one or more lobes by *Streptococcus pneumoniae*, mainly Types 1, 2 and 3. The infection leads to production of watery inflammatory exudate in the alveoli. This accumulates and fills the lobule then overflows into adjacent lobules, spreading the microbes. It is of sudden onset and pleuritic pain accompanies inflammation of the visceral pleura. If not treated by antibacterial drugs the disease goes through a series of stages followed by resolution and reinflation of the lobes in 2 to 3 weeks.

Complications of lobar pneumonia

Incomplete resolution. If the fibrous exudate, formed as the infection subsides, is not completely cleared it may become permanently solid, tough, leathery and airless, reducing the surface area for gaseous exchange.

Pleural effusion and empyema. When infection spreads to the pleura, inflammatory exudate accumulates (*effusion*) in the pleural cavity and pus is formed (*empyema*). Healing may lead to formation of fibrous adhesions which prevent normal expansion of the lung.

Spread of infection. This may be to local tissues or cause:

- pericarditis
- acute endocarditis
- meningitis
- acute otitis media
- arthritis.

Lung abscess. This may develop but only rarely when antimicrobial drugs are available.

Cardiac complications. These include endocarditis or toxic myocarditis that may lead to heart failure, especially in elderly people.

Bronchopneumonia

Infection is spread from the bronchi to terminal bronchioles and alveoli. As these become inflamed, fibrous exudate accumulates and there is an influx of leukocytes. Small foci of consolidation develop. There is frequently incomplete resolution with fibrosis. Bronchiectasis is a common complication leading to further acute attacks, lung fibrosis and progressive destruction of lung substance. Bronchopneumonia occurs most commonly in infancy and old age, and death is fairly common, especially when the condition complicates debilitating diseases. Predisposing factors include:

- debility due to, e.g., cancer, uraemia, cerebral haemorrhage, congestive heart failure, malnutrition, hypothermia
- chronic bronchitis
- bronchiectasis
- cystic fibrosis
- general anaesthetics which depress respiratory and ciliary activity
- acute viral infections
- inhalation of gastric contents in, e.g., unconsciousness, very deep sleep, following excessive alcohol consumption, drug overdose
- inhalation of infected material from the paranasal sinuses or upper respiratory tract.

Microbes causing bronchopneumonia

Staphylococcus aureus. Infection is usually preceded by influenza, measles, whooping cough or chronic lung disease. Incomplete resolution may cause abscess formation, with rupture into the pleural cavity, empyema and possibly pneumothorax. Pleural adhesions may form during healing and limit lung expansion.

Friedländer's bacillus (*Klebsiella pneumoniae*). This commensal is sometimes present in the upper respiratory tract, especially where there is advanced dental caries. It commonly causes pneumonia in men over 50 years and is often associated with diabetes mellitus and alcoholism.

Legionella pneumonophila. These microbes are widely distributed in water tanks, shower heads and air conditioning systems, and are therefore commonly found in institutions such as hospitals and hotels. They may cause a severe form of pneumonia (*Legionnaires' disease*), complicated by gastrointestinal disturbances, headache, mental confusion and renal failure.

Streptococcus pyogenes. Infection is usually preceded by influenza or measles. In very severe cases death may occur within a few days.

Pseudomonas pyocyanea. This organism causes a type of pneumonia acquired by cross-infection in hospitals, especially in patients with mechanically assisted ventilation or tracheostomy. It is resistant to many antibacterial agents and multiplies at room temperature in, e.g., water, soap solution, eye drops, ointments, weak antiseptics.

***Streptococcus pneumoniae* (pneumococcus).** This is a commensal in the respiratory tract which may cause lobar pneumonia or bronchopneumonia, usually preceded by virus infection. It affects mainly debilitated bed-ridden patients when there is stagnation of mucus in the respiratory passages.

Other organisms. Some viruses, protozoa and fungi may cause pneumonia in people whose general resistance is lowered or whose immune systems are depressed by, e.g., drugs.

Lung abscess

Local suppuration and necrosis within the lung substance is most commonly caused by: *Streptococcus viridans, Streptococcus pyogenes, Streptococcus pneumoniae, Staphylococcus aureus.*

Sources of infection

Inhalation. Infected matter from the paranasal sinuses, gums and the upper respiratory passages may be inhaled. An important predisposing factor is inhalation of regurgitated gastric contents that may occur during coma, emergency anaesthesia, very deep sleep, following alcohol consumption, drug overdose or sniffing volatile gases from, e.g., glue (*aspiration pneumonia*). The hydrochloric acid and food particles cause severe irritation of the upper respiratory tract, allowing bacteria already present to invade the tissues and spread to the lungs.

Pneumonia. Lung abscess may complicate pneumonia, especially when the latter is caused by *Staphylococcus aureus, Streptococcus pneumoniae* or Friedländer's bacillus.

Septic embolism. Thrombophlebitis and right-sided endocarditis are the main sources of septic emboli that cause lung abscess.

Traumatic penetration of the lung. Pathogenic microbes may enter the lung when both skin and lung are penetrated, e.g. in compound fracture of rib, stab wound, gunshot wound, during surgery.

Local spread of infection. Microbes may spread from the pleural cavity, oesophagus, spine or a subphrenic abscess. Recovery from lung abscess may be complete or lead to complications, e.g.:

- chronic suppuration
- septic emboli may spread to other parts of the body, e.g. the brain, causing cerebral abscess or meningitis
- subpleural abscesses may spread and cause empyema and possibly bronchopleural fistula formation
- erosion of a pulmonary blood vessel, leading to haemorrhage.

Tuberculosis

This infection is caused by one of two forms of mycobacteria.

Mycobacterium tuberculosis. Humans are the main host. The microbes cause pulmonary tuberculosis and are spread either by droplet infection from an individual with active tuberculosis, or in dust contaminated by infected sputum.

Mycobacterium bovis. Animals are the main host. The microbes are usually spread to humans by untreated milk from infected cows, causing infection of the alimentary tract. In Britain the incidence has been greatly reduced by the elimination of bovine tuberculosis and the pasteurisation of milk. It is still a significant infection in many countries.

Phases of pulmonary tuberculosis

Primary tuberculosis

When microbes are inhaled they colonise a lung bronchiole, usually towards the apex of the lung. There may be no evidence of clinical disease during the initial stage of non-specific inflammation. Later, cell-mediated T-lymphocytes respond to the microbes (antigens) and the individual becomes *sensitised*. Macrophages surround the microbes at the site of infection, forming *Ghon foci* (tubercles). Some macrophages containing live microbes are spread in lymph and infect hilar lymph nodes. *Primary complexes* are formed, consisting of Ghon foci plus infected hilar lymph nodes. Necrosis (caseation) may reduce the core of foci to a cheese-like substance consisting of dead macrophages, dead lung tissue and live and dead microbes. Primary tuberculosis is usually asymptomatic. There are various outcomes.

- The disease may be permanently arrested, the foci becoming fibrosed and calcified.
- Microbes may survive in the foci and become the source of *postprimary infection* months or years later.
- The disease may spread:
  - throughout the lung, forming multiple small foci; to the respiratory passages, causing bronchopneumonia or bronchiectasis; to the pleura causing pleurisy, with or without effusion
  - to other parts of the body via lymph and blood leading to wide spread of the infection and the development of numerous small foci throughout the body (*miliary tuberculosis*).

Weight loss and malaise develop insidiously, and night sweats are common.

Secondary (postprimary) tuberculosis

This phase occurs only in people *previously sensitised* by a primary lesion, usually situated in the apex of one or both lungs. It may be caused by a new infection or by reactivation of infection by microbes surviving in Ghon foci. As sensitisation has already occurred, T-lymphocytes stimulate an immediate immune reaction, followed by phagocytosis. The subsequent course of the disease is variable, e.g.:

- it may be arrested, healing occurring with fibrosis and calcification of the foci
- foci, containing live microbes, may be walled off by fibrous tissue, becoming a potential source of future infection
- live microbes in foci may break out through the fibrous walls and cause further infection
- pleurisy with or without effusion or empyema may develop

- haemoptysis (expectoration of blood-stained sputum) may occur if a small blood vessel is eroded and bleeds into the respiratory tract
- caseous material containing live microbes may be expectorated, leaving cavities in the lung, and become a source of infection of:
  - the other lung, bronchi, trachea and larynx
  - the alimentary tract when microbes are swallowed
- microbes may spread in blood and lymph, leading to widespread infection and the development of numerous small foci throughout the body (miliary tuberculosis).

Bovine tuberculosis follows the same course but primary complexes develop in the intestines.

Pneumoconioses (occupational lung diseases)

This group of lung diseases is caused by inhaling organic or inorganic atmospheric pollutants. To cause pneumoconiosis, particles must be so small that they are carried in inspired air to the level of the respiratory bronchioles and alveoli where they can only be cleared by phagocytosis. Larger particles are trapped by mucus higher up the tract and expelled by ciliary action and coughing. Other contributory factors include:

- high concentration of pollutants in the air
- long exposure to pollutants
- reduced numbers of macrophages and ineffectual phagocytosis
- cigarette smoking.

Coal workers' pneumoconiosis

This is caused by inhaling dust from soft bituminous coal. It occurs in two forms.

Simple pneumoconiosis
The particles of coal dust lodge mainly in the upper two-thirds of the lungs and are ingested by macrophages inside the alveoli. Some macrophages remain in the alveoli and some move out into the surrounding tissues and adhere to the outside of the alveolar walls, respiratory bronchioles, blood vessels and to the visceral pleura. Macrophages are unable to digest inorganic particles and when they die they are surrounded by fibrous tissue. Fibrosis is progressive during exposure to coal dust but tends to stop when exposure stops. Early in the disease there may be few clinical signs unless emphysema develops or there is concurrent chronic bronchitis.

Pneumoconiosis with progressive massive fibrosis
This develops in a small number of cases, sometimes after the worker is no longer exposed to coal dust. Masses of fibrous tissue develop and progressively encroach on the blood vessels and bronchioles. Large parts of the lung are destroyed and emphysema is extensive, leading to pulmonary oedema, pulmonary hypertension and right-sided cardiac failure. The reasons for the severity of the disease are not clear. One factor may be hypersensitivity to antigens released by the large number of dead macrophages. About 40% of the patients have tuberculosis.

Silicosis

This may be caused by long-term exposure to dust containing silicon compounds. High-risk industries are:

- quarrying granite, slate, sandstone
- mining hard coal, gold, tin, copper
- stone masonry and sand blasting
- glass and pottery work.

When silica particles are inhaled they accumulate in the alveoli. The particles are ingested by macrophages, some of which remain in the alveoli and some move out into the connective tissues around respiratory bronchioles and blood vessels and close to the pleura. Progressive fibrosis is stimulated which eventually obliterates the blood vessels and respiratory bronchioles. Fibrous adhesions form between the two layers of pleura, and eventually fix the lung to the chest wall. The relationship between the presence of silicon and the production of excess fibrous tissue is not clear. It may be that:

- inflammation is caused by silicic acid which gradually forms when silicon compounds dissolve
- there is an immune reaction in which silicon is the antigen
- fibrosis is stimulated by enzymes released when macrophages containing silicon die.

Silicosis appears to predispose to the development of tuberculosis which rapidly progresses to tubercular bronchopneumonia and possibly to miliary tuberculosis. Gradual destruction of lung tissue leads to pulmonary hypertension and right-sided heart failure.

Asbestos-related diseases

Disease caused by inhaling asbestos fibres usually develop after 10 to 20 years' exposure but sometimes after only 2 years. Asbestos miners and workers involved in making and using some products containing asbestos are at risk. The types associated with disease are crocidolite (blue asbestos), chrysotile (white asbestos) and amosite (brown asbestos).

Asbestosis

This occurs when asbestos fibres are inhaled in dust. In spite of their large size the particles penetrate to the level of respiratory bronchioles and alveoli. Macrophages accumulate in the alveoli and the shorter fibres are ingested. The larger fibres form *asbestos bodies*, consisting of fibres surrounded by macrophages, protein material and iron deposits. Their presence in sputum indicates exposure to asbestos but not necessarily that there is asbestosis. The macrophages that have engulfed fibres move out of the alveoli and accumulate round respiratory bronchioles and blood vessels, stimulating the formation of fibrous tissue. There is progressive destruction of lung tissue, with the development of dyspnoea, chronic hypoxia, pulmonary hypertension and right-sided cardiac failure. The link between inhaled asbestos and fibrosis is not clear. It may be that asbestos stimulates the macrophages to secrete enzymes that promote fibrosis or that it stimulates an immune reaction causing fibrosis.

Pleural mesothelioma

The majority of cases of this malignant tumour of the pleura are linked with previous exposure to asbestos dust, e.g. asbestos workers and people living near asbestos mines and factories. Mesothelioma may develop after widely varying duration of exposure to asbestos, from 3 months to 60 years, and is usually associated with crocidolite fibres (blue asbestos). The latent period between exposure and the appearance of symptoms may range from 10 to 40 years. The tumour involves both layers of pleura and as it grows it obliterates the pleural cavity, compressing the lung. Lymph and blood-spread metastases are commonly found in the hilar and mesenteric lymph nodes, the other lung, liver, thyroid and adrenal glands, bone, skeletal muscle and brain.

Byssinosis

This is caused by the inhalation of fibres of cotton, flax and hemp over a period of years. The fibres cause bronchial irritation and possibly the release of histamine-like substances. At first, breathless attacks similar to asthma occur only when the individual is at work. Later, they become more persistent and chronic bronchitis and emphysema may develop, leading to chronic hypoxia, pulmonary hypertension and right-sided heart failure.

Table 10.3 Conditions caused by inhaled contaminants

Disease	Contaminant
Farmer's lung	Mouldy hay
Bagassosis	Mouldy sugar waste
Bird handler's lung	Moulds in bird droppings
Malt worker's lung	Mouldy barley

Extrinsic allergic alveolitis

This group of conditions is caused by inhaling materials contaminated by moulds and fungi, e.g. those in Table 10.3. The contaminants act as antigens causing antigen/antibody reactions in the walls of the alveoli. There is excess fluid exudate and the accumulation of platelets, lymphocytes and plasma cells. The alveolar walls become thick and there is progressive fibrosis, leading to pulmonary hypertension and right-sided heart failure.

Chemically induced lung diseases

Paraquat (1,1-dimethyl-4,4 bipyridylium chloride)

Within hours of ingestion of this weedkiller it is blood-borne to the lungs and begins to cause irreversible damage. The alveolar membrane becomes swollen, pulmonary oedema develops and alveolar epithelium is destroyed. The kidneys are also damaged and death may be due to combined respiratory and renal failure or cardiac failure.

Cytotoxic drugs (busulphan, bleomycin, methotrexate)

These and other drugs used in cancer treatment may cause inflammation that heals by fibrosis of interstitial tissue in the lungs and is followed by alveolar fibrosis.

Oxygen toxicity

The lungs may be damaged by a high concentration of oxygen administered for several days, e.g. in intensive care units, to premature babies in incubators. The mechanisms involved are unknown but effects include:

- progressive decrease in lung compliance
- pulmonary oedema
- fibrosis of lung tissue
- breakdown of capillary walls.

In severe cases pneumonia may develop followed by pulmonary hypertension and right-sided heart failure.

Retinopathy of prematurity. This affects premature babies requiring high-concentration oxygen therapy. The oxygen may stimulate immature retinal blood vessels to constrict causing fibrosis, retinal detachment and blindness (p. 211).

Bronchial carcinoma

Primary bronchial carcinoma is a common form of malignancy. The tumour usually develops in a main bronchus, forming a large friable mass that projects into the lumen sometimes causing obstruction. Mucus then collects and predisposes to development of infection. As the tumour grows it may erode a blood vessel, causing haemoptysis.

The cause is not known but there is a strong positive association with cigarette smoking and the inhalation of other people's smoke (passive smoking).

Spread of bronchial cancer

This does not follow any particular pattern or sequence. The modes of spread are infiltration of local tissues and the transport of tumour fragments in blood and lymph. If blood or lymph vessels are eroded, fragments may spread while the tumour is quite small. A metastatic tumour may, therefore, cause symptoms before the primary in the lung has been detected.

Local spread. This may be within the lung, to the other lung or to mediastinal structures, e.g. blood vessels, nerves, oesophagus.

Lymphatic spread. Tumour fragments spread along lymph vessels to successive lymph nodes in which they may cause metastatic tumours. Fragments may enter lymph draining from a tumour or gain access to a larger vessel when its walls have been eroded by a growing tumour. Early symptoms may be due to pressure caused by enlarged lymph nodes in the thorax.

Blood spread. Tumour cells usually enter the blood when a blood vessel is eroded by local spread of the tumour. The most common sites of bloodborne metastases are the liver, brain, adrenal glands, bones and kidneys.

Lung collapse (Fig. 10.28)

The clinical effects of collapse of all or part of a lung depend on how much of the lung is affected. Fairly large sections of a single lung can be out of action without obvious symptoms. The term *atelectasis* is often used to described lung collapse. There are four main causes of this condition:

- obstruction of an airway (absorption collapse)
- impaired surfactant function
- pressure collapse
- alveolar hypoventilation.

Obstruction of an airway (absorption collapse)

The amount of lung affected depends on the size of the obstructed air passage. Distal to the obstruction air is trapped and absorbed, the lung collapses and secretions

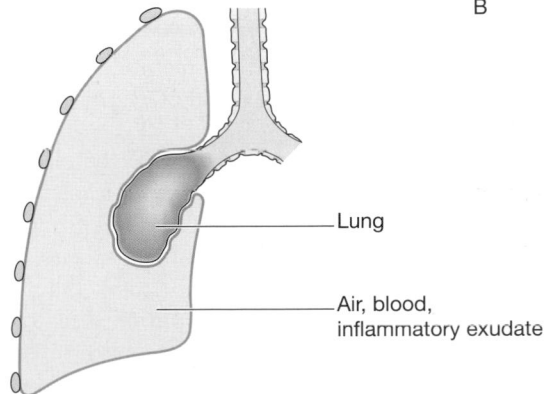

Figure 10.28 Collapse of a lung: A. Absorption collapse. B. Pressure collapse.

267

collect. These may become infected, causing abscess formation. Short-term obstruction is usually followed by reinflation of the lung without lasting ill-effects. Prolonged obstruction leads to progressive fibrosis and permanent collapse. Sudden obstruction may be due to inhalation of a foreign body or a mucus plug formed during an asthmatic attack or in chronic bronchitis. Gradual obstruction may be due to a bronchial tumour or pressure on a bronchus by, e.g., enlarged mediastinal lymph nodes, aortic aneurysm.

Impaired surfactant function

Premature babies, born before the 34th week, are unable to expand their lungs by their own respiratory effort because their lungs are too immature to produce surfactant (p. 249). Surfactant coats the inner surface of each alveolus and reduces surface tension, allowing alveolar expansion during inspiration. These babies need to be mechanically ventilated until their lungs begin to produce surfactant. This problem is called *respiratory disease of the newborn* (RDN).

In the condition called *adult respiratory distress syndrome* (ARDS), dilution of surfactant by fluid collecting in the alveoli (pulmonary oedema) causes surfactant efficiency to be reduced and atelectasis follows. These patients are often gravely ill already, and collapse of substantial areas of lung contributes to the mortality rate of around 50%.

Pressure collapse

When air or fluid enters the pleural cavity the negative pressure becomes positive, preventing lung expansion. The collapse usually affects only one lung and may be partial or complete. There is no obstruction of the airway.

Pneumothorax

In this condition there is air in the pleural cavity. It may occur spontaneously or be the result of trauma.

Spontaneous pneumothorax. This may be either primary or secondary. *Primary spontaneous pneumothorax* is of unknown cause and occurs in fit and healthy people, usually males between 20 and 40 years. *Secondary spontaneous pneumothorax* occurs when air enters the pleural cavity after the visceral pleura ruptures due to lung disease, e.g. emphysema, asthma, pulmonary tuberculosis, bronchial cancer.

Traumatic pneumothorax. This is due to a penetrating injury, e.g. compound fracture of rib, stab or gunshot wound, surgery.

Tension pneumothorax. This occurs as a complication when a flap or one-way valve develops between the lungs and the pleural cavity. Air enters the pleural cavity during inspiration but cannot escape on expiration and steadily accumulates. This causes shift of the mediastinum and compression of the other lung resulting in severe respiratory distress and is often fatal.

Haemothorax

This is blood in the pleural cavity. It may be caused by:

- penetrating chest injury involving blood vessels
- ruptured aortic aneurysm
- erosion of a blood vessel by a malignant tumour.

Pleural effusion

This is excess fluid in the pleural cavity and may be caused by:

- increased hydrostatic pressure, e.g. heart failure, increased blood volume
- increased capillary permeability due to local inflammation, e.g. pneumonia, pulmonary tuberculosis, bronchial cancer, mesothelioma
- decreased plasma osmotic pressure, e.g. nephrotic syndrome (p. 352), cirrhosis of the liver (p. 335)
- impaired lymphatic drainage, e.g. malignant tumour involving the pleura.

Fibrous adhesions which limit reinflation may form between the layers of pleura, following haemothorax and pleural effusion.

Alveolar hypoventilation

In the normal individual breathing quietly at rest there will always be some atelectatic lobules within the lungs due to the low tidal volume. These lobules will re-expand without difficulty at the next deep inspiration. Another common cause of hypoventilation atelectasis occurs postoperatively, particularly after chest and upper abdominal surgery, when pain restricts thoracic expansion. Postoperative atelectasis predisposes to chest infections, because mucus collects in the underventilated airways and is not expectorated.

Introduction to nutrition

Before discussing the digestive system it is necessary to have an understanding of the nutritional needs of the body, i.e. the dietary constituents and their functions within the body.

A *nutrient* is any substance that is digested, absorbed and utilised to promote body function. These substances are:

- carbohydrates
- proteins
- fats
- vitamins
- mineral salts
- water.

Many foods contain a number of nutrients, e.g. potatoes and bread are mainly carbohydrate but both contain protein and some vitamins. Foods are described as carbohydrate or protein because they contain a higher proportion of one or the other. *Fibre* consists of indigestible material. It is not a nutrient, as it is not digested, absorbed or utilised, but it has many beneficial effects on the digestive tract.

The *diet* is the selection of foods eaten by an individual. A *balanced diet* is essential for health. It provides the appropriate amounts of all nutrients in the correct proportions to meet the requirements of the body cells. An *essential nutrient* is a substance that cannot be made by the body and must therefore be included in the diet.

270

THE BALANCED DIET

Learning outcome

After studying this section, you should be able to:

- list the constituent food groups of a balanced diet.

A balanced diet contains all nutrients required for health in appropriate proportions, and is normally achieved by eating a variety of foods. If any nutrient is eaten in excess, or is deficient, health may be adversely affected. For example, a calorie-rich diet can lead to obesity, and an iron-deficient one to anaemia. Ensuring a balanced diet requires a certain amount of knowledge and planning. Recommendations for daily food intake sort foods of similar origins and nutritive values into food groups, and advise that a certain number of servings from each group be eaten daily (Fig. 11.1). If this plan is followed, the resulting dietary intake is likely to be well balanced.

The five main food groups are:

- bread, rice, cereal and pasta
- fruit and vegetables
- meat and fish
- dairy products, e.g. milk and cheese
- fats, oils and sweets.

Bread, rice, cereal and pasta

Most (50–60%) of the daily calorie requirements should come from these sources. In practice this means eating 6–11 servings from this food group every day. These foods contain large amounts of complex carbohydrates, which provide sustained energy release, as well as fibre.

one serving = one slice of bread, one small bread roll, two large crackers, 1 oz cereal

Fruit and vegetables

It is recommended that at least five portions should be eaten daily. Fruit and vegetables are high in vitamins, minerals and fibre, and (provided they have not been, for example, fried) are low in fat.

one serving = a medium apple, orange or banana; 100 g cooked/raw vegetables or tinned/fresh/cooked fruit; one wedge of melon; 125 ml fruit or vegetable juice

Meat, fish and alternatives

Current dietary habits in developed countries mean that too much of the daily calorific requirements are met from this group of foods (which includes eggs and nuts) and from high-fat foods. Although these foods are high in protein, and some vitamins and minerals, only 2–3 servings daily are recommended because they have a high fat content.

one serving = one egg, 30 g peanut butter, 80 g lean cooked meat

Dairy products

This group includes milk, cheese and yoghurt, and is high in calcium and vitamins. 2–3 servings per day are recommended. Dairy foods are often high in fat.

1 serving = 250 ml milk or yoghurt; 50 g cheese

Fats, oils and sweets

These foods provide high numbers of calories with little other nutritional value and should be used sparingly, if at all.

Certain groups of individuals may require a diet different from the principles outlined above. For example, pregnant and lactating women have higher energy

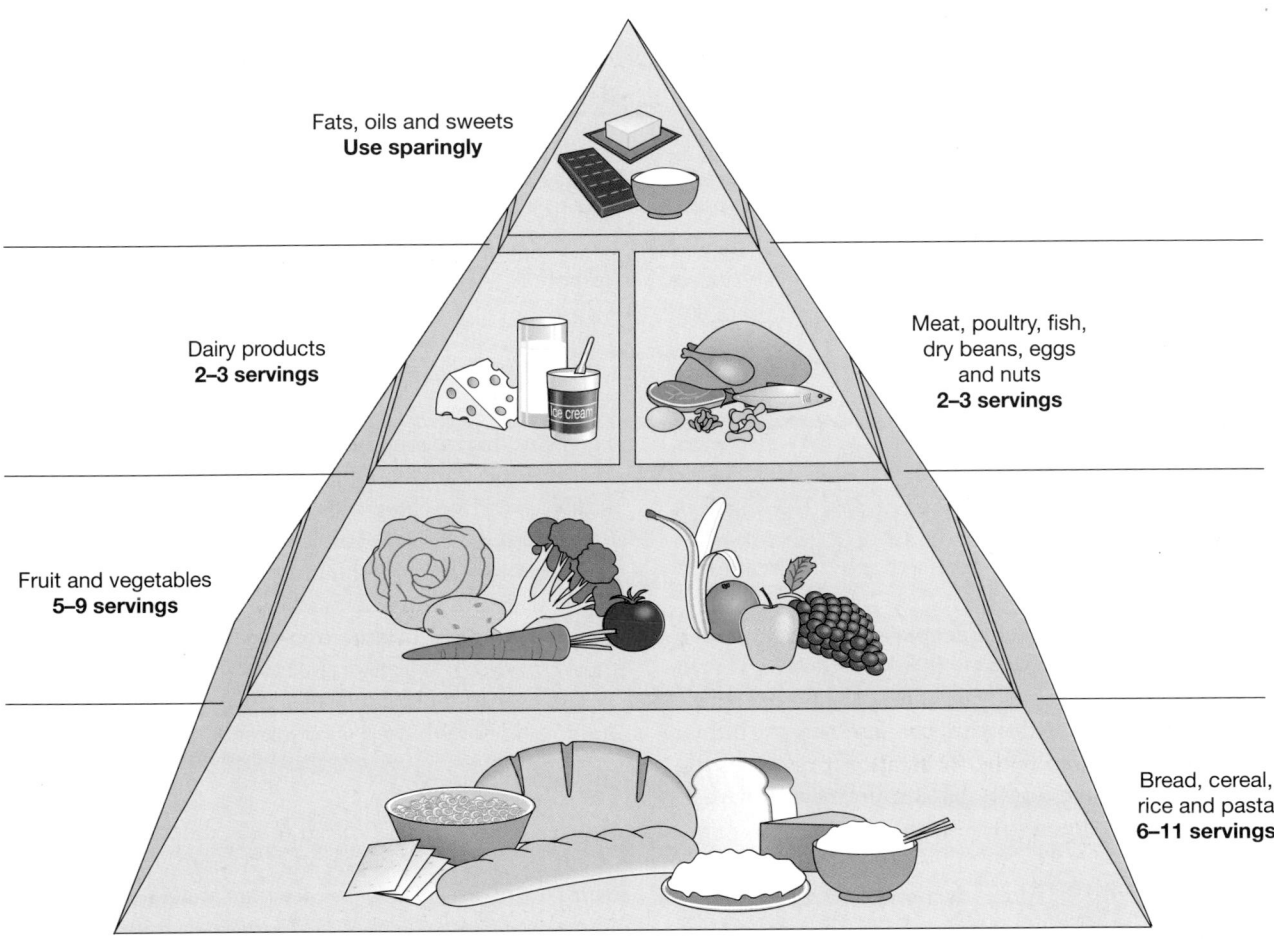

Figure 11.1 The main food groups and their recommended proportions within a balanced diet.

requirements to support the growing baby and milk production. Menstruating women need higher iron levels in their diet than non-menstruating women to compensate for blood loss during menstruation. Babies and growing children have higher fat requirements than adults because they have higher growth and metabolic rates. In some gastrointestinal disorders there is intolerance of certain foods which restricts that person's dietary choices, e.g. coeliac disease (p. 332).

Details of digestion, absorption and utilisation of nutrients are presented in Chapter 12. Structures and chemistry of carbohydrates, proteins and fats are described in Chapter 2.

CARBOHYDRATES

Learning outcomes

After studying this section, you should be able to:

- describe the main mono-, di- and polysaccharides
- list the nutritional function of digestible carbohydrates.

These are found in a wide variety of foods, e.g. sugar, jam, cereals, bread, biscuits, pasta, convenience foods, fruit and vegetables. They consist of carbon, hydrogen and oxygen, the hydrogen and oxygen being in the same proportion as in water. Carbohydrates are classified according to the complexity of the chemical substances of which they are formed.

Monosaccharides

Carbohydrates are digested in the alimentary canal and when absorbed they are in the form of monosaccharides. Examples include glucose (see Fig. 2.7, p. 23), fructose and galactose. These are, chemically, the simplest form in which a carbohydrate can exist. They are made up of single units or molecules which, if they were broken down further, would cease to be sugars.

Disaccharides

These consist of two monosaccharide molecules chemically combined to form sugars, e.g. sucrose (see Fig. 2.7), maltose and lactose.

Polysaccharides

These consist of complex molecules made up of large numbers of monosaccharide molecules in chemical combination, e.g. starches, glycogen, cellulose and dextrins.

Not all polysaccharides can be digested by human beings; e.g. cellulose and other substances present in vegetables, fruit and some cereals pass through the alimentary canal almost unchanged.

Functions of digestible carbohydrates

These include:

- provision of rapidly available energy and heat
- 'protein sparing'; i.e., when there is an adequate supply of carbohydrate in the diet, protein does not need to be used to provide energy and heat
- provision of a store of energy when carbohydrate is eaten in excess of the body's needs as it is converted to fat and deposited in the fat depots, e.g. under the skin.

PROTEINS OR NITROGENOUS FOODS

Learning outcomes

After studying this section, you should be able to:

- describe the structure of amino acids, including essential and non-essential amino acids
- list the nutritional functions of dietary proteins.

Proteins are broken down into their constituent amino acids by digestion and it is in this form that they are absorbed through the intestinal wall. Dietary protein is the main source of nitrogen that can be used in the body. If it is absent from the diet the body goes into *negative nitrogen balance*. This is because amino acids are constantly being used to form enzymes, hormones and cell proteins and the turnover of cells is accompanied by the formation of nitrogenous waste materials that are excreted by the kidneys.

Amino acids (see Fig. 2.8)

These are composed of the elements carbon, hydrogen, oxygen and nitrogen. Some contain minerals such as iron, copper, zinc, iodine, sulphur and phosphate. They are divided into two categories, *essential* and *non-essential*.

Essential amino acids cannot be synthesised in the body, therefore they must be included in the diet. *Non-essential amino acids* are those which can be synthesised in the body. The essential and non-essential amino acids are shown in Box 11.1.

The nutritional value of a protein depends on the amino acids of which it is composed.

Complete proteins

This term is given to protein foods which contain all the essential amino acids in the proportions required to maintain health. They are derived almost entirely from animal sources and include meat, fish, milk, eggs, soya beans and milk products (excluding butter).

Box 11.1 Essential and non-essential amino acids

Essential amino acids	Non-essential amino acids
Isoleucine	Alanine
Leucine	Arginine
Lysine	Asparagine
Methionine	Aspartic acid
Phenylalanine	Cysteine
Threonine	Cystine
Tryptophan	Glutamic acid
Valine	Glutamine
Histidine	Glycine
	Hydroxyproline
	Proline
	Serine
	Tyrosine

Protein quality

The nutritional value of a protein (its *quality*) is measured by how well it meets the nutritional needs of the body. High-quality protein is usually of animal origin, easily digested and contains all essential amino acids in the proportions required by the body. One way of measuring a protein's quality is to feed it to animals and measure how much is retained in the body for growth and repair; this is called the *biological value* (BV). A balanced diet, containing all the amino acids required, may be achieved by eating a range of foods containing low-quality proteins, provided that deficiencies in amino acid content of any one of the constituent proteins of the diet is supplied by another. A balanced vegetarian diet, which consists primarily of lower-quality protein, e.g. vegetables, cereals and pulses, is based on this principle.

Functions of proteins

Amino acids are used for:

- growth and repair of body cells and tissues
- synthesis of enzymes, plasma proteins, antibodies (immunoglobulins) and some hormones
- provision of energy. Normally a secondary function, this becomes important only when there is not enough carbohydrate in the diet and fat stores are depleted.

When protein is eaten in excess of the body's needs, the nitrogenous part is detached, i.e. it is deaminated, and excreted by the kidneys. The remainder is converted to fat for storage in the fat depots, e.g. in the fat cells of adipose tissue (p. 316).

FATS

Learning outcomes

After studying this section, you should be able to:

- outline the main sources of dietary fat
- list the functions of fats in the body.

Fats (see Fig. 2.9, p. 24) consist of carbon, hydrogen and oxygen, but they differ from carbohydrates in that the hydrogen and oxygen are not in the same proportions as in water. Fats are divided into two groups, *saturated* and *unsaturated*.

Saturated or *animal fat*, containing mainly saturated fatty acids and glycerol, is found in milk, cheese, butter, eggs, meat and oily fish such as herring, cod and halibut. All animal sources of protein contain some saturated fat.

Cholesterol is synthesised in the body and is also obtained in the diet from full fat dairy products, fatty meat and egg yolk.

Unsaturated or *vegetable fat*, containing mainly unsaturated fatty acids and glycerol, is found in some margarine and in most vegetable oils.

Linoleic, linolenic and arachidonic acids are polyunsaturated fatty acids that are essential in the diet because they cannot be synthesised in the body. They are the precursors of prostaglandins, thromboxanes and leukotrienes (p. 226).

Functions of fats

These include:

- provision of a source of chemical energy and heat
- support of certain body organs, e.g. the kidneys, the eyes
- transport and storage of the fat-soluble vitamins: A, D, E, K
- constituent of nerve sheaths and of sebum, the secretion of sebaceous glands in the skin
- formation of cholesterol and steroid hormones
- storage of energy as fat in adipose tissue under the skin and in the mesentery, when eaten in excess of requirements
- insulation—as a subcutaneous layer it reduces heat loss through the skin
- satiety value—when gastric contents (chyme) containing fat enter the duodenum, the emptying time of the stomach is prolonged, postponing the return of hunger.

VITAMINS

Learning outcomes

After studying this section, you should be able to:

- outline the sources and functions of the fat-soluble vitamins: A, D, E and K
- describe the sources and functions of the water-soluble vitamins: the vitamin B complex and C.

273

Vitamins are chemical compounds required in very small quantities which are essential for normal metabolism and health. They are found widely distributed in food and are divided into two main groups:

- fat-soluble vitamins: A, D, E and K
- water-soluble vitamins: B complex, C.

Fat-soluble vitamins

Vitamin A (retinol)

This vitamin is found in such foods as cream, egg yolk, liver, fish oil, milk, cheese and butter. It is absent from vegetable fats and oils but is added to margarine during manufacture. It can be formed in the body from certain carotenes, the main dietary sources of which are green vegetables, fruit and carrots. Vitamin A and carotene are only absorbed from the small intestine satisfactorily if fat absorption is normal. Although some is synthesised in the body the daily dietary requirement is 600 to 700 μg. The main roles of vitamin A in the body are:

- generation of the light-sensitive pigment rhodopsin (visual purple) in the retina of the eye
- cell growth and differentiation; this is especially important in fast-growing cells, such as the epithelial cells covering both internal and external body surfaces
- promotion of immunity and defence against infection
- promotion of growth, e.g. in bones.

The first sign of vitamin A deficiency is night blindness due to defective retinal pigment. Other consequences include xerophthalmia, which is drying and thickening of the conjunctiva and, ultimately, there is ulceration and destruction of the conjunctiva. This is a common cause of blindness in developing countries. Atrophy and keratinisation of other epithelial tissues leads to increased incidence of infections of the ear, and the respiratory, genitourinary and alimentary tracts. Immunity is compromised and bone development may be slow and faulty.

Vitamin D

Vitamin D_3 is found mainly in animal fats such as eggs, butter, cheese, fish liver oils. Humans and other animals can synthesise vitamin D by the action of the ultraviolet rays of the sun on a form of cholesterol in the skin (7-dehydrocholesterol).

Vitamin D regulates calcium and phosphate metabolism by increasing their absorption in the gut and stimulating their retention by the kidneys. It therefore promotes the calcification of bones and teeth.

Deficiency causes *rickets* in children and *osteomalacia* in adults, due to deficient absorption and utilisation of calcium and phosphate. The daily requirement is 10 μg and stores in fat and muscle are such that deficiency may not be apparent for several years.

Vitamin E

This is a group of eight substances called *tocopherols*. They are found in nuts, egg yolk, wheat germ, whole cereal, milk and butter.

Vitamin E is an antioxidant, which means that it protects body constituents such as membrane lipids from being destroyed in oxidative reactions. Deficiency is rare, because of the widespread occurrence of this vitamin in foods, and is usually seen only in premature babies and in conditions associated with impaired fat absorption, e.g. cystic fibrosis. Haemolytic anaemia occurs, as abnormal red blood cell membranes rupture. White blood cells can likewise be affected, and vitamin E supplements boost immune function. Neurological abnormalities such as ataxia and visual disturbances may occur if the deficiency is severe. Recently, vitamin E has been shown to protect against coronary artery disease. Recommended daily intake is 10 mg for men and 8 mg for women, but this should be increased in high-fat diets.

Vitamin K

The sources of vitamin K are fish, liver, leafy green vegetables and fruit. It is synthesised in the large intestine by microbes and significant amounts are absorbed. Absorption is dependent upon the presence of bile salts in the small intestine. The normal daily requirement is 1 μg/kg body weight and only a small amount is stored in the liver and spleen.

Vitamin K is required by the liver for the production of prothrombin and factors VII, IX and X, all essential for the clotting of blood (p. 67). Deficiency therefore prevents normal blood coagulation. It may occur in adults when there is obstruction to the flow of bile, severe liver damage and in malabsorption conditions, such as *coeliac disease*. Newborn infants may be given vitamin K because their intestines are sterile and require several weeks to become colonised with vitamin K-producing bacteria.

Water-soluble vitamins

Vitamin B complex

This is a group of water-soluble vitamins that promote activity of enzymes at various stages in the chemical breakdown (catabolism) of nutrients to release energy.

Vitamin B_1 (thiamine). This vitamin is present in nuts, yeast, egg yolk, liver, legumes, meat and the germ of cereals. It is rapidly destroyed by heat. The daily requirement is 0.8 to 1 mg and the body stores only about 30 mg. Thiamine is essential for the complete aerobic release of energy from carbohydrate. When it is absent there is accumulation of lactic and pyruvic acids, which may lead to accumulation of tissue fluid (oedema) and heart failure. Thiamine is also important for nervous system function because of the dependency of these tissues on glucose for fuel.

Deficiency causes *beriberi* which occurs mainly in countries where polished rice is the chief constituent of the diet. In beriberi there is:

- severe muscle wasting
- stunted growth in children
- polyneuritis, causing degeneration of motor, sensory and some autonomic nerves
- susceptibility to infections.

If untreated, death occurs due to cardiac failure or severe microbial infection.

The main cause of thiamine deficiency in developed countries is chronic alcohol abuse, where the diet is usually poor. Neurological symptoms include memory loss, ataxia and visual disturbances; sometimes these are reversed with oral thiamine supplements.

Vitamin B$_2$ (riboflavine). Riboflavine is found in yeast, green vegetables, milk, liver, eggs, cheese and fish roe. The daily requirement is 1.1 to 1.3 mg and only small amounts are stored in the body. It is concerned with carbohydrate and protein metabolism, especially in the eyes and skin. Deficiency leads to:

- blurred vision, cataract formation and corneal ulceration
- cracking of the skin, commonly around the mouth (angular stomatitis)
- lesions of intestinal mucosa.

Folic acid. This is found in liver, kidney, fresh leafy green vegetables and yeast. It is synthesised by bacteria in the large intestine, and significant amounts derived from this source are believed to be absorbed. The daily requirement is 200 µg, and, as only a small amount is stored in the body, deficiency is evident within a short time. It is essential for DNA synthesis, and when lacking mitosis (cell division) is impaired. This manifests particularly in rapidly dividing tissues such as blood, and folate deficiency therefore leads to a type of megaloblastic anaemia (p. 70), which is reversible with folate supplements. Deficiency at conception and during early pregnancy is linked to an increased incidence of spina bifida (p. 189).

Niacin (nicotinic acid). This is found in liver, cheese, yeast, whole cereals, eggs, fish and nuts; in addition, the body can synthesise it from the amino acid tryptophan. It is associated with energy-releasing reactions in cells. In fat metabolism it inhibits the production of cholesterol and assists in fat breakdown. Deficiency occurs mainly in areas where maize is the chief constituent of the diet because niacin in maize is in an unusable form. The daily requirement is 12 to 17 mg.

Pellagra develops within 6 to 8 weeks of severe deficiency. It is characterised by:

- redness of the skin in parts exposed to light, especially in the neck
- anorexia, nausea, dysphagia and inflammation of the lining of the mouth
- delirium, mental disturbance and dementia.

Vitamin B$_6$ (pyridoxine). This is found in egg yolk, peas, beans, soya beans, yeast, meat and liver. The daily requirement is about 1.2 to 1.4 mg and dietary deficiency is rare, although certain drugs, e.g. alcohol and antituberculous drugs, antagonise the vitamin and can induce deficiency states. It is associated with amino acid metabolism, including the synthesis of non-essential amino acids and molecules such as haem and nucleic acids.

Vitamin B$_{12}$ (cyanocobalamin). Vitamin B$_{12}$ consists of a number of *cobalamin compounds* (containing cobalt). It is found in liver, meat, eggs, milk and fermented liquors. The normal daily requirement is 1.5 µg.

Like folic acid, vitamin B$_{12}$ is essential for DNA synthesis, and deficiency also leads to a megaloblastic anaemia, which is correctable with supplements. However, vitamin B$_{12}$ is also required for formation and maintenance of myelin, the fatty substance that surrounds and protects some nerves. Deficiency accordingly causes peripheral neuropathy and/or spinal cord degeneration. Such neurological changes are irreversible. The presence of intrinsic factor in the stomach is essential for vitamin B$_{12}$ absorption and deficiency is usually associated with insufficient intrinsic factor (p. 70).

Pantothenic acid. This is found in many foods and is associated with amino acid metabolism. The daily safe intake is 3 to 7 mg and no deficiency diseases have been identified.

Biotin. This is found in yeast, egg yolk, liver, kidney and tomatoes and is synthesised by microbes in the intestine. It is associated with the metabolism of carbohydrates. The daily safe intake is 10 to 200 µg. Deficiency is rare.

Vitamin C (ascorbic acid)

This is found in fresh fruit, especially blackcurrants, oranges, grapefruit and lemons, and also in rosehips and green vegetables. The vitamin is very soluble in water and is easily destroyed by heat, so cooking may be a factor in the development of *scurvy*.

The daily requirement is 40 mg and after 2 to 3 months, deficient intake becomes apparent.

Vitamin C is associated with protein metabolism, especially the laying down of collagen fibres in connective tissue.

Vitamin C, like vitamin E, acts as an antioxidant, protecting body molecules from damaging oxidative reactions. When deficiency occurs, collagen production is affected, leading to fragility of blood vessels, delayed wound healing and poor bone repair. Gums become swollen and spongy and the teeth loosen in their sockets.

Summary of the vitamins

Tables 11.1 and 11.2 summarise the vitamins: their chemical names, sources, stability, functions, deficiency diseases and daily adult requirements.

MINERAL SALTS

Learning outcomes

After studying this section, you should be able to:

- list the commonest mineral salts required by the body
- describe their functions.

Mineral salts (inorganic compounds) are necessary within the body for all body processes, usually in only small quantities.

Calcium

This is found in milk, cheese, eggs, green vegetables and some fish. An adequate supply should be obtained in a normal, well-balanced diet, although requirements are higher in pregnant women and growing children. 99% of body calcium is found in the bones, where it is an essential

Table 11.1 Summary – fat-soluble vitamins (DoH 1991)

Vitamin	Chemical name	Source	Stability	Functions	Effects of deficiency	Daily recommended intake (adults)
A	Retinol (carotene provitamin in plants)	Milk, butter, cheese, egg yolk, fish, liver oils, green and yellow vegetables	Some loss at high temperatures and long exposure to light and air	Maintains healthy epithelial tissues and cornea. Formation of rhodopsin (visual purple)	Keratinisation Xerophthalmia Stunted growth Night blindness	600–700 µg
D	Calciferol	Fish, liver, oils, milk, cheese, egg yolk, irradiated 7-dehydrocholesterol in human skin	Very stable	Facilitates the absorption and use of calcium and phosphate in the maintenance of healthy bones and teeth	Rickets (children) Osteomalacia (adults)	10 µg
E	Tocopherols	Egg yolk, milk, butter, green vegetables, nuts	Stable in heat but oxidised by exposure to air	Antioxidant Promotes immune function	Anaemia Ataxia Visual disturbances	3–4 mg*
K	Phylloquinone	Leafy vegetables, fish, liver, fruit	Destroyed by light, strong acids and alkalis	Formation of prothrombin and factors VII, IX and X in the liver	Slow blood clotting Haemorrhages in the newborn	60–70 µg*

Bile is necessary for the absorption of these vitamins. Mineral oils interfere with absorption.
*Daily safe intake (DoH 1991). Data for recommended intake not available.

Table 11.2 Summary – water-soluble vitamins (DoH 1991)

Vitamin	Chemical name	Source	Stability	Functions	Effects of deficiency	Daily recommended intake (adults)
B_1	Thiamine	Yeast, liver, germ of cereals, nuts, pulses, rice polishings, egg yolk, liver, legumes	Destroyed by heat	Metabolism of carbohydrates and nutrition of nerve cells	General fatigue and loss of muscle tone Ultimately leads to beriberi Stunted growth	0.8–1 mg
B_2	Riboflavine	Liver, yeast, milk, eggs, green vegetables, kidney, fish roe	Destroyed by light and alkalis	Carbohydrate and protein metabolism Healthy skin and eyes	Angular stomatitis Dermatitis Eye lesions	1–1.3 mg
B_6	Pyridoxine	Meat, liver, vegetables, bran of cereals, egg yolk, beans	Stable	Protein metabolism	Very rare	1.2–1.4 mg
B_{12}	Cobalamins	Liver, milk, moulds, fermenting liquors, egg	Destroyed by heat	DNA synthesis	Megaloblastic anaemia Degeneration of nerve fibres of the spinal cord	1.5 µg
B	Folic acid	Dark green vegetables, liver, kidney, eggs Synthesised in colon	Destroyed by heat and moisture	DNA synthesis Normal development of spinal cord in early pregnancy	Anaemia Increased incidence of spina bifida	200 µg
B	Niacin (nicotinic acid)	Yeast, offal, fish, pulses, wholemeal cereals Synthesised in the body from tryptophan	Fairly stable	Necessary for cell respiration Inhibits production of cholesterol	Prolonged deficiency causes pellagra, i.e. dermatitis, diarrhoea, dementia	12–17 mg
B	Pantothenic acid	Liver, yeast, egg yolk, fresh vegetables	Destroyed by excessive heat and freezing	Associated with amino acid metabolism	Unknown	3–7 mg*
B	Biotin	Yeasts, liver, kidney, pulses, nuts	Stable	Carbohydrates and fat metabolism	Dermatitis, conjunctivitis Hypercholesterolaemia	10–200 µg*
C	Ascorbic acid	Citrus fruits, currants, berries, green vegetables, potatoes, liver and glandular tissue in animals	Destroyed by heat, ageing, acids, alkalis, chopping, salting, drying	Formation of collagen Maturation of RBCs Antioxidant	Multiple haemorrhages Slow wound healing Anaemia Gross deficiency causes scurvy	40 mg

*Daily safe intake (DoH 1991). Data for recommended intake not available.

structural component. Calcium is also involved in the coagulation of blood and the mechanism of muscle contraction.

Phosphate

Sources of phosphate include cheese, oatmeal, liver and kidney. If there is sufficient calcium in the diet it is unlikely that there will be a phosphate deficiency.

It is associated with calcium and vitamin D in the hardening of bones and teeth; 85% of body phosphate is found in these sites. Phosphates are an essential part of systems of energy storage inside cells as adenosine triphosphate (ATP, Fig. 2.12, p. 25).

Sodium

Sodium is found in most foods, especially fish, meat, eggs, milk, artificially enriched bread and as cooking and table salt. The normal intake of sodium chloride per day varies from 5 to 20 g and the daily requirement is 1.6 g. Excess is excreted in the urine.

It is the most commonly occurring *extracellular cation* and is associated with:

- contraction of muscles
- transmission of nerve impulses along axons
- maintenance of the electrolyte balance in the body.

Potassium

This substance is to be found widely distributed in all foods, especially fruit and vegetables. The normal intake of potassium chloride is 3.5 g per day and this is in excess of potassium requirements.

It is the most commonly occurring *intracellular cation* and is involved in many chemical activities inside cells including:

- contraction of muscles
- transmission of nerve impulses
- maintenance of the electrolyte balance in the body.

Iron

Iron, as a soluble compound, is found in liver, kidney, beef, egg yolk, wholemeal bread and green vegetables. In normal adults about 1 mg of iron is lost from the body daily. The normal daily diet contains more, i.e. 9 to 15 mg, but only 5–15% of intake is absorbed. Iron is essential for the formation of *haemoglobin* in the red blood cells. It is also necessary for oxidation of carbohydrate and in the synthesis of some hormones and neurotransmitters.

Iron deficiency is a relatively common condition, and causes anaemia if iron stores become sufficiently depleted. Menstruating and pregnant women have increased iron requirements, as do young people experiencing growth spurts. Iron deficiency anaemia may also occur in chronic bleeding, e.g. peptic ulcer disease.

Iodine

Iodine is found in salt-water fish and in vegetables grown in soil containing iodine. In some parts of the world where iodine is deficient in soil very small quantities are added to table salt. The daily requirement of iodine depends upon the individual's metabolic rate. Some people have a higher normal metabolic rate than others and their iodine requirements are greater. The daily requirement is 140 µg.

It is essential for the formation of *thyroxine* and *tri-iodothyronine*, two hormones secreted by the thyroid gland (p. 220).

FIBRE

> **Learning outcome**
>
> After studying this section, you should be able to:
>
> - describe the sources and functions of dietary fibre.

Fibre is the indigestible part of the diet that comes from plants and meat. It consists of bran, cellulose and other polysaccharides. It is widely distributed in wholemeal flour, the husks of cereals and in vegetables. Dietary fibre is partly digested by microbes in the large intestine with gas (flatus) formation. The daily requirement of fibre is not less than 20 g.

Functions of dietary fibre

Fibre:

- provides bulk to the diet and helps to satisfy the appetite
- stimulates peristalsis (muscular activity) of the alimentary tract
- attracts water, increasing bulk and softness of faeces
- increases frequency of defecation preventing constipation
- prevents some gastrointestinal disorders, e.g. diverticular disease (p. 328).

WATER (see Fig. 2.4, p. 20)

Learning outcomes

After studying this section, you should be able to:

- explain the distribution of water within the body
- describe the functions of water within the body.

Water makes up about 70% of the body weight in men and about 60% in women.

A man weighing 65 kg contains about 40 litres of water, 28 of which are intracellular and 12 extracellular. Extracellular water consists of 2 to 3 litres in plasma and the remainder, interstitial fluid (see Fig. 2.16, p. 28).

A large amount of water is lost each day in faeces, sweat and urine. Under normal circumstances this is balanced by intake in food and to satisfy thirst. Dehydration with serious consequences may occur if intake does not balance loss.

Functions of water

These include:

- provision of the moist internal environment which is required by all living cells in the body, i.e. all the cells except the superficial layers of the skin, the nails, the hair and outer hard layer of the teeth
- participation in all the chemical reactions which occur inside and outside the body cells
- dilution and moistening of food (see saliva, p. 292)
- regulation of body temperature — as a constituent of sweat, which is secreted onto the skin, it evaporates, cooling the body surface (p. 365)
- a major constituent of blood and tissue fluid, it transports some substances in solution and some in suspension round the body
- dilution of waste products and poisonous substances in the body
- providing the medium for the excretion of waste products, e.g. urine and faeces.

DISORDERS OF NUTRITION

Learning outcome

After studying this section, you should be able to:

■ describe the main consequences of malnutrition, malabsorption and obesity.

The importance of nutrition is increasingly recognised as essential for health, and illness often alters nutritional requirements.

Malnutrition

This may be due to:

■ protein–energy malnutrition (PEM)
■ vitamin deficiencies (Tables 11.1 and 11.2)
■ both PEM and vitamin deficiencies.

Protein–energy malnutrition (Fig. 11.2)

This is the result of inadequate intake of protein, carbohydrate and fat. Infants and young children are especially susceptible as they need sufficient nutrients to grow and develop normally. If dietary intake is inadequate, it is not uncommon for vitamin deficiency to develop at the same time. Poor nutrition, or malnutrition, reduces the ability to combat other illness and infection.

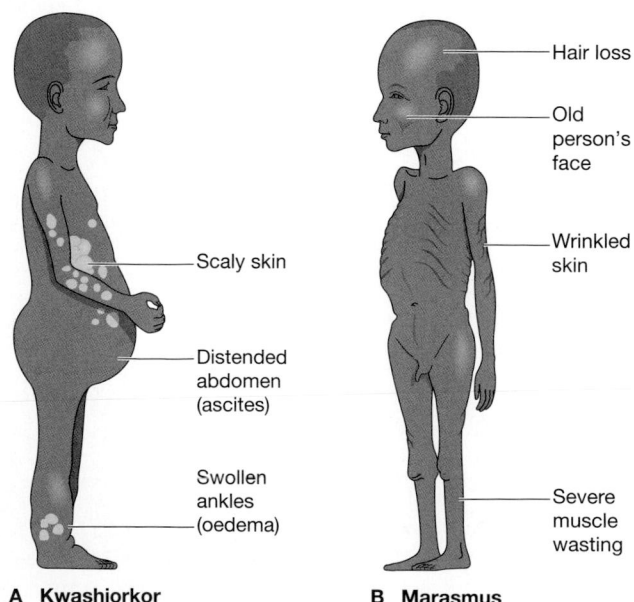

A **Kwashiorkor**   B **Marasmus**

Figure 11.2 Features of protein–energy malnutrition.

Kwashiorkor

This is mainly caused by protein deficiency, and occurs in infants and children in some developing countries and when there has been serious drought and crop failure. Reduced plasma proteins lead to ascites and oedema (p. 118) in the lower limbs that masks emaciation. There is severe liver damage. Growth stops and there is loss of weight and loss of pigmentation of skin and hair accompanied by listlessness, apathy and irritability.

Marasmus

This is caused by deficiency of both protein and carbohydrate. It is characterised by severe emaciation due to breakdown (catabolism) of muscle and fat. Growth is retarded, the skin becomes wrinkled and hair is lost.

Malabsorption

The causes of malabsorption vary widely, from short-term problems such as gastrointestinal infections to chronic conditions such as cystic fibrosis. Malabsorption may be specific for one nutrient, e.g. vitamin B_{12} in pernicious anaemia (p. 70), or it may apply across a spectrum of nutrients, e.g. in tropical sprue (p. 332).

Obesity

This is a very common nutritional disorder in which there is accumulation of excess body fat. Clinically, obesity is present when body weight is 120% of that recommended for the height, age and sex of the individual. It occurs when energy intake exceeds energy expenditure, e.g. in inactive individuals eating more calories than they need for daily energy requirements.

Obesity predisposes to:

■ gallstones (p. 336)
■ cardiovascular diseases, e.g. ischaemic heart disease (p. 121), hypertension (p. 126)
■ hernias (p. 329)
■ varicose veins (p. 116)
■ osteoarthritis (p. 426)
■ type II (non-insulin-dependent) diabetes mellitus
■ increased incidence of postoperative complications.

Phenylketonuria

(See p. 185.)

12

The digestive system

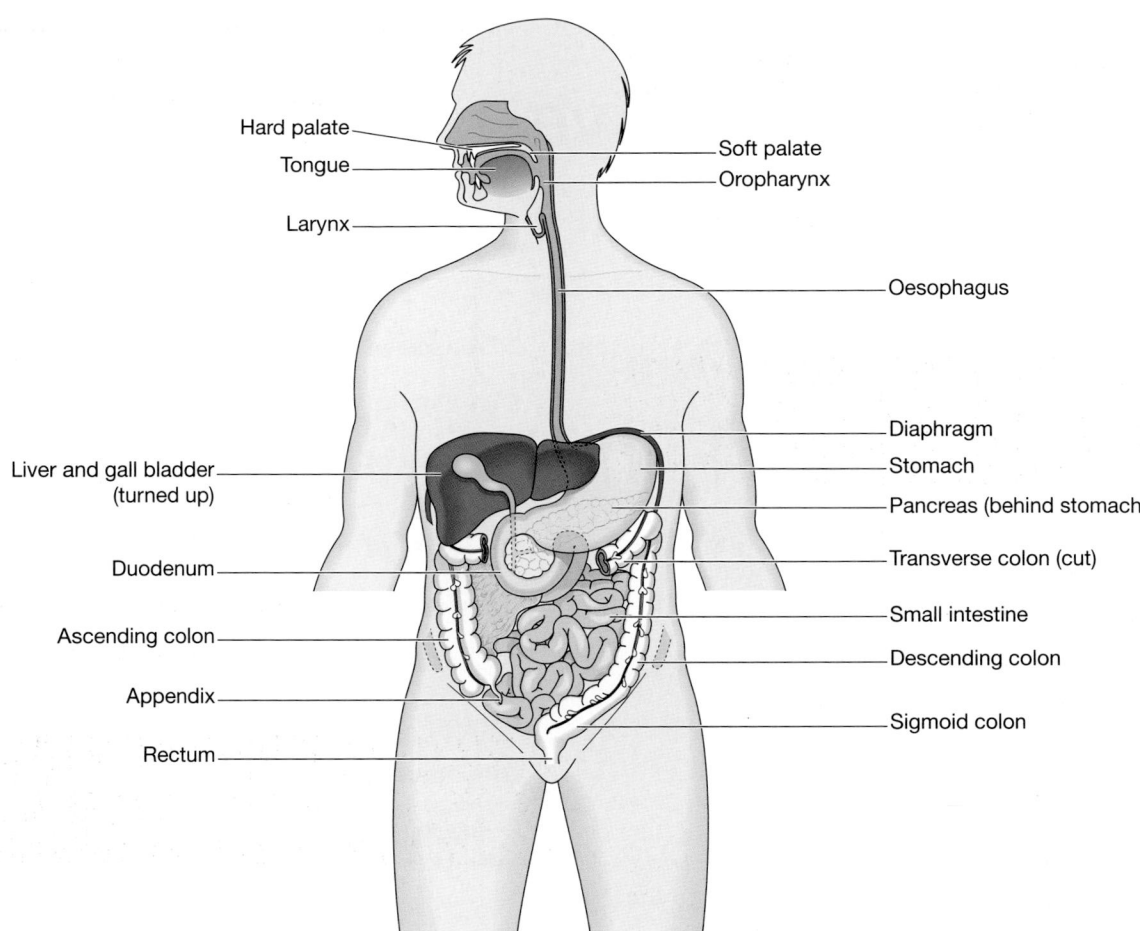

Figure 12.1 The organs of the digestive system.

The digestive system is the collective name used to describe the *alimentary canal*, some *accessory organs* and a variety of *digestive processes* which take place at different levels in the canal to prepare food eaten in the diet for absorption. The alimentary canal begins at the mouth, passes through the thorax, abdomen and pelvis and ends at the anus (Fig. 12.1). It has a general structure which is modified at different levels to provide for the processes occurring at each level (Fig. 12.2). The complex of digestive processes gradually breaks down the foods eaten until they are in a form suitable for absorption. For example, meat, even when cooked, is chemically too complex to be absorbed from the alimentary canal. It therefore goes through a series of changes which release its constituent nutrients: amino acids, mineral salts, fat and vitamins. Chemical substances or *enzymes* (p. 26) which effect these changes are secreted into the canal by specialised glands, some of which are in the walls of the canal and some outside the canal, but with ducts leading into it.

After absorption, nutrients are used to synthesise body constituents. They provide the raw materials for the manufacture of new cells, hormones and enzymes, and the energy needed for these and other processes and for the disposal of waste materials.

The activities in the digestive system can be grouped under five main headings.

Ingestion. This is the process of taking food into the alimentary tract.

Propulsion. This moves the contents along the alimentary tract.

Digestion. This consists of:

- *mechanical breakdown* of food by, e.g. mastication (chewing)
- *chemical digestion* of food by enzymes present in secretions produced by glands and accessory organs of the digestive system.

Absorption. This is the process by which digested food substances pass through the walls of some organs of the alimentary canal into the blood and lymph capillaries for circulation round the body.

Elimination. Food substances which have been eaten but cannot be digested and absorbed are excreted by the bowel as faeces.

ORGANS OF THE DIGESTIVE SYSTEM (Fig. 12.1)

Learning outcomes

After studying this section, you should be able to:

- list the main organs of the alimentary tract
- list the accessory organs of digestion.

Alimentary tract

This is a long tube through which food passes. It commences at the mouth and terminates at the anus, and the various parts are given separate names, although structurally they are remarkably similar. The parts are:

- mouth
- pharynx
- oesophagus
- stomach
- small intestine
- large intestine
- rectum and anal canal.

Accessory organs

Various secretions are poured into the alimentary tract, some by glands in the lining membrane of the organs, e.g. gastric juice secreted by glands in the lining of the stomach, and some by glands situated outside the tract. The latter are the accessory organs of digestion and their secretions pass through ducts to enter the tract. They consist of:

- 3 pairs of salivary glands
- pancreas
- liver and the biliary tract.

The organs and glands are linked physiologically as well as anatomically in that digestion and absorption occur in stages, each stage being dependent upon the previous stage or stages.

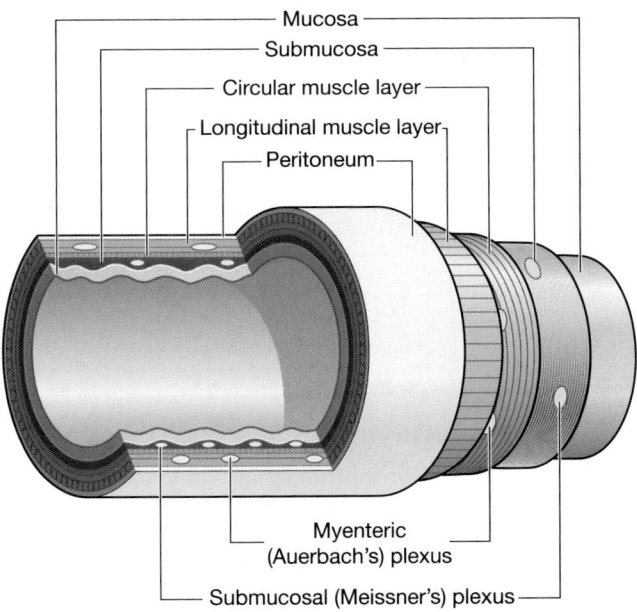

Figure 12.2 General structure of the alimentary canal.

BASIC STRUCTURE OF THE ALIMENTARY CANAL (Fig. 12.2)

Learning outcomes

After studying this section, you should be able to:

- describe the distribution of the peritoneum
- explain the function of smooth muscle in the walls of the alimentary canal
- discuss the structures of the alimentary mucosa
- outline the nerve and blood supply of the alimentary canal.

The layers of the walls of the alimentary canal follow a consistent pattern from the oesophagus onwards. This basic structure does not apply so obviously to the mouth and the pharynx, which are considered later in the chapter.

In the different organs from the oesophagus onwards, modifications of structure are found which are associated with special functions. The basic structure is described here and any modifications in structure and function are described in the appropriate section.

283

A

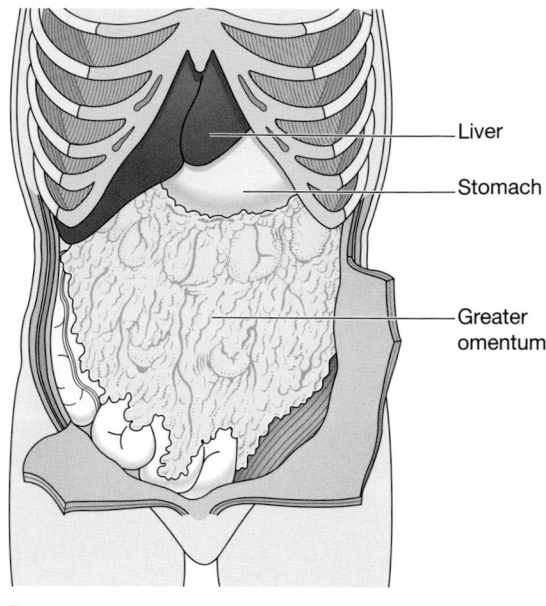

B

Figure 12.3 A. The peritoneal cavity (gold), the abdominal organs of the digestive system and the pelvic organs. B. The greater omentum.

The walls of the alimentary tract are formed by four layers of tissue:

- adventitia or outer covering
- muscle layer
- submucosal layer
- mucosa—lining.

Adventitia (outer covering)

In the thorax this consists of *loose fibrous tissue* and in the abdomen the organs are covered by a serous membrane called *peritoneum*.

Peritoneum

The peritoneum is the largest serous membrane of the body (Fig. 12.3A). It consists of a closed sac, containing a small amount of serous fluid, within the abdominal cavity. It is richly supplied with blood and lymph vessels, and contains a considerable number of lymph nodes. It provides a physical barrier to local spread of infection, and can isolate an infective focus such as appendicitis, preventing involvement of other abdominal structures. It has two layers:

- the *parietal layer*, which lines the abdominal wall
- the *visceral layer*, which covers the organs (viscera) within the abdominal and pelvic cavities.

The arrangement of the peritoneum is such that the organs are invaginated into the closed sac from below, behind and above so that they are at least partly covered by the visceral layer. This means that:

- pelvic organs are covered only on their superior surface
- the stomach and intestines, deeply invaginated from behind, are almost completely surrounded by peritoneum and have a double fold (the *mesentery*) that attaches them to the posterior abdominal wall. The fold of peritoneum enclosing the stomach extends beyond the greater curvature of the stomach, and hangs down in front of the abdominal organs like an apron (Fig. 12.3B). This is the *greater omentum*, and it stores fat, which provides both insulation and a long-term energy store
- the pancreas, spleen, kidneys and adrenal glands are invaginated from behind but only their anterior surfaces are covered and are therefore *retroperitoneal*
- the liver is invaginated from above and is almost completely covered by peritoneum which attaches it to the inferior surface of the diaphragm
- the main blood vessels and nerves pass close to the posterior abdominal wall and send branches to the organs between folds of peritoneum.

The parietal peritoneum lines the anterior abdominal wall.

The two layers of peritoneum are actually in contact and friction between them is prevented by the presence

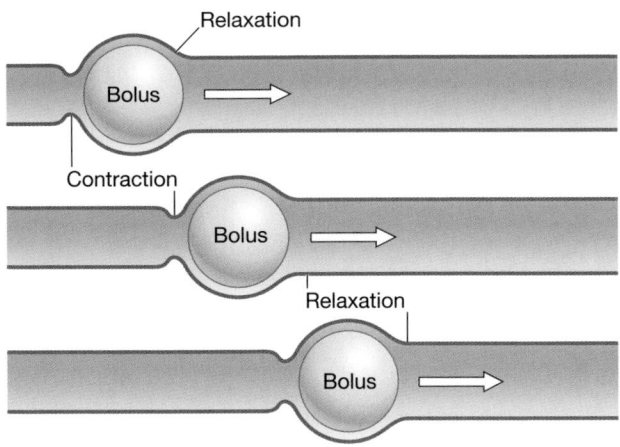

Figure 12.4 Movement of a bolus by peristalsis.

Figure 12.5 Columnar epithelium with goblet cells.

of serous fluid secreted by the peritoneal cells, thus the *peritoneal cavity* is only a *potential cavity*. A similar arrangement is seen with the membranes covering the lungs, the pleura (p. 251). In the male it is completely closed but in the female the uterine tubes open into it and the ovaries are the only structures inside (Ch. 19).

Muscle layer

With some exceptions this consists of two layers of *smooth (involuntary) muscle*. The muscle fibres of the outer layer are arranged longitudinally, and those of the inner layer encircle the wall of the tube. Between these two muscle layers are blood vessels, lymph vessels and a plexus (network) of sympathetic and parasympathetic nerves, called the *myenteric* or *Auerbach's plexus*. These nerves supply the adjacent smooth muscle and blood vessels.

Contraction and relaxation of these muscle layers occurs in waves which push the contents of the tract onwards. This type of contraction of smooth muscle is called *peristalsis* (Fig. 12.4). Muscle contraction also mixes food with the digestive juices. Onward movement of the contents of the tract is controlled at various points by *sphincters* consisting of an increased number of circular muscle fibres. They also act as valves preventing backflow in the tract. The control allows time for digestion and absorption to take place.

Submucosa

This layer consists of loose connective tissue with some elastic fibres. Within this layer are plexuses of blood vessels and nerves, lymph vessels and varying amounts of lymphoid tissues. The blood vessels consist of arterioles, venules and capillaries. The nerve plexus is the *submucosal* or *Meissner's plexus*, consisting of sympathetic and parasympathetic nerves which supply the mucosal lining.

Mucosa

This consists of three layers of tissue:

- *mucous membrane* formed by columnar epithelium is the innermost layer and has three main functions: *protection, secretion* and *absorption*
- *lamina propria* consisting of loose connective tissue, which supports the blood vessels that nourish the inner epithelial layer, and varying amounts of lymphoid tissue that has a protective function
- *muscularis mucosa*, a thin outer layer of smooth muscle that provides involutions of the mucosa layer, e.g. gastric glands, villi.

Mucous membrane

In parts of the tract which are subject to great wear and tear or mechanical injury this layer consists of *stratified squamous epithelium* with mucus-secreting glands just below the surface. In areas where the food is already soft and moist and where secretion of digestive juices and absorption occur, the mucous membrane consists of *columnar epithelial cells* interspersed with mucus-secreting goblet cells (Fig. 12.5). Mucus lubricates the walls of the tract and protects them from digestive enzymes. Below the surface in the regions lined with columnar epithelium are collections of specialised cells, or glands, which pour their secretions into the lumen of the tract. The secretions include:

- *saliva* from the salivary glands
- *gastric juice* from the gastric glands
- *intestinal juice* from the intestinal glands
- *pancreatic juice* from the pancreas
- *bile* from the liver.

285

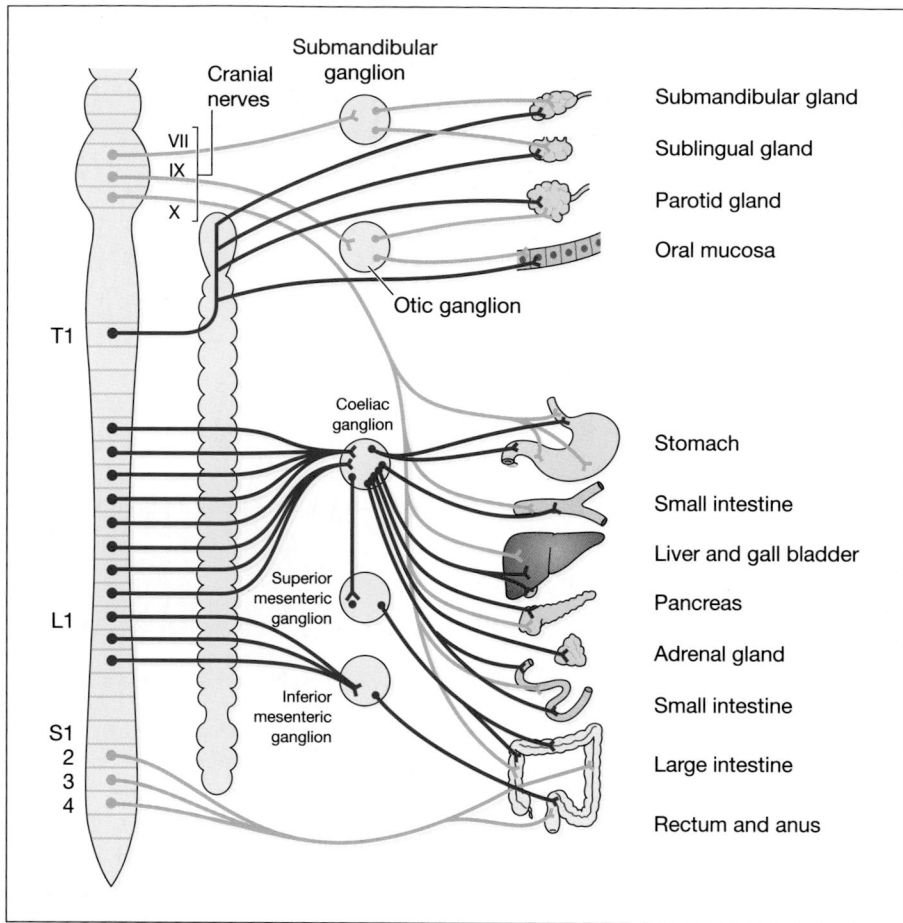

Figure 12.6 Autonomic nerve supply to the digestive system. Parasympathetic – blue; sympathetic – red.

These are *digestive juices* and they contain the enzymes which chemically break down food. Under the epithelial lining are varying amounts of lymphoid tissue.

Nerve supply

The alimentary tract is supplied by nerves from both divisions of the autonomic nervous system, i.e. parasympathetic and sympathetic, and in the main their actions are antagonistic (Fig. 12.6). In the normal healthy state one influence may outweigh the other according to the needs of the body as a whole at a particular time.

The parasympathetic supply. This supply to most of the alimentary tract is provided by one pair of cranial nerves, the *vagus nerves*. Stimulation causes smooth muscle contraction and the secretion of digestive juices. The most distal part of the tract is supplied by sacral nerves.

The sympathetic supply. This is provided by numerous nerves which emerge from the spinal cord in the thoracic

and lumbar regions. These form plexuses in the thorax, abdomen and pelvis, from which nerves pass to the organs of the alimentary tract. Their action is to reduce smooth muscle contraction and glandular secretion.

Within the walls of the canal there are two nerve plexuses from which both sympathetic and parasympathetic fibres are distributed (Fig. 12.2).

The myenteric or Auerbach's plexus lies between the two layers of smooth muscle that it supplies, and influences peristalsis.

The submucosal or Meissner's plexus lies in the submucosa and supplies the mucous membrane and secretory glands.

Blood supply

Arterial blood supply

In the thorax. The oesophagus is supplied by paired *oesophageal arteries*, branches from the thoracic aorta.

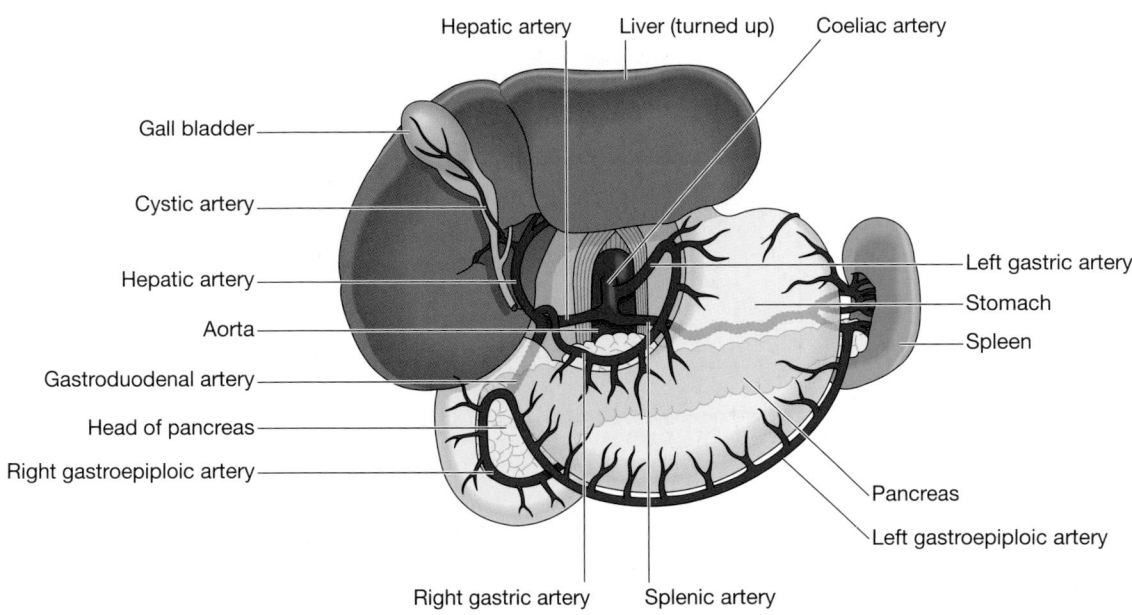

Figure 12.7 Branches of the coeliac artery and the organs they supply. The pancreas is shown behind the stomach.

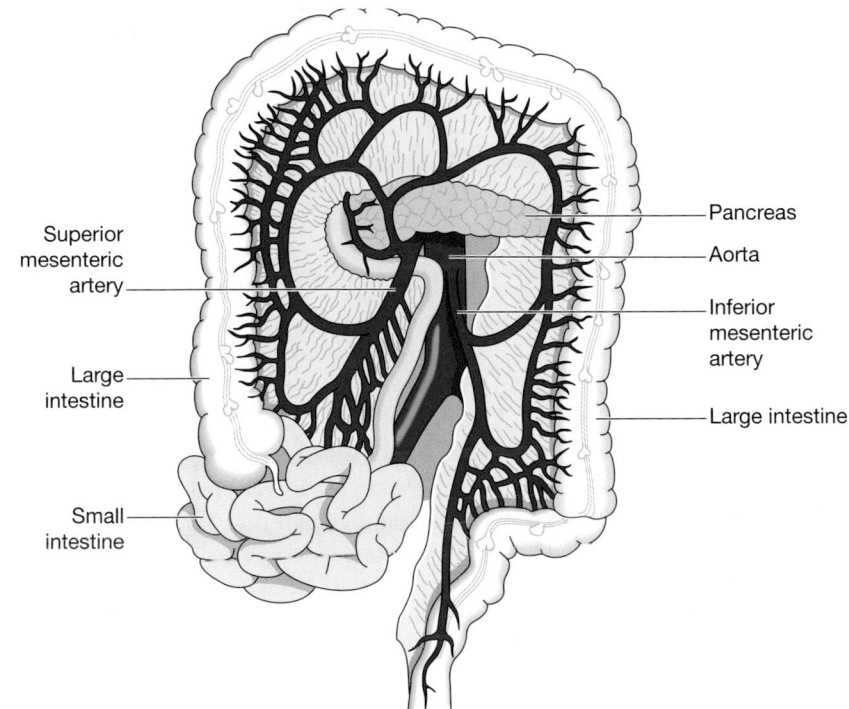

Figure 12.8 Blood supply to the small and large intestines.

In the abdomen and pelvis. The alimentary tract, pancreas, liver and biliary tract are supplied by the unpaired branches from the aorta: the *coeliac artery* and the *superior* and *inferior mesenteric arteries* (Figs 12.7 and 12.8).

The *coeliac artery* divides into three branches which supply the stomach, duodenum, pancreas, spleen, liver, gall bladder and bile ducts. They are:

- left gastric artery
- splenic artery
- hepatic artery.

The *superior mesenteric artery* supplies the whole of the small intestine, the caecum, ascending colon and most of the transverse colon.

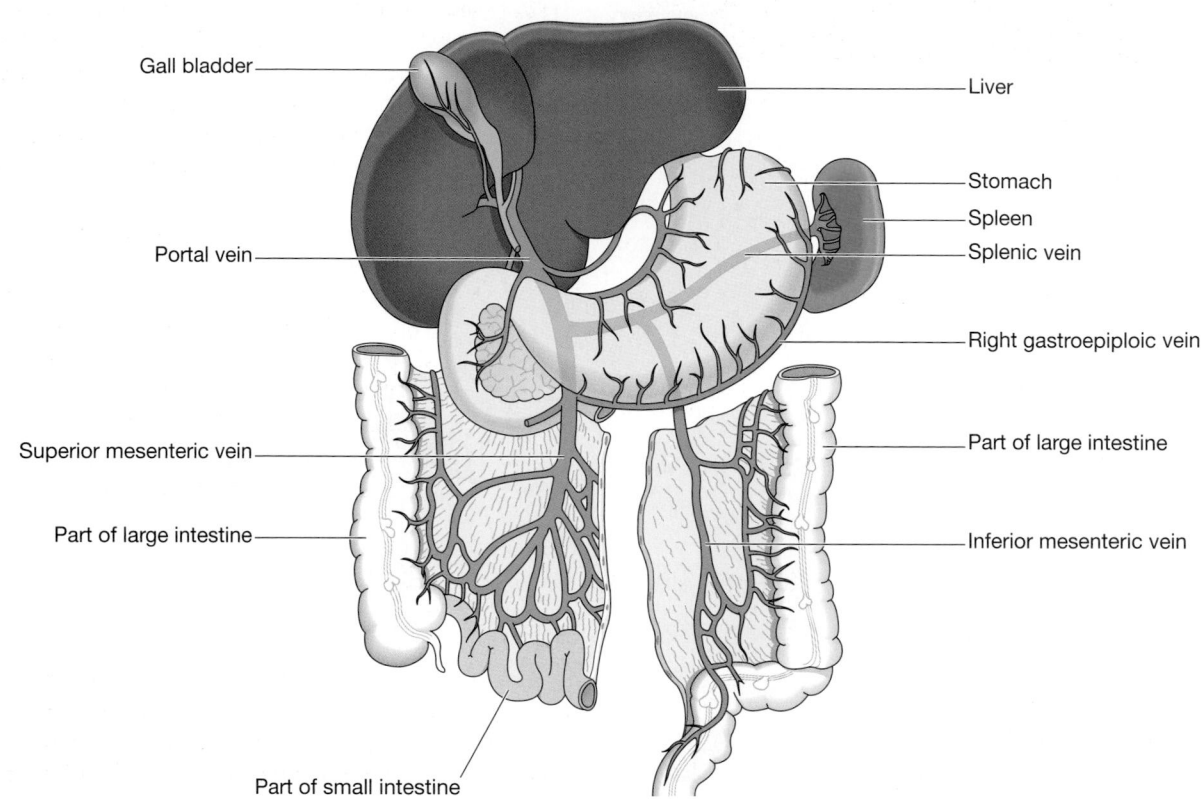

Gall bladder

Liver

Portal vein

Stomach

Spleen

Splenic vein

Right gastroepiploic vein

Superior mesenteric vein

Part of large intestine

Part of large intestine

Inferior mesenteric vein

Part of small intestine

Figure 12.9 Venous drainage from the abdominal organs of the digestive system.

The *inferior mesenteric artery* supplies a small part of the transverse colon, the descending colon, sigmoid colon and most of the rectum.

The distal part of the rectum and the anus are supplied by the *middle* and *inferior rectal arteries*, branches of the internal iliac arteries.

The arteries supplying the stomach and intestines pass between the layers of peritoneum from the posterior abdominal wall to the organs.

Venous drainage

In the thorax. Venous blood from the oesophagus passes in the oesophageal veins to the *azygos* and *hemi-azygos veins*. The azygos vein joins the superior vena cava near the heart, and the hemiazygos joins the left brachiocephalic vein.

Some blood from the lower part of the oesophagus drains into the *left gastric vein*. There are anastomotic vessels between the azygos, hemiazygos and left gastric veins.

In the abdomen and pelvis. The veins that drain blood from the lower part of the oesophagus, the stomach, pancreas, small intestine, large intestine and most of the rectum join to form the *portal vein* (Fig. 12.9). This blood, containing a high concentration of absorbed nutritional materials, is conveyed first to the liver then to the inferior vena cava. The circulation of blood in liver lobules is described later (p. 308).

Blood from the lower part of the rectum and the anal canal drains into the *internal iliac veins*. This blood is delivered directly into the inferior vena cava, hence bypassing the hepatic portal circulation.

MOUTH (Fig. 12.10)

Learning outcomes

After studying this section, you should be able to:

- list the principal structures associated with the mouth

- describe the structure of the mouth

- describe the structure and function of the tongue

- describe the structure and function of the teeth

- outline the arrangement of normal primary and secondary dentition.

The mouth or oral cavity is bounded by muscles and bones:

Anteriorly — by the lips
Posteriorly — it is continuous with the oropharynx
Laterally — by the muscles of the cheeks
Superiorly — by the bony hard palate and muscular soft palate
Inferiorly — by the muscular tongue and the soft tissues of the floor of the mouth.

The oral cavity is lined throughout with *mucous membrane*, consisting of *stratified squamous epithelium* containing small mucus-secreting glands.

The part of the mouth between the gums (alveolar ridges) and the cheeks is the *vestibule* and the remainder of the cavity is the *mouth proper*. The mucous membrane lining of the cheeks and the lips is reflected on to the gums or *alveolar ridges* and is continuous with the skin of the face.

The *palate* forms the roof of the mouth and is divided into the anterior *hard palate* and the posterior *soft palate* (Fig. 12.1). The bones forming the hard palate are the maxilla and the palatine bones. The soft palate is muscular, curves downwards from the posterior end of the hard palate and blends with the walls of the pharynx at the sides.

The *uvula* is a curved fold of muscle covered with mucous membrane, hanging down from the middle of the free border of the soft palate. Originating from the upper end of the uvula there are four folds of mucous membrane, two passing downwards at each side to form membranous arches. The posterior folds, one on each side, are the *palatopharyngeal arches* and the two anterior folds are the *palatoglossal arches*. On each side, between the arches, is a collection of lymphoid tissue called the *palatine tonsil*.

Tongue

The tongue is a voluntary muscular structure which occupies the floor of the mouth. It is attached by its base to the *hyoid bone* (see Fig. 10.4, p. 242) and by a fold of its mucous membrane covering, called the *frenulum*, to the floor of the mouth (Fig. 12.11). The superior surface consists of stratified squamous epithelium, with numerous *papillae* (little projections), containing nerve endings of the sense of taste, sometimes called the *taste buds*. There are three varieties of papillae (Fig. 12.12).

Vallate papillae, usually between 8 and 12 altogether, are arranged in an inverted V shape towards the base of the tongue. These are the largest of the papillae and are the most easily seen.

289

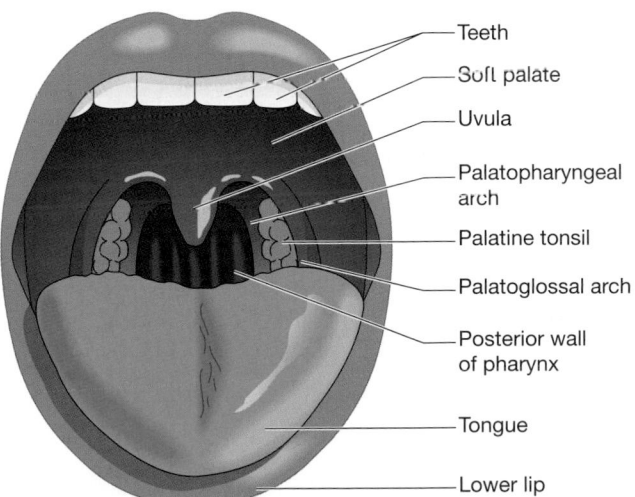

Figure 12.10 Structures seen in the widely open mouth.

Teeth
Soft palate
Uvula
Palatopharyngeal arch
Palatine tonsil
Palatoglossal arch
Posterior wall of pharynx
Tongue
Lower lip

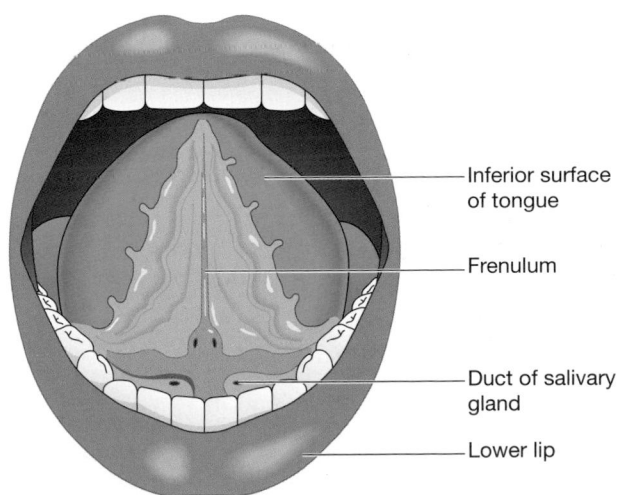

Figure 12.11 The inferior surface of the tongue.

Inferior surface of tongue
Frenulum
Duct of salivary gland
Lower lip

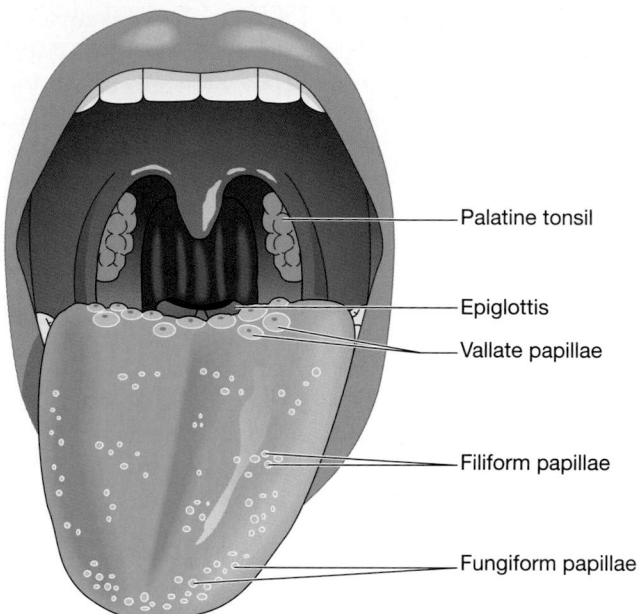

Figure 12.12 Locations of the papillae of the tongue and related structures.

Fungiform papillae are situated mainly at the tip and the edges of the tongue and are more numerous than the vallate papillae.

Filiform papillae are the smallest of the three types. They are most numerous on the surface of the anterior two-thirds of the tongue.

Blood supply

The main arterial blood supply to the tongue is by the *lingual branch* of the *external carotid artery*. Venous drainage is by the *lingual vein* which joins the *internal jugular vein*.

Nerve supply

The nerves involved are:

- the *hypoglossal nerves* (12th cranial nerves) which supply the voluntary muscle tissue
- the *lingual branch of the mandibular nerves* which are the nerves of somatic (ordinary) sensation, i.e. pain, temperature and touch
- the *facial* and *glossopharyngeal nerves* (7th and 9th cranial nerves) which are the nerves of the special sensation of taste.

Functions of the tongue

The tongue plays an important part in:

- mastication (chewing)
- deglutition (swallowing)
- speech (p. 245)
- taste (p. 207).

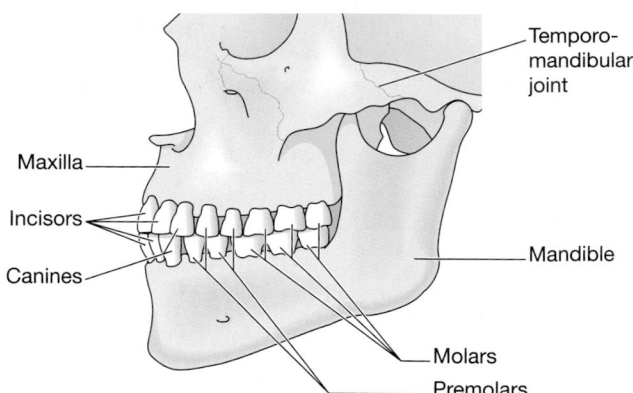

Figure 12.13 The permanent teeth and the jaw bones.

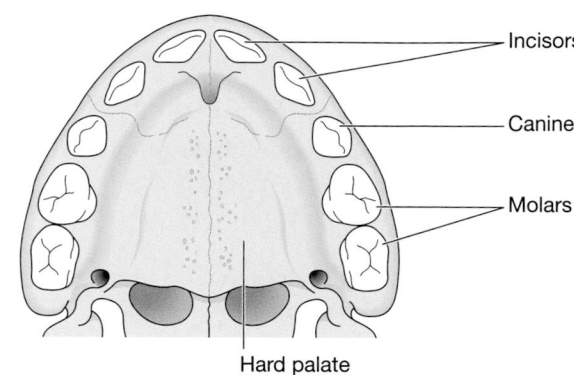

Figure 12.14 The roof of the mouth and the deciduous teeth – viewed from below.

Nerve endings of the sense of taste are present in the papillae and widely distributed in the epithelium of the tongue, soft palate, pharynx and epiglottis.

Teeth

The teeth are embedded in the alveoli or sockets of the alveolar ridges of the mandible and the maxilla (Fig. 12.13). Each individual has two sets, or *dentitions*, the *temporary* or *deciduous teeth* and the *permanent teeth* (Figs 12.14 and 12.15). At birth the teeth of both dentitions are present in immature form in the mandible and maxilla.

There are 20 temporary teeth, 10 in each jaw. They begin to erupt when the child is about 6 months old, and should all be present after 24 months (Table 12.1).

The permanent teeth begin to replace the deciduous teeth in the 6th year of age and this dentition, consisting of 32 teeth, is usually complete by the 24th year.

Functions of the teeth

The *incisor* and *canine* teeth are the cutting teeth and are used for biting off pieces of food, whereas the *premolar*

Table 12.1 Deciduous and permanent dentitions

Jaw	Molars	Premolars	Canine	Incisors	Incisors	Canine	Premolars	Molars
Deciduous teeth								
Upper	2	–	1	2	2	1	–	2
Lower	2	–	1	2	2	1	–	2
Permanent teeth								
Upper	3	2	1	2	2	1	2	3
Lower	3	2	1	2	2	1	2	3

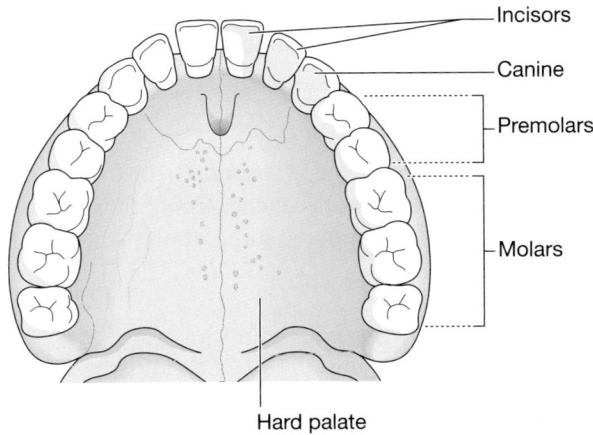

Hard palate

Figure 12.15 The roof of the mouth and the permanent teeth – viewed from below.

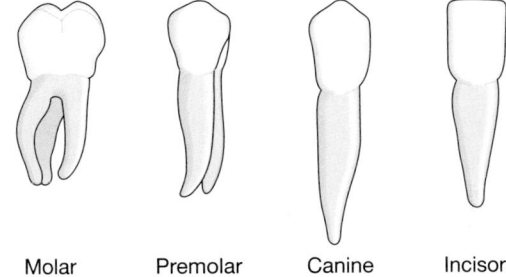

Molar   Premolar   Canine   Incisor

Figure 12.16 The shapes of the permanent teeth.

and *molar* teeth, with broad, flat surfaces, are used for grinding or chewing food (Fig. 12.16).

Structure of a tooth (Fig. 12.17)

Although the shapes of the different teeth vary, the structure is the same and consists of:

- *the crown* — the part which protrudes from the gum
- *the root* — the part embedded in the bone
- *the neck* — the slightly narrowed region where the crown merges with the root.

In the centre of the tooth is the *pulp cavity* containing blood vessels, lymph vessels and nerves, and surrounding this is a hard ivory-like substance called *dentine*. Outside the dentine of the crown is a thin layer of very hard substance, the *enamel*. The root of the tooth, on the other hand, is covered with a substance resembling bone, called *cement*, which fixes the tooth in its socket. Blood vessels and nerves pass to the tooth through a small foramen at the apex of each root.

Blood supply

Most of the arterial blood supply to the teeth is by branches of the *maxillary arteries*. The venous drainage is by a number of veins which empty into the *internal jugular veins*.

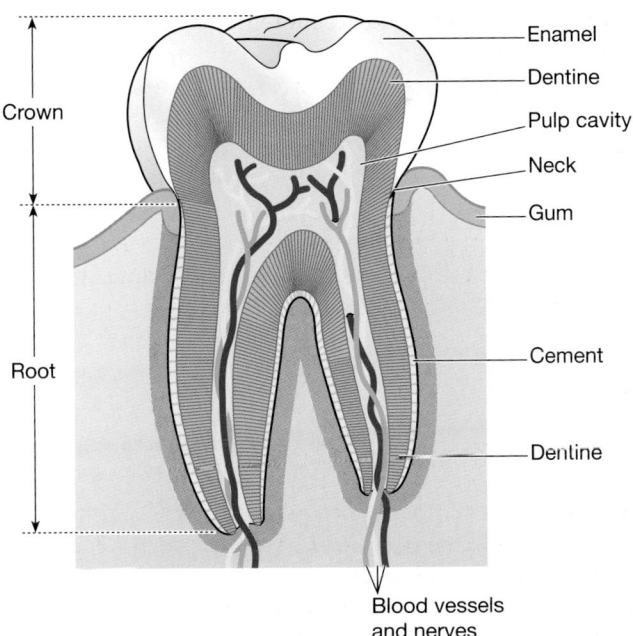

Enamel
Dentine
Pulp cavity
Neck
Gum
Cement
Dentine
Blood vessels and nerves
Crown
Root

Figure 12.17 A section of a tooth.

291

Nerve supply

The nerve supply to the upper teeth is by branches of the *maxillary nerves* and to the lower teeth by branches of the *mandibular nerves*. These are both branches of the *trigeminal nerves* (5th cranial nerves) (see p. 166).

SALIVARY GLANDS (Fig. 12.18)

Learning outcomes

After studying this section, you should be able to:

- describe the structure and the function of the principal salivary glands
- explain the role of saliva in digestion.

Salivary glands pour their secretions into the mouth. There are three pairs: the parotid glands, the submandibular glands and the sublingual glands.

Parotid glands

These are situated one on each side of the face just below the external acoustic meatus (see Fig. 8.1, p. 192). Each gland has a *parotid duct* opening into the mouth at the level of the second upper molar tooth.

Submandibular glands

These lie one on each side of the face under the angle of the jaw. The two *submandibular ducts* open on the floor of the mouth, one on each side of the frenulum of the tongue.

Sublingual glands

These glands lie under the mucous membrane of the floor of the mouth in front of the submandibular glands. They have numerous small ducts that open into the floor of the mouth.

Structure of the salivary glands

The glands are all surrounded by a *fibrous capsule*. They consist of a number of *lobules* made up of small acini lined with *secretory cells* (Fig. 12.18B). The secretions are poured into ductules which join up to form larger ducts leading into the mouth.

Nerve supply

The glands are supplied by parasympathetic and sympathetic nerve fibres. Parasympathetic stimulation increases secretion, whereas sympathetic stimulation decreases it.

Blood supply

Arterial supply is by various branches from the *external carotid arteries* and venous drainage is into the *external jugular veins*.

Composition of saliva

Saliva is the combined secretions from the salivary glands and the small mucus-secreting glands of the lining of the oral cavity. About 1.5 litres of saliva is produced daily and it consists of:

292

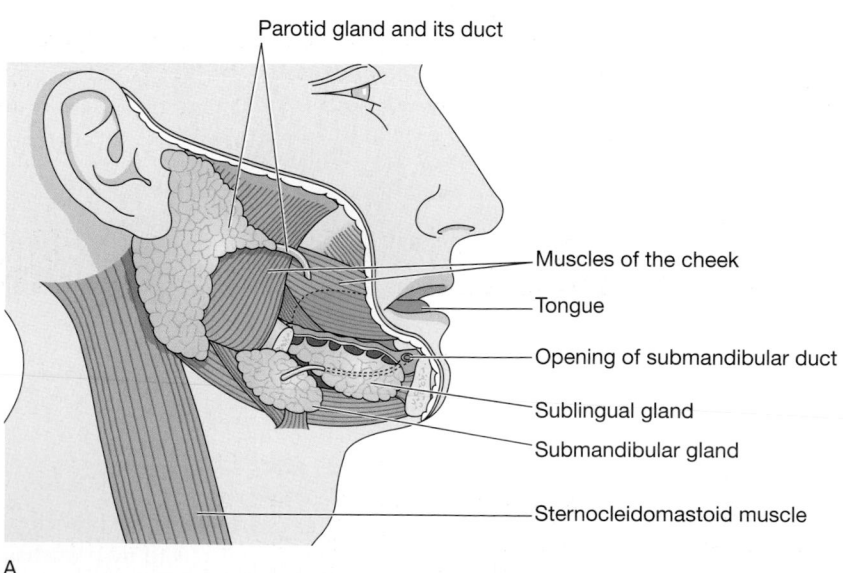

Parotid gland and its duct

Muscles of the cheek

Tongue

Opening of submandibular duct

Sublingual gland

Submandibular gland

Sternocleidomastoid muscle

A

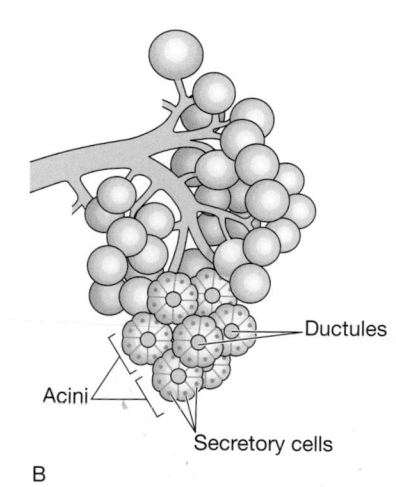

Ductules

Acini

Secretory cells

B

Figure 12.18 A. The position of the salivary glands. B. Enlargement of part of a gland.

- water
- mineral salts
- enzyme: salivary amylase
- mucus
- lysozyme
- immunoglobulins
- blood-clotting factors.

Secretion of saliva

Secretion of saliva is under autonomic nerve control. Parasympathetic stimulation causes vasodilatation and profuse secretion of watery saliva with a relatively low content of enzymes and other organic substances. Sympathetic stimulation causes vasoconstriction and secretion of small amounts of saliva rich in organic material, especially from the submandibular glands. Reflex secretion occurs when there is food in the mouth and the reflex can easily become *conditioned* so that the sight, smell and even the thought of food stimulates the flow of saliva.

Functions of saliva

Chemical digestion of polysaccharides. Saliva contains the enzyme amylase that begins the breakdown of complex sugars, reducing them to the disaccharide maltose. The optimum pH for the action of salivary amylase is 6.8 (slightly acid). Salivary pH ranges from 5.8 to 7.4 depending on the rate of flow; the higher the flow rate, the higher is the pH. Enzyme action continues during swallowing until terminated by the strongly acidic pH (1.5 to 1.8) of the gastric juices, which degrades the amylase.

Lubrication of food. Dry food entering the mouth is moistened and lubricated by saliva before it can be made into a bolus ready for swallowing.

Cleansing and lubricating. An adequate flow of saliva is necessary to cleanse the mouth and keep its tissues soft, moist and pliable. It helps to prevent damage to the mucous membrane by rough or abrasive foodstuffs.

Non-specific defence. Lysozyme, immunoglobulins and clotting factors combat invading microbes.

Taste. The taste buds are stimulated only by chemical substances in solution. Dry foods stimulate the sense of taste only after thorough mixing with saliva. The senses of taste and smell are closely linked in the enjoyment, or otherwise, of food.

PHARYNX

Learning outcome

After studying this section, you should be able to:

- describe the structure of the pharynx.

The pharynx is divided for descriptive purpose into three parts, the nasopharynx, oropharynx and laryngopharynx (see. p. 243). The nasopharynx is important in respiration. The oropharynx and laryngopharynx are passages common to both the respiratory and the digestive systems. Food passes from the oral cavity into the pharynx then to the oesophagus below, with which it is continuous. The walls of the pharynx are built of three layers of tissue.

The lining membrane (mucosa) is stratified squamous epithelium, continuous with the lining of the mouth at one end and with the oesophagus at the other.

The middle layer consists of fibrous tissue which becomes thinner towards the lower end and contains blood and lymph vessels and nerves.

The outer layer consists of a number of involuntary *constrictor* muscles which are involved in swallowing. When food reaches the pharynx swallowing is no longer under voluntary control.

Blood supply

The blood supply to the pharynx is by several branches of the *facial arteries*. Venous drainage is into the *facial veins* and the *internal jugular veins*.

Nerve supply

This is from the *pharyngeal plexus* and consists of parasympathetic and sympathetic nerves. Parasympathetic supply is mainly by the *glossopharyngeal* and *vagus nerves* and sympathetic from the *cervical ganglia*.

OESOPHAGUS (Fig. 12.19)

Learning outcomes

After studying this section, you should be able to:

- describe the location of the oesophagus
- outline the structure of the oesophagus
- explain the mechanisms involved in swallowing, and the route taken by a bolus.

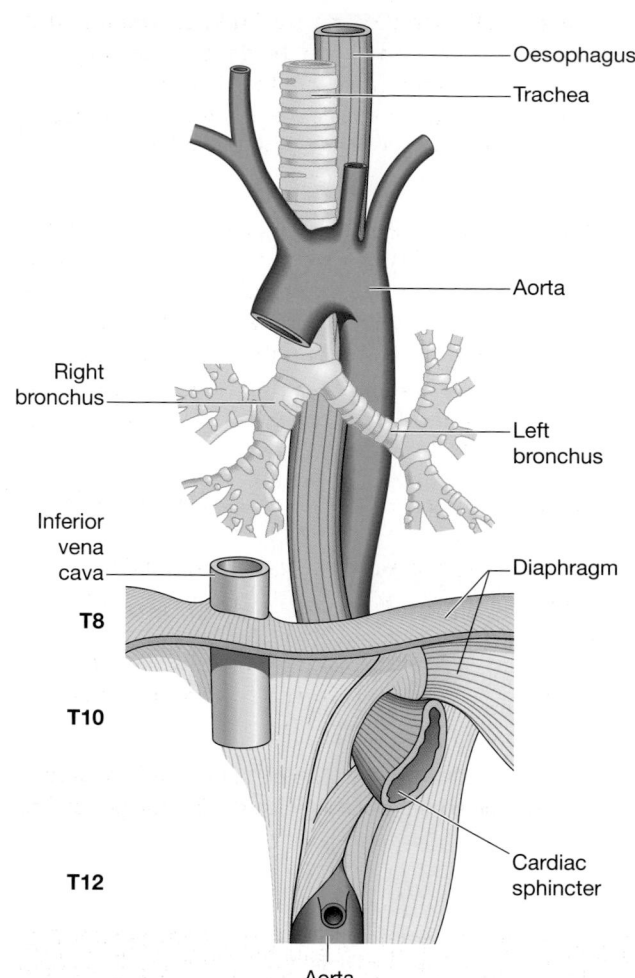

Figure 12.19 The oesophagus and some related structures.

The oesophagus is about 25 cm long and about 2 cm in diameter and lies in the median plane in the thorax in front of the vertebral column behind the trachea and the heart. It is continuous with the pharynx above and just below the diaphragm it joins the stomach. It passes between muscle fibres of the diaphragm behind the central tendon at the level of the 10th thoracic vertebra. Immediately the oesophagus has passed through the diaphragm it curves upwards before opening into the stomach. This sharp angle is believed to be one of the factors which prevents the regurgitation (backward flow) of gastric contents into the oesophagus. The upper and lower ends of the oesophagus are closed by sphincter muscles. The upper *cricopharyngeal sphincter* prevents air passing into the oesophagus during inspiration and the aspiration of oesophageal contents. The *cardiac* or *lower oesophageal sphincter* prevents the reflux of acid gastric contents into the oesophagus. There is no thickening of the circular muscle in this area and this sphincter is therefore

'physiological', i.e. this region can act as a sphincter without the presence of the anatomical features. When intra-abdominal pressure is raised, e.g. during inspiration and defaecation, the tone of the lower sphincter muscle increases. There is an added pinching effect by the contracting muscle fibres of the diaphragm.

Structure

There are four layers of tissue as shown in Figure 12.2. As the oesophagus is almost entirely in the thorax the outer covering, the adventitia, consists of *elastic fibrous tissue*. The proximal third is lined by stratified squamous epithelium and the distal third by columnar epithelium. The middle third is lined by a mixture of the two.

Blood supply
Arterial. The thoracic region of the oesophagus is supplied mainly by the oesophageal arteries, branches from the aorta. The abdominal region is supplied by branches from the inferior phrenic arteries and the left gastric branch of the coeliac artery.

Venous drainage. From the thoracic region venous drainage is into the azygos and hemiazygos veins. The abdominal part drains into the left gastric vein. There is a venous plexus at the distal end that links the upward and downward venous drainage, i.e. the general and portal circulations.

Nerve supply
Sympathetic and parasympathetic nerves terminate in the myenteric and submucosal plexuses. Parasympathetic fibres are branches of the vagus nerves (Fig. 12.6).

Functions of the mouth, pharynx and oesophagus

Formation of a bolus. When food is taken into the mouth it is masticated or chewed by the teeth and moved round the mouth by the tongue and muscles of the cheeks (Fig. 12.20). It is mixed with saliva and formed into a soft mass or *bolus* ready for *deglutition* or swallowing. The length of time that food remains in the mouth depends, to a large extent, on the consistency of the food. Some foods need to the chewed longer than others before the individual feels that the mass is ready for swallowing.

Deglutition or swallowing (Fig. 12.21). This occurs in three stages after mastication is complete and the bolus has been formed. It is initiated voluntarily but completed by a reflex (involuntary) action.

into the mouth; and the larynx is lifted up and forward so that its opening is occluded by the overhanging epiglottis preventing entry into the airway.

3. The presence of the bolus in the pharynx stimulates a wave of peristalsis which propels the bolus through the oesophagus to the stomach.

Peristaltic waves pass along the oesophagus only after swallowing (Fig. 12.4). Otherwise the walls are relaxed. Ahead of a peristaltic wave, the cardiac sphincter guarding the entrance to the stomach relaxes to allow the descending bolus to pass into the stomach. Usually, constriction of the cardiac sphincter prevents reflux of gastric acid into the oesophagus. Other factors preventing gastric reflux include:

■ the attachment of the stomach to the diaphragm by the peritoneum
■ the maintenance of an acute angle between the oesophagus and the fundus of the stomach, i.e. an acute cardio-oesophageal angle
■ increased tone of the cardiac sphincter when intra-abdominal pressure is increased and the pinching effect of diaphragm muscle fibres.

The walls of the oesophagus are lubricated by mucus which assists the passage of the bolus during the peristaltic contraction of the muscular wall.

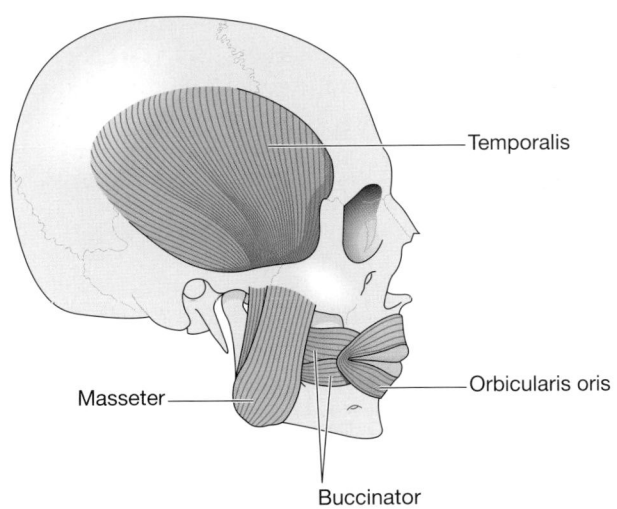

Masseter —
Temporalis —
Orbicularis oris —
Buccinator —

Figure 12.20 The muscles used in chewing.

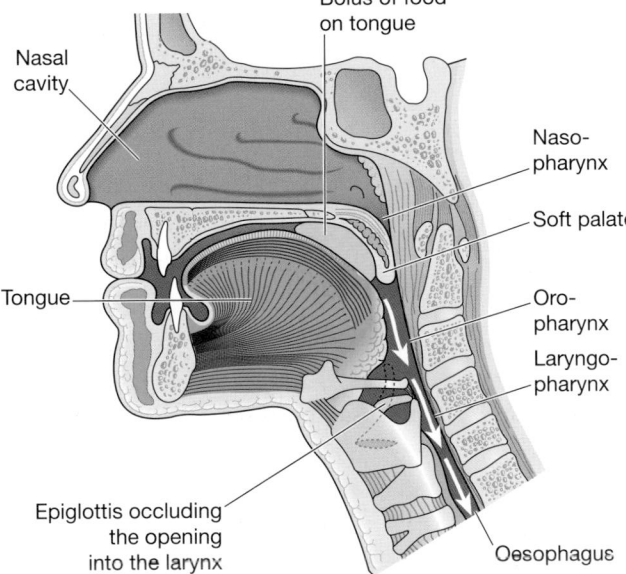

Nasal cavity —
Bolus of food on tongue —
Naso-pharynx —
Soft palate —
Tongue —
Oro-pharynx —
Laryngo-pharynx —
Epiglottis occluding the opening into the larynx —
Oesophagus —

Figure 12.21 Section of the face and neck showing the positions of structures during swallowing.

1. The mouth is closed and the voluntary muscles of the tongue and cheeks push the bolus backwards into the pharynx.
2. The muscles of the pharynx are stimulated by a reflex action initiated in the walls of the oropharynx and coordinated in the medulla and lower pons in the brain stem. Contraction of these muscles propels the bolus down into the oesophagus. All other routes that the bolus could possibly take are closed. The soft palate rises up and closes off the nasopharynx; the tongue and the pharyngeal folds block the way back

295

STOMACH

Learning outcomes

After studying this section, you should be able to:

■ describe the location of the stomach with reference to surrounding structures
■ explain the physiological significance of the layers of the stomach wall
■ discuss the digestive functions of the stomach.

The stomach is a J-shaped dilated portion of the alimentary tract situated in the epigastric, umbilical and left hypochondriac regions of the abdominal cavity.

Organs associated with the stomach (Fig. 12.22)

Anteriorly — left lobe of liver and anterior abdominal wall

Posteriorly — abdominal aorta, pancreas, spleen, left kidney and adrenal gland

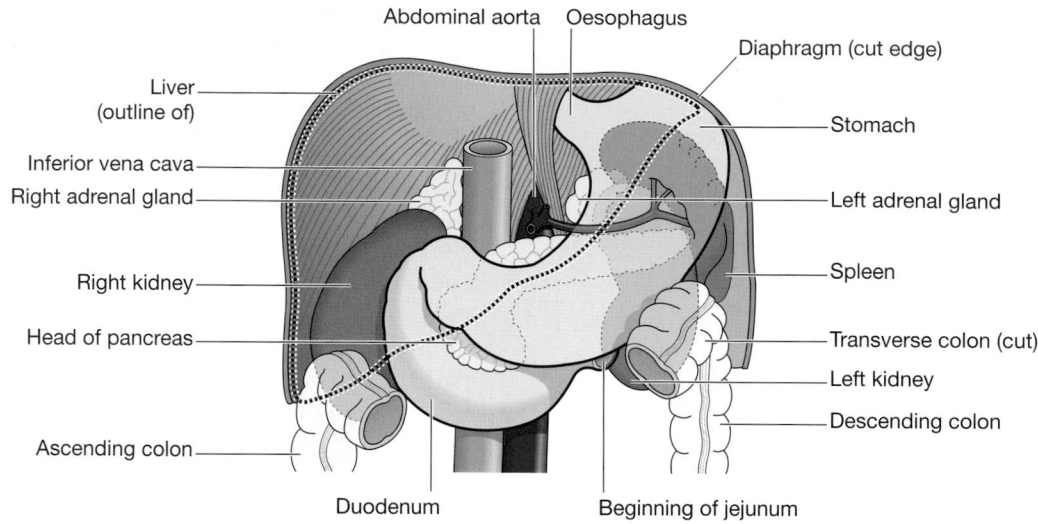

Figure 12.22 The stomach and its associated structures.

Superiorly — diaphragm, oesophagus and left lobe of liver
Inferiorly — transverse colon and small intestine
To the left — diaphragm and spleen
To the right — liver and duodenum

Structure of the stomach (Fig. 12.23)

The stomach is continuous with the oesophagus at the *cardiac sphincter* and with the duodenum at the *pyloric sphincter*. It has two curvatures. The *lesser curvature* is short, lies on the posterior surface of the stomach and is the downwards continuation of the posterior wall of the oesophagus. Just before the pyloric sphincter it curves upwards to complete the J shape. Where the oesophagus joins the stomach the anterior region angles acutely upwards, curves downwards forming the *greater curvature* then slightly upwards towards the pyloric sphincter.

The stomach is divided into three regions: the fundus, the body and the antrum. At the distal end of the pyloric antrum is the pyloric sphincter, guarding the opening between the stomach and the duodenum. When the stomach is inactive the pyloric sphincter is relaxed and open and when the stomach contains food the sphincter is closed.

Walls of the stomach

The four layers of tissue that comprise the basic structure of the alimentary canal (Fig. 12.2) are found in the stomach but with some modifications.

Muscle layer (Fig. 12.24). This consists of three layers of smooth muscle fibres:

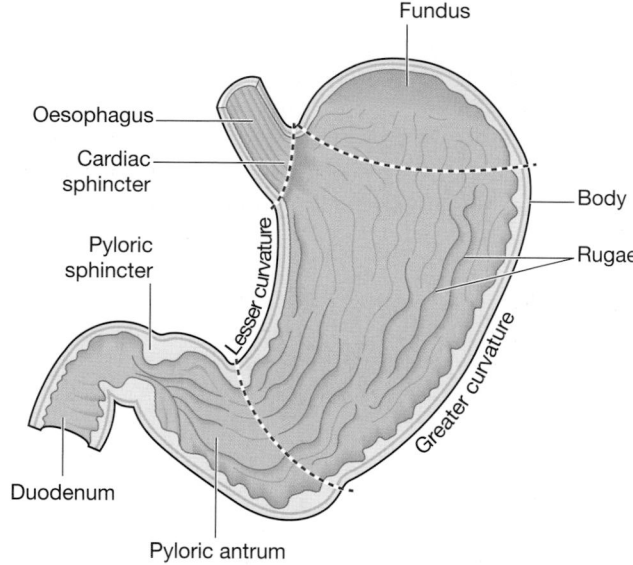

Figure 12.23 Longitudinal section of the stomach.

- an outer layer of longitudinal fibres
- a middle layer of circular fibres
- an inner layer of oblique fibres.

In this respect, the stomach is different from other regions of the alimentary tract as it has three layers of muscle instead of two (Fig. 12.2).

This arrangement allows for the churning motion characteristic of gastric activity, as well as peristaltic movement. Circular muscle is strongest in the pyloric antrum and sphincter.

296

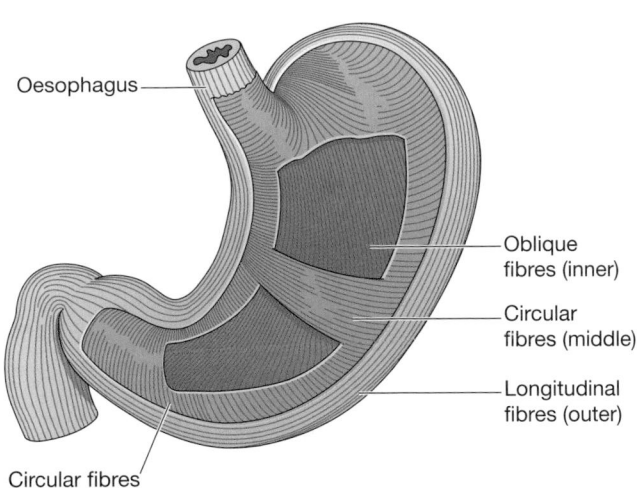

Figure 12.24 The muscle fibres of the stomach wall. Sections have been removed to show the three layers.

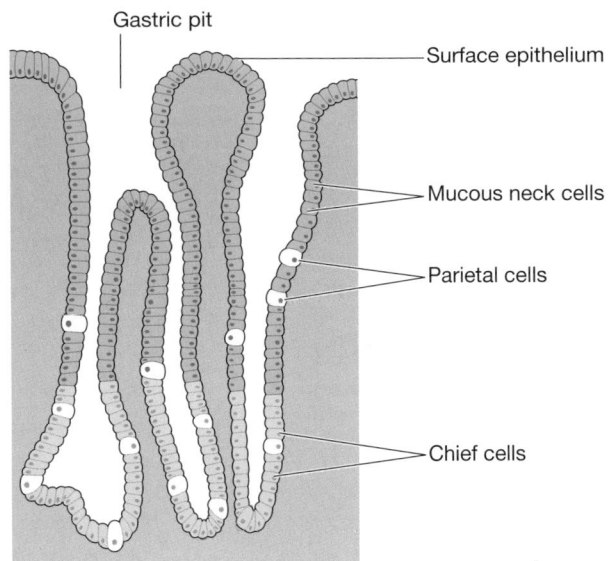

Figure 12.25 Structure of gastric glands.

Mucosa. When the stomach is empty the mucous membrane lining is thrown into longitudinal folds or *rugae*, and when full the rugae are 'ironed out' and the surface has a smooth, velvety appearance. Numerous *gastric glands* are situated below the surface in the mucous membrane. They consist of specialised cells that secrete *gastric juice* into the stomach.

Blood supply

Arterial blood is supplied to the stomach by branches of the coeliac artery and venous drainage is into the portal vein. Figures 12.7 and 12.9 give details of the names of these vessels.

Nerve supply

The sympathetic supply to the stomach is mainly from the *coeliac plexus* and the parasympathetic supply is from the *vagus nerves*. Sympathetic stimulation reduces the motility of the stomach and the secretion of gastric juice; vagal stimulation has the opposite effect (Fig. 12.6).

Gastric juice and functions of the stomach

Stomach size varies with the volume of food it contains, which may be 1.5 litres or more in an adult. When a meal has been eaten the food accumulates in the stomach in layers, the last part of the meal remaining in the fundus for some time. Mixing with the gastric juice takes place gradually and it may be some time before the food is sufficiently acidified to stop the action of salivary amylase.

Gastric muscle contraction consists of a churning movement that breaks down the bolus and mixes it with gastric juice, and peristaltic waves that propel the stomach contents towards the pylorus. When the stomach is active the pyloric sphincter closes. Strong peristaltic contraction of the pyloric antrum forces gastric contents, after they are sufficiently liquefied, through the pylorus into the duodenum in small spurts.

Gastric juice

About 2 litres of gastric juice are secreted daily by special secretory glands in the mucosa (Fig. 12.25). It consists of:

- water ⎱ secreted by gastric glands
- mineral salts ⎰
- mucus secreted by goblet cells in the glands and on the stomach surface
- hydrochloric acid ⎱ secreted by *parietal*
- intrinsic factor ⎰ *cells* in the gastric glands
- inactive enzyme precursors: pepsinogens secreted by *chief cells* in the glands.

Functions of gastric juice

- *Water* further liquefies the food swallowed.
- *Hydrochloric acid*:
  - acidifies the food and stops the action of salivary amylase
  - kills ingested microbes
  - provides the acid environment needed for effective digestion by pepsins.

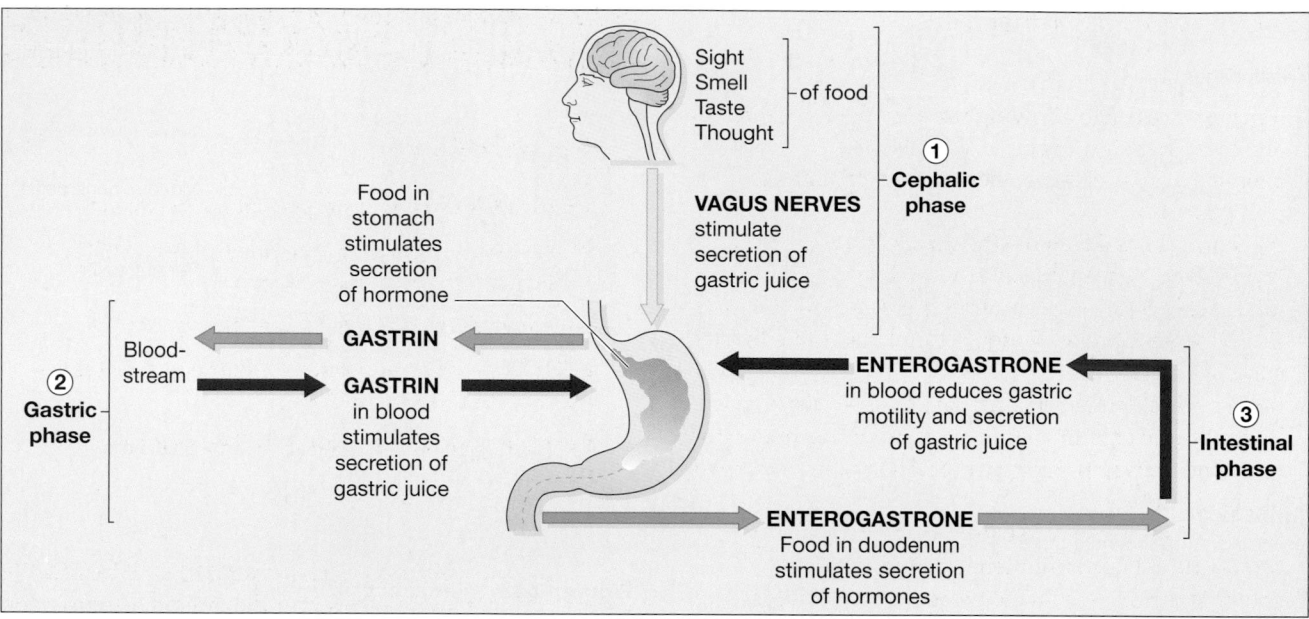

Figure 12.26 The three phases of secretion of gastric juice.

- *Pepsinogens* are activated to *pepsins* by hydrochloric acid and by pepsins already present in the stomach. They begin the digestion of proteins, breaking them into smaller molecules. Pepsins act most effectively at pH 1.5 to 3.5.
- *Intrinsic factor* (a protein) is necessary for the absorption of vitamin B_{12} from the ileum.
- *Mucus* prevents mechanical injury to the stomach wall by lubricating the contents. It prevents chemical injury by acting as a barrier between the stomach wall and the corrosive gastric juice. Hydrochloric acid is present in potentially damaging concentrations and pepsins digest protein.

Secretion of gastric juice

There is always a small quantity of gastric juice present in the stomach, even when it contains no food. This is known as *fasting juice*. Secretion reaches its maximum level about 1 hour after a meal then declines to the fasting level after about 4 hours.

There are three phases of secretion of gastric juice (Fig. 12.26).

1. *Cephalic phase*. This flow of juice occurs *before* food reaches the stomach and is due to reflex stimulation of the vagus nerves initiated by the sight, smell or taste of food. When the vagus nerves have been cut (vagotomy) this phase of gastric secretion stops.
2. *Gastric phase*. When stimulated by the presence of food the *enteroendocrine cells* in the pyloric antrum and duodenum secrete *gastrin*, a hormone which passes directly into the circulating blood. Gastrin, circulating in the blood which supplies the stomach, stimulates the gastric glands to produce more gastric juice. In this way the secretion of digestive juice is continued after the completion of the meal and the end of the cephalic phase. Gastrin secretion is suppressed when the pH in the pyloric antrum falls to about 1.5.
3. *Intestinal phase*. When the partially digested contents of the stomach reach the small intestine, a hormone complex *enterogastrone** is produced by endocrine cells in the intestinal mucosa, which slows down the secretion of gastric juice and reduces gastric motility. Two of the hormones forming this complex are *secretin* and *cholecystokinin* (CCK).

By slowing the emptying rate of the stomach, the contents of the duodenum become more thoroughly mixed with bile and pancreatic juice. This phase of gastric secretion is most marked when the meal has had a high fat content.

The rate at which the stomach empties depends to a large extent on the type of food eaten. A carbohydrate meal leaves the stomach in 2 to 3 hours, a protein meal remains longer and a fatty meal remains in the stomach longest.

---

* Enterogastrone has been described as any hormone or combination of hormones released by the intestine that inhibits gastric secretion.

Functions of the stomach

These include:

- temporary storage allowing time for the digestive enzymes, pepsins, to act
- chemical digestion—pepsins convert proteins to polypeptides
- mechanical breakdown—the three smooth muscle layers enable the stomach to act as a churn, gastric juice is added and the contents are liquefied to *chyme*
- limited absorption of water, alcohol and some lipid-soluble drugs
- non-specific defence against microbes—provided by hydrochloric acid in gastric juice. Vomiting may be a response to ingestion of gastric irritants, e.g. microbes or chemicals
- preparation of iron for absorption further along the tract—the acid environment of the stomach solubilises iron salts, which is required before iron can be absorbed
- production of intrinsic factor needed for absorption of vitamin B_{12} in the terminal ileum
- regulation of the passage of gastric contents into the duodenum. When the chyme is sufficiently acidified and liquefied, the pyloric antrum forces small jets of gastric contents through the pyloric sphincter into the duodenum.

SMALL INTESTINE (Figs 12.27 and 12.28)

Learning outcomes

After studying this section, you should be able to:

- describe the location of the small intestine, with reference to surrounding structures
- sketch a villus, naming its component parts
- discuss the digestive functions of the small intestine and its secretions
- explain how nutrients are absorbed in the small intestine.

The small intestine is continuous with the stomach at the pyloric sphincter and leads into the large intestine at the *ileocaecal valve*. It is a little over 5 metres long and lies in the abdominal cavity surrounded by the large intestine. In the small intestine the chemical digestion of food is completed and most of the absorption of nutrients takes place.

The small intestine comprises three main sections continuous with each other.

The *duodenum* is about 25 cm long and curves around the head of the pancreas. Secretions from the gall bladder and pancreas are released into the duodenum through a common structure, the hepatopancreatic ampulla, and

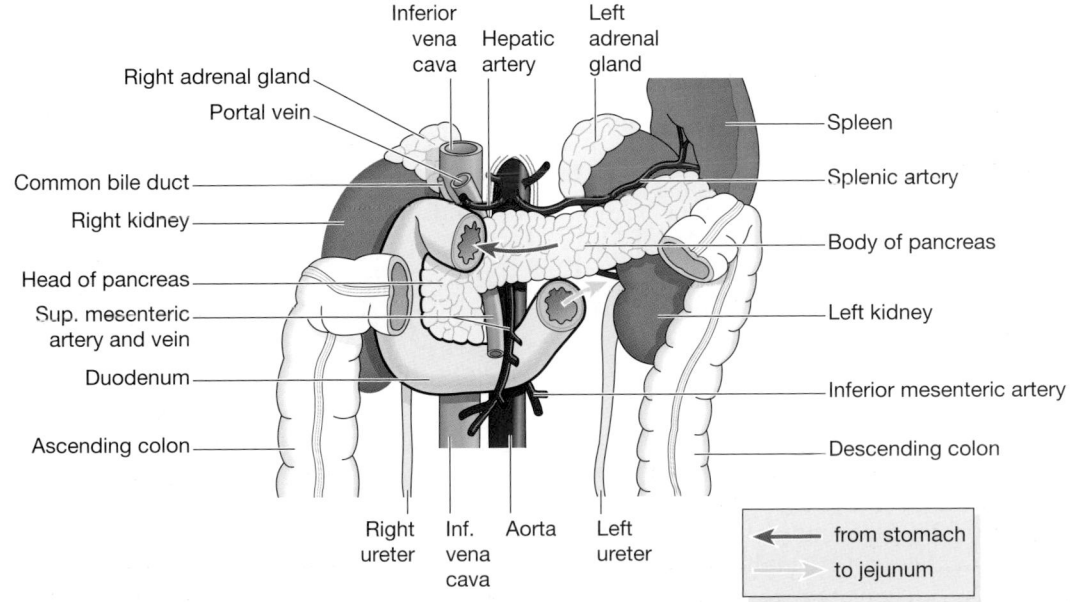

Figure 12.27 The duodenum and its associated structures.

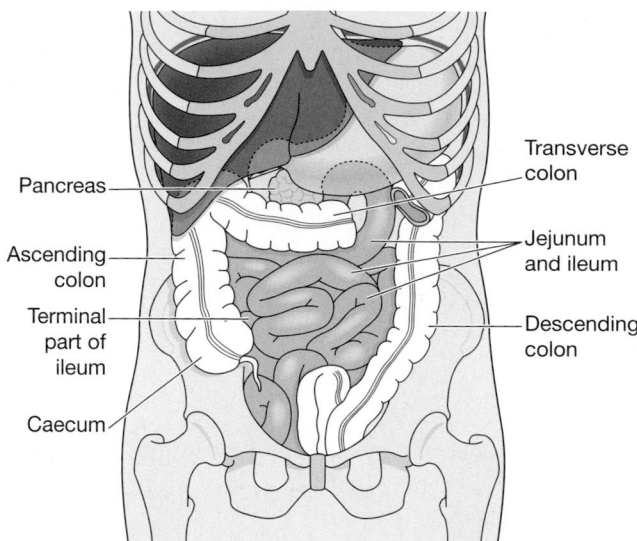

Figure 12.28 The jejunum and ileum and their related structures.

the opening into the duodenum is guarded by the hepatopancreatic sphincter (of Oddi) (Fig. 12.42).

The *jejunum* is the middle section of the small intestine and is about 2 metres long.

The *ileum*, or terminal section, is about 3 metres long and ends at the ileocaecal valve, which controls the flow of material from the ileum to the *caecum*, the first part of the large intestine, and prevents regurgitation.

Structure of the small intestine

The walls of the small intestine are composed of the four layers of tissue shown in Figure 12.2. Some modifications of the peritoneum and mucosa (mucous membrane lining) are described below.

Peritoneum. A double layer of peritoneum called the *mesentery* attaches the jejunum and ileum to the posterior abdominal wall (Fig. 12.3A). The attachment is quite short in comparison with the length of the small intestine, therefore it is fan-shaped. The large blood vessels and nerves lie on the posterior abdominal wall and the branches to the small intestine pass between the two layers of the mesentery.

Mucosa. The surface area of the small intestine mucosa is greatly increased by permanent circular folds, villi and microvilli.

The *permanent circular folds*, unlike the rugae of the stomach, are not smoothed out when the small intestine is distended (Fig. 12.29). They promote mixing of chyme as it passes along.

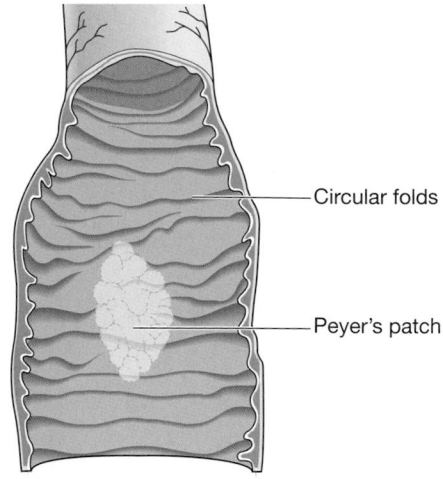

Figure 12.29 Section of a small piece of small intestine (opened out), showing the permanent circular folds.

The *villi* are tiny finger-like projections of the mucosal layer into the intestinal lumen, about 0.5 to 1 mm long (Fig. 12.30). Their walls consist of columnar epithelial cells, or *enterocytes*, with tiny *microvilli* (1 μm long) on their free border. *Goblet cells* that secrete mucus are interspersed between the enterocytes. These epithelial cells enclose a network of blood and lymph capillaries. The lymph capillaries are called *lacteals* because absorbed fat gives the lymph a milky appearance. Absorption and some final stages of digestion of nutrients take place in the enterocytes before entering the blood and lymph capillaries.

The *intestinal glands* are simple tubular glands situated below the surface between the villi. The cells of the glands migrate upwards to form the walls of the villi replacing those at the tips as they are rubbed off by the intestinal contents. The entire epithelium is replaced every 3 to 5 days. During migration the cells form digestive enzymes that lodge in the microvilli and, together with intestinal juice, complete the chemical digestion of carbohydrates, protein and fats.

Numerous *lymph nodes* are found in the mucosa at irregular intervals throughout the length of the small intestine. The smaller ones are known as *solitary lymphatic follicles*, and about 20 or 30 larger nodes situated towards the distal end of the ileum are called *aggregated lymphatic follicles* (Peyer's patches). These lymphatic tissues, packed with defensive cells, are strategically placed to neutralise ingested antigens (Ch. 15).

Blood supply (Figs 12.8 and 12.9)

The *superior mesenteric artery* supplies the whole of the small intestine, and venous drainage is by the *superior mesenteric vein* which joins other veins to form the portal vein.

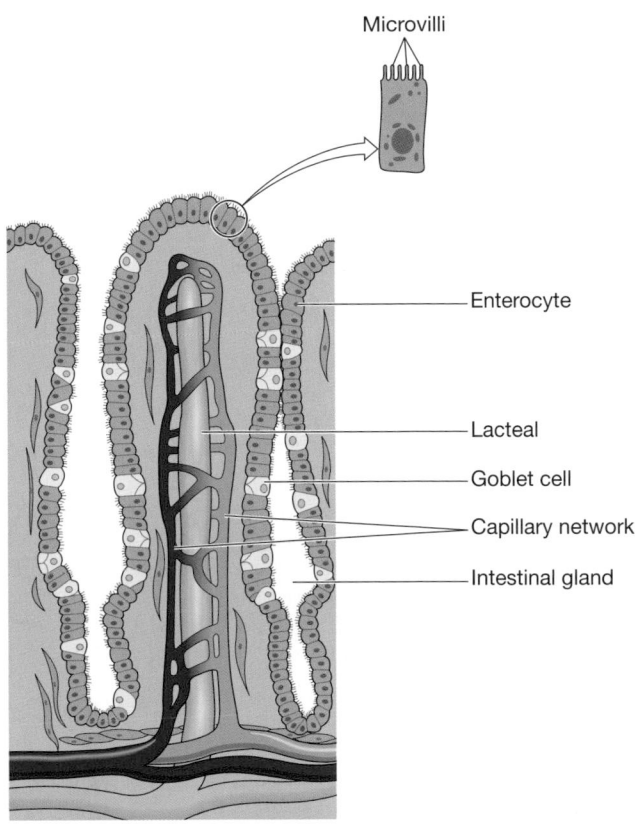

Microvilli

Enterocyte

Lacteal

Goblet cell

Capillary network

Intestinal gland

Figure 12.30 A highly magnified view of one complete villus in the small intestine.

Nerve supply

Innervation of the small intestine is both sympathetic and parasympathetic (Fig. 12.6).

Intestinal juice

About 1500 ml of intestinal juice are secreted daily by the glands of the small intestine. It consists of:

- water
- mucus
- mineral salts
- enzyme: enterokinase (enteropeptidases).

The pH of intestinal juice is usually between 7.8 and 8.0.

Functions of the small intestine

The functions are:

- onward movement of its contents which is produced by peristalsis
- secretion of intestinal juice
- completion of chemical digestion of carbohydrates, protein and fats in the enterocytes of the villi

- protection against infection by microbes that have survived the antimicrobial action of the hydrochloric acid in the stomach, by the solitary lymph follicles and aggregated lymph follicles
- secretion of the hormones cholecystokinin (CCK) and secretin
- absorption of nutrients.

Chemical digestion in the small intestine

When acid chyme passes into the small intestine it is mixed with *pancreatic juice, bile* and *intestinal juice*, and is in contact with the enterocytes of the villi. In the small intestine the digestion of all the nutrients is completed:

- carbohydrates are broken down to monosaccharides
- proteins are broken down to amino acids
- fats are broken down to fatty acids and glycerol.

Pancreatic juice

Pancreatic juice enters the duodenum at the hepatopancreatic ampulla and consists of:

- water
- mineral salts
- enzymes:
  - amylase
  - lipase
- inactive enzyme precursors:
  - trypsinogen
  - chymotrypsinogen
  - procarboxypeptidase.

Pancreatic juice is alkaline (pH 8) because it contains significant quantities of bicarbonate ions, which are alkaline in solution. When acid stomach contents enter the duodenum they are mixed with pancreatic juice and bile and the pH is raised to between 6 and 8. This is the pH at which the pancreatic enzymes, amylase and lipase, act most effectively.

Functions

Digestion of proteins. Trypsinogen and chymotrypsinogen are inactive enzyme precursors activated by *enterokinase* (enteropeptidase), an enzyme in the microvilli, which converts them into the active proteolytic enzymes *trypsin* and *chymotrypsin*. These enzymes convert polypeptides to tripeptides, dipeptides and amino acids. It is important that they are produced as inactive precursors and are activated only upon arrival in the duodenum, otherwise they would digest the pancreas.

Digestion of carbohydrates. *Pancreatic amylase* converts *all digestible* polysaccharides (starches) not acted upon by salivary amylase to disaccharides.

Digestion of fats. *Lipase* converts fats to fatty acids and glycerol. To aid the action of lipase, *bile salts* emulsify fats, i.e. reduce the size of the globules, increasing their surface area.

Control of secretion

The secretion of pancreatic juice is stimulated by secretin and CCK, produced by endocrine cells in the walls of the duodenum. The presence in the duodenum of acid material from the stomach stimulates the production of these hormones.

Bile

Bile, secreted by the liver, is unable to enter the duodenum when the hepatopancreatic sphincter is closed; therefore it passes from the *hepatic duct* along the *cystic duct* to the gall bladder where it is stored (Fig. 12.42).

Bile has a pH of 8 and between 500 and 1000 ml are secreted daily. It consists of:

- water
- mineral salts
- mucus
- bile salts
- bile pigments, mainly bilirubin
- cholesterol.

Functions

- The bile salts, *sodium taurocholate* and *sodium glycocholate*, emulsify fats in the small intestine.
- The bile pigment, *bilirubin*, is a waste product of the breakdown of erythrocytes and is excreted in the bile rather than in the urine because of its low solubility in water. Bilirubin is altered by microbes in the large intestine. Some of the resultant *urobilinogen*, which is highly water soluble, is reabsorbed and then excreted in the urine, but most is converted to *stercobilin* and excreted in the faeces.
- Fatty acids are insoluble in water, which makes them very difficult to absorb through the intestinal wall. Bile salts make fatty acids soluble, enabling both these and fat-soluble vitamins (e.g. vitamin K) to be readily absorbed.
- Stercobilin colours and deodorises the faeces.

Release from the gall bladder

When a meal has been eaten the hormone CCK is secreted by the duodenum during the intestinal phase of secretion of gastric juice (p. 298). This stimulates contraction of the gall bladder and relaxation of the hepatopancreatic sphincter, enabling the bile and pancreatic juice to pass into the duodenum together. A more marked activity is noted if chyme entering the duodenum contains a high proportion of fat.

Intestinal secretions

The principal constituents of intestinal secretions are:

- water
- mucus
- mineral salts
- enzyme: enterokinase (enteropeptidase).

Most of the digestive enzymes in the small intestine are contained in the enterocytes of the walls of the villi. Digestion of carbohydrate, protein and fat is completed by direct contact between these nutrients and the microvilli and within the enterocytes.

The enzymes involved in completing the chemical digestion of food in the enterocytes of the villi are:

- peptidases
- lipase
- sucrase, maltase and lactase.

Chemical digestion associated with enterocytes

Alkaline intestinal juice (pH 7.8 to 8.0) assists in raising the pH of the intestinal contents to between 6.5 and 7.5.

Enterokinase activates pancreatic peptidases such as trypsin which convert some polypeptides to amino acids and some to smaller peptides. The final stage of breakdown to amino acids of all peptides occurs inside the enterocytes.

Lipase completes the digestion of emulsified fats to *fatty acids* and *glycerol* partly in the intestine and partly in the enterocytes.

Sucrase, maltase and *lactase* complete the digestion of carbohydrates by converting disaccharides such as sucrose, maltose and lactose to monosaccharides inside the enterocytes.

Control of secretion

Mechanical stimulation of the intestinal glands by chyme is believed to be the main stimulus for the secretion of intestinal juice, although the hormone secretin may also be involved.

Absorption of nutrients (Fig. 12.31)

Absorption of nutrients occurs by two possible processes:

- *Diffusion*. Monosaccharides, amino acids, fatty acids and glycerol diffuse slowly down their concentration gradients into the enterocytes from the intestinal lumen.
- *Active transport*. Monosaccharides, amino acids, fatty acids and glycerol may be actively transported into the villi; this is faster than diffusion. Disaccharides, dipeptides and tripeptides are also actively transported into the enterocytes where their digestion is completed before transfer into the capillaries of the villi.

Monosaccharides and amino acids pass into the capillaries in the villi and fatty acids and glycerol into the lacteals.

Some proteins are absorbed unchanged, e.g. antibodies present in breast milk and oral vaccines, such as poliomyelitis vaccine. The extent of protein absorption is believed to be limited.

Other nutrients such as vitamins, mineral salts and water are also absorbed from the small intestine into the blood capillaries. Fat-soluble vitamins are absorbed into the lacteals along with fatty acids and glycerol. Vitamin B_{12} combines with intrinsic factor in the stomach and is actively absorbed in the terminal ileum.

The surface area through which absorption takes place in the small intestine is greatly increased by the *circular folds* of mucous membrane and by the very large number of *villi* and *microvilli* present. It has been calculated that the surface area of the small intestine is about five times that of the whole body.

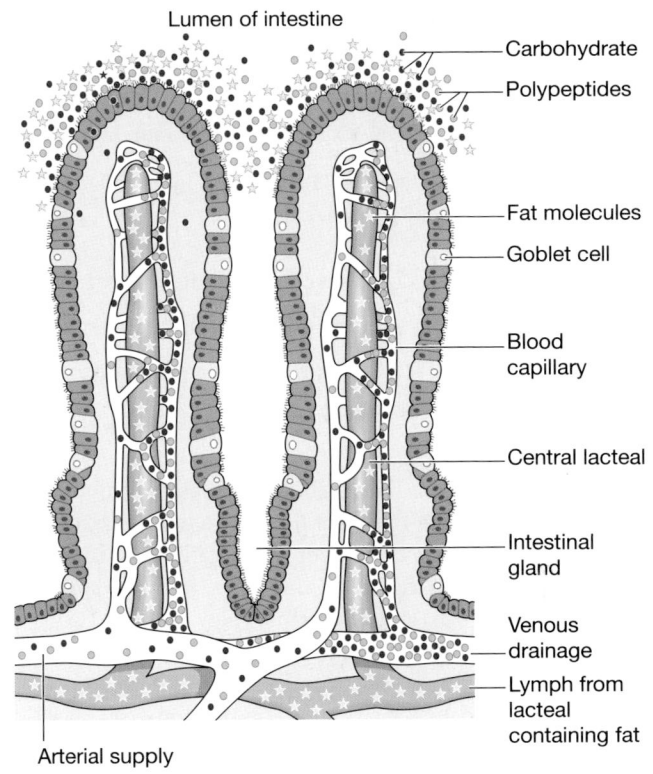

Figure 12.31 The absorption of nutrients.

Large amounts of fluid enter the alimentary tract each day (Fig. 12.32). Of this, only about 500 ml is not absorbed by the small intestine, and passes into the large intestine.

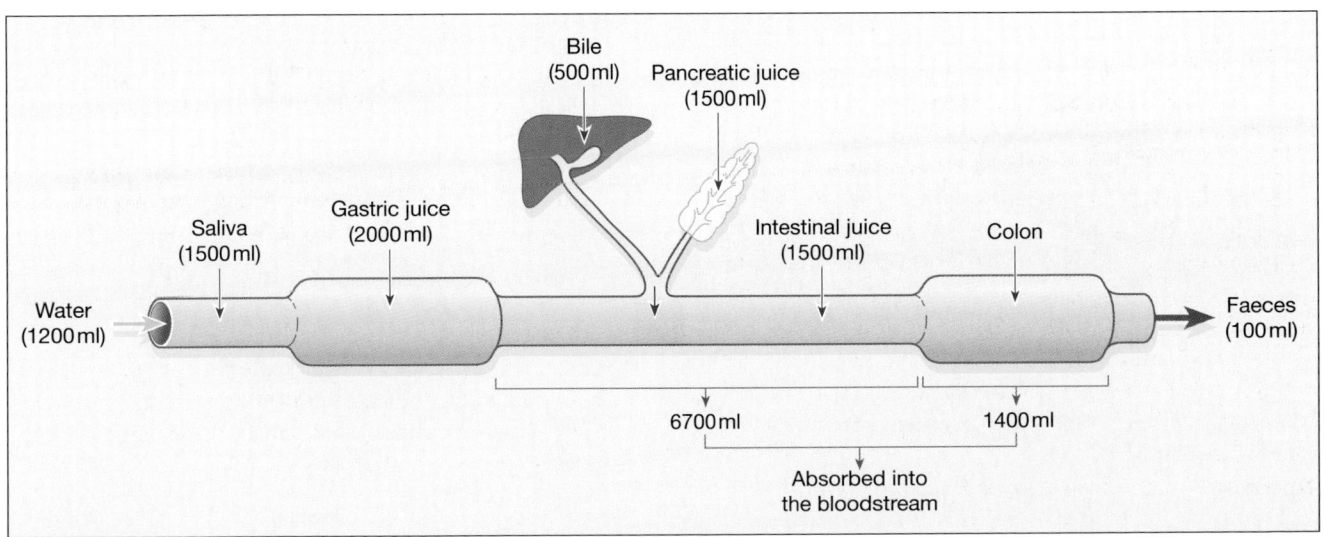

Figure 12.32 Average volumes of fluid ingested, secreted, absorbed and eliminated from the gastrointestinal tract daily.

LARGE INTESTINE (COLON), RECTUM AND ANAL CANAL

Learning outcomes

After studying this section, you should be able to:

■ identify the different sections of the large intestine

■ describe the structure and functions of the large intestine, the rectum and the anal canal.

The large intestine. This is about 1.5 metres long, beginning at the *caecum* in the right iliac fossa and terminating at the *rectum* and *anal canal* deep in the pelvis. Its lumen is larger than that of the small intestine. It forms an arch round the coiled-up small intestine (Fig. 12.33).

For descriptive purposes the colon is divided into the caecum, ascending colon, transverse colon, descending colon, sigmoid colon, rectum and anal canal.

The caecum. This is the first part of the colon. It is a dilated region which has a blind end inferiorly and is continuous with the ascending colon superiorly. Just below the junction of the two the *ileocaecal valve* opens from the ileum. The *vermiform appendix* is a fine tube, closed at one end, which leads from the caecum. It is usually about 13 cm long and has the same structure as the walls of the colon but contains more lymphoid tissue (Fig. 12.34).

The ascending colon. This passes upwards from the caecum to the level of the liver where it curves acutely to the left at the *hepatic flexure* to become the transverse colon.

The transverse colon. This is a loop of colon which extends across the abdominal cavity in front of the duodenum and the stomach to the area of the spleen where it forms the *splenic flexure* and curves acutely downwards to become the descending colon.

The descending colon. This passes down the left side of the abdominal cavity then curves towards the midline. After it enters the true pelvis it is known as the sigmoid colon.

The sigmoid colon. This part describes an S-shaped curve in the pelvis then continues downwards to become the rectum.

The rectum. This is a slightly dilated section of the colon about 13 cm long. It leads from the sigmoid colon and terminates in the anal canal.

The anal canal. This is a short passage about 3.8 cm long in the adult and leads from the rectum to the exterior. Two sphincter muscles control the anus; the *internal sphincter*, consisting of smooth muscle fibres, is under the control of the autonomic nervous system and the *external sphincter*, formed by skeletal muscle, is under voluntary control (Fig. 12.35).

Structure

The four layers of tissue described in the basic structure of the gastrointestinal tract (Fig. 12.2) are present in the colon, the rectum and the anal canal. The arrangement of the longitudinal muscle fibres is modified in the colon.

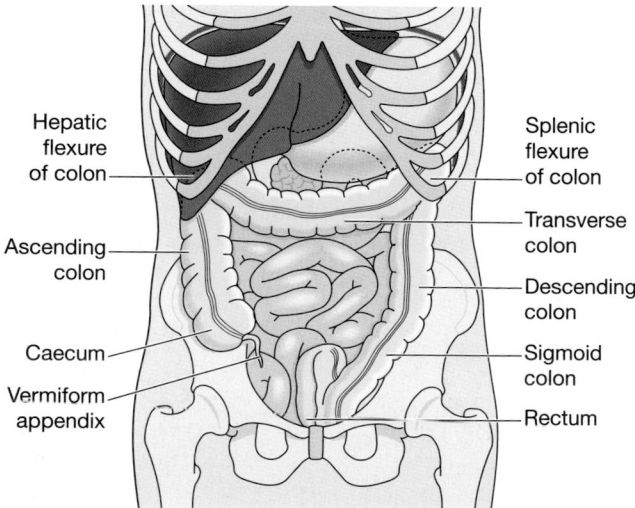

Figure 12.33 The parts of the large intestine (colon) and their positions.

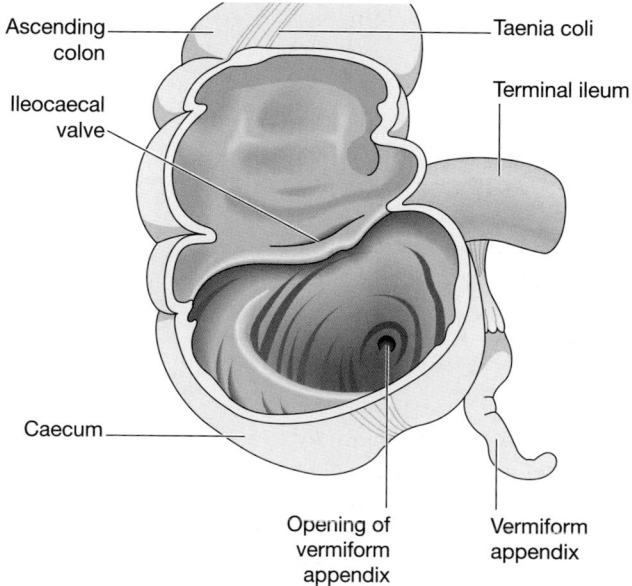

Figure 12.34 Interior of the caecum.

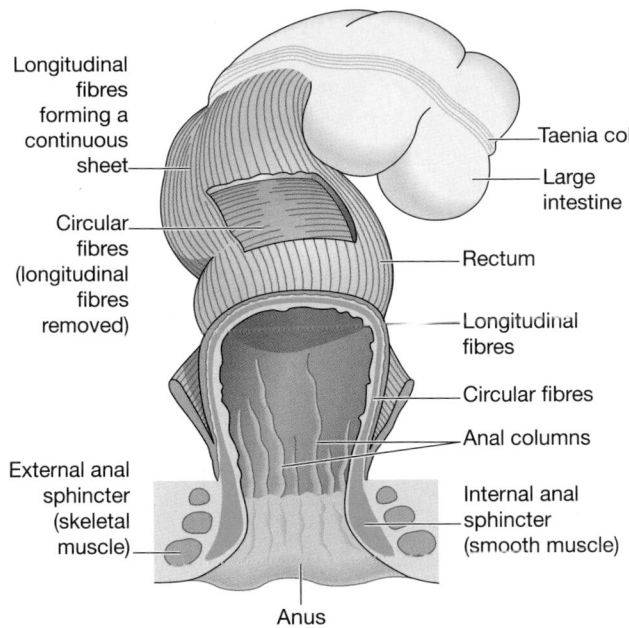

Longitudinal fibres forming a continuous sheet

Circular fibres (longitudinal fibres removed)

External anal sphincter (skeletal muscle)

Taenia coli

Large intestine

Rectum

Longitudinal fibres

Circular fibres

Anal columns

Internal anal sphincter (smooth muscle)

Anus

Figure 12.35 Arrangement of muscle fibres in the colon, rectum and anus. Sections have been removed to show the layers.

They do not form a smooth continuous layer of tissue but are collected into three bands, called *taeniae coli*, situated at regular intervals round the colon. They stop at the junction of the sigmoid colon and the rectum. As these bands of muscle tissue are slightly shorter than the total length of the colon they give a sacculated or puckered appearance to the organ (Fig. 12.35).

The longitudinal muscle fibres spread out as in the basic structure and completely surround the rectum and the anal canal. The anal sphincters are formed by thickening of the circular muscle layer.

In the submucosal layer there is more lymphoid tissue than in any other part of the alimentary tract, providing non-specific defence against invasion by resident and other microbes.

In the mucosal lining of the colon and the upper region of the rectum are large numbers of goblet cells forming simple tubular glands, which secrete mucus. They are not present beyond the junction between the rectum and the anus.

The lining membrane of the anus consists of stratified squamous epithelium continuous with the mucous membrane lining of the rectum above and which merges with the skin beyond the external anal sphincter. In the upper section of the anal canal the mucous membrane is arranged in 6 to 10 vertical folds, the *anal columns*. Each column contains a terminal branch of the superior rectal artery and vein.

Blood supply

Arterial supply is mainly by the superior and inferior mesenteric arteries (Fig. 12.8).

The *superior mesenteric artery* supplies the caecum, ascending and most of the transverse colon.

The *inferior mesenteric artery* supplies the remainder of the colon and the proximal part of the rectum.

The distal section of the rectum and the anus are supplied by branches from the *internal iliac arteries*.

Venous drainage is mainly by the *superior* and *inferior mesenteric veins* which drain blood from the parts supplied by arteries of the same names. These veins join the splenic and gastric veins to form the portal vein (Fig. 12.9). Veins draining the distal part of the rectum and the anus join the *internal iliac veins*.

Functions of the large intestine, rectum and anal canal

Absorption

The contents of the ileum which pass through the ileocaecal valve into the caecum are fluid, even though some water has been absorbed in the small intestine. In the large intestine absorption of water continues until the familiar semisolid consistency of faeces is achieved. Mineral salts, vitamins and some drugs are also absorbed into the blood capillaries from the large intestine.

Microbial activity

The large intestine is heavily colonised by certain types of bacteria, which synthesise vitamin K and folic acid. They include *Escherichia coli, Enterobacter aerogenes, Streptococcus faecalis* and *Clostridium perfringens (welchii)*. These microbes are *commensals* in humans. They may become pathogenic if transferred to another part of the body, e.g. *Escherichia coli* may cause cystitis if it gains access to the urinary bladder.

Gases in the bowel consist of some of the constituents of air, mainly nitrogen, swallowed with food and drink and as a feature of some anxiety states. Hydrogen, carbon dioxide and methane are produced by bacterial fermentation of unabsorbed nutrients, especially carbohydrate. Gases pass out of the bowel as *flatus*.

Large numbers of microbes are present in the faeces.

Mass movement

The large intestine does not exhibit peristaltic movement as it is seen in other parts of the digestive tract. Only at fairly long intervals (about twice an hour) does a wave of strong peristalsis sweep along the transverse colon forcing its contents into the descending and sigmoid colons. This is known as *mass movement* and it is often precipitated by the entry of food into the stomach. This combination of stimulus and response is called the *gastrocolic reflex*.

Defaecation

Usually the rectum is empty, but when a mass movement forces the contents of the sigmoid colon into the rectum the nerve endings in its walls are stimulated by stretch. In the infant defaecation occurs by reflex (involuntary) action. However, sometime in the second or third year of life the ability to override the defaecation reflex is developed. In practical terms this acquired voluntary control means that the brain can inhibit the reflex until such time as it is convenient to defaecate. The external anal sphincter is under conscious control through the *pudendal nerve*. Thus defaecation involves involuntary contraction of the muscle of the rectum and relaxation of the internal anal sphincter. Contraction of the abdominal muscles and lowering of the diaphragm increase the intra-abdominal pressure (Valsalva's manoeuvre) and so assist the process of defaecation. When defaecation is voluntarily postponed the feeling of fullness and need to defaecate tends to fade until the next mass movement occurs and the reflex is initiated again. Repeated suppression of the reflex may lead to constipation.

Constituents of faeces. The faeces consist of a semi-solid brown mass. The brown colour is due to the presence of stercobilin (p. 310 and Fig. 12.41).

Even though absorption of water takes place in the large intestine, water still makes up about 60 to 70% of the weight of the faeces. The remainder consists of:

- fibre (indigestible cellular plant and animal material)
- dead and live microbes
- epithelial cells from the walls of the tract
- fatty acids
- mucus secreted by the epithelial lining of the large intestine.

Mucus helps to lubricate the faeces and an adequate amount of roughage in the diet ensures that the contents of the colon are sufficiently bulky to stimulate defaecation.

PANCREAS (Fig. 12.36)

Learning outcome

After studying this section, you should be able to:

- differentiate between the structures and functions of the exocrine and endocrine pancreas.

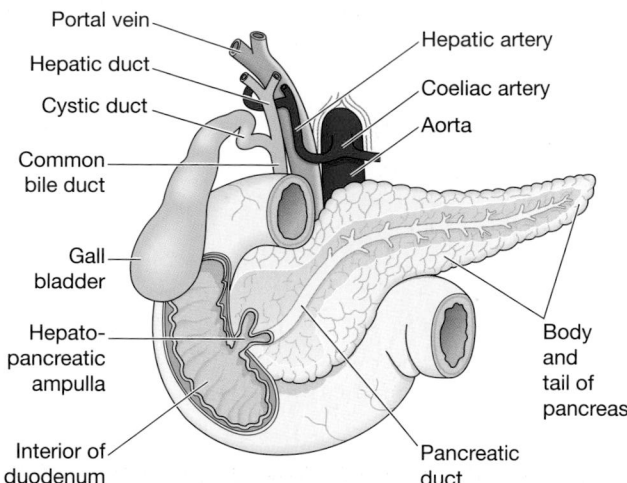

Figure 12.36 The pancreas in relation to the duodenum and biliary tract; part of the anterior wall of the duodenum has been removed.

The pancreas is a pale grey gland weighing about 60 grams. It is about 12 to 15 cm long and is situated in the epigastric and left hypochondriac regions of the abdominal cavity (see Figs 3.36 and 3.37, p. 51). It consists of a broad head, a body and a narrow tail. The head lies in the curve of the duodenum, the body behind the stomach and the tail lies in front of the left kidney and just reaches the spleen. The abdominal aorta and the inferior vena cava lie behind the gland.

The pancreas is both an exocrine and endocrine gland.

The exocrine pancreas

This consists of a large number of *lobules* made up of small alveoli, the walls of which consist of secretory cells. Each lobule is drained by a tiny duct and these unite eventually to form the *pancreatic duct*, which extends the whole length of the gland and opens into the duodenum. Just before entering the duodenum the pancreatic duct joins the *common bile duct* to form the *hepatopancreatic ampulla*. The duodenal opening of the ampulla is controlled by the *hepatopancreatic sphincter* (of Oddi).

The function of the exocrine pancreas is to produce *pancreatic juice* containing enzymes that digest carbohydrates, proteins and fats (p. 301).

The endocrine pancreas

Distributed throughout the gland are groups of specialised cells called the pancreatic islets (of Langerhans). The islets have no ducts so the hormones diffuse directly into the blood.

The function of the endocrine pancreas is to secrete the hormones insulin and glucagon, which are principally concerned with control of blood glucose levels.

Blood supply

The splenic and mesenteric arteries supply arterial blood to the pancreas and the venous drainage is by the veins of the same names that join other veins to form the portal vein (Figs 12.7 and 12.9).

Nerve supply

As in the alimentary tract, parasympathetic stimulation increases the secretion of pancreatic juice and sympathetic stimulation depresses it.

LIVER

Learning outcomes

After studying this section, you should be able to:

- describe the location of the liver in the abdominal cavity
- describe the structure of a liver lobule
- list the functions of the liver.

The liver is the largest gland in the body, weighing between 1 and 2.3 kg. It is situated in the upper part of the abdominal cavity occupying the greater part of the right hypochondriac region, part of the epigastric region and extending into the left hypochondriac region.

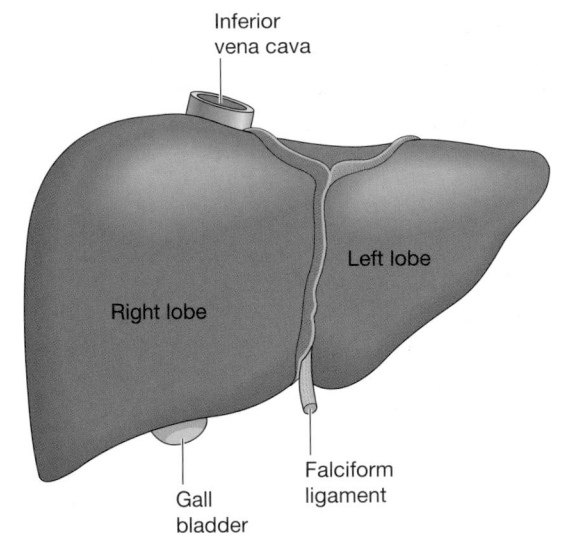

Figure 12.37 The liver: anterior view.

Its upper and anterior surfaces are smooth and curved to fit the under surface of the diaphragm (Fig. 12.37); its posterior surface is irregular in outline (Fig. 12.38).

Organs associated with the liver

Superiorly and anteriorly	— diaphragm and anterior abdominal wall
Inferiorly	— stomach, bile ducts, duodenum, hepatic flexure of the colon, right kidney and adrenal gland
Posteriorly	— oesophagus, inferior vena cava, aorta, gall bladder, vertebral column and diaphragm
Laterally	— lower ribs and diaphragm

307

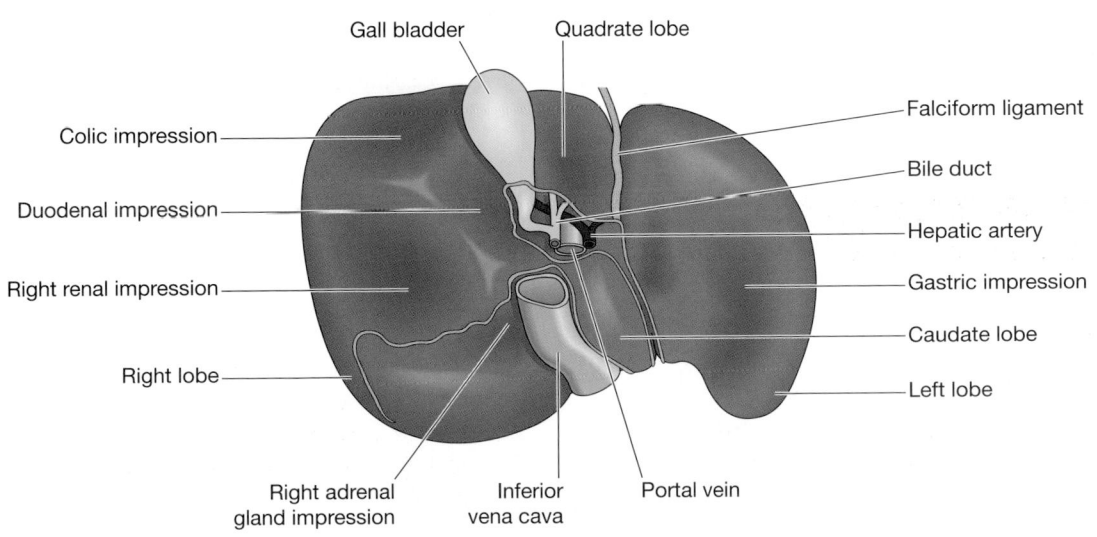

Figure 12.38 The liver, turned up to show the posterior surface.

The liver is enclosed in a thin inelastic capsule and incompletely covered by a layer of peritoneum. Folds of peritoneum form supporting ligaments attaching the liver to the inferior surface of the diaphragm. It is held in position partly by these ligaments and partly by the pressure of the organs in the abdominal cavity.

The liver has four lobes. The two most obvious are the large *right lobe* and the smaller, wedge-shaped, *left lobe*. The other two, the *caudate* and *quadrate* lobes, are areas on the posterior surface (Fig. 12.38).

The portal fissure

This is the name given to the region on the posterior surface of the liver where various structures enter and leave the gland.

The *portal vein* enters, carrying blood from the stomach, spleen, pancreas and the small and large intestines.

The *hepatic artery* enters, carrying arterial blood. It is a branch from the coeliac artery which is a branch from the abdominal aorta.

Nerve fibres, sympathetic and parasympathetic, enter here.

The *right* and *left hepatic ducts* leave, carrying bile from the liver to the gall bladder.

Lymph vessels leave the liver, draining some lymph to abdominal and some to thoracic nodes.

Blood supply (Figs 12.7 and 12.9)

The hepatic artery and the portal vein take blood to the liver. Hepatic veins, varying in number, leave the posterior surface and immediately enter the inferior vena cava just below the diaphragm.

Structure

The lobes of the liver are made up of tiny lobules just visible to the naked eye (Fig. 12.39A). These lobules are hexagonal in outline and are formed by cubical-shaped cells, the *hepatocytes*, arranged in pairs of columns radiating from a central vein. Between two pairs of columns of cells there are *sinusoids* (blood vessels with incomplete walls) containing a mixture of blood from the tiny branches of the portal vein and hepatic artery (Fig. 12.39B). This arrangement allows the arterial blood and portal venous blood (with a high concentration of nutrients) to mix and come into close contact with the liver cells. Amongst the cells lining the sinusoids are hepatic macrophages (Kupffer cells) whose function is to ingest and destroy any foreign particles present in the blood flowing through the liver.

Blood drains from the sinusoids into *central* or *centrilobular veins*. These then join with veins from other lobules, forming larger veins, until eventually they become the hepatic veins which leave the liver and empty into

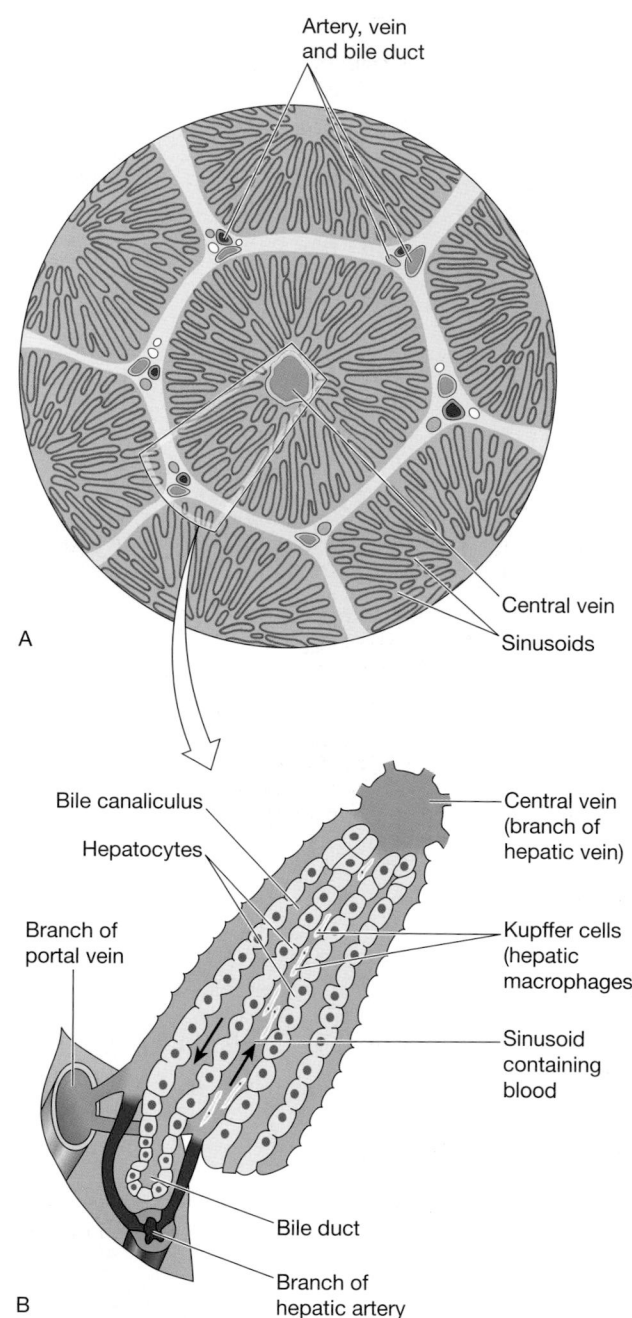

Figure 12.39 A. A magnified transverse section of a liver lobule. B. Direction of the flow of blood and bile in a liver lobule.

the inferior vena cava just below the diaphragm. Figure 12.40 shows the system of blood flow through the liver. One of the functions of the liver is to secrete *bile*. In Figure 12.39B it is seen that *bile canaliculi* run between the columns of liver cells. This means that each column of hepatocytes has a blood sinusoid on one side and a bile canaliculus on the other. The canaliculi join up to form larger bile canals until eventually they form the *right and left hepatic ducts* which drain bile from the liver.

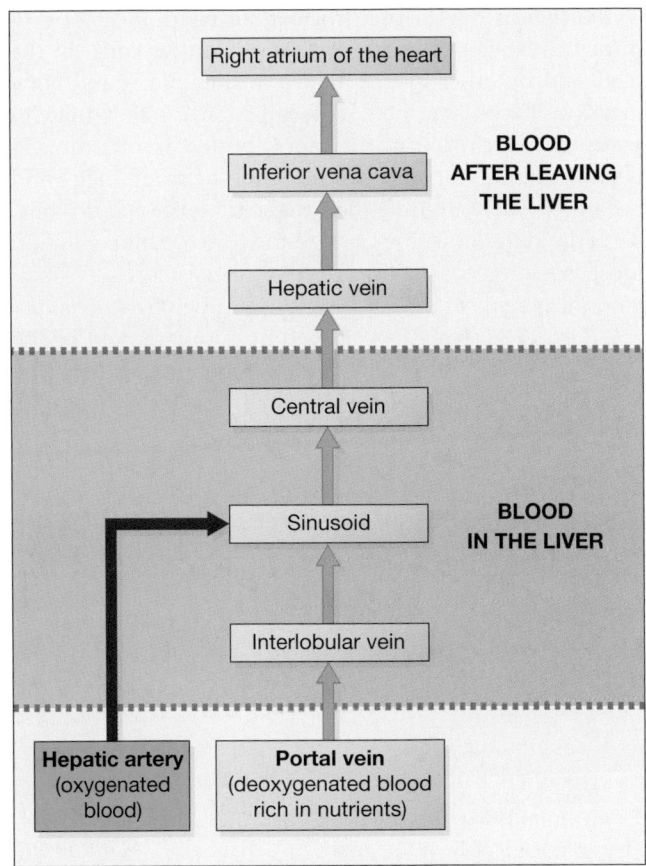

Figure 12.40 Scheme of blood flow through the liver.

Lymphoid tissue and a system of lymph vessels are present in each lobule.

Functions of the liver

The liver is an extremely active organ. Some of its functions have already been described, and they will only be mentioned here.

Carbohydrate metabolism. *Conversion of glucose to glycogen* in the presence of insulin, and converting liver glycogen back to glucose in the presence of glucagon. These changes are important regulators of the blood glucose level. After a meal the blood in the portal vein has a high glucose content and insulin converts some to glycogen for storage. Glucagon converts this glycogen back to glucose as required, to maintain the blood glucose level within relatively narrow limits.

$$\text{glucose} \underset{\text{glucagon}}{\overset{\text{insulin}}{\rightleftharpoons}} \text{glycogen}$$

Fat metabolism. *Desaturation of fat*, i.e. converts stored fat to a form in which it can be used by the tissues to provide energy.

Protein metabolism. *Deamination of amino acids*

- removes the nitrogenous portion from the amino acids not required for the formation of new protein; *urea* is formed from this nitrogenous portion which is excreted in urine.
- breaks down genetic material of worn-out cells of the body to form *uric acid* which is excreted in the urine.

Transamination—removes the nitrogenous portion of amino acids and attaches it to other carbohydrate molecules forming new non-essential amino acids (Fig. 12.46). *Synthesis of plasma proteins* and most of the *blood clotting factors* from the available amino acids occurs in the liver.

Breakdown of erythrocytes and defence against microbes. This is carried out by phagocytic Kupffer cells (hepatic macrophages) in the sinusoids.

Detoxification of drugs and noxious substances. These include ethanol (alcohol) and toxins produced by microbes.

Metabolism of ethanol. This follows consumption of alcoholic drinks.

Inactivation of hormones. These include insulin, glucagon, cortisol, aldosterone, thyroid and sex hormones.

Synthesis of vitamin A from carotene. Carotene is the provitamin found in some plants, e.g. carrots and green leaves of vegetables.

Production of heat. The liver uses a considerable amount of energy, has a high metabolic rate and produces a great deal of heat. It is the main heat-producing organ of the body.

Secretion of bile. The hepatocytes synthesise the constituents of bile from the mixed arterial and venous blood in the sinusoids. These include bile salts, bile pigments and cholesterol.

Storage. The substances include:

- fat-soluble vitamins: A, D, E, K
- iron, copper
- some water-soluble vitamins, e.g. riboflavine, niacin, pyridoxine, folic acid and vitamin B_{12}.

309

Composition of bile

About 500 ml of bile are secreted by the liver daily. Bile consists of:

- water
- mineral salts
- mucus
- bile pigments, mainly bilirubin
- bile salts, which are derived from the primary bile acids, cholic acid and chenodeoxycholic acid
- cholesterol.

The bile acids, *cholic* and *chenodeoxycholic acid*, are synthesised by hepatocytes from cholesterol, conjugated (combined) with either glycine or taurine, then secreted into bile as sodium or potassium salts. In the small intestine they emulsify fats, aiding their digestion. In the terminal ileum most of the bile salts are reabsorbed and return to the liver in the portal vein. This *enterohepatic circulation*, or recycling of bile salts, ensures that large amounts of bile salts enter the small intestine daily from a relatively small bile acid pool (Fig. 12.41).

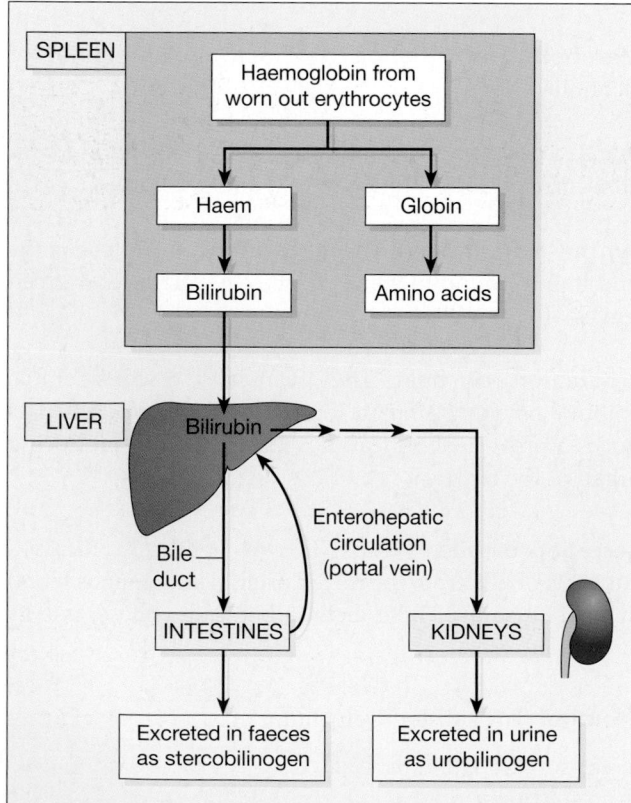

Figure 12.41 Fate of bilirubin from breakdown of worn-out erythrocytes.

Bilirubin is one of the products of haemolysis of erythrocytes by hepatic macrophages (Kupffer cells) in the liver and by other macrophages in the spleen and bone marrow. In its original form bilirubin is insoluble in water and is carried in the blood bound to albumin. In hepatocytes it is conjugated with glucuronic acid and becomes water soluble before being excreted in bile. Bacteria in the intestine change the form of bilirubin and most is excreted as *stercobilinogen* in the faeces. A small amount is reabsorbed and excreted in urine as *urobilinogen* (Fig. 12.41). Jaundice is yellow pigmentation of the tissues, seen in the skin and conjunctiva, caused by excess blood bilirubin (p. 337).

BILIARY TRACT

Learning outcomes

After studying this section, you should be able to:

- describe the route taken by bile from the liver, to the gall bladder, and then to the duodenum
- outline the structure and functions of the gall bladder.

Bile ducts (Fig. 12.42)

The *right and left hepatic ducts* join to form the *common hepatic duct* just outside the portal fissure. The hepatic duct passes downwards for about 3 cm where it is joined at an acute angle by the *cystic duct* from the gall bladder. The cystic and hepatic ducts together form the *common bile duct* which passes downwards behind the head of the pancreas to be joined by the main pancreatic duct at the *hepatopancreatic ampulla*. The opening of the combined ducts into the duodenum is controlled by the *hepatopancreatic sphincter* (sphincter of Oddi). The common bile duct is about 7.5 cm long and has a diameter of about 6 mm.

Structure

The walls of the bile ducts have the same layers of tissue as those described in the basic structure of the alimentary canal (Fig. 12.2). In the cystic duct the mucous membrane lining is arranged in irregularly situated circular folds which have the effect of a *spiral valve*. Bile passes through the cystic duct twice—once on its way into the gall bladder and again when it is expelled from the gall bladder to the common bile duct and thence to the duodenum.

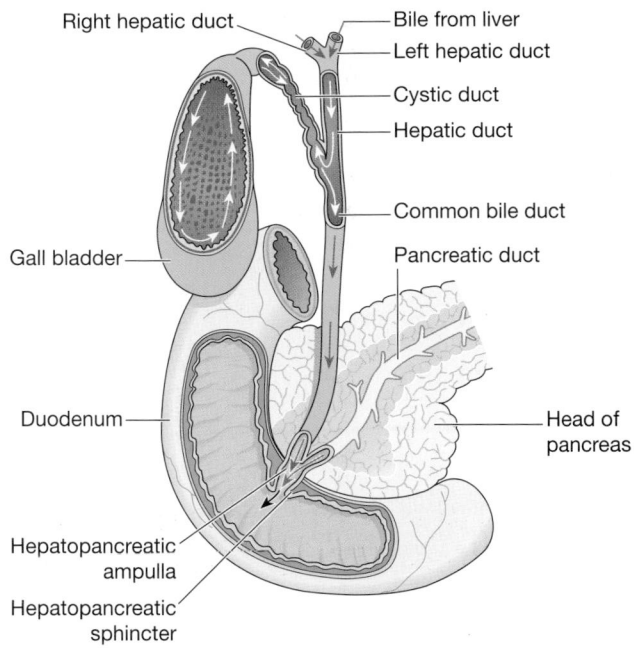

Right hepatic duct
Bile from liver
Left hepatic duct
Cystic duct
Hepatic duct
Common bile duct
Pancreatic duct
Gall bladder
Duodenum
Head of pancreas
Hepatopancreatic ampulla
Hepatopancreatic sphincter

Figure 12.42 Direction of the flow of bile from the liver to the duodenum.

Gall bladder

The gall bladder is a pear-shaped sac attached to the posterior surface of the liver by connective tissue. It has a *fundus* or expanded end, a *body* or main part and a *neck* which is continuous with the cystic duct.

Structure

The gall bladder has the same layers of tissue as those described in the basic structure of the alimentary canal, with some modifications.

Peritoneum covers only the inferior surface. The gall bladder is in contact with the posterior surface of the right lobe of the liver and is held in place by the visceral peritoneum of the liver.

Muscle layer. There is an additional layer of oblique muscle fibres.

Mucous membrane displays small rugae when the gall bladder is empty that disappear when it is distended with bile.

Blood supply

The *cystic artery*, a branch of the hepatic artery, supplies blood to the gall bladder. Blood is drained away by the *cystic vein* which joins the portal vein.

Nerve supply

Nerve impulses are conveyed by sympathetic and parasympathetic nerve fibres. There are the same autonomic plexuses as those described in the basic structure (Fig. 12.2).

Functions of the gall bladder

These include:

- reservoir for bile
- concentration of the bile by up to 10- or 15-fold, by absorption of water through the walls of the gall bladder
- release of stored bile.

When the muscle wall of the gall bladder contracts bile passes through the bile ducts to the duodenum. Contraction is stimulated by:

- the hormone *cholecystokinin* (CCK), secreted by the duodenum
- the presence of fat and acid chyme in the duodenum.

Relaxation of the hepatopancreatic sphincter (of Oddi) is caused by CCK and is a reflex response to contraction of the gall bladder.

SUMMARY OF DIGESTION AND ABSORPTION OF NUTRIENTS

> **Learning outcomes**
>
> After studying this section, you should be able to:
>
> - list the principal digestive enzymes, their sites of action, their substrates and their products
> - describe the sites of absorption of the main nutrient groups.

Table 12.2 summarises the main digestive processes to which the principal nutrient groups are subjected, the locations in the gastrointestinal tract where these processes occur and the enzymes responsible for them.

Table 12.2 Summary showing the sites of digestion and absorption of nutrients

	Mouth	Stomach	Small intestine		Large intestine
			Digestion	Absorption	
Carbohydrate	*Salivary amylase*: cooked starches to disaccharides	*Acid* denatures and stops action of salivary amylase	*Pancreatic amylase*: cooked and uncooked starches to disaccharides *Sucrase* *Maltase* *Lactase* (in enterocytes): disaccharides to monosaccharides (mainly glucose)	Into blood capillaries of villi	—
Proteins	—	*Acid*: pepsinogen to pepsin *Pepsin*: proteins to polypeptides	*Enterokinase* (in intestinal mucosa): chymotrypsinogen and trypsinogen (from pancreas) to chymotrypsin and trypsin *Chymotrypsin and trypsin*: polypeptides to di- and tripeptides *Peptidases* (in enterocytes): di- and tripeptides to amino acids	Into blood capillaries of villi	—
Fats	—	—	*Bile* (from liver): bile salts emulsify fats *Pancreatic lipase*: fats to fatty acids and glycerol *Lipases* (in enterocytes): fats to fatty acids and glycerol	Into the lacteals of the villi	—
Water	—	Small amount absorbed here	—	Most absorbed here	Remainder absorbed here
Vitamins	—	Intrinsic factor secreted for vitamin B_{12} absorption	—	Water-soluble vitamins absorbed into capillaries; fat-soluble ones into lacteals of villi	Bacteria synthesise vitamin K in colon; absorbed here

METABOLISM

Learning outcomes

After studying this section, you should be able to:

- discuss general principles of metabolism, including anabolism, catabolism, units of energy and metabolic rate

- compare and contrast the metabolic rates of the body's main energy sources (carbohydrate, protein and fat)

- describe in simple terms the central metabolic pathways; glycolysis, Krebs cycle and oxidative phosphorylation.

Metabolism constitutes all the chemical reactions that occur in the body, using absorbed nutrients to:

- provide energy by chemical oxidation of nutrients
- make new or replacement body substances.

Two types of processes are involved.

Catabolism. This process breaks down large molecules into smaller ones releasing *chemical energy* that is stored as adenosine triphosphate (ATP), and *heat*. Heat is used to maintain core body temperature at the optimum level for chemical activity (36.8°C). Excess heat is lost through the skin and excreta (p. 365).

Anabolism. This is building up, or synthesis, of large molecules from smaller ones and requires a source of energy, usually ATP.

Anabolism and catabolism usually involve a series of chemical reactions, known as *metabolic pathways*. These permit controlled, efficient and gradual transfer of energy from ATP rather than large intracellular 'explosions'. Metabolic pathways are switched on and off by hormones, providing control of metabolism and meeting individual requirements.

Both processes occur continually in all cells maintaining an energy balance. Very active tissues, such as muscle or liver, need an adequate energy supply to support their requirements.

Energy

The energy produced in the body may be measured and expressed in units of work (*joules*) or units of heat (kilocalories).

A kilocalorie (kcal) is the amount of heat required to raise the temperature of 1 litre of water by 1 degree Celsius (1°C). On a daily basis, the body's collective metabolic processes generate a total of about 3 million kilocalories.

1 kcal = 4184 joules (J) = 4.184 kilojoules (kJ)

The nutritional value of carbohydrates, protein and fats eaten in the diet may be expressed in *kilojoules per gram* or kcal per gram.

1 gram of carbohydrate provides 17 kilojoules (4 kcal)
1 gram of protein provides 17 kilojoules (4 kcal)
1 gram of fat provides 38 kilojoules (9 kcal)

Energy balance

Body weight remains constant when energy intake in the form of nutrients is equal to energy use. When intake exceeds requirement, body weight increases. Conversely, body weight decreases when nutrient intake does not meet energy requirements.

Metabolic rate

The metabolic rate is the rate at which energy is released from the fuel molecules inside cells. As most of the processes involved require oxygen and produce carbon dioxide as waste, the metabolic rate can be estimated by measuring oxygen uptake or carbon dioxide excretion.

The *basal metabolic rate* (BMR) is the rate of metabolism when the individual is at rest in a warm environment and is in the *post-absorptive state*, i.e. has not had a meal for at least 12 hours. In this state the release of energy is sufficient to meet only the essential needs of vital organs, such as the heart, lungs, nervous system and kidneys. The post-absorptive state is important because the intake of food, especially protein, stimulates an increase in metabolic rate, possibly due to increased energy utilisation by the liver. This is called the *specific dynamic action* (SDA) of food. In measuring the BMR, the surface area of the body is taken into account because energy in the form of heat is lost through the skin. Surface area in square metres is calculated from the height and weight of the individual. Some of the wide variety of factors that affect the metabolic rate are shown in Table 12.3.

Most foods contain a mixture of different amounts of carbohydrate, protein, fat, minerals, vitamins, fibre and water. Carbohydrates, proteins and fats are the sources of energy and they are obtained from the variety of food, usually in the following proportions:

protein	10–15%
fat	15–30%
carbohydrate	55–75%

313

Table 12.3 Factors affecting metabolic rate

Factor	Effect on metabolic rate
Age	Gradually reduced with age
Gender	Higher in men than women
Height, weight	Relatively higher in small people
Pregnancy, menstruation, lactation	Increased
Ingestion of food	Increased
Muscular activity	Increased
Elevated body temperature	Increased
Excess thyroid hormones	Increased
Starvation	Decreased

Central metabolic pathways

Much of the metabolic effort of cells is concerned with energy production to fuel cellular activities. Certain common pathways are central to this function. Fuel molecules enter these central energy-producing pathways and in a series of steps, during which a series of intermediate molecules are formed and energy is released, these fuel molecules are chemically broken down. The end results of these processes are energy production and carbon dioxide and water (called metabolic water) formation. Much of the energy is stored as ATP, although some is lost as heat. The carbon dioxide is excreted through the lungs.

The preferred fuel molecule is glucose, but alternatives should glucose be unavailable include amino acids, fatty acids, glycerol and occasionally nucleic acids. Each of these may enter the central energy-producing pathways and be converted to energy, carbon dioxide and water. There are three central metabolic pathways (Fig. 12.48):

- glycolysis
- the citric acid or Krebs cycle
- oxidative phosphorylation.

Products from glycolysis enter the citric acid cycle, and products from the citric acid cycle proceed to oxidative phosphorylation. The fates of the different fuel molecules entering the central metabolic pathways are discussed in the following sections.

Metabolism of carbohydrate

Erythrocytes and neurones can use only glucose for fuel and therefore maintenance of blood glucose levels is needed to provide a constant energy source to these cells. Most other cells can also use other sources of fuel.

Digested carbohydrate, mainly glucose, is absorbed into the blood capillaries of the villi of the small intestine. It is transported by the portal circulation to the liver, where it is dealt with in several ways (Fig. 12.43):

- Glucose may be oxidised to provide the chemical energy, in the form of ATP, necessary for the considerable metabolic activity which takes place in the liver (p. 309).
- Some glucose may remain in the circulating blood to maintain the normal blood glucose of about 2.5 to 5.3 millimoles per litre (mmol/l) (45 to 95 mg/100 ml).
- Some glucose, if in excess of the above requirements, may be converted to the insoluble polysaccharide, *glycogen*, in the liver and in skeletal muscles. *Insulin* is the hormone necessary for this change to take place. The formation of glycogen inside cells is a means of storing carbohydrate without upsetting the osmotic equilibrium. Before it can be used to maintain blood levels or to provide ATP it must be broken down again into its constituent glucose units. Liver

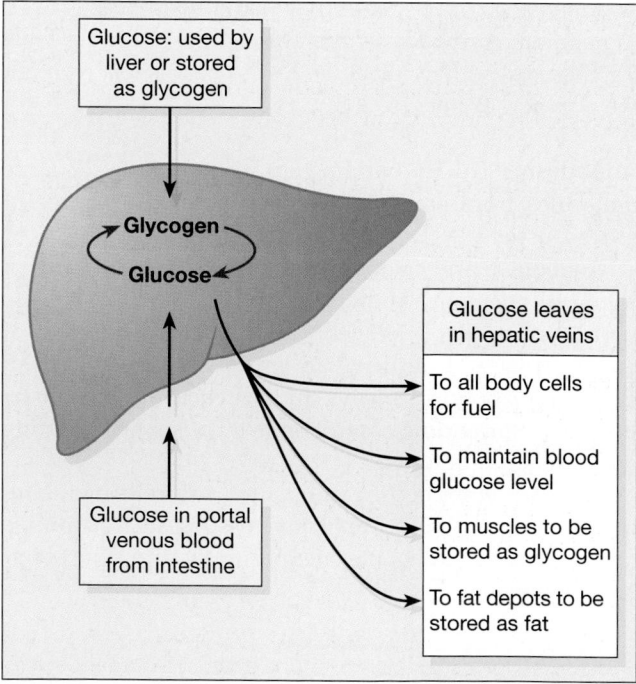

Figure 12.43 Summary of the source, distribution and use of glucose.

glycogen constitutes a store of glucose used for liver activity and to maintain the blood glucose level. Muscle glycogen provides the glucose requirement of muscle activity. *Adrenaline, thyroxine* and *glucagon* are the main hormones associated with the breakdown of glycogen to glucose.

■ Carbohydrate in excess of that required to maintain the blood glucose level and glycogen level in the tissues is converted to fat and stored in the fat depots.

All the cells of the body require energy to carry out their metabolic processes including multiplication of cells for replacement of worn out cells, contraction of muscle fibres and synthesis of secretions produced by glandular tissues. The oxidation of carbohydrate and fat provides most of the energy required by the body. When glycogen stores are low and more glucose is needed, the body can make glucose from non-carbohydrate sources, e.g. amino acids, glycerol. This is called *gluconeogenesis* (formation of new glucose).

Carbohydrate and energy release (Fig. 12.44)

Glucose is broken down in the body giving energy, carbon dioxide and metabolic water. Catabolism of glucose occurs in a series of steps with a little energy being released at each stage. The total number of ATP molecules which may be generated from the complete breakdown of one molecule of glucose is 38, but for this to be achieved the process must occur in the presence of oxygen (aerobically). In the absence of oxygen (anaerobically) this number is greatly reduced; the process is therefore significantly less efficient.

Aerobic respiration (catabolism). Aerobic catabolism of glucose can occur only if the oxygen supply is adequate, and is the process by which energy is released during prolonged, manageable exercise. When exercise levels become very intense, the energy requirements of the muscle outstrip the oxygen supply, and anaerobic breakdown then occurs. Such high levels of activity can be sustained for only short periods, because there is accumulation of wastes (mainly lactic acid) and reduced efficiency of the energy production process.

The first stage of glucose catabolism is glycolysis. This is an anaerobic process that takes place in the cytoplasm of the cell. Through a number of intermediate steps one glucose molecule is converted to two molecules of pyruvic acid, with the net production of two molecules of ATP. The remainder of the considerable energy stores locked up in the original molecule of glucose is released only if there is enough oxygen to allow the pyruvic acid molecules to enter the biochemical

Figure 12.44 Oxidation of glucose.

roundabout called the citric acid cycle (Fig. 12.44). This takes place in the mitochondria of the cell and is oxygen dependent. For every two molecules of pyruvic acid entering the citric acid cycle, a further two molecules of ATP are formed. This is far short of the maximum 38 ATP molecules that can be formed. The remaining 34 molecules of ATP come from the third energy-generating process, oxidative phosphorylation, a process dependent on hydrogen atoms released during earlier stages of glucose breakdown. Oxidative phosphorylation, like the citric acid cycle, can occur only in the presence of oxygen and takes place in the mitochondria.

Anaerobic catabolism. When oxygen levels in the cell are low, the molecule of glucose still undergoes glycolysis and is split into two molecules of pyruvic acid, because glycolysis is an anaerobic process. However, the pyruvic acid does not enter the citric acid cycle or progress to oxidative phosphorylation; instead it is converted anaerobically to lactic acid. Build-up of lactic acid causes the pain and cramps of overexercised muscles. When oxygen levels are restored, lactic acid is reconverted to pyruvic acid, which may then enter the citric acid cycle.

Fate of the end products of carbohydrate metabolism

Lactic acid. Some of the lactic acid produced by anaerobic catabolism of glucose may be oxidised in the cells to carbon dioxide and water but first it must be changed back to pyruvic acid. If complete oxidation does not take place, lactic acid passes to the liver in the circulating blood where it is converted to glucose and may then take any of the pathways open to glucose (Fig. 12.43).

Carbon dioxide. This is excreted from the body as a gas by the lungs.

Metabolic water. This is added to the considerable amount of water already present in the body; excess is excreted as urine by the kidneys.

Metabolism of protein

Dietary protein consists of a number of amino acids (p. 272). About *20 amino acids* have been named and nine of these are described as *essential* because they cannot be synthesised in the body. The remainder are described as *non-essential* amino acids because they can be synthesised by many tissues. The enzymes involved in this process are called *transaminases*. Digestion breaks down the protein of the diet to its constituent amino acids in preparation for transfer into the blood capillaries of the villi in the wall of the small intestine. In the portal circulation amino acids are transported to the liver then into the general circulation, thus making them available to all the cells and tissues of the body. Different cells choose from those available the particular amino acids required for building or repairing their specific type of tissue and for synthesising their secretions, e.g. antibodies, enzymes or hormones.

Amino acids not required for building and repairing body tissues cannot be stored and are broken down in the liver.

- The *nitrogenous part*, the amino group (NH_2) is converted to ammonia (NH_3) and then combined with carbon dioxide forming *urea* by the process of *deamination* and excreted in the urine.
- The remaining part is used to provide energy, as glucose by gluconeogenesis, or stored as fat, if in excess of immediate requirements.

Amino acid pool (Fig. 12.45)

A small pool of amino acids is maintained within the body. This is the source from which the different cells of the body draw the amino acids they need to synthesise their own materials, e.g. new cells, secretions such as enzymes, hormones and plasma proteins.

Sources of amino acids

Exogenous. These are derived from the protein eaten in the diet.

Figure 12.45 Sources and use of amino acids in the body.

Endogenous. These are obtained from the breakdown of body protein. In an adult about 80 to 100 g of protein are broken down and replaced each day. Intestinal mucosa has the most rapid turnover of cells.

Loss of amino acids

Deamination. Amino acids not needed by the body are deaminated, mainly in the liver. The nitrogenous part, or amino group (NH_2) is converted to ammonia (NH_3^+) and then to urea before being excreted by the kidneys. The remainder is used to provide energy and heat.

Excretion. The faeces contain a considerable amount of protein consisting of desquamated cells from the lining of the alimentary tract.

Endogenous and exogenous amino acids are mixed in the 'pool' and the body is said to be in *nitrogen balance* when the rate of removal from the pool is equal to the additions to it. Unlike carbohydrates, the body has no capacity for the storage of amino acids except for this relatively small pool. Figure 12.46 depicts what happens to amino acids in the body.

Amino acids and energy release (Fig. 12.48)

Proteins, in the form of amino acids, are potential fuel molecules that are used by the body only when other energy sources are low, e.g. in starvation. To supply the amino acids for use as fuel the body breaks down muscle, its main protein source. Some amino acids can be converted directly to glucose, which enters glycolysis. Other amino acids are changed to intermediate compounds of

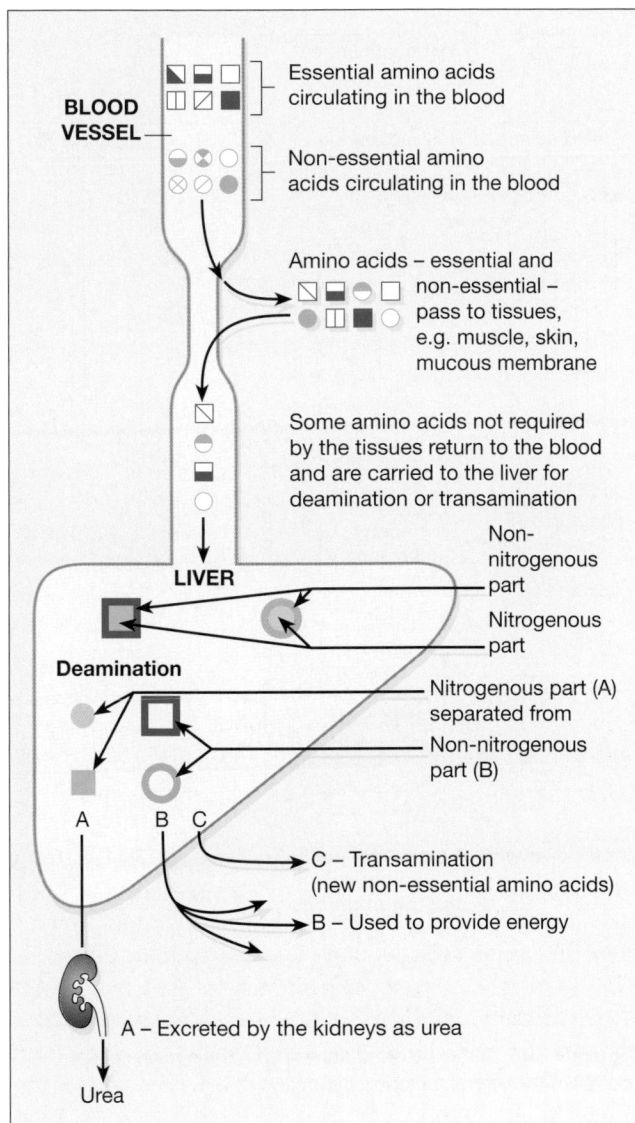

Figure 12.46 The fate of amino acids in the body.

the central metabolic pathways, e.g. acetyl coenzyme A or oxaloacetic acid, and therefore enter the system at a later stage.

Metabolism of fat (Fig. 12.47)

Fat is synthesised from carbohydrates and proteins which are taken into the body in excess of its needs and stored in the fat depots, i.e. under the skin, in the omentum or around the kidneys.

Fats which have been digested and absorbed as fatty acids and glycerol into the *lacteals* are transported via the cisterna chyli and the thoracic duct to the bloodstream and so, by a circuitous route, to the liver. Fatty acids and

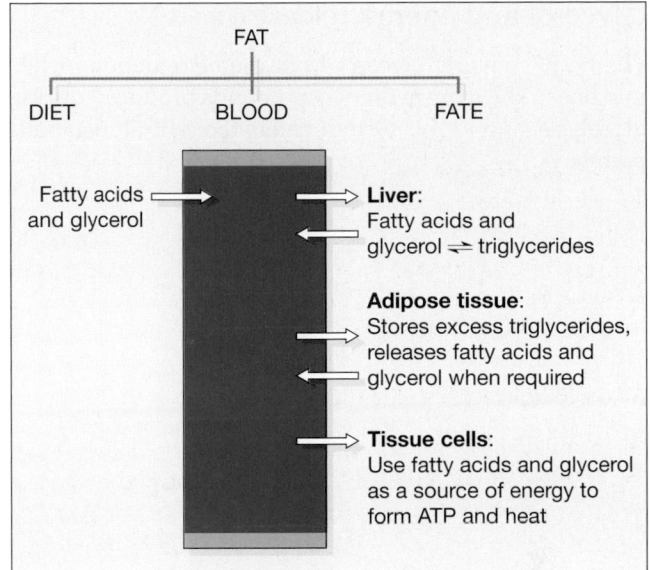

Figure 12.47 Sources, distribution and use of fats in the body.

glycerol circulating in the blood are used by the cells of organs and glands to provide energy and in the synthesis of some of their secretions. In the liver some fatty acids and glycerol are used to provide energy and heat, and some are recombined forming *triglycerides*, the form in which fat is stored. A triglyceride consists of three fatty acids chemically combined with a glycerol molecule (see Fig. 2.9, p. 24). When required, triglycerides are converted back to fatty acids and glycerol and used to provide energy. The end products of fat metabolism are energy, heat, carbon dioxide and water.

Fatty acids and energy release

When body tissues are deprived of glucose, as occurs in starvation, low-calorie diets or in uncontrolled diabetes mellitus, the body uses alternative energy sources, mainly fat stores. Fatty acids may be converted to acetyl coenzyme A, and enter the energy production pathway in that form. One consequence of this is accumulation of ketone bodies, which are produced in the liver from acetyl coenzyme A when levels are too high for processing through the citric acid cycle (Fig. 12.48). Ketone bodies then enter the blood and can be used by other body tissues, including the brain (which is usually glucose dependent) as a source of fuel. However, at high concentrations, ketones are toxic, particularly in the brain. In uncontrolled diabetes mellitus, insulin deficiency results in very high blood sugar levels (hyperglycaemia). Accumulating ketones are excreted by the lungs and give a sweet acetone-like smell to the breath. Ketones are also excreted in the urine (ketonuria).

Glycerol and energy release (Fig. 12.48)

The body converts glycerol from the degradation of fats into one of the intermediary compounds produced during glycolysis, and in this form it enters the central metabolic pathways.

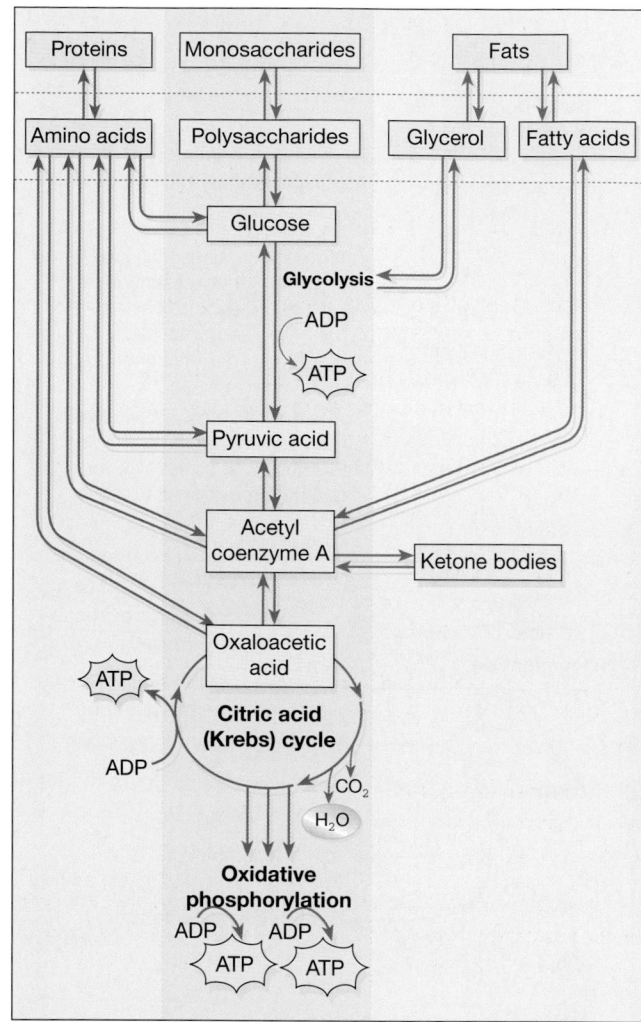

Figure 12.48 Summary of the fates of the three main energy sources in the central metabolic pathways.

DISEASES OF THE MOUTH

Learning outcomes

After studying this section, you should be able to:

■ discuss the main inflammatory and infectious conditions of the mouth

■ describe briefly the site and effects of oral squamous cell carcinoma

■ distinguish between cleft lip and cleft palate, including describing the anatomical abnormalities involved.

Inflammatory and infectious conditions

Physical damage

Injury may be caused to tissues in and around the mouth by foods and other substances taken into the mouth, if they are:

■ excessively hot or cold
■ abrasive
■ corrosive.

Corrosive chemicals are the most likely to cause serious tissue damage and acute inflammation. The outcome depends on the extent and depth of the injury.

Thrush (oral candidiasis)

This acute fungal infection of the epithelium of the mouth is caused by the yeast *Candida albicans*. In adults it causes infection mainly in debilitated people and in those whose immunity is suppressed by steroids, antibiotics or cytotoxic drugs. In babies it may be a severe infection, sometimes causing epidemics in nurseries by cross-infection. It occurs most commonly in bottle-fed babies. *Chronic thrush* may develop, affecting the roof of the mouth in people who wear dentures. The fungus survives in the fine grooves on the upper surface of the denture and repeatedly reinfects the epithelium.

Angular cheilitis

Painful cracks develop in folds of tissue at the corners of the mouth, usually occurring in elderly debilitated people, especially if they do not wear their dentures and the folds remain moist. The usual causal organisms are *Candida albicans* and *Staphylococcus aureus*.

Dietary deficiency of iron and vitamins in the B group predispose to this condition.

Acute gingivitis (Vincent's infection)

This is an acute infection with severe ulceration of the lips, gums, mouth, throat and the palatine tonsil. It is caused by two commensal organisms acting together, *Borrelia vincenti* and a fusiform bacillus. Both organisms may be present in the mouth and only cause the disease in the presence of:

■ malnutrition
■ debilitating disease
■ poor mouth hygiene
■ injury caused by previous infection.

Aphthous stomatitis (recurrent oral ulceration)

Extremely painful ulcers occur singly or in crops inside the mouth. They are often found in association with iron and vitamin B group deficiency but a link has not been established.

Viral infections

Acute herpetic gingivostomatitis
This is caused by *Herpes simplex* virus and is the commonest oral virus infection. It is characterised by extensive and very painful ulceration.

Secondary or recurrent herpes lesions (cold sores)
Lesions, caused by *Herpes simplex* virus, occur round the nose and on the lips. After an outbreak the viruses remain dormant within the cells. Later outbreaks, usually at the same site, are precipitated by a variety of stimuli including failing immune response in old age.

Tumours of the mouth

Squamous cell carcinoma
This is the most common type of malignant tumour in the mouth and carries a poor prognosis. The usual sites are the lower lip and the edge of the tongue. Ulceration occurs frequently and there is early spread to surrounding tissues and cervical lymph nodes.

Developmental defects

Cleft palate and cleft lip (harelip)
During embryonic development, the roof of the mouth (hard palate) develops as two separate (right and left)

319

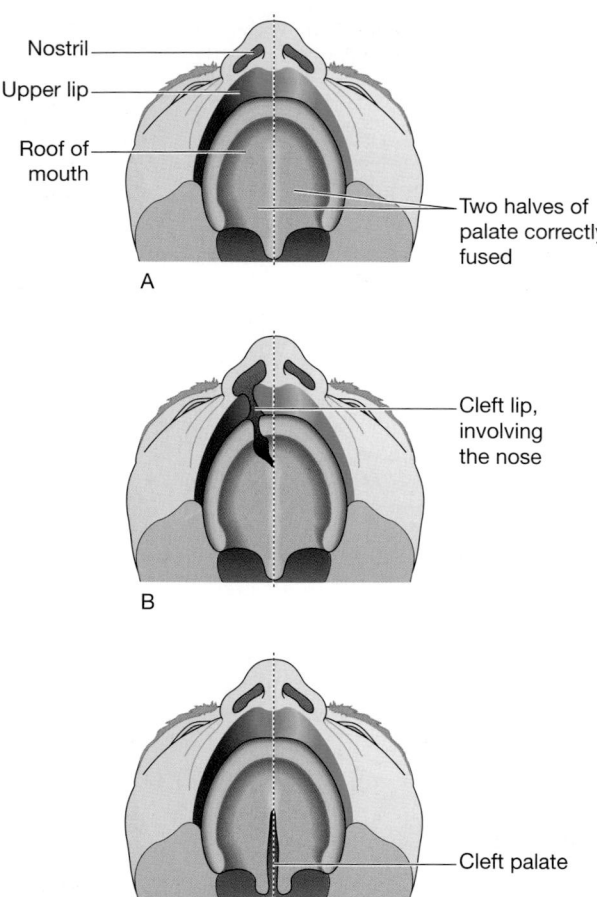

Figure labels: Nostril, Upper lip, Roof of mouth — A; Two halves of palate correctly fused. Cleft lip, involving the nose — B. Cleft palate — C.

Figure 12.49 Cleft lip and cleft palate: A. Normal hard palate. B. Cleft lip. C. Cleft palate.

halves; this occurs from the lips anteriorly to the uvula posteriorly. Before birth, these two halves fuse along the midline. If fusion is incomplete, a cleft (division) occurs, which may be very minor, or it may be substantial. *Cleft lip* (Fig. 12.49B) may be merely a minor notch in the upper lip, or substantial when the lip is completely split in one or two places and the nose is involved. In *cleft palate*, there is a gap between the two halves of the palate, which creates a channel of communication between the mouth and the nasal cavity (Fig. 12.49C). Factors believed to play a causative part in these conditions include genetic abnormalities, and fetal exposure to detrimental factors such as hypoxia, certain drugs or poor nutrition, between weeks 7 and 10 of pregnancy.

Speech development, and the activities of eating and drinking, cannot take place normally until the defect has been surgically repaired.

DISEASES OF THE PHARYNX

Tonsillitis and diphtheria are described on pages 258 and 259.

DISEASES OF THE SALIVARY GLANDS

Learning outcomes

After studying this section, you should be able to:

- outline the pathophysiology of mumps
- explain the nature of salivary calculi
- describe the commonest tumours of the salivary glands.

Mumps

This is an acute inflammatory condition of the salivary glands, especially the parotids. It is caused by the mumps virus, one of the parainfluenza group. The virus is inhaled in infected droplets and during the 18- to 21-day incubation period viruses multiply elsewhere in the body before spreading to the salivary glands. The virus is present in saliva for about 7 days before and after symptoms appear so infection may spread to others during this 2-week period. They may also spread to:

- the pancreas, causing pancreatitis
- the testes, causing orchitis after puberty and sometimes atrophy of the glands and sterility
- the brain, causing meningitis or meningoencephalitis.

In developed countries, children are usually vaccinated against mumps in their preschool years.

Calculus formation

Calculi (stones) are formed in the salivary glands by the crystallisation of mineral salts in saliva. They may partially or completely block the ducts, leading to swelling of the gland, a predisposition to infection and, in time, atrophy. The causes are not known.

Tumours of the salivary glands

Mixed tumours (pleomorphic salivary adenoma)

This benign tumour consists of epithelial and connective tissue cells and occurs mainly in the parotid gland. A second tumour may develop in the same gland several years after the first has been removed. It rarely undergoes malignant change.

Carcinoma

Malignant tumours may occur in any salivary gland or duct. Some forms have a tendency to infiltrate nerves in the surrounding tissues, causing severe pain. Lymph spread is to the cervical nodes.

DISEASES OF THE OESOPHAGUS

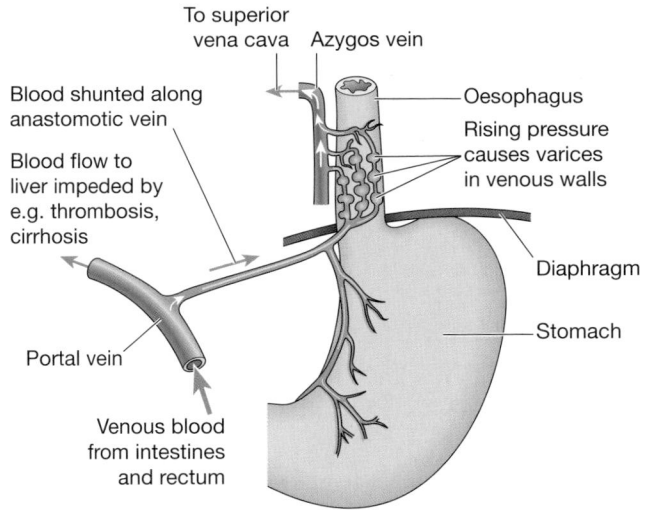

Figure 12.50 Oesophageal varices.

Learning outcomes

After studying this section, you should be able to:

- explain how oesophageal varices develop

- discuss the main inflammatory conditions of the oesophagus

- list the likely causes of oesophageal rupture

- describe the main oesophageal tumours

- define oesophageal atresia and tracheo-oesophageal fistula.

Oesophageal varices (Fig. 12.50)

In conditions such as cirrhosis or venous thrombosis, blood flow into the liver via the portal vein is obstructed and blood pressure within the portal system rises (portal hypertension). This forces blood from the portal vein into anastomotic veins, which redirect (shunt) blood into the systemic venous circulation, bypassing the liver. Fifty per cent or more of the portal blood may be shunted into anastomotic veins, leading to rising pressure in these veins too. One route taken by the shunted blood is into veins of the distal oesophagus, which become distended and weakened by the abnormally high volume of blood. *Varices* develop when the weakest regions of the vessel wall bulge outwards into the lumen of the oesophagus, and, being thin walled and fragile, they are easily eroded by swallowed foodstuffs. Bleeding may be slight, but chronic, leading to iron deficiency anaemia; however, sudden rupture can cause life-threatening haemorrhage.

Inflammatory and infectious conditions

Peptic reflux oesophagitis

This condition, the commonest cause of indigestion, is caused by persistent regurgitation of acid gastric juice into the oesophagus, causing irritation and painful ulceration. Haemorrhage occurs when blood vessels are eroded. Persistent reflux leads to chronic inflammation and if damage is extensive, secondary healing with fibrosis occurs. Shrinkage of ageing fibrous tissue may cause stricture of the oesophagus. Reflux of gastric contents is associated with:

- increase in the intra-abdominal pressure, e.g. in pregnancy, constipation and obesity
- high acid content of gastric juice
- low levels of secretion of the hormone gastrin, leading to reduced sphincter action at the lower end of the oesophagus
- the presence of hiatus hernia (p. 330).

Swallowing caustic materials

When swallowed, caustic materials burn the walls of the oesophagus causing an inflammatory reaction. The extent of the damage depends on the concentration and amount swallowed. Following severe injury, healing causes fibrosis, and there is a risk of oesophageal stricture developing later, as the fibrous tissue shrinks.

Microbial infections

Infections are relatively rare and are usually spread from the mouth or pharynx. The microbes most commonly involved are *Candida albicans*, which causes thrush, and herpes viruses. Bottle-fed babies and adults with diminished immunity are most susceptible.

Achalasia

This problem tends to occur in young adults. The cardiac sphincter is constricted and, because of this obstruction blocking the passage of ingested materials into the stomach, the oesophagus becomes dilated and the muscle layer hypertrophies. Autonomic nerve supply to the oesophageal muscle is abnormal, but the cause of the condition is not known.

The condition may lead to dysphagia, regurgitation of gastric contents and possibly aspiration pneumonia.

Oesophageal rupture

This may occur, usually at the distal end, if the oesophagus is suddenly distended:

- during a vomiting attack
- by ingestion of foreign bodies
- by passage of an instrument.

Gastric contents pass into the mediastinum, causing acute inflammation. The cause of weakness in the wall of the oesophagus is not known.

Tumours of the oesophagus

Benign tumours occur rarely.

Malignant tumours

These occur more often in males than females. The most common sites are the distal end of the oesophagus and at the levels of the larynx and bifurcation of the trachea. The tumours are mainly of two types, either of which may eventually lead to oesophageal obstruction.

Scirrhous (fibrous) tumours. These spread round the circumference and along the oesophagus. They cause thickening of the wall and loss of elasticity.

Soft tissue tumours. These grow into the lumen and spread along the wall.

The causes of malignant change are not known but may be associated with diet and regular consumption of very hot food.

Spread of a malignant tumour at the level of the bifurcation of the trachea may ulcerate the wall of the oesophagus, the trachea or a bronchus, leading to aspiration pneumonia. Other local spread may involve adjacent mediastinal structures, such as lymph nodes. Death is usually due to oesophageal obstruction before metastasis occurs.

Congenital abnormalities

The most common congenital abnormalities of the oesophagus are:

- *oesophageal atresia* in which the lumen is narrow or blocked
- *tracheo-oesophageal fistula* in which there is an opening between the oesophagus and the trachea through which milk or regurgitated gastric contents are aspirated.

One or both abnormalities may be present. The causes of these developmental deficiencies are not known.

DISEASES OF THE STOMACH

Learning outcomes

After studying this section, you should be able to:

- compare the main features of chronic and acute gastritis

- discuss the pathophysiology of peptic ulcer disease

- describe the main tumours of the stomach and their consequences

- define the term congenital pyloric stenosis.

Gastritis

This is a common condition which occurs when an imbalance between the corrosive action of gastric juice and the protective effect of mucus on the gastric mucosa develops. The amount of mucus in the stomach is insufficient to protect the surface epithelium from the destructive effects of hydrochloric acid. It may be acute or chronic.

Acute gastritis

Gastritis occurs with varying degrees of severity. The most severe form is *acute haemorrhagic gastritis*. When the surface epithelium of the stomach is exposed to acid gastric juice the cells absorb hydrogen ions which increase their internal acidity, disrupt their metabolic processes and trigger the inflammatory reaction. The causes of acute gastritis include:

- regular prolonged use of aspirin and other anti-inflammatory drugs, especially the non-steroids
- regular excessive alcohol consumption
- food poisoning caused by, e.g., *Staphylococcus aureus, Salmonella paratyphi* or viruses
- heavy cigarette smoking
- treatment with cytotoxic drugs and ionising radiation
- ingestion of corrosive poisons, acids and alkalis
- regurgitation of bile into the stomach.

The outcome depends on the extent of the damage. In many cases recovery is uneventful after the cause is removed. In the most severe forms there is ulceration of the mucosa that may be followed by haemorrhage, perforation of the stomach wall and peritonitis. Where there has been extensive tissue damage, healing is by fibrosis causing reduced elasticity and peristalsis.

Chronic gastritis

Chronic gastritis is a milder longer-lasting form. It may follow repeated acute attacks or be an autoimmune disease and is more common in later life.

Helicobacter-associated gastritis

The microbe *Helicobacter pylori* is known to be associated with gastric conditions, especially chronic gastritis and peptic ulcer disease. Antibodies to this microbe develop in early adulthood although lesions of gastritis occur later in life.

Autoimmune chronic gastritis

This is a progressive form of the disease. Destructive inflammatory changes that begin on the surface of the mucous membrane may extend to affect its whole thickness, including the gastric glands. When this stage is reached, the secretion of digestive enzymes, hydrochloric acid and intrinsic factor are markedly reduced. The antigens are the gastric parietal cells and the *intrinsic factor* they secrete. When these cells are destroyed as a result of this abnormal autoimmune condition, the inflammation subsides. The initial causes of the autoimmunity are not known but there is a familial predisposition and an association with chronic thyroiditis, thyrotoxicosis and atrophy of the adrenal glands. Secondary effects include:

- pernicious anaemia due to lack of intrinsic factor (p. 70)
- impairment of digestion due to lack of enzymes
- microbial infection due to lack of hydrochloric acid.

Peptic ulceration

Ulceration of the gastrointestinal mucosa is caused by disruption of the normal balance of the corrosive effect of gastric juice and the protective effect of mucus on the gastric epithelial cells. It may be viewed as an extension of the cell damage found in acute gastritis. The most common sites for ulcers are the stomach and the first few centimetres of the duodenum. More rarely they occur in the oesophagus, following reflux of gastric juice, and round the anastomosis of the stomach and small intestine, following gastrectomy. The underlying causes are not known but, if factors associated with the maintenance of healthy mucosa are defective, acid gastric juice gains access to the epithelium, causing the initial cell damage that leads to ulceration. The main factors are: normal blood supply, mucus secretion and cell replacement.

Blood supply

Reduced blood flow and ischaemia may be caused by excessive cigarette smoking and stress, either physical or mental. In a stressful situation there is an increase in the secretion of the hormones noradrenaline and adrenaline and these cause constriction of the blood vessels supplying the alimentary tract.

Secretion of mucus

The composition and the amount of mucus may be altered, e.g.:

- by regular and prolonged use of aspirin and other anti-inflammatory drugs
- by the reflux of bile acids and salts
- in chronic gastritis.

Epithelial cell replacement

There is normally a rapid turnover of gastric and intestinal epithelial cells. This may be reduced:

- by raised levels of steroid hormones, e.g. in response to stress or when they are used as drugs
- in chronic gastritis
- by irradiation and the use of cytotoxic drugs.

In peptic ulcer disease, the alimentary tract is commonly colonised by the bacterium *Helicobacter pylori*, a causative agent in this disorder.

Acute peptic ulcers

These lesions involve tissue to the depth of the submucosa and the lesions may be single or multiple. They are found in many sites in the stomach and in the first few centimetres of the duodenum. The underlying causes are unknown but their development is often associated with severe stress, e.g. severe illness, shock, burns, severe emotional disturbance and following surgery. Healing without the formation of fibrous tissue usually occurs when the cause of the stress is removed.

Chronic peptic ulcers

These ulcers penetrate through the epithelial and muscle layers of the stomach wall and may include the adjacent pancreas or liver. In the majority of cases they occur singly in the pyloric antrum of the stomach and in the duodenum. Occasionally there are two ulcers facing each other in the duodenum, called kissing ulcers. Healing occurs with the formation of fibrous tissue and subsequent shrinkage may cause:

- stricture of the lumen of the stomach
- stenosis of the pyloric sphincter
- adhesions to adjacent structures, e.g. pancreas, liver, transverse colon.

Complications of peptic ulcers

Haemorrhage. Acid gastric juice may cause the development of many tiny ulcers, or *gastric erosions*, leading to multiple capillary bleeding points and possibly iron deficiency anaemia (p. 69).

When a major artery is eroded a serious and possibly life-threatening haemorrhage may occur, causing:

- shock (p. 111)
- haematemesis — vomiting of blood
- melaena — blood in the faeces.

Perforation. When an ulcer erodes through the full thickness of the wall of the stomach or duodenum their contents enter the peritoneal cavity, causing acute peritonitis (p. 325).

Infected inflammatory material may collect under the diaphragm, forming a *subphrenic abscess* and the infection may spread through the diaphragm to the pleural cavity.

Pyloric stenosis. Fibrous tissue formed as an ulcer in the pyloric region heals and may cause narrowing of the pylorus, obstructing outflow from the stomach and resulting in persistent vomiting.

Development of a malignant tumour. This may complicate gastric ulceration.

Tumours of the stomach

Benign tumours of the stomach occur rarely.

Malignant tumours

This is a relatively common form of malignancy and it occurs more frequently in men than women. The local growth of the tumour gradually destroys the normal tissue so that achlorhydria (reduced hydrochloric acid secretion) and pernicious anaemia are frequently secondary features. The causes have not been established but there appears to be:

- a familial predisposition
- an association with diet — high-salt diets and regular consumption of smoked or pickled foods increase the risk
- the presence of other diseases, e.g. chronic gastritis, chronic ulceration and pernicious anaemia.

Spread of gastric carcinoma

Local spread. These tumours spread locally to the remainder of the stomach, to the oesophagus, duodenum, omentum, liver and pancreas. The spleen is seldom affected.

As the tumour grows, the surface may ulcerate and become infected, especially when achlorhydria develops.

Lymphatic spread. This occurs early in the disease. At first the spread is within the lymph channels in the stomach wall, and then to lymph nodes round the stomach, in the mesentery, omentum and walls of the small intestine and colon.

Blood spread. The common sites for blood-spread metastases are the liver, lungs, brain and bones.

Peritoneal spread. When a tumour includes the full thickness of the stomach wall, small groups of cells may break off and spread throughout the peritoneal cavity. Metastases may develop in any tissue in the abdominal or pelvic cavity where the fragments settle.

Congenital pyloric stenosis

In this condition there is spasmodic constriction of the pyloric sphincter, characteristic projective vomiting and failure to put on weight. In an attempt to overcome the spasms, hypertrophy of the muscle of the pyloric antrum develops, causing obstruction of the pylorus 2 to 3 weeks after birth. The reason for the excess stimulation or neuromuscular abnormality of the pylorus is not known but there is a familial tendency and it is more common in males.

DISEASES OF THE INTESTINES

Learning outcomes

After studying this section, you should be able to:

- describe appendicitis and its consequences
- discuss the principal infectious disease of the intestines
- compare and contrast the two commonest forms of inflammatory bowel disease: Crohn's disease and ulcerative colitis
- distinguish between diverticulitis and diverticulosis
- describe the main tumours of the intestines
- describe the abnormalities present in hernia, volvulus and intussusception
- list the main causes of intestinal obstruction
- compare the causes and outcomes of primary and secondary malabsorption.

Diseases of the small and large intestines will be described together because they have certain characteristics in common and some conditions affect both.

Appendicitis

The lumen of the appendix is very small and there is little room for swelling when it becomes inflamed. The initial cause of inflammation is not always clear. Microbial infection is commonly superimposed on obstruction by, e.g., hard faecal matter (faecoliths), kinking or a foreign body. Inflammatory exudate, with fibrin and phagocytes, causes swelling and ulceration of the mucous membrane lining. In the initial stages, the pain of appendicitis is usually located in the central area of the abdomen. After a few hours, the pain shifts and is localised to the region above the appendix (the right iliac fossa) (see also p. 174). In mild cases the inflammation subsides and healing takes place. In more severe cases microbial growth progresses, leading to suppuration, abscess formation and further congestion. The rising pressure inside the appendix occludes first the veins, then the arteries and ischaemia develops, followed by gangrene and rupture.

Complications of appendicitis

Peritonitis. The peritoneum becomes acutely inflamed, the blood vessels dilate and excess serous fluid is secreted. It occurs as a complication of appendicitis when:

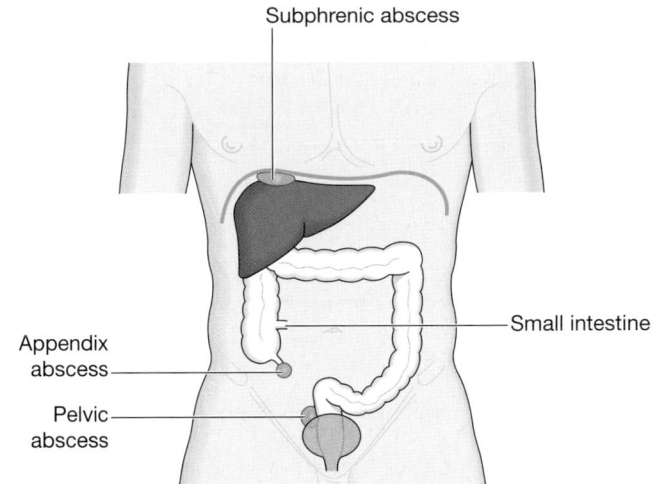

Figure 12.51 Abscess formation; complication of appendicitis.

- microbes spread through the wall of the appendix and infect the peritoneum
- an appendix abscess ruptures and pus enters the peritoneal cavity
- the appendix becomes gangrenous and ruptures, discharging its contents into the peritoneal cavity.

Abscess formation. The most common abscesses are (Fig. 12.51):

- subphrenic abscess, between the liver and diaphragm, from which infection may spread upwards to the pleura, pericardium and mediastinal structures
- pelvic abscess from which infection may spread to adjacent structures.

Fibrous adhesions. When healing takes place fibrous tissue forms and later shrinkage may cause:

- stricture or obstruction of the bowel
- limitation of the movement of a loop of bowel which may twist around the adhesion, causing a type of bowel obstruction called a *volvulus* (p. 330).

Microbial diseases (Fig. 12.52)

Typhoid fever

This type of enteritis is caused by the microbe *Salmonella typhi*, ingested in food and water. Humans are its only host so the source of contamination is an individual who is either suffering from the disease or is a carrier.

After ingestion of microbes there is an incubation period of about 14 days before signs of the disease

325

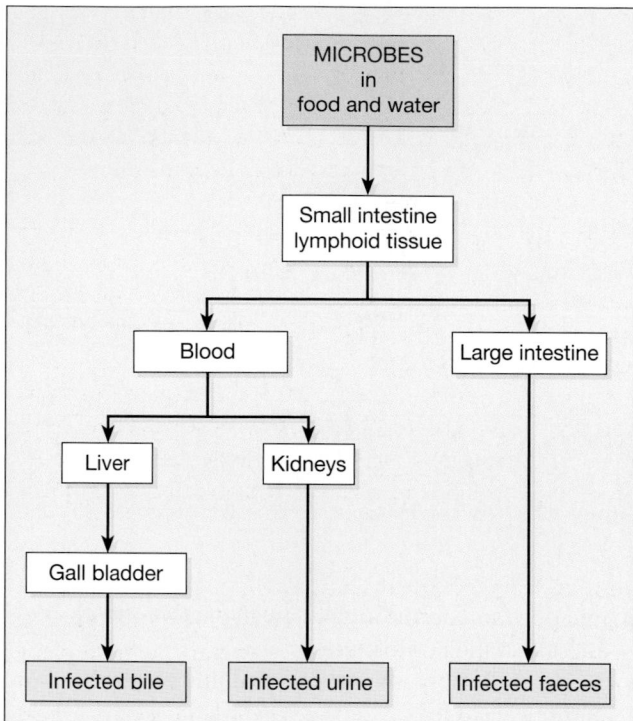

Figure 12.52 The routes of excretion of microbes in enteric fever.

appear. During this period the microbes invade lymphoid tissue in the walls of the small and large intestine, especially the aggregated lymph follicles (Peyer's patches) and solitary lymph nodes. The microbes then enter the blood vessels and spread to the liver, spleen and gall bladder. In the bacteraemic period acute inflammation develops with necrosis of intestinal lymphoid tissue and ulceration of overlying mucosa. Other effects of *Salmonella typhi* or their endotoxins include:

- typhoid cholecystitis in which the microbes multiply in the gall bladder and are excreted in bile, reinfecting the intestine
- red spots on the skin, especially of the chest and abdomen
- enlargement of the spleen
- myocardial damage and endocarditis
- liver and kidney damage
- reduced resistance to other infections, especially of the respiratory tract, e.g. laryngitis, bronchitis, pneumonia.

Uncomplicated recovery takes place in about 5 weeks with healing of intestinal ulcers and very little fibrosis.

Complications

- The ulcers may penetrate a blood vessel, causing haemorrhage, or erode the intestinal wall, leading to acute peritonitis.

- The individual may become a carrier. When this happens the typhoid fever becomes a chronic, asymptomatic infection of the biliary and urinary tracts. Microbes continue to be excreted indefinitely in urine and faeces. Contamination of food and water by carriers is the usual source of infection.

Paratyphoid fever

This disease is caused by *Salmonella paratyphi A* or *B* spread in the same way as typhoid fever, i.e. in food and drink contaminated by infected urine or faeces. The infection, causing inflammation of the intestinal mucosa, is usually confined to the ileum. Other parts of the body are not usually affected but occasionally chronic infection of the urinary and biliary tracts occurs and the individual becomes an asymptomatic carrier, excreting the microbes in urine and faeces.

Other salmonella infections

Salmonella typhimurium and *S. enteritidis* are the most common infecting microbes in this group. In addition to humans their hosts are domestic animals and birds. The microbes may be present in meat, poultry, eggs and milk, causing infection if cooking does not achieve sterilisation. Mice and rats also carry the organisms and may contaminate food before or after cooking.

The infection is usually of short duration but may be accompanied by acute abdominal pain and diarrhoea, causing dehydration and electrolyte imbalance. In children and debilitated elderly people the infection may be severe or even fatal. Chronic infection of the biliary and urinary tracts may develop and the individual becomes a carrier, excreting the organisms in urine and faeces (Fig. 12.52).

Escherichia coli (E. coli) food poisoning

Common sources for these organisms include undercooked meat and unpasteurised milk; adequate cooking kills *E. coli*. The severity of the disease depends on the type of *E. coli* responsible; some types are more virulent than others and outbreaks of *E. coli* food poisoning can cause fatalities, particularly in the elderly.

Staphylococcal food poisoning

This is not an infection in the true sense. Acute gastroenteritis is caused by toxins produced by the *Staphylococcus aureus* before ingestion of the contaminated food. The organisms are usually killed by cooking but the toxins can withstand higher temperatures and remain unchanged.

There is usually short-term acute inflammation with violent vomiting and diarrhoea, causing dehydration and electrolyte imbalance. In most cases complete recovery occurs within 24 hours.

Clostridium perfringens (*Cl. welchii*) food poisoning

These microbes, although normally present in the intestines of humans and animals, cause food poisoning when ingested in large numbers. Meat may be contaminated at any stage between slaughter and the consumer. Outbreaks of food poisoning are associated with large-scale cooking, e.g. in institutions. The spores survive the initial cooking and if the food is cooled slowly they enter the vegetative phase and multipy between the temperatures of 50°C and 20°C. Following refrigeration the microbes multiply if the food is reheated slowly. After being eaten, microbes that remain vegetative die and release endotoxins that cause gastroenteritis.

Campylobacter food poisoning

These Gram-negative bacilli are a common cause of gastroenteritis accompanied by fever, acute pain and sometimes bleeding. They affect mainly young adults and children under 5 years. The microbes are present in the intestines of birds and animals and are spread in undercooked poultry and meat. They may also be spread in water and milk. Pets, such as cats and dogs, may be a source of infection.

Cholera

Cholera is caused by *Vibrio cholerae* and is spread by contaminated water, food, hands and fomites. The only known hosts are humans. A very powerful toxin is produced by the bacteria, which stimulates the intestinal glands to secrete large quantities of water, bicarbonate and chloride. This leads to persistent diarrhoea, severe dehydration and electrolyte imbalance, and may cause death due to hypovolaemic shock. The microbes occasionally spread to the gall bladder where they multiply. They are then excreted in bile and faeces. This carrier state usually lasts for a maximum of about 4 years providing a reservoir for spread of infection.

Dysentery

Bacillary dysentery
This infection of the colon is caused by bacteria of the *Shigella* group. The severity of the condition depends on the organisms involved. In Britain it is usually a relatively mild condition caused by *Shigella sonnei*. Outbreaks may reach epidemic proportions, especially in institutions. Children and elderly debilitated adults are particularly susceptible. The only host is humans and the organisms are spread by faecal contamination of food, drink, hands and fomites.

The intestinal mucosa becomes inflamed, ulcerated and oedematous with excess mucus secretion. In severe infections, the acute diarrhoea, containing blood and excess mucus, causes dehydration, electrolyte imbalance and anaemia. When healing occurs the mucous membrane is fully restored. Occasionally a chronic infection develops and the individual becomes a carrier, excreting the microbes in faeces. *Shigella dysenteriae* causes the most severe type of infection. It occurs mainly in tropical countries.

Amoebic dysentery
This disease is caused by *Entamoeba histolytica*. The only known hosts are humans and it is spread by faecal contamination of food, water, hands and fomites. Before ingestion the amoebae are inside resistant cysts. When these reach the colon they grow and divide and invade the mucosal cells, causing inflammation and ulceration. Further development of the disease may result in destruction of the mucosa over a large area and sometimes perforation occurs. Diarrhoea containing mucus and blood is persistent and debilitating.

The disease may progress in a number of ways.

- Healing may produce fibrous adhesions, causing partial or complete obstruction.
- The amoebae may spread to the liver, causing amoebic hepatitis and abscesses.
- Chronic dysentery may develop with intermittent diarrhoea and amoebae in the faeces.

Although most infected people do not develop symptoms they may become carriers.

Inflammatory bowel disease (Table 12.4)

Crohn's disease (regional ileitis)

This chronic inflammatory condition of the alimentary tract usually occurs in young adults. The terminal ileum and the rectum are most commonly affected but the disease may be more widespread. There is chronic patchy inflammation with oedema of the full thickness of the intestinal wall, causing partial obstruction of the lumen, sometimes described as *skip lesions*. There are periods of remission of varying duration. The cause of Crohn's

Table 12.4 Comparison of the main features of Crohn's disease and ulcerative colitis

	Crohn's disease	Ulcerative colitis
Incidence	Usually between 20 and 40 years of age; both sexes affected equally; smokers at higher risk	Usually between 20 and 40 years of age; more women affected than men; smoking not a risk factor
Main sites of lesions	Anywhere in digestive tract from mouth to anus; common in terminal ileum	Rectum always involved, with variable spread along colon
Tissue involved	Entire thickness of the wall inflamed and thickened	Only mucosa involved
Nature of lesions	'Skip' lesions, i.e. diseased areas interspersed with regions of normal tissue; ulcers and fistulae common	Continuous lesion; mucosa is red and inflamed
Prognosis	In severe cases, surgery may improve condition, but relapse rate very high	Surgical removal of entire colon cures the condition

disease is not entirely clear but it may be that immunological abnormality renders the individual susceptible to infection, especially by viruses. Complications include:

- secondary infections, occurring when inflamed areas ulcerate
- fibrous adhesions and subsequent intestinal obstruction caused by the healing process
- fistulae between intestinal lesions and adjacent structures, e.g. loops of bowel, surface of the skin (p. 378)
- peri-anal fistula formation
- megaloblastic anaemia due to malabsorption of vitamin B_{12} and folic acid
- cancer of the small or large intestine.

Ulcerative colitis

This is a chronic inflammatory disease of the mucosa of the colon and rectum which may ulcerate and become infected. It usually occurs in young adults and begins in the rectum and sigmoid colon. From there it may spread to involve a variable proportion of the colon and, sometimes, the entire colon. There are periods of remission lasting weeks, months or years. The cause is not known but there is an association with arthritis, iritis, some skin lesions, haemolytic anaemia and some drug sensitivities. In long-standing cases cancer sometimes develops.

Fulminating ulcerative colitis

This is also called *toxic megacolon*. The colon loses its muscle tone and dilates, the wall becomes thinner and

perforation, which may be fatal, may follow. There is a sudden onset of acute diarrhoea, with severe blood loss, leading to dehydration, electrolyte imbalance, perforation, hypovolaemic shock and possibly death.

Diverticular disease

Diverticula are small pouches of mucosa that protrude into the peritoneal cavity through the circular muscle fibres of the colon between the taeniae coli (Fig. 12.53). The walls consist of mucous membrane with a covering of visceral peritoneum. They occur at the weakest points of the intestinal wall, i.e. where the blood vessels enter, most commonly in the sigmoid colon. *Diverticulitis* arises when faeces impact in the diverticula and the walls become inflamed and oedematous as secondary infection develops. This reduces the blood supply causing ischaemic pain. Occasionally, rupture occurs resulting in peritonitis.

The causes of *diverticulosis* (presence of diverticuli) are not known but it is associated with low-residue diet and abnormally active peristalsis. In Western countries diverticulosis is fairly common after the age of 60 but diverticulitis affects only a small proportion.

Tumours of the small and large intestines

Benign and malignant tumours of the small intestine are rare, compared with their occurrence in the stomach and colon.

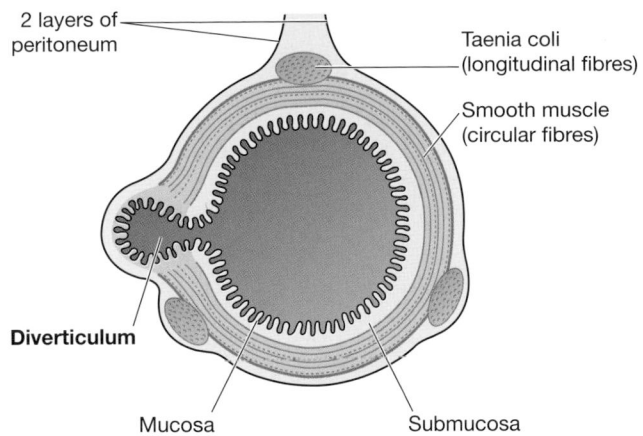

Figure 12.53 Diverticular disease; cross-section of bowel showing one diverticulum.

Labels: 2 layers of peritoneum; Taenia coli (longitudinal fibres); Smooth muscle (circular fibres); Diverticulum; Mucosa; Submucosa.

Benign tumours

Benign neoplasms may form a broad-based mass or develop a pedicle. Occasionally those with pedicles twist upon themselves, causing ischaemia, necrosis and possibly gangrene. Malignant changes may occur.

Malignant tumours

Small intestine. Malignant tumours tend not to obstruct the lumen and may remain unnoticed until symptoms caused by metastases appear. The most common sites of metastases are local lymph nodes, the liver, lungs and brain.

The colon. This is the most common site of malignancy in the alimentary tract in Western countries. The tumour may be:

- a soft friable mass, projecting into the lumen of the colon with a tendency to ulceration, infection and haemorrhage
- a hard fibrous mass encircling the colon, causing reduced elasticity and peristalsis and narrowing of the lumen
- a gelatinous mucoid mass that thickens the wall and tends to ulcerate and become infected.

The most important factor for colorectal cancer is thought to be diet. In cultures eating a high-fibre, low-fat diet, the disease is virtually unknown, whereas in Western countries, where large quantities of red meat and insufficient fibre are eaten, the disease is much more common. Slow movement of bowel contents may result in the conversion of as yet unknown substances that are present into carcinogenic agents. Predisposing diseases include ulcerative colitis and some benign tumours.

Local spread of intestinal tumours occurs early but may not be evident until there is severe ulceration and haemorrhage or obstruction. Spread can be outwards through the wall into the peritoneal cavity and adjacent structures.

Lymph-spread metastases occur in mesenteric lymph nodes, the peritoneum and other abdominal and pelvic organs. Pressure caused by enlarged lymph nodes may cause obstruction or damage other structures.

Blood-spread metastases are most common in the liver, brain and bones.

Carcinoid tumours (argentaffinomas)

These tumours are considered, on clinical evidence, to be benign but they spread into the tissues around their original site. They grow very slowly and rarely metastasise. The parent cells are hormone-secreting cells widely dispersed throughout the body, not situated in endocrine glands. Some of these tumours secrete hormones while others do not. They are called APUD cells, an acronym for some of their chemical characteristics. The cells react with silver compounds, hence the name argentaffinomas. Common sites in the intestines for these *apudomas* are the appendix, ileum, stomach, colon and rectum. The tumours are frequently multiple and may spread locally, causing obstruction.

Carcinoid syndrome. This is the name given to the effects of the variety of substances secreted by apudomas in the intestine and elsewhere. The secretions include serotonin (5-hydroxytryptamine), histamine and bradykinin, and the effects include flushing attacks, tachycardia, sweating, anxiety and diarrhoea.

Hernias

A hernia is a protrusion of bowel through a weak point in the musculature of the anterior abdominal wall or an existing opening (Fig. 12.54A). It occurs when there are intermittent increases in intra-abdominal pressure, most commonly in men who lift heavy loads at work. The underlying causes of the abdominal wall weakness are not known. Possible outcomes include:

- spontaneous reduction, i.e. the loop of bowel slips back to its correct place when the intra-abdominal pressure returns to normal
- manual reduction, i.e. by applying slight pressure over the abdominal swelling
- strangulation, when the venous drainage from the herniated loop of bowel is impaired, causing congestion, ischaemia and gangrene. In addition there is intestinal obstruction.

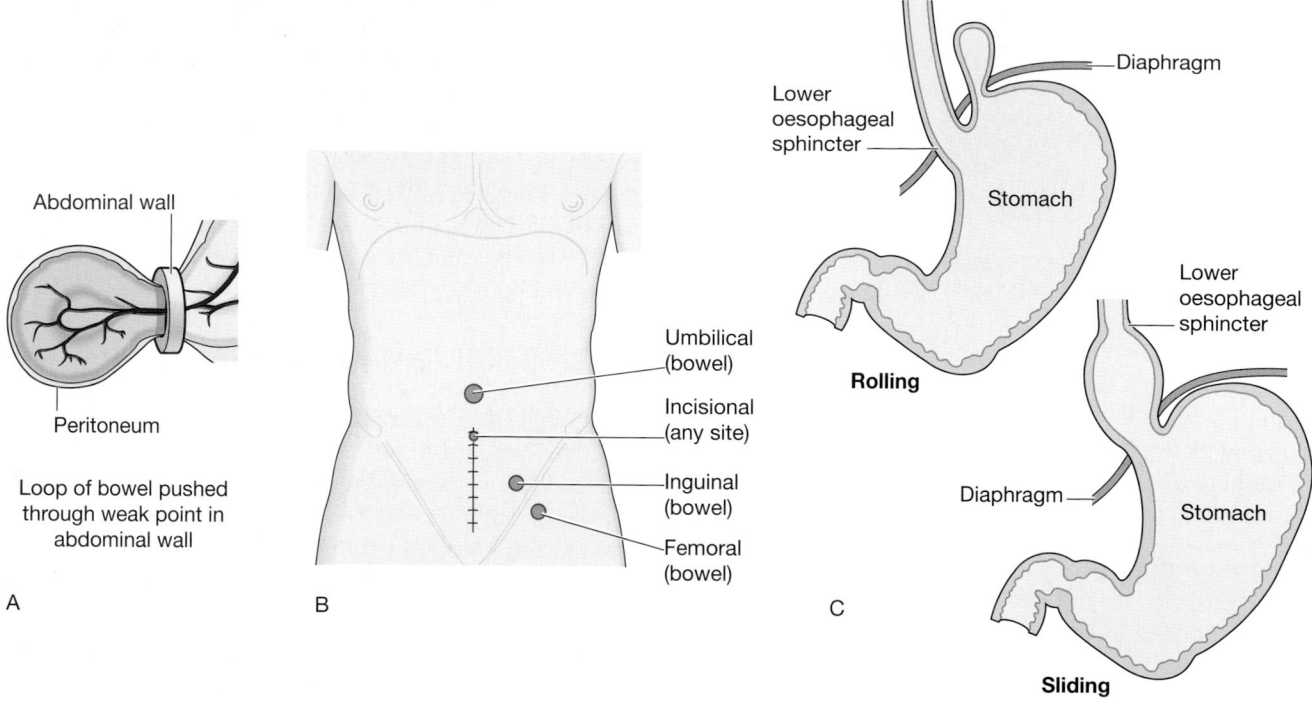

Figure 12.54 Hernias: A. Strangulated hernia formation. B. Common sites of herniation. C. Hiatus hernia.

Sites of hernias (Fig. 12.54B)

Inguinal hernia. The weak point is the inguinal canal which contains the spermatic cord in the male and the round ligament in the female. It occurs more commonly in males than in females.

Femoral hernia. The weak point is the femoral canal through which the femoral artery, vein and lymph vessels pass from the pelvis to the thigh.

Umbilical hernia. The weak point is the umbilicus where the umbilical blood vessels from the placenta enter the fetus.

Incisional hernia. This is caused by repeated stretching of the fibrous tissue formed during the repair of a surgical wound.

Diaphragmatic or hiatus hernia (Fig. 12.54C) This is the protrusion of a part of the fundus of the stomach through the oesophageal opening in the diaphragm. The main complication is irritation caused by reflux of acid gastric juice, especially when the individual lies flat or bends down. The long-term effects may be oesophagitis, fibrosis and narrowing of the oesophagus, causing dysphagia. Strangulation does not occur.

Sliding hiatus hernia. An unusually short oesophagus that ends above the diaphragm pulls a part of the stomach upwards into the thorax. The abnormality may be congenital or be caused by shrinkage of fibrous tissue formed during healing of a previous oesophageal injury. The sliding movement of the stomach in the oesophageal opening is due to normal shortening of the oesophagus by muscular contraction during swallowing.

Rolling hiatus hernia. An abnormally large opening in the diaphragm allows a pouch of stomach to 'roll' upwards into the thorax beside the oesophagus. This is associated with obesity and increased intra-abdominal pressure.

Peritoneal hernia. A loop of bowel may herniate through the foramen of Winslow, the opening in the lesser omentum that separates the greater and lesser peritoneal sacs.

Volvulus

This occurs when a loop of bowel twists through 180°, cutting off its blood supply, causing gangrene and obstruction. It occurs in parts of the intestine that are attached to the posterior abdominal wall by a long double fold of visceral peritoneum, the mesentery. The most common site in adults is the sigmoid colon and in children the small intestine. The causes are unknown but predisposing factors include:

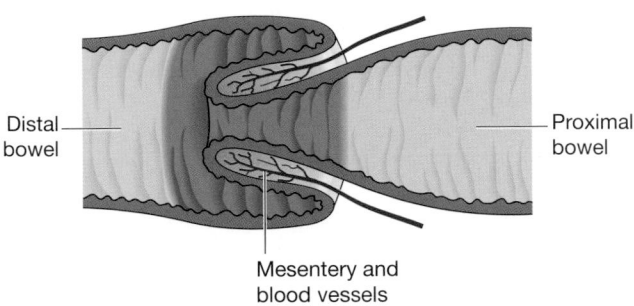

Distal bowel

Proximal bowel

Mesentery and blood vessels

Figure 12.55 Intussusception.

- an unusually long mesocolon or mesentery
- heavy loading of the pelvic colon with faeces
- a slight twist of a loop of bowel, causing gas and fluid to accumulate and promote further twisting
- adhesions formed following surgery or peritonitis.

Intussusception

In this condition a length of intestine is invaginated into itself (Fig. 12.55). It occurs most commonly in children when a piece of terminal ileum is pushed through the ileocaecal valve. In a child, infection, usually by viruses, causes swelling of the lymphoid tissue in the intestinal wall. The overlying mucosa bulges into the lumen, creating a partial obstruction and a rise in pressure inside the intestine proximal to the swelling. Strong peristaltic waves develop in an attempt to overcome the partial obstruction. These push the swollen piece of bowel into the lumen of the section immediately distal to it, creating the intussusception. The pressure on the veins in the invaginated portion is increased, causing congestion, further swelling, ischaemia and possibly gangrene. Complete intestinal obstruction may occur. In adults tumours that bulge into the lumen, e.g. polypi, together with the strong peristalsis, may be the cause.

Intestinal obstruction

This is not a disease in itself. The following is a summary of the main causes of obstruction with some examples.

Mechanical causes of obstruction

These include:

- constriction of the intestine by, e.g., strangulated hernia, intussusception, volvulus, peritoneal adhesions; partial obstruction may suddenly become complete

- stenosis and thickening of the intestinal wall, e.g. in diverticulosis, Crohn's disease and malignant tumours; there is usually a gradual progression from partial to complete obstruction
- obstruction by, e.g., a large gallstone or a tumour growing into the lumen
- pressure on the intestine from outside, e.g. a large tumour in any pelvic or abdominal organ, such as a uterine fibroid; this type is most likely to occur inside the confined space of the bony pelvis.

Neurological causes of obstruction

Partial or complete loss of peristaltic activity produces the effects of obstruction. *Paralytic ileus* is the most common form but the paralysis may be more widespread. The cause is either excessive sympathetic stimulation or lack of parasympathetic stimulation. The mechanisms are not clear but there are well-recognised predisposing conditions including:

- general peritonitis, especially when large amounts of exotoxin are released from dead microbes
- following surgery when there has been a considerable amount of handling of the intestines
- severe intestinal infection, especially if there is acute toxaemia, e.g. following ruptured appendix.

Secretion of water and electrolytes continues although intestinal mobility is lost and absorption impaired. This causes distension and electrolyte imbalance, leading to hypovolaemic shock. Growth and multiplication of microbes may also occur.

Vascular causes of obstruction

When the blood supply to a segment of bowel is cut off, ischaemia is followed by infarction, gangrene and obstruction. The causes may be:

- atheromatous changes in the blood vessel walls, with thrombosis
- embolism
- mechanical obstruction of the bowel, e.g. strangulated hernia.

Malabsorption

Impaired absorption of nutrient materials and water from the intestines is not a disease in itself. It is the result of diseases causing one or more of the following changes:

- atrophy of the villi of the mucosa of the small intestine

331

- incomplete digestion of food
- interference with the transport of absorbed nutrients from the small intestine to the blood.

Primary malabsorption

Disease of the intestinal mucous membrane

Atrophy of the villi is the main cause, varying in severity from minor abnormality to almost complete loss of function. The most common underlying diseases are coeliac disease and tropical sprue.

Coeliac disease (idiopathic steatorrhoea). This disease is believed to be due to a genetically determined abnormal immunological reaction to the protein *gluten*, present in wheat. When it is removed from the diet, recovery is complete. There is marked villous atrophy and malabsorption characterised by the passage of loose, pale coloured, fatty stools.

There may be abnormal immune reaction to other antigens. Atrophy of the spleen is common and malignant lymphoma of the small intestine may develop. It often presents in infants after weaning but can affect any age.

Tropical sprue. In this disease there is partial villous atrophy with malabsorption, chronic diarrhoea, severe wasting and pernicious anaemia due to deficient absorption of vitamin B_{12} and folic acid. The cause is unknown but it may be that bacterial growth in the small intestine is a factor. The disease is endemic in subtropical and tropical countries except Africa south of the Sahara. After leaving the endemic area most people suffering from sprue recover, but others may not develop symptoms until months or even years later.

Secondary malabsorption

This is associated with incomplete digestion of food, impaired transport of absorbed nutrients and following extensive small bowel resection.

Defective digestion

This occurs in a variety of conditions:

- disease of the liver and pancreas
- following a resection of small intestine
- following surgery if microbes grow in a blind end of intestine.

Impaired transport of nutrients

This occurs when there is:

- lymphatic obstruction by, e.g., lymph node tumours, removal of nodes at surgery, tubercular disease of lymph nodes

- impairment of mesenteric blood flow by, e.g., arterial or venous thrombosis, pressure caused by a tumour
- obstruction of blood flow through the liver, e.g. in cirrhosis of liver.

DISEASES OF THE PANCREAS

Learning outcomes

After studying this section, you should be able to:

- compare and contrast the causes and effects of acute and chronic pancreatitis
- explain the effects of cystic fibrosis
- outline the main pancreatic tumours and their consequences.

Acute pancreatitis

Proteolytic enzymes produced by the pancreas are secreted in inactive forms, which are not activated until they reach the intestine; this protects the pancreas from digestion by its own enzymes. If these precursor enzymes are activated while still in the pancreas, pancreatitis results. The severity of the disease is directly related to the amount of pancreatic tissue destroyed.

Mild forms may damage only those cells near the ducts.

Severe forms cause widespread damage with necrosis and haemorrhage. Common complications include infection, suppuration, and local venous thrombosis. Pancreatic enzymes, especially amylase, enter and circulate in the blood, causing similar damage to other structures. In severe cases there is a high mortality rate.

The causes of acute pancreatitis are not clear but known predisposing factors are gallstones and alcoholism. When a gallstone obstructs the hepatopancreatic ampulla there is reflux of bile into the pancreas and the spread of infection from cholangitis. Other associated conditions include:

- cancer of the ampulla or head of pancreas
- virus infections, notably mumps
- chronic renal failure
- renal transplantation
- hyperparathyroidism
- hypothermia
- drugs, e.g. corticosteroids, cytotoxic agents
- diabetes mellitus
- cholecystitis.

Chronic pancreatitis

This is due to repeated attacks of acute pancreatitis or may arise gradually without evidence of pancreatic disease. It is frequently associated with fibrosis and distortion of the main pancreatic duct.

There is obstruction of the tiny acinar ducts by protein material secreted by the acinar cells. This eventually leads to the formation of cysts which may rupture into the peritoneal cavity. Intact cysts may cause obstruction of the:

- common bile duct, causing jaundice
- portal vein, causing venous congestion in the organs drained by its tributaries.

The causes of these changes are not known but they are associated mainly with heavy wine drinking.

Cystic fibrosis (mucoviscidosis)

This is one of the most common genetic diseases, affecting 1 in 2500 babies. It is estimated that almost 20% of people carry the abnormal recessive gene which must be present in *both parents* to cause the disease.

The secretions of all exocrine glands have abnormally high viscosity but the most severely affected are those of the pancreas, intestines, biliary tract, lungs and the reproductive system in the male. Sweat glands secrete abnormally large amounts of salt during excessive sweating. In the pancreas highly viscous mucus is secreted by the walls of the ducts and causes obstruction, parenchymal cell damage, the formation of cysts and defective enzyme secretion. In the newborn, intestinal obstruction may be caused by a plug of meconium and viscid mucus, leading to perforation and meconium peritonitis which is often fatal. In less acute cases there may be impairment of protein and fat digestion resulting in malabsorption, steatorrhoea and failure to thrive in infants. In older children:

- digestion of food and absorption of nutrients is impaired
- there may be obstruction of bile ducts in the liver, causing cirrhosis
- bronchitis, bronchiectasis and pneumonia may develop.

The life span of affected individuals is likely to be less than 40 years; the main treatments offered are aimed at controlling pulmonary infection. Chronic lung disease and *cor pulmonale* are the commonest causes of death.

Tumours of the pancreas

Benign tumours of the pancreas are very rare.

Malignant tumours

These are relatively common and affect men more than women. They occur most frequently in the head of the pancreas, obstructing the flow of bile and pancreatic juice into the duodenum. Jaundice and acute pancreatitis usually develop. Weight loss is the result of impaired digestion and absorption of fat. Tumours in the body and tail of the gland rarely cause symptoms until the disease is advanced. Metastases are often recognised before the primary tumour. The causes of the malignant changes are not known but it is believed that there may be an association with:

- cigarette smoking
- diet high in fats and carbohydrates
- diabetes mellitus.

DISEASES OF THE LIVER

Learning outcomes

After studying this section, you should be able to:

- compare and contrast the causes, forms and effects of chronic and acute hepatitis
- describe the main non-viral inflammatory conditions of the liver
- discuss the causes and consequences of liver failure
- describe the main liver tumours.

New liver cells develop only when needed to replace damaged cells. Capacity for regeneration is considerable and damage is usually extensive before it is evident. The effects of disease or toxic agents are seen when:

- regeneration of hepatocytes (liver cells) does not keep pace with damage, leading to hepatocellular failure
- there is a gradual replacement of damaged cells by fibrous tissue, leading to portal hypertension.

In most liver disease both conditions are present.

Acute hepatitis

Areas of necrosis develop as groups of hepatocytes die and the eventual outcome depends on the size and number of these areas. Causes of the damage may be a variety of conditions, including:

- viral infections
- toxic substances
- circulatory disturbances.

Viral hepatitis

Virus infections are the commonest cause of acute liver injury and include Type A, Type B and Type C. The types are distinguished serologically, i.e. by the antibodies produced to combat the infection. The severity of the ensuing disease caused by the different virus types varies considerably but the pattern is similar. The viruses enter the liver cells, causing degenerative changes by mechanisms not yet understood. An inflammatory reaction ensues, accompanied by production of an exudate containing lymphocytes, plasma cells and granulocytes. There is reactive hyperplasia of the hepatic macrophages (Kupffer cells) in the walls of the sinusoids.

As groups of cells die, necrotic areas of varying sizes develop, phagocytes remove the necrotic material and the lobules collapse. The basic lobule framework (Fig. 12.40) becomes distorted and blood vessels develop kinks. These changes interfere with the circulation of blood to the remaining hepatocytes and the resultant hypoxia causes further damage. Fibrous tissue develops in the damaged area, and adjacent hepatocytes proliferate. The effect of these changes on the overall functioning of the liver depends on the size of the necrotic areas, the amount of fibrous tissue formed and the extent to which the blood and bile channels are distorted.

Type A virus (infectious hepatitis)

This virus has only one known serological type. It occurs endemically, affecting mainly children, causing a mild illness. Infection is spread by hands, food, water and fomites contaminated by infected faeces. The incubation period is 15 to 40 days and the viruses are excreted in the faeces for 7 to 14 days before clinical symptoms appear and for about 7 days after. Antibodies develop and immunity persists after recovery. Subclinical disease may occur but carriers do not develop.

Type B virus (serum hepatitis)

This virus has a number of serological types. Infection occurs at any age, but mostly in adults. The incubation period is 50 to 180 days. The virus enters the blood and is spread by blood and blood products. People at greatest risk of infection are those who come in contact with blood and blood products in their daily work, e.g. people in the health, ambulance and fire services. The virus is also spread by body fluids, i.e. saliva, semen, vaginal secretions and from mother to fetus. Others at risk include intravenous drug addicts and male homosexuals. Antibodies are formed and immunity persists after recovery. Infection usually leads to severe illness lasting 2 to 6 weeks, often followed by a protracted convalescence. Carriers may, or may not, have had clinical disease. Type B virus may cause massive liver necrosis and death. In less severe cases recovery may be complete. In chronic hepatitis which may develop, live viruses continue to circulate in the blood and other body fluids. The condition may predispose to liver cancer.

Hepatitis C

This virus is spread by blood and blood products. It is prevalent in IV drug users and also occurs as a complication of blood transfusion. The infection can be asymptomatic as a carrier state occurs. When hepatitis develops, it is often recurrent and may result in chronic liver disease, especially cirrhosis.

Toxic substances

Many drugs undergo chemical change in the liver before excretion in bile or by other organs. They may damage the liver cells in their original form or while in various intermediate stages. Some substances always cause liver damage (predictably toxic) while others only do so when hypersensitivity develops (unpredictably toxic). In both types the extent of the damage depends on the size of the dose and/or the duration of exposure (Box 12.1).

Box 12.1 Some hepatotoxic substances

Predictable group (dose related)	Unpredictable group (individual idiosyncrasy)
Chloroform	Phenothiazine compounds
Tetracyclines	Halothane
Cytotoxic drugs	Methyldopa
Anabolic steroids	Phenylbutazone
Alcohol	Indomethacin
Paracetamol	Chlorpropamide
Some hydrocarbons	Thiouracil
Some fungi	Sulphonamides

Circulatory disturbances

The intensely active hepatocytes are particularly vulnerable to damage by hypoxia which is usually due to deficient blood supply caused by:

- fibrosis in the liver following inflammation
- compression of the portal vein, hepatic artery or vein by a tumour
- acute general circulatory failure and shock
- venous congestion caused by acute or chronic right-sided heart failure.

Chronic hepatitis

This is defined as any form of hepatitis which persists for more than 6 months. It may be caused by viruses or drugs, but in some cases the cause is unknown.

Chronic persistent hepatitis

This is a mild, persistent inflammation following acute viral hepatitis. There is usually little or no fibrosis.

Chronic active hepatitis

This is a continuing progressive inflammation with cell necrosis and the formation of fibrous tissue that may lead to cirrhosis of the liver. There is distortion of the liver blood vessels and hypoxia, leading to further hepatocyte damage. This condition is commonly associated with Type B virus hepatitis, with some forms of autoimmunity and unpredictable drug reactions.

Non-viral inflammation of the liver

Pyogenic

Ascending cholangitis. Infection, usually by *Escherichia coli*, may spread from the biliary tract. The most common predisposing factor is obstruction of the common bile duct by gallstones.

Liver abscess. Septic emboli from septic foci in the abdomen and pelvis may lodge in branches of the portal vein and cause multiple abscesses or infect the vein, causing *portal pylephlebitis*. Common sources of this type of infection are acute appendicitis, diverticulitis and inflamed haemorrhoids.

Cirrhosis of the liver

This is the result of long-term inflammation caused by a wide variety of agents. The most common causes are:

- alcohol abuse
- hepatitis B and C virus infections
- the effects of bile retained in hepatocytes due to obstruction of bile flow or chronic inflammation
- congenital metabolic abnormalities.

As the inflammation subsides, destroyed liver tissue is replaced by fibrous tissue. There is hyperplasia of hepatocytes adjacent to the damaged area, in an attempt to compensate for the destroyed cells. This leads to the formation of nodules consisting of hepatocytes confined within sheets of fibrous tissue.

As the condition progresses there is the development of portal hypertension, leading to congestion in the organs drained by the tributaries of the portal vein, to ascites and possibly to the development of oesophageal varices (p. 321).

Liver failure may occur when hyperplasia is unable to keep pace with cell destruction and there is increased risk of liver cancer developing.

Liver failure

This occurs when liver function is reduced to such an extent that other body activities are impaired. It may be acute or chronic and may be the outcome of a wide variety of disorders, e.g.:

- acute viral hepatitis
- extensive necrosis due to poisoning, e.g. some drug overdoses, hepatotoxic chemicals, adverse drug reactions
- cirrhosis of the liver
- following some medical procedures, e.g. abdominal paracentesis, portacaval shunt operations.

Liver failure has serious effects on other parts of the body.

Hepatic encephalopathy

The cells affected are the astrocytes in the brain. The condition is characterised by apathy, disorientation, muscular rigidity, delirium and coma. Several factors may be involved, e.g.:

- Nitrogenous bacterial metabolites absorbed from the colon, which are normally detoxified in the liver, reach the brain via the blood
- Other metabolites, normally present in trace amounts, e.g. ammonia, may reach toxic concentrations and change the permeability of the cerebral blood vessels and the effectiveness of the blood–brain barrier
- Hypoxia and electrolyte imbalance.

Blood coagulation defects

The liver fails to synthesise substances needed for blood clotting, i.e. prothrombin, fibrinogen and factors II, V, VII, IX and X. Platelet production is impaired but the cause is unknown. Purpura and bleeding may occur.

Oliguria and renal failure

Portal hypertension may cause the development of oesophageal varices. If these rupture, bleeding may lead to a fall in blood pressure sufficient to reduce the renal blood flow, causing progressive oliguria and renal failure.

Oedema and ascites

These may be caused by the combination of two factors.

- Portal hypertension raises the capillary hydrostatic pressure in the organs drained by the tributaries of the portal vein (Fig. 12.9).
- Diminished production of serum albumin and clotting factors reduces the plasma osmotic pressure.

Together these changes cause the movement of excess fluid into the interstitial spaces where it causes *oedema*. Eventually free fluid accumulates in the peritoneal cavity and the resultant *ascites* may be severe.

Anaemia

This is usually due to the combined effect of a number of factors:

- upset in the metabolism of folic acid and vitamin B_{12}
- chronic blood loss from oesophageal varices, causing iron deficiency anaemia
- increased breakdown of red blood cells in the congested spleen, causing haemolytic anaemia.

Jaundice

The following factors may cause jaundice as liver failure develops:

- inability of the hepatocytes to conjugate and excrete bilirubin
- obstruction to the movement of bile through the bile channels by fibrous tissue that has distorted the structural framework of liver lobules.

Tumours of the liver

Benign tumours of the liver are very rare.

Malignant tumours

In many cases cancer of the liver is associated with cirrhosis but the relationship between them is not clear. It may be that both cirrhosis and cancer are caused by the same

agents or that the carcinogenic action of other agents is promoted by cirrhotic changes. Malignancy develops in a number of cases of acute hepatitis caused by Type B virus. The most common sites of metastases are the abdominal lymph nodes, the peritoneum and the lungs.

Secondary malignant tumours in the liver are common, especially from primary tumours in the gastrointestinal tract, the lungs and the breast. The metastases tend to grow rapidly and are often the cause of death.

DISEASES OF THE GALL BLADDER AND BILE DUCTS

Learning outcomes

After studying this section, you should be able to:

- describe the causes and consequences of gallstones
- compare and contrast acute and chronic cholecystitis
- briefly outline the common sites and consequences of biliary tract tumours
- discuss the main causes and effects of jaundice.

Gallstones (cholelithiasis)

Gallstones consist of deposits of the constituents of bile, most commonly cholesterol. Many small stones or one large stone may form. The causes are not clear but predisposing factors include:

- changes in the composition of bile that affect the solubility of its constituents
- high levels of blood and dietary cholesterol
- cholecystitis
- diabetes mellitus when associated with high blood cholesterol levels
- haemolytic disease
- female gender
- obesity
- long-term use of oral contraceptives
- several pregnancies in young women especially when accompanied by obesity.

Complications

Biliary colic. If a gallstone gets stuck in the cystic or common bile duct there is strong peristaltic contraction of the smooth muscle in the wall of the duct (spasm) in an effort to move the stone onwards. The severe pain associated with biliary colic is due to ischaemia of the duct wall over the stone during the smooth muscle spasm.

Inflammation. Gallstones cause irritation and inflammation of the walls of the gall bladder and the cystic and common bile ducts. There may be superimposed microbial infection.

Impaction. Blockage of the cystic duct by a gallstone leads to distension of the gall bladder and *cholecystitis*. This does not cause jaundice because bile from the liver can still pass directly into the duodenum. Obstruction of the common bile duct leads to retention of bile, jaundice and *cholangitis* (infection of the bile ducts).

Acute cholecystitis

This is usually a complication of gallstones or an exacerbation of chronic cholecystitis, especially if there has been partial or intermittent obstruction of the cystic duct. Inflammation develops followed by secondary microbial infections spread from a focus of infection elsewhere in the body, e.g. they may be blood-borne or pass directly from the adjacent colon. Those most commonly involved are *Escherichia coli* and *Streptococcus faecalis*. In severe cases there may be fibrinous exudate into the gall bladder, suppuration, gangrene, perforation, peritonitis, local abscess formation, disruption of gall bladder activity, gallstone formation and the infection may spread to the bile ducts and the liver.

Chronic cholecystitis

The onset is usually insidious, sometimes following repeated acute attacks. Gallstones are usually present and there may be accompanying biliary colic. Pain is due to the spasmodic contraction of muscle, causing ischaemia when the gall bladder is packed with gallstones. There is usually secondary infection with suppuration. Ulceration of the tissues between the gall bladder and the duodenum or colon may occur with fistula formation and, later, fibrous adhesions.

Tumours of the biliary tract

Benign tumours are rare.

Malignant tumours
These are relatively rare but when they do occur the most common sites are:

- the neck of the gall bladder
- the junction of the cystic and bile ducts
- the ampulla of the bile duct.

Local spread to the liver, the pancreas and other adjacent organs is common. Lymph and blood spread lead to widespread metastases. Early sites include the liver, lungs, abdominal lymph nodes and the peritoneum.

Jaundice

This is not a disease in itself. It is a sign of abnormal bilirubin metabolism and excretion. Bilirubin, produced from the breakdown of haemoglobin, is usually conjugated in the liver and excreted in the bile. Conjugation, the process of adding certain groups to the bilirubin molecule, makes it water soluble and greatly enhances its removal from the blood, an essential step in excretion.

Unconjugated bilirubin, which is fat soluble, has a toxic effect on brain cells. However, it is unable to cross the blood–brain barrier until the plasma level rises above 340 μmol/l, but when it does it may cause neurological damage, fits and mental handicap. Serum bilirubin may rise to 34 μmol/l before the yellow colouration of jaundice is evident in the skin and conjunctiva (normal 3 to 13 μmol/l).

Jaundice develops when there is an abnormality at some stage in the metabolic sequence caused by one or more factors, e.g.:

- excess haemolysis of red blood cells with the production of more bilirubin than the liver can deal with
- abnormal liver function that may cause:
  - incomplete uptake of unconjugated bilirubin by hepatocytes
  - ineffective conjugation of bilirubin
  - interference with bilirubin secretion into the bile
- obstruction to the flow of bile from the liver to the duodenum.

Types of jaundice

Whatever stage in bilirubin processing is affected, the end result is rising blood bilirubin levels.

Haemolytic jaundice
This is due to increased haemolysis of red blood cells in the spleen. The amount of bilirubin is increased and if hypoxia develops the efficiency of hepatocyte activity is reduced.

Neonatal haemolytic jaundice occurs in many babies, especially in prematurity where the normal high haemolysis is coupled with shortage of conjugating enzymes in the hepatocytes.

Obstructive jaundice

Obstruction to the flow of bile in the biliary tract is caused by, e.g.:

- gallstones
- tumour of the head of the pancreas
- fibrosis of the bile ducts, following inflammation or injury by cholangitis or the passage of gallstones.

Effects include:

- pruritus caused by the irritating effects of bile salts on the skin
- pale faeces due to absence of stercobilin (p. 310)
- dark urine due to the presence of increased amounts of bilirubin.

Hepatocellular jaundice

This is the result of damage to the liver by, e.g.:

- viral infection
- toxic substances, such as drugs
- amoebiasis (amoebic dysentery)
- cirrhosis of the liver.

The damaged hepatocytes may be unable to remove unconjugated bilirubin from the blood, or conjugate bilirubin, or secrete conjugated bilirubin into bile canaliculi.

13

The urinary system

The urinary system is one of the excretory systems of the body. It consists of the following structures:

- 2 *kidneys*, which secrete urine
- 2 *ureters*, which convey the urine from the kidneys to the urinary bladder
- 1 *urinary bladder* where urine collects and is temporarily stored
- 1 *urethra* through which the urine is discharged from the urinary bladder to the exterior.

Figure 13.1 shows an overview of the urinary system.

The urinary system plays a vital part in maintaining homeostasis of water and electrolyte concentrations within the body. The kidneys produce urine that contains metabolic waste products, including the nitrogenous compounds urea and uric acid, excess ions and some drugs.

The main functions of the kidneys are:

- formation and secretion of urine
- production and secretion of erythropoietin, the hormone responsible for controlling the rate of formation of red blood cells (p. 63)
- production and secretion of renin, an important enzyme in the control of blood pressure (p. 223).

Urine is stored in the bladder and excreted by the process of *micturition*.

KIDNEYS

Learning outcomes

After studying this section you should be able to:

- identify the organs associated with the kidneys
- outline the gross structure of the kidneys
- describe the structure of a nephron
- explain the processes involved in the formation of urine
- explain how body water and electrolyte balance is maintained.

The kidneys (Fig. 13.2) lie on the posterior abdominal wall, one on each side of the vertebral column, behind the peritoneum and below the diaphragm. They extend from the level of the 12th thoracic vertebra to the 3rd lumbar vertebra, receiving some protection from the lower rib cage. The right kidney is usually slightly lower than the left, probably because of the considerable space occupied by the liver.

Kidneys are bean-shaped organs, about 11 cm long, 6 cm wide, 3 cm thick and weigh 150 g. They are embedded in, and held in position by, a mass of fat. A sheath of fibroelastic *renal fascia* encloses the kidney and the renal fat.

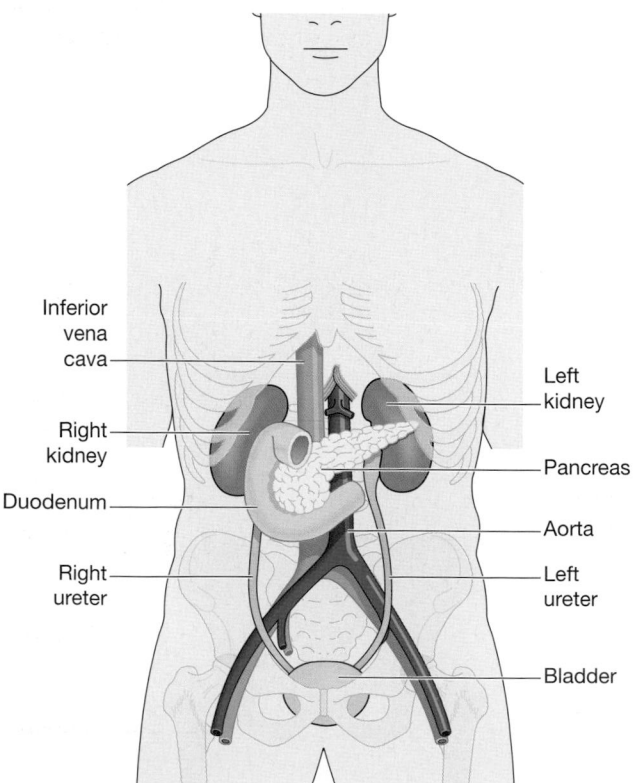

Figure 13.1 The parts of the urinary system (excluding the urethra) and some associated structures.

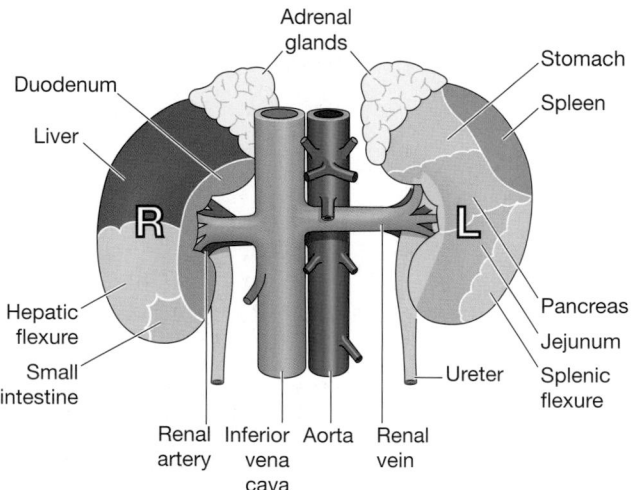

Figure 13.2 Anterior view of the kidneys showing the areas of contact with associated structures.

Organs associated with the kidneys

(Figs 13.1, 13.2 and 13.3)

As the kidneys lie on either side of the vertebral column each is associated with a different group of structures.

Right kidney

Superiorly — the right adrenal gland
Anteriorly — the right lobe of the liver, the duodenum and the hepatic flexure of the colon
Posteriorly — the diaphragm, and muscles of the posterior abdominal wall

Left kidney

Superiorly — the left adrenal gland
Anteriorly — the spleen, stomach, pancreas, jejunum and splenic flexure of the colon
Posteriorly — the diaphragm and muscles of the posterior abdominal wall

Gross structure of the kidney

There are three areas of tissue which can be distinguished when a longitudinal section of the kidney is viewed with the naked eye (Fig. 13.4):

- a *fibrous capsule*, surrounding the kidney
- the *cortex*, a reddish-brown layer of tissue immediately below the capsule and outside the pyramids

- the *medulla*, the innermost layer, consisting of pale conical-shaped striations, the *renal pyramids*.

The hilum is the concave medial border of the kidney where the renal blood and lymph vessels, the ureter and nerves enter.

The renal pelvis is the funnel-shaped structure which acts as a receptacle for the urine formed by the kidney (Fig. 13.4). It has a number of distal branches called *calyces*, each of which surrounds the apex of a renal pyramid. Urine formed in the kidney passes through a *papilla* at the apex of a pyramid into a minor calyx, then into a major calyx before passing through the pelvis into the ureter. The walls of the pelvis contain smooth muscle and are lined with transitional epithelium. Peristalsis of the smooth muscle originating in pacemaker cells in the walls of the calyces propels urine through the pelvis and ureters to the bladder. This is an intrinsic property of the smooth muscle, and is not under nerve control.

Microscopic structure of the kidney

The kidney is composed of about 1 million functional units, the *nephrons*, and a smaller number of *collecting tubules*. The collecting tubules transport urine through the pyramids to the renal pelvis giving them their striped appearance. The tubules are supported by a small amount of connective tissue, containing blood vessels, nerves and lymph vessels.

341

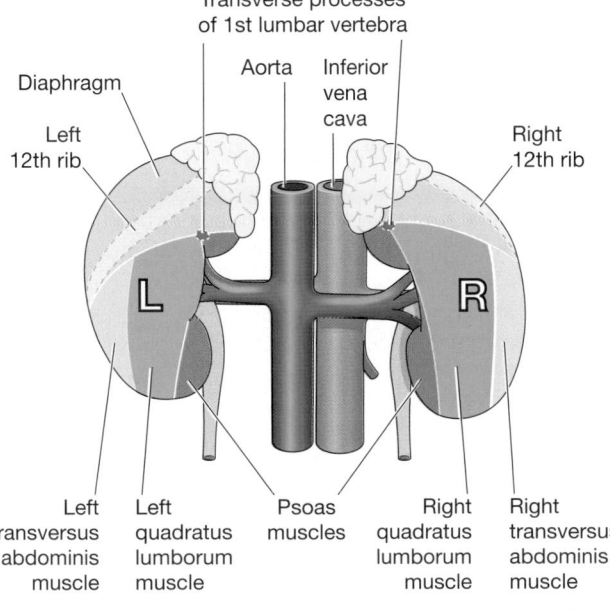

Figure 13.3 Posterior view of the kidneys showing the areas of contact with associated structures.

Figure 13.4 A longitudinal section of the right kidney.

Figure 13.5 A nephron and associated blood vessels.

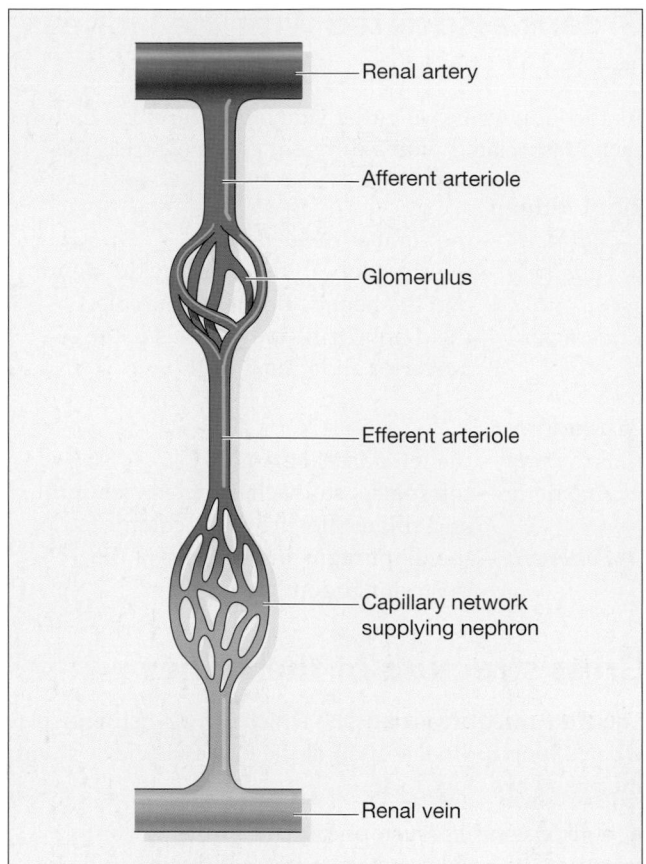

Figure 13.6 The series of blood vessels in the kidney.

The nephron (Fig. 13.5)

The nephron consists of a tubule closed at one end, the other end opening into a collecting tubule. The closed or blind end is indented to form the cup-shaped *glomerular capsule* (Bowman's capsule) which almost completely encloses a network of arterial capillaries, the *glomerulus*. Continuing from the glomerular capsule the remainder of the nephron is about 3 cm long and is described in three parts:

- the *proximal convoluted tubule*
- the *medullary loop* (loop of Henle)
- the *distal convoluted tubule*, leading into a *collecting duct*.

The collecting ducts unite, forming larger ducts that empty into the minor calyces.

After entering the kidney at the hilum the renal artery divides into smaller arteries and arterioles. In the cortex an arteriole, the *afferent arteriole*, enters each glomerular

capsule then subdivides into a cluster of capillaries, forming the glomerulus. Between the capillary loops there are connective tissue phagocytic *mesangial cells*, which are part of the reticuloendothelial system (p. 66). The blood vessel leading away from the glomerulus is the *efferent arteriole*; it breaks up into a second capillary network to supply oxygen and nutrients to the remainder of the nephron. Venous blood drained from this capillary bed eventually leaves the kidney in the renal vein which empties into the inferior vena cava (Fig. 13.6). The blood pressure in the glomerulus is higher than in other capillaries because the diameter of the afferent arteriole is greater than that of the efferent arteriole.

The walls of the glomerulus and the glomerular capsule consist of a single layer of *flattened epithelial cells* (Fig. 13.7). The glomerular walls are more permeable than those of other capillaries. The remainder of the nephron and the collecting tubule are formed by a single layer of highly specialised cells.

The nerve supply to the blood vessels of the kidney consists of sympathetic and parasympathetic nerves. The presence of both branches of the autonomic nervous system permits control of renal blood vessel diameter and renal blood flow independently of autoregulation.

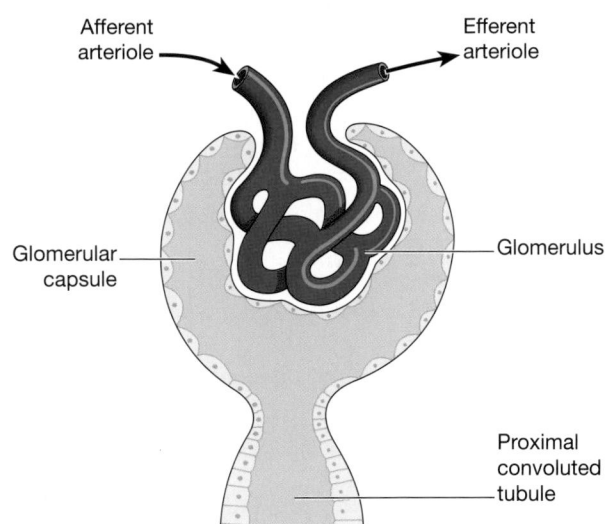

Figure 13.7 The glomerulus and glomerular capsule.

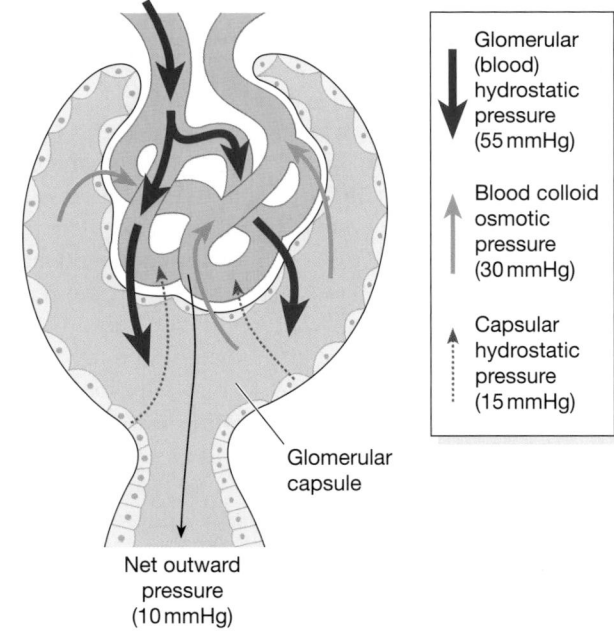

Figure 13.8 Filtration in the nephron.

Functions of the kidney

Formation of urine

The kidneys form urine which passes through the ureters to the bladder for storage prior to excretion. The composition of urine reflects the activities of the nephrons in the maintenance of homeostasis. Waste products of protein metabolism are excreted, electrolyte balance is maintained and the pH (acid–base balance) is maintained by the excretion of hydrogen ions. There are three processes involved in the formation of urine:

- simple filtration
- selective reabsorption
- secretion.

Simple filtration (Fig. 13.8)

Filtration takes place through the semipermeable walls of the glomerulus and glomerular capsule. Water and a large number of small molecules pass through, although some are reabsorbed later. Blood cells, plasma proteins and other large molecules are unable to filter through and remain in the capillaries (see Box 13.1). The filtrate in the glomerulus is very similar in composition to plasma with the important exception of plasma proteins.

Filtration is assisted by the difference between the blood pressure in the glomerulus and the pressure of the filtrate in the glomerular capsule. Because the diameter of the efferent arteriole is less than that of the afferent arteriole, a *capillary hydrostatic pressure* of about 7.3 kPa (55 mmHg) builds up in the glomerulus. This pressure is opposed by the *osmotic pressure* of the blood, about 4 kPa (30 mmHg), and by *filtrate hydrostatic pressure* of about

> **Box 13.1 Constituents of glomerular filtrate and glomerular capillaries**
>
> | **Blood constituents in glomerular filtrate** | **Blood constituents remaining in the glomerulus** |
> | --- | --- |
> | Water | Leukocytes |
> | Mineral salts | Erythrocytes |
> | Amino acids | Platelets |
> | Ketoacids | Plasma proteins |
> | Glucose | Some drugs |
> | Hormones | |
> | Creatinine | |
> | Urea | |
> | Uric acid | |
> | Toxins | |
> | Some drugs | |

343

2 kPa (15 mmHg) in the glomerular capsule. The net *filtration pressure* is, therefore:

7.3 – (4 + 2) = 1.3 kPa, or
55 – (30 + 15) = 10 mmHg.

The volume of filtrate formed by both kidneys each minute is called the *glomerular filtration rate* (GFR). In a healthy adult the GFR is about 125 ml/min; i.e. 180 litres of dilute filtrate are formed each day by the two kidneys. Most of the filtrate is reabsorbed with less than 1%, i.e. 1 to 1.5 litres, excreted as urine. The difference in volume and concentration is due to selective reabsorption of some constituents of the filtrate and tubular secretion of others.

Autoregulation of filtration. Renal blood flow is protected by a mechanism called *autoregulation* whereby renal blood flow is maintained at a constant pressure across a wide range of systolic blood pressures (from 80 to 200 mmHg). Autoregulation operates independently of nervous control; i.e. if the nerve supply to the renal blood vessels is interrupted, autoregulation continues to operate. It is therefore a property inherent in renal blood vessels; it may be stimulated by changes in blood pressure in the renal arteries or by fluctuating levels of certain metabolites, e.g. prostaglandins.

In severe shock when the systolic blood pressure falls below 80 mmHg, autoregulation fails and renal blood flow and the hydrostatic pressure decrease, impairing filtration within the nephrons.

Selective reabsorption (Fig. 13.9)

Selective reabsorption is the process by which the composition and volume of the glomerular filtrate are altered during its passage through the convoluted tubules, the medullary loop and the collecting tubule. The general purpose of this process is to reabsorb into the blood those filtrate constituents needed by the body to maintain fluid and electrolyte balance and the pH of the blood. Active transport is carried out at carrier sites in the epithelial membrane using chemical energy to transport substances against their concentration gradients (p. 34).

Some constituents of glomerular filtrate (e.g. glucose, amino acids) do not normally appear in urine because they are completely reabsorbed unless they are present in blood in excessive quantities. The kidneys' maximum capacity for reabsorption of a substance is the *transport maximum*, or renal threshold, e.g. normal blood glucose level is 2.5 to 5.3 mmol/l (45 to 95 mg/100 ml). If the level rises above the transport maximum of about 9 mmol/l (160 mg/100 ml) glucose appears in the urine because all the carrier sites are occupied and the mechanism for active transfer out of the tubules is overloaded. Other substances reabsorbed by active transport include amino acids and sodium, calcium, potassium, phosphate and chloride.

Some ions, e.g. sodium and chloride, can be absorbed by both active and passive mechanisms depending on the site in the nephron.

The transport maximum, or renal threshold, of some substances varies according to the body's need for them at the time, and in some cases reabsorption is regulated by hormones.

Parathyroid hormone from the parathyroid glands and *calcitonin* from the thyroid gland together regulate reabsorption of calcium and phosphate.

Antidiuretic hormone (ADH) from the posterior lobe of the pituitary gland increases the permeability of the distal convoluted tubules and collecting tubules, increasing water reabsorption (Fig. 13.10).

Aldosterone, secreted by the adrenal cortex, increases the reabsorption of sodium and excretion of potassium (Fig. 13.11).

Nitrogenous waste products, such as urea and uric acid, are reabsorbed only to a slight extent.

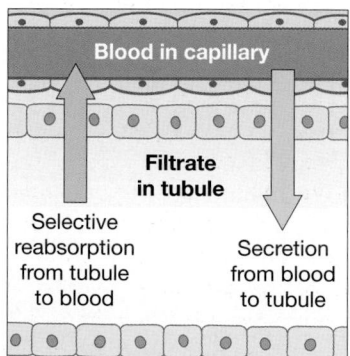

Figure 13.9 Directions of selective reabsorption and secretion in the nephron.

Figure 13.10 Negative feedback regulation of secretion of antidiuretic hormone (ADH).

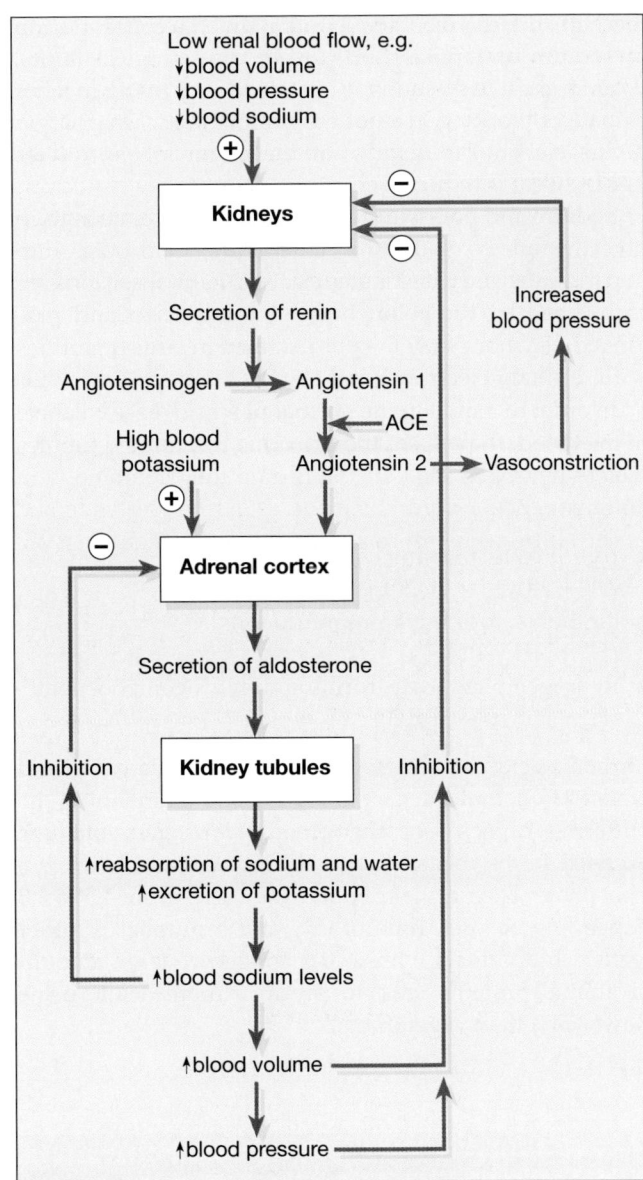

Figure 13.11 Negative feedback regulation of aldosterone secretion. ACE = angiotensin converting enzyme.

Substances that are not normal blood constituents are not reabsorbed. If the blood passes through the glomerulus too quickly for filtration to clear such substances from the blood, the tubules secrete them into the filtrate.

Secretion (Fig. 13.9)

Filtration occurs as the blood flows through the glomerulus. Substances not required and foreign materials, e.g. drugs including penicillin and aspirin, may not be cleared from the blood by filtration because of the short time it remains in the glomerulus. Such substances are cleared by *secretion into the convoluted tubules* and excreted from the body in the urine. Tubular secretion of hydrogen

(H^+) ions is important in maintaining homeostasis of blood pH.

Composition of urine

Water	96%
Urea	2%
Uric acid	
Creatinine	
Ammonia	
Sodium	
Potassium	2%
Chlorides	
Phosphates	
Sulphates	
Oxalates	

Urine is clear and amber in colour due to the presence of urobilin, a bile pigment altered in the intestine, reabsorbed then excreted by the kidneys (see Fig. 12.43, p. 314). The specific gravity is between 1020 and 1030, and the pH is around 6 (normal range of 4.5 to 8). A healthy adult passes 1000 to 1500 ml per day. The amount of urine produced and the specific gravity vary according to the fluid intake and the amount of solute excreted. During sleep and muscular exercise urine production is decreased.

Water balance and urine output

Water is taken into the body through the alimentary tract and a small amount (called 'metabolic water') is formed by the metabolic processes. Water is excreted in saturated expired air, as a constituent of the faeces, through the skin as sweat and as the main constituent of urine. The amount lost in expired air and in the faeces is fairly constant and the amount of sweat produced is associated with the maintenance of normal body temperature (p. 365).

The balance between fluid intake and output is therefore controlled by the kidneys. The minimum urinary output, i.e., the smallest volume required to excrete the body's waste products, is about 500 ml per day. The amount produced in excess of this is controlled mainly by *antidiuretic hormone* (ADH) released into the blood by the posterior lobe of the pituitary gland. There is a close link between the posterior pituitary and the hypothalamus in the brain (see Fig. 9.3A and B, p. 216).

Sensory nerve cells in the hypothalamus (*osmoreceptors*) detect changes in the osmotic pressure of the blood. Nerve impulses from the osmoreceptors stimulate the posterior lobe of the pituitary gland to release ADH. When the osmotic pressure is raised, ADH output is increased and as a result, water reabsorption by the cells in distal convoluted tubules and collecting ducts is increased, reducing the blood osmotic pressure and ADH

345

output. This feedback mechanism maintains the blood osmotic pressure (and therefore sodium and water concentrations) within normal limits (Fig. 13.10).

The feedback mechanism may be opposed when there is an excessive amount of a dissolved substance in the blood. For example, in diabetes mellitus when the blood glucose level is above the transport maximum of the renal tubules, excess water is excreted with the excess glucose. This *polyuria* may lead to dehydration in spite of increased production of ADH but it is usually accompanied by acute thirst and increased water intake.

Electrolyte balance

Changes in the concentration of electrolytes in the body fluids may be due to changes in:

- the body water content, or
- electrolyte levels.

There are several mechanisms that maintain the balance between water and electrolyte concentration.

Sodium and potassium concentration

Sodium is the most common cation (positively charged ion) in extracellular fluid and potassium is the most common intracellular cation.

Sodium is a constituent of almost all foods and it is often added to food during cooking. This means that intake is usually in excess of the body's needs. It is excreted mainly in urine and sweat.

Sodium is a normal constituent of urine and the amount excreted is regulated by the hormone *aldosterone*, secreted by the adrenal cortex. Cells in the afferent arteriole of the nephron are stimulated to produce the enzyme *renin* by sympathetic stimulation, low blood volume or by low arterial blood pressure. Renin converts the plasma protein *angiotensinogen*, produced by the liver, to *angiotensin 1*. *Angiotensin converting enzyme* (ACE), formed in small quantities in the lungs, proximal convoluted tubules and other tissues, converts angiotensin 1 into angiotensin 2 which is a very potent vasoconstrictor and increases blood pressure. Renin and raised blood potassium levels also stimulate the adrenal gland to secrete aldosterone (Fig. 13.11). Water is reabsorbed with sodium and together they increase the blood volume, leading to reduced renin secretion through the negative feedback mechanism (Fig. 13.11). When *sodium reabsorption* is increased *potassium excretion* is increased, indirectly reducing intracellular potassium.

The amount of sodium excreted in sweat is insignificant except when sweating is excessive. This may occur when there is pyrexia, a high environmental temperature or during sustained physical exercise. Normally the renal mechanism described above maintains the concentration of sodium and potassium within physiological limits. When excessive sweating is sustained, e.g. living in a hot climate or working in a hot environment, acclimatisation occurs in about 7 to 10 days and the amount of electrolytes lost in sweat is reduced.

Sodium and potassium occur in high concentrations in digestive juices — sodium in gastric juice and potassium in pancreatic and intestinal juice. Normally these ions are reabsorbed by the colon but following acute and prolonged diarrhoea they may be excreted in large quantities with resultant electrolyte imbalance.

In order to maintain the normal pH (acid–base balance) of the blood, the cells of the proximal convoluted tubules secrete hydrogen ions. In the filtrate they combine with buffers (p. 22):

- bicarbonate, forming carbonic acid
  ($H^+ + HCO_3^- \rightarrow H_2CO_3$)
- ammonia, forming ammonium ions
  ($H^+ + NH_3 \rightarrow NH_4^+$)
- hydrogen phosphate, forming dihydrogen phosphate
  ($H^+ + HPO_4^{2-} \rightarrow H_2PO_4^-$).

Carbonic acid is converted to carbon dioxide (CO_2) and water (H_2O), and the CO_2 is reabsorbed maintaining the buffering capacity of the blood. Hydrogen ions are excreted in the urine as ammonium salts and hydrogen phosphate. The normal pH of urine varies from 4.5 to 7.8 depending on diet, time of day and a number of other factors. Individuals whose diet contains a large amount of animal proteins tend to produce more acidic urine (lower pH) than vegetarians.

URETERS

Learning outcome

After studying this section you should be able to:

- outline the structure and function of the ureters.

The ureters are the tubes that convey urine from the kidneys to the urinary bladder (Fig. 13.12). They are about 25 to 30 cm long with a diameter of about 3 mm.

The ureter is continuous with the funnel-shaped renal pelvis. It passes downwards through the abdominal cavity, behind the peritoneum in front of the psoas muscle into the pelvic cavity, and passes obliquely through the posterior wall of the bladder (Fig. 13.13). Because of this

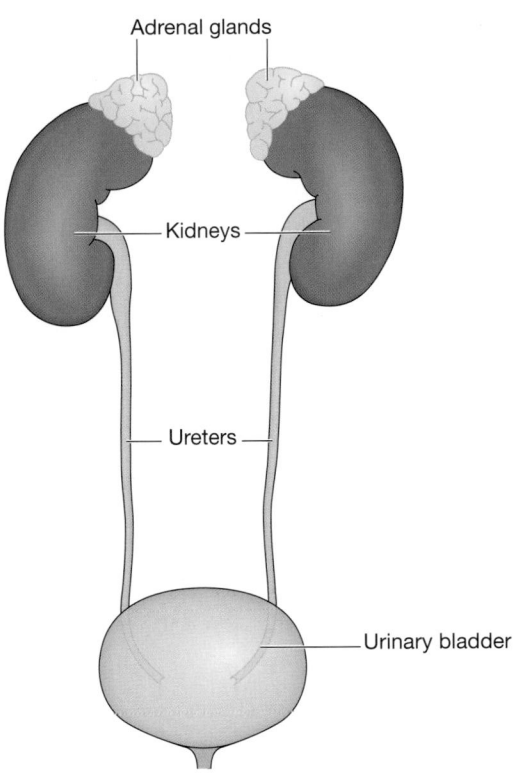

Figure 13.12 The ureters and their relationship to the kidneys and bladder.

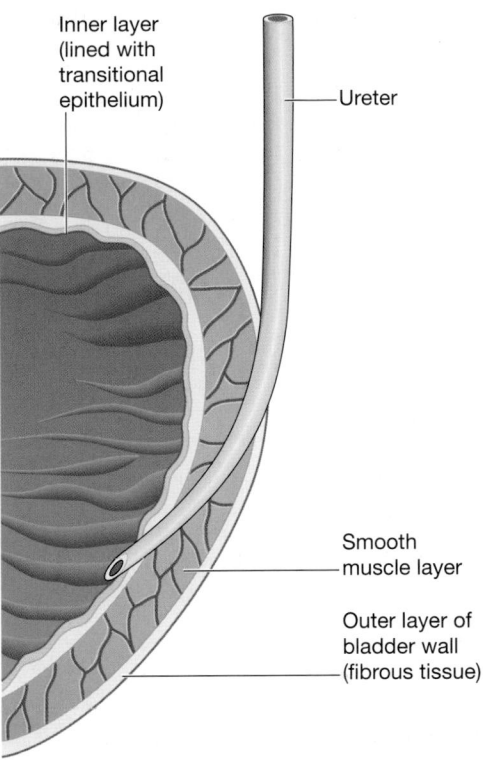

Figure 13.13 The position of the ureter where it passes through the bladder wall.

347

arrangement, when urine accumulates and the pressure in the bladder rises, the ureters are compressed and the openings occluded. This prevents reflux of urine into the ureters (towards the kidneys) as the bladder fills and during micturition, when pressure increases as the muscular bladder wall contracts.

Structure

The ureters consist of three layers of tissue:

- an outer covering of *fibrous tissue*, continuous with the fibrous capsule of the kidney
- a middle *muscular layer* consisting of interlacing smooth muscle fibres that form a syncytium spiralling round the ureter, some in clockwise and some in anticlockwise directions and an additional outer longitudinal layer in the lower third
- an inner layer, the *mucosa*, lined with transitional epithelium.

Function

The ureters propel the urine from the kidneys into the bladder by peristaltic contraction of the smooth muscle layer. This is an intrinsic property of the smooth muscle and is not under autonomic nerve control. The waves of contraction originate in a pacemaker in the minor calyces. Peristaltic waves occur several times per minute, increasing in frequency with the volume of urine produced, and send little spurts of urine into the bladder.

URINARY BLADDER

Learning outcome

After studying this section you should be able to:

- describe the structure of the bladder.

The urinary bladder is a reservoir for urine. It lies in the pelvic cavity and its size and position vary, depending on the amount of urine it contains. When distended, the bladder rises into the abdominal cavity.

Organs associated with the bladder

Organs associated with the bladder in the female		
Anteriorly	—	the symphysis pubis
Posteriorly	—	the uterus and upper part of the vagina
Superiorly	—	the small intestine
Inferiorly	—	the urethra and the muscles forming the pelvic floor

Organs associated with the bladder in the male		
Anteriorly	—	the symphysis pubis
Posteriorly	—	the rectum and seminal vesicles
Superiorly	—	the small intestine
Inferiorly	—	the urethra and prostate gland

Figure 13.14 The pelvic organs associated with the bladder and the urethra in: A. The female. B. The male.

Structure (Fig. 13.15)

The bladder is roughly pear-shaped, but becomes more oval as it fills with urine. It has anterior, superior and posterior surfaces. The posterior surface is the *base*. The bladder opens into the urethra at its lowest point, *the neck*.

The *peritoneum* covers only the superior surface before it turns upwards as the parietal peritoneum, lining the anterior abdominal wall. Posteriorly it surrounds the uterus in the female and the rectum in the male.

The bladder wall is composed of three layers:

- the outer layer of loose connective tissue, containing blood and lymphatic vessels and nerves, covered on the upper surface by the peritoneum
- the middle layer, consisting of a mass of interlacing smooth muscle fibres and elastic tissue loosely arranged in three layers. This is called the *detrusor muscle* and it empties the bladder when it contracts
- the mucosa, lined with transitional epithelium (p. 36).

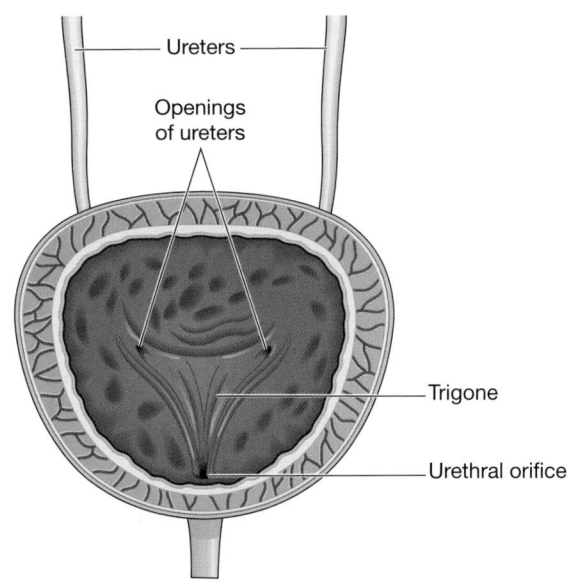

Figure 13.15 Section of the bladder showing the trigone.

When the bladder is empty the inner lining is arranged in folds, or rugae, and these gradually disappear as the bladder fills. The bladder is distensible but when it contains 300 to 400 ml the awareness of the desire to urinate is initiated. The total capacity is rarely more than about 600 ml.

The three orifices in the bladder wall form a triangle or *trigone* (Fig. 13.15). The upper two orifices on the posterior wall are the openings of the ureters. The lower orifice is the point of origin of the urethra. Where the urethra commences is a thickening of the smooth muscle layer forming the *internal urethral sphincter*. This sphincter is not under voluntary control.

URETHRA

Learning outcome

After studying this section you should be able to:

■ outline the structure and function of the urethra in males and females.

The urethra is a canal extending from the neck of the bladder to the exterior, at the external urethral orifice. Its length differs in the male and in the female. The male urethra is associated with the urinary and the reproductive systems, and is described in Chapter 19.

The female urethra is approximately 4 cm long. It runs downwards and forwards behind the symphysis pubis and opens at the *external urethral orifice* just in front of the vagina. The external urethral orifice is guarded by the *external urethral sphincter* which is under voluntary control. Except during the passage of urine, the walls of the urethra are in close apposition.

The male urethra is described in detail in Chapter 19, but in both sexes the basic structure is the same. Its walls consist of three layers of tissue.

■ the *muscle layer*, continuous with that of the bladder. At its origin there is the *internal urethral sphincter*, consisting mainly of elastic tissue and smooth muscle fibres, under autonomic nerve control. Slow and continuous contraction of this sphincter keeps the urethra closed. In the middle third there is skeletal muscle surrounding the urethra, under voluntary nerve control, that forms the *external urethral sphincter*
■ the *submucosa,* a spongy layer containing blood vessels and nerves
■ the *mucosa*, which is continuous with that of the bladder in the upper part. In the lower part the lining consists of stratified squamous epithelium, continuous externally with the skin of the vulva.

MICTURITION

Learning outcome

After studying this section you should be able to:

■ compare and contrast the process of micturition in babies and adults.

The urinary bladder acts as a reservoir for urine. When 300 to 400 ml of urine have accumulated, afferent autonomic nerve fibres in the bladder wall sensitive to stretch are stimulated. In the infant this initiates a *spinal reflex action* (see p. 159) and micturition occurs (Fig. 13.16). Micturition occurs when autonomic efferent fibres convey impulses to the bladder causing contraction of the detrusor muscle and relaxation of the internal urethral sphincter.

When the nervous system is fully developed the micturition reflex is stimulated but sensory impulses pass upwards to the brain and there is an awareness of the desire to pass urine. By conscious effort, reflex contraction

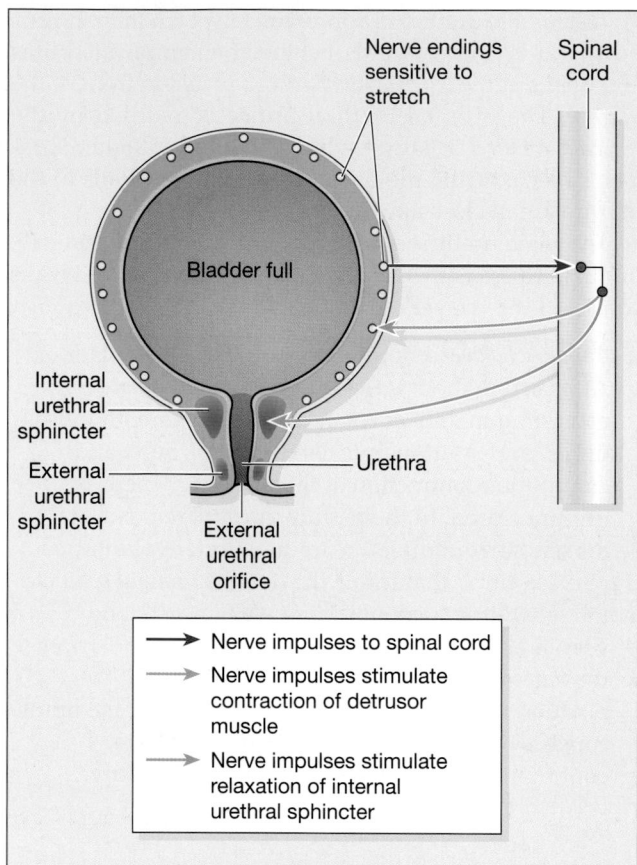

Figure 13.16 Simple reflex control of micturition when conscious effort cannot override the reflex action.

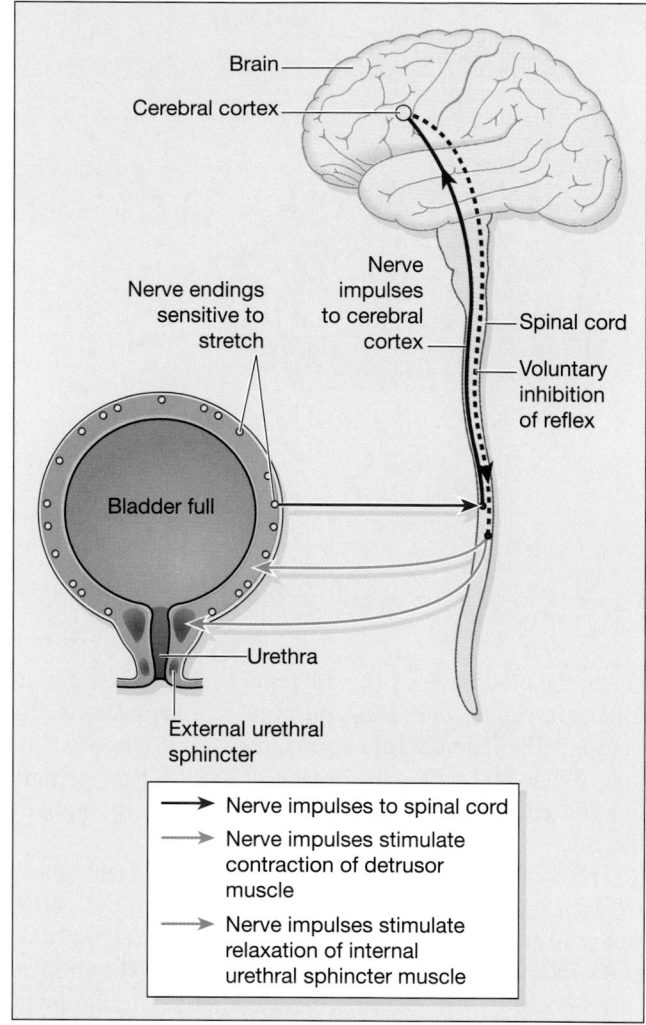

Figure 13.17 Control of micturition when conscious effort overrides the reflex action.

of the bladder wall and relaxation of the internal sphincter can be inhibited for a limited period of time (Fig. 13.17).

In adults, micturition occurs when the detrusor muscle contracts, and there is reflex relaxation of the internal sphincter and voluntary relaxation of the external sphincter. It can be assisted by increasing the pressure within the pelvic cavity, achieved by lowering the diaphragm and contracting the abdominal muscles (Valsalva's manoeuvre). Over-distension of the bladder is

extremely painful, and when this stage is reached there is a tendency for involuntary relaxation of the external sphincter to occur and a small amount of urine to escape, provided there is no mechanical obstruction.

DISEASES OF THE KIDNEYS

Learning outcomes

After studying this section you should be able to:

- outline the principal causes and effects of glomerulonephritis

- describe the effects of systemic conditions, e.g. diabetes mellitus and hypertension on kidney function

- discuss the sources and consequences of kidney infections

- explain the causes and implications of acute and chronic renal failure

- describe the pathogenesis of kidney stones

- list common congenital abnormalities of the kidneys

- outline the development and spread of common tumours of the kidney.

Glomerulonephritis (GN)

This term suggests inflammatory conditions of the glomerulus, but there are several types of GN and inflammatory changes are not always present. In many cases immune complexes damage the glomeruli. These are formed when antigens and antibodies combine either within the kidney or elsewhere in the body, and they circulate in the blood. When immune complexes lodge in the walls of the glomeruli they often cause an inflammatory response that impairs glomerular function. Other immune mechanisms are also implicated in GN.

Classification of GN is complex and based on a number of features: the cause, immunological characteristics and findings on microscopy. Microscopic distinction is based on:

- the extent of damage:
  - *diffuse:* affecting all glomeruli
  - *focal:* affecting some glomeruli
- appearance:
  - *proliferative:* increased number of cells in the glomeruli
  - *membranous:* thickening of the glomerular basement membrane.

Examples of some different types of GN and their features are shown in Table 13.1.

351

Table 13.1 Some types of glomerulonephritis and their features

Type	Presenting features	Other features
Diffuse proliferative GN	Acute nephritis Haematuria Proteinuria	Deposition of immune complexes in all glomeruli stimulates the inflammatory response Often follows 1 to 4 weeks after a β-haemolytic streptococcal infection of the tonsils, pharynx, middle ear or skin; or more rarely by a variety of other microbes Prognosis: good in children, less good in adults, up to 40% develop hypertension or chronic renal failure
Focal proliferative GN	Acute nephritis Haematuria Proteinuria	An inflammatory response develops in parts of some glomeruli Usually accompanied by a systemic disease, e.g. systemic lupus erythematosus (SLE), Henoch–Schönlein purpura, infective endocarditis Prognosis: variable
Membranous GN	Nephrotic syndrome Haematuria Proteinuria	Deposition of immune complexes in the glomerular basement membrane stimulates the inflammatory response Cause is often unknown, but sometimes secondary to infections, tumours, drugs, SLE Prognosis: variable, but most cases progress to chronic renal failure as sclerosis of glomeruli progresses
Minimal change GN	Nephrotic syndrome Haematuria Proteinuria	Immune complexes are not involved Commonest cause of nephrotic syndrome in children, usually occurring between the ages of 1 to 4 years and often following a chest infection Prognosis: good in children, but recurrences are common in adults

Effects of glomerulonephritis

These depend on the type and are listed below.

Haematuria. This is usually painless and not accompanied by other symptoms. When microscopic, it may be found on routine urinalysis when red blood cells have passed from the damaged glomeruli into the filtrate.

Asymptomatic proteinuria. This may also be found on routine urinalysis and when it is of a low level does not cause nephrotic syndrome. It occurs as protein passes through the damaged glomeruli into the filtrate.

Acute nephritis. This is characterised by the presence of:

- anuria or oliguria
- hypertension
- haematuria
- fluid retention
- uraemia.

Loin pain, headache and malaise are also common.

Nephrotic syndrome. (See below.)

Chronic renal failure. This occurs when nephrons are progressively and irreversibly damaged after the renal reserve is lost.

Nephrotic syndrome

This is not a disease in itself but is an important feature of several kidney diseases. The main characteristics are:

- marked proteinuria
- hypoalbuminaemia
- generalised oedema
- hyperlipidaemia.

When glomeruli are damaged, the permeability of the glomerular membrane is increased and plasma proteins pass through in the filtrate. Albumin is the main protein lost because it is the most common and is the smallest of the plasma proteins. When the daily loss exceeds the rate of production by the liver there is a significant fall in the total plasma protein level. The consequent low plasma osmotic pressure leads to widespread oedema and reduced plasma volume (see Fig. 5.57, p. 119). This reduces the renal blood flow and stimulates the renin–angiotensin–aldosterone mechanism, causing increased reabsorption of water and sodium from the renal tubules. The reabsorbed water further reduces the osmotic pressure, increasing the oedema. The key factor is the loss of albumin across the glomerular membrane and as long as this continues the vicious circle is perpetuated

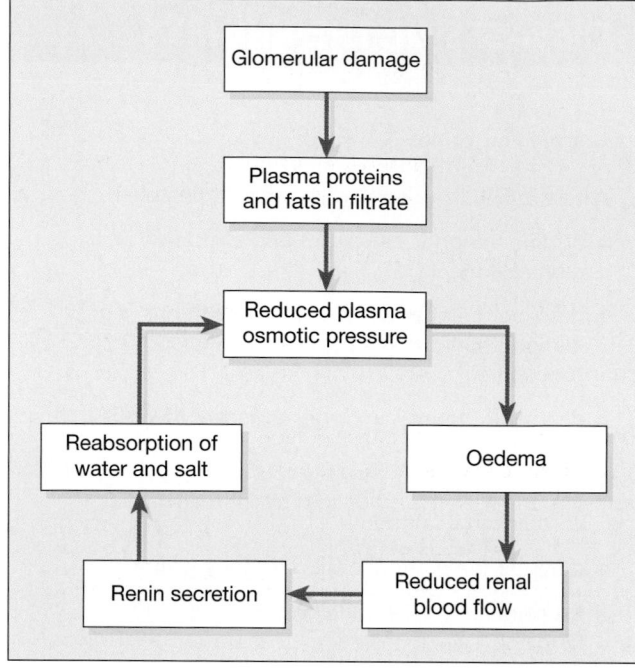

Figure 13.18 Stages of development of nephrotic syndrome.

(Fig. 13.18). Levels of nitrogenous waste products, i.e. uric acid, urea and creatinine, usually remain normal. Hyperlipidaemia, especially hypercholesterolaemia, also occurs but the cause is unknown.

The nephrotic syndrome occurs in a number of diseases. In children the most common cause is minimal-change glomerulonephritis. In adults it may complicate:

- most forms of glomerulonephritis
- diabetes mellitus
- systemic lupus erythematosus
- infections, e.g. malaria, infective endocarditis, syphilis, hepatitis B
- drugs treatment, e.g. penicillamine, gold, captopril, phenytoin.

Diabetic kidney

Renal failure is the cause of death in 10% of all diabetics and up to 50% of cases of the insulin-dependent (type I) diabetes mellitus (p. 236). There is damage to large and small blood vessels in many parts of the body. The effects include:

- progressive glomerulosclerosis followed by atrophy of the tubules
- acute pyelonephritis with papillary necrosis
- atheroma of the renal arteries and their branches, leading to renal ischaemia and hypertension (Ch. 5)
- nephrotic syndrome.

Hypertension and the kidneys

Essential and secondary hypertension (p. 126) both affect the kidneys when there is renal arteriosclerosis and arteriolosclerosis, causing ischaemia. The reduced blood flow stimulates the renin–angiotensin–aldosterone mechanism (Fig. 13.11), raising the blood pressure still further.

Essential hypertension

Benign hypertension. This causes gradual and progressive sclerosis and fibrosis of the glomeruli, leading to renal failure or, more commonly, to malignant hypertension.

Malignant hypertension. This causes rapidly developing arteriolosclerosis which spreads to the glomeruli with subsequent destruction of nephrons, leading to:

- further rise in blood pressure
- reduction in renal blood flow and the amount of filtrate
- increased permeability of the glomeruli, with the passage of plasma proteins and red blood cells into the filtrate resulting in proteinuria and haematuria
- progressive oliguria and renal failure.

Secondary hypertension

This is caused by long-standing kidney diseases such as chronic glomerulonephritis and pyelonephritis and leads to chronic renal ischaemia, further hypertension and renal failure.

Acute pyelonephritis

This is an acute microbial infection of the renal pelvis and calyces, spreading to the kidney substance causing formation of small abscesses. The infection may travel up the urinary tract from the perineum or be blood-borne. It is accompanied by fever, malaise and loin pain.

Ascending infection

Upward spread of microbes from the bladder (see cystitis, p. 357) is the most common cause of this condition. Reflux of infected urine into the ureters when the bladder contracts during micturition predisposes to upward spread of infection to the renal pelves and kidney substance.

Blood-borne infection

The source of microbes may be from septicaemia or elsewhere in the body, e.g. respiratory tract infections, infected wounds or abscesses.

When the infection spreads into the kidney tissue it causes suppuration and destruction of nephrons. The prognosis depends on the amount of healthy kidney remaining after the infection subsides. Necrotic tissue is eventually replaced by fibrous tissue but there may be some hypertrophy of healthy nephrons. There are a number of outcomes: healing, recurrence, especially if there is a structural abnormality of the urinary tract, and chronic pyelonephritis. Perinephric abscess and papillary necrosis are complications, usually if the condition is untreated.

Chronic pyelonephritis

This usually follows repeated attacks of acute pyelonephritis with scar tissue formation. It is usually associated with reflux of urine from the bladder to the ureter enabling microbes to gain access to the kidneys. A congenital abnormality of the angle of insertion of the ureter into the bladder often predisposes to the reflux of urine but it is sometimes caused by an obstruction that develops later in life. The progressive loss of functioning nephrons leads to chronic renal failure and uraemia. Concurrent hypertension is common.

Acute renal failure

There is a sudden and severe reduction in the glomerular filtration rate and kidney function that is usually reversible over days or weeks when treated. This occurs as a complication of a variety of conditions not necessarily associated with the kidneys. The causes of acute renal failure are classified as:

- *prerenal*: the result of reduced renal blood flow, especially severe and prolonged shock
- *renal*, or parenchymal: damage to the kidney itself due to, e.g., acute tubular necrosis, glomerulonephritis
- *post-renal*: obstruction to the outflow of urine, e.g. tumour of the bladder, uterus or cervix, large calculus in the renal pelvis.

Acute tubular necrosis (ATN)

This is the most common cause of acute renal failure. There is severe damage to the tubular epithelial cells caused by ischaemia or nephrotoxicity.

Ischaemic ATN

This is caused by severe and prolonged shock due to, e.g., haemorrhage, severe trauma, marked dehydration, acute intestinal obstruction, prolonged and complicated surgical procedures, extensive burns.

Nephrotoxic ATN

This is caused by:

- toxic chemicals, e.g. carbon tetrachloride (used in dry cleaning), chromic acid, ethylene glycol (antifreeze), mercurial compounds, ionising radiation
- drugs, e.g. trilene, aminoglycosides, paracetamol overdose
- endogenous substances, e.g. myoglobin (from damaged muscle), haemoglobin (from incompatible blood transfusion).

Oliguria (less than 400 ml of urine per day in adults), *severe oliguria* (less than 100 ml of urine per day in adults) or *anuria* (absence of urine) may last for a few weeks, followed by diuresis. There is reduced glomerular filtration and tubular selective reabsorption and secretion, leading to:

- generalised and pulmonary oedema
- accumulation of urea (uraemia) and other metabolic waste products
- electrolyte imbalance which may be exacerbated by the retention of potassium (hyperkalaemia) released from cells following severe injury and extensive tissue damage elsewhere in the body
- acidosis due to disrupted excretion of hydrogen ions.

Profound diuresis (the diuretic phase) occurs during the healing process when the epithelial cells of the tubules have regenerated but are still incapable of selective reabsorption and secretion. Diuresis may lead to acute dehydration, complicating the existing high plasma urea, acidosis and electrolyte imbalance. If the patient survives the initial acute phase, a considerable degree of renal function is usually restored over a period of months.

Chronic renal failure

This is reached when irreversible damage to nephrons is so severe that 75% of renal function has been lost and the kidneys cannot function effectively. The main causes are glomerulonephritis, diabetes mellitus, chronic pyelonephritis and hypertension. The effects are reduced glomerular filtration rate, selective reabsorption and secretion, and glomerular fibrosis, which interferes with blood flow. These changes have a number of effects on the body.

- *Uraemia* develops after about 7 days of anuria because of the reduced glomerular filtration rate and impaired tubular secretion of urea. Increased blood urea usually leads to confusion and mental disorientation.
- *Polyuria* is caused by defective reabsorption of water in spite of the reduced glomerular filtration rate (GFR) (Table 13.2). This may cause nocturia, thirst and polydipsia.
- *Fixed specific gravity.* The specific gravity of the urine is similar to that of glomerular filtrate, i.e. about 1.010 (normal = 1.020 to 1.030). It remains low and fixed because of defective tubular reabsorption of water.
- *Acidosis.* Control of the pH of body fluids is lost mainly because the tubules fail to remove hydrogen ions by forming ammonia and hydrogen phosphates.
- *Electrolyte imbalance* occurs as tubular reabsorption and secretion are impaired.
- *Anaemia* caused by deficiency of the hormone erythropoietin occurs when the chronic state extends over a period of months and is usually exacerbated by dialysis. It results in fatigue, dyspnoea and cardiac failure.
- *Hypertension* is often a consequence if not the cause of renal failure.

Anorexia, nausea and very deep (Kussmaul's) respirations occur as uraemia progresses. In the later stages there may also be hiccoughs, vomiting, muscle twitching, confusion, drowsiness and coma.

Renal calculi

Calculi (stones) form in the kidneys and bladder when urinary constituents normally in solution are precipitated. The solutes involved are oxalates, phosphates, urates and uric acid, and stones usually consist of more than one substance, deposited in layers. They are more

Table 13.2 Polyuria in chronic renal failure		
	Normal kidney	**End-stage kidney**
GFR	125 ml/min or 180 l/day	10 ml/min or 14 l/day
Reabsorption of water	>99%	Approx. 30%
Urine output	<1 ml/min or 1.5 l/day	Approx. 7 ml/min or 10 l/day

common in males and after 30 years of age. Most originate in collecting tubules or in renal papillae. They then pass into the renal pelvis where they may increase in size. Some become too large to pass through the ureter and may obstruct the outflow of urine causing renal failure. Others pass to the bladder and are either excreted or increase in size and obstruct the urethra. Sometimes stones originate in the bladder, usually in developing countries and often in children. Predisposing factors include:

- *Dehydration*. This leads to increased reabsorption of water from the tubules but does not change solute reabsorption, resulting in a reduced volume of highly concentrated filtrate in the collecting tubules.
- *pH of urine*. When the normally acid filtrate becomes alkaline some substances may be precipitated, e.g. phosphates. This occurs when the kidney buffering system is defective, and in some infections.
- *Infection*. Necrotic material and pus provide foci upon which solutes in the filtrate may be deposited and the products of infection may alter the pH of the urine. Infection sometimes leads to alkaline urine (see above).
- *Metabolic conditions*. These include hyperparathyroidism and gout.

Small calculi

These may pass through or become impacted in a ureter and damage the epithelium, leading to haematuria then fibrosis and stricture. In ureteric obstruction, usually unilateral, there is spasmodic contraction of the ureter, causing acute intermittent ischaemic pain (*renal colic*) as the ureter contracts over the stone. Stones reaching the bladder may be passed in urine or increase in size and eventually obstruct the urethra. Consequences include retention of urine and bilateral hydronephrosis, infection proximal to the blockage, pyelonephritis and severe kidney damage.

Large calculi (staghorn calculus)

One large stone may form, filling the renal pelvis and the calyces (Fig. 13.19). It causes stagnation of urine, predisposing to infection, hydronephrosis and occasionally kidney tumours. It may cause chronic renal failure.

Congenital abnormalities of the kidneys

Misplaced (ectopic) kidney

One or both kidneys may develop in abnormally low positions. Misplaced kidneys function normally if the

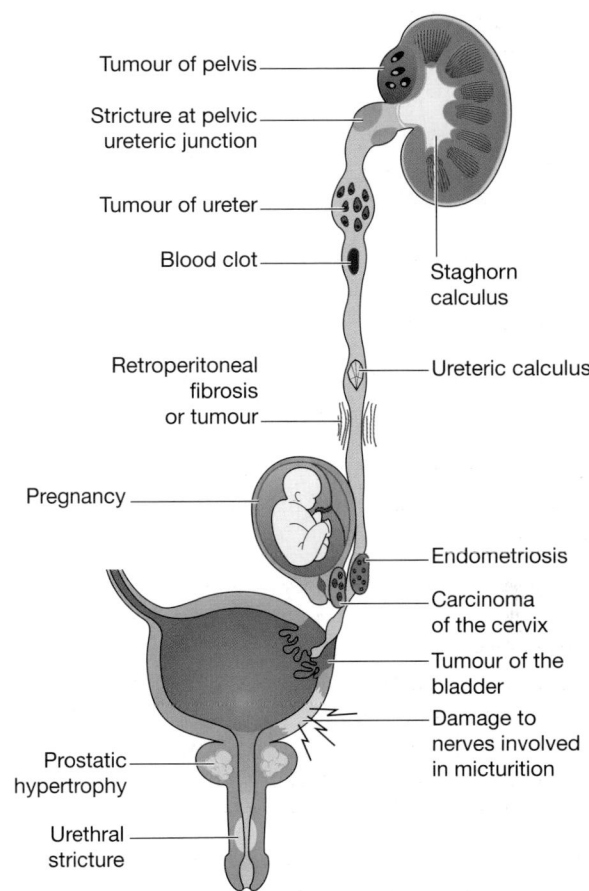

Figure 13.19 Summary of obstructions of the urinary tract.

blood vessels are long enough to provide an adequate blood supply but a kidney in the pelvis may cause problems during pregnancy as the expanding uterus compresses renal blood vessels or the ureters. If the ureters become kinked there is increased risk of infection as there is a tendency for reflux and backflow to the kidney. There may also be difficulties during parturition (childbirth).

Polycystic disease

This disease, caused by genetic abnormality, occurs in infantile and adult forms. The *infantile form* is very rare and the child usually dies soon after birth.

Adult polycystic kidney disease. This inherited condition usually becomes apparent at between 30 and 50 years of age. Both kidneys are affected. Dilatations (cysts) form at the junction of the distal convoluted and collecting tubules. The cysts slowly enlarge and pressure causes ischaemia and necrosis of nephrons, resulting in their destruction. The disease is progressive and secondary hypertension and chronic renal failure usually develop. Death may be due to chronic renal failure, cardiac failure, cerebral haemorrhage or subarachnoid haemorrhage due to increased incidence of berry aneurysms of the circulus arteriosus. Other associated abnormalities include polycystic liver disease and cysts in the spleen and pancreas.

Tumours of the kidney

Benign tumours of the kidney are relatively uncommon.

Malignant tumours

Renal clear cell carcinoma (Grawitz's tumour or hypernephroma)

This is a tumour of tubular epithelium and is more common after 50 years of age, especially in males. Local spread involves the renal vein and leads to early blood-spread of tumour fragments, most commonly to the lungs and bones. The causes are not known but cigarette smoking is believed to be a predisposing factor.

Nephroblastoma (Wilms' tumour)

This is one of the most common malignant tumours in children, usually occurring in the first 3 years. It is usually unilateral but rapidly becomes very large and invades the renal blood vessels, causing early blood-spread of the malignancy to the lungs. It is believed that the cell abnormalities occur before birth but the cause is not known.

DISEASES OF THE RENAL PELVIS, URETERS, BLADDER AND URETHRA

Learning outcomes

After studying this section you should be able to:

- describe the causes and implications of urinary obstruction

- explain the pathological features of urinary tract infections

- outline the characteristics of the main bladder tumours

- discuss the principal causes of urinary incontinence.

These structures are considered together because their combined functions are to collect and store urine prior to excretion from the body. Obstruction and infection are the main causes of dysfunction.

Obstruction to the outflow of urine

Hydronephrosis

This is dilatation of the renal pelvis and calyces caused by accumulation of urine. It leads to destruction of the nephrons, fibrosis and atrophy of the kidney. One or both kidneys may be involved, depending on the cause and site. When there is an abnormality of the bladder or urethra both kidneys are affected whereas an obstruction above the bladder is more common and affects only one kidney (Fig. 13.19).

Complete sustained obstruction

In this condition hydronephrosis develops quickly, pressure in the nephrons rises and urine production stops. The most common causes are a large calculus or tumour. The outcome depends on whether one or both kidneys are involved (homeostasis can be maintained by one kidney).

Partial or intermittent obstruction

This may lead to progressive hydronephrosis caused by, e.g.:

- a succession of renal calculi in a ureter, eventually moved onwards by peristalsis
- a calculus that partially blocks the ureter
- constriction of a ureter or the urethra by fibrous tissue, following epithelial inflammation caused by the passage of a stone or by infection
- a tumour in the urinary tract or in the abdominal or pelvic cavity
- enlarged prostate gland in the male.

Spinal lesions

The immediate effect of transverse spinal cord lesions that damage the nerve supply to the bladder is that micturition does not occur. When the bladder fills the rise in pressure causes overflow incontinence, back pressure into the ureters and hydronephrosis. Reflex micturition is usually re-established after a time, but loss of voluntary control may be irreversible. Pressure on the spinal cord and other abnormalities, e.g. spina bifida, can also impair micturition.

Complications of urinary tract obstruction

Infection. Stasis of urine predisposes to infection and pyelonephritis. The microbes usually spread upwards in the urinary tract or are sometimes bloodborne.

Calculus formation. Infection and urinary stasis predispose to calculus formation when:

- the pH of urine changes from acid to alkaline, promoting the precipitation of some solutes, e.g. phosphates
- cell debris and pus provide foci upon which solutes in the urine may be deposited.

Infections of the urinary tract

Infection of any part of the tract may spread upwards causing pyelonephritis (p. 353) and severe kidney damage.

Ureteritis

Inflammation of a ureter is usually due to the upward spread of infection in cystitis.

Acute cystitis

This is inflammation of the bladder and may be due to:

- spread of microbes that are commensals of the bowel (*Escherichia coli* and *Streptococcus faecalis*) from the perineum, especially in women because of the short wide urethra, its proximity to the anus and the moist perineal conditions
- a mixed infection of coliform and other organisms which may follow the passage of a urinary catheter or other instrument
- inflammation in the absence of microbes, e.g. following radiotherapy or passage of a catheter or other instrument.

The effects are inflammation, with oedema and small haemorrhages of the mucosa, which may be accompanied by *haematuria*. There is hypersensitivity of the sensory nerve endings in the bladder wall, which are stimulated before the bladder has filled leading to *frequency of micturition* and *dysuria* (a burning sensation on micturition). The urine may appear cloudy and have an unpleasant smell. Lower abdominal pain often accompanies cystitis.

Predisposing factors. The most important predisposing factors are coliform microbes in the perineal region and stasis of urine in the bladder. During sexual intercourse there may be trauma to the urethra and transfer of microbes from the perineum, especially in the female. Hormones associated with pregnancy cause relaxation of perineal muscle and relaxation and kinking of the ureters. Towards the end of pregnancy pressure caused by the fetus may obstruct the outflow of urine. In the male, prostatitis provides a focus of local infection or an enlarged prostate gland may cause progressive urethral obstruction.

Chronic cystitis

This may follow repeated attacks of acute cystitis. It occurs most commonly in males over 60 years of age when compression of the urethra by an enlarged prostate gland prevents the bladder from emptying completely. Calculus formation is common, especially if the normally acid urine becomes alkaline due to microbial action or kidney damage.

Urethritis

This is inflammation of the urethra. A common cause is *Neisseria gonorrhoeae* (gonococcus) spread by sexual intercourse directly to the urethra in the male and indirectly from the perineum in the female. Many cases of urethritis have no known cause, i.e. *non-specific urethritis* (Ch. 19).

Tumours of the bladder

It is not always clear whether bladder tumours are benign or malignant. Tumours are often multiple and recurrence is common. The causes of both types are not known but predisposing factors include cigarette smoking, taking high doses of analgesics over a long period and exposure to chemicals used in some industries, e.g. manufacture of aniline dyes, rubber industry, benzidine-based industries.

Papillomas

These tumours arise from transitional epithelium and are usually benign. They consist of a stalk with fine-branching fronds which tend to break off, causing painless bleeding and haematuria. Papillomas commonly recur, even when they are benign. Although the cells are well differentiated some papillomas behave as carcinomas and invade surrounding blood and lymph vessels.

Solid tumours

These are all malignant to some degree. At an early stage the more malignant and solid tumours rapidly invade the bladder wall and spread in lymph and blood to other parts of the body. If the surface ulcerates there may be haemorrhage and necrosis.

Urinary incontinence

In this condition there is involuntary passage of urine due to defective voluntary control of the external urethral sphincter.

Stress incontinence

This is leakage of urine when intra-abdominal pressure is raised, e.g. on coughing, laughing, sneezing or lifting. It usually affects women when there is weakness of the muscles of the pelvic floor or pelvic ligaments, e.g. after childbirth or as part of the ageing process.

Retention and overflow incontinence

This occurs when there is:

- retention of urine due to obstruction of urinary outflow, e.g. enlarged prostate or urethral stricture
- a neurological abnormality affecting the nerves involved in micturition, e.g. stroke, spinal cord injury or multiple sclerosis.

The bladder becomes distended and when the pressure inside overcomes the resistance of the urethral sphincter, urine dribbles from the urethra. The individual may be unable to initiate and/or maintain micturition.

Urge incontinence

Leakage of urine follows a sudden and intense urge to void and may be due to a urinary tract infection, calculus, tumour or sudden stress.

Protection and survival

4

14

The skin

The skin completely covers the body and is continuous with the membranes lining the body orifices. It:

- protects the underlying structures from injury and from invasion by microbes
- contains sensory (*somatic*) nerve endings of pain, temperature and touch
- is involved in the regulation of body temperature.

Structure of the skin

Learning outcome

After studying this section you should be able to:

- describe the structure of the skin.

The skin has a surface area of about 1.5 to 2 m² in adults and it contains glands, hair and nails. There are two main layers:

- epidermis
- dermis.

Between the skin and underlying structures there is a layer of subcutaneous fat.

Epidermis (Fig. 14.1)

The epidermis is the most superficial layer of the skin and is composed of *stratified keratinised squamous epithelium* (see Fig. 3.12, p. 36) which varies in thickness in different parts of the body. It is thickest on the palms of the hands and soles of the feet. There are no blood vessels or nerve endings in the epidermis, but its deeper layers are bathed in interstitial fluid from the dermis, which provides oxygen and nutrients, and is drained away as lymph.

There are several layers (strata) of cells in the epidermis which extend from the deepest *germinative layer* to the surface *stratum corneum* (a thick horny layer). The cells on the surface are flat, thin, non-nucleated, dead cells, or *squames*, in which the cytoplasm has been replaced by the fibrous protein *keratin*. These cells are constantly being rubbed off and replaced by cells which originated in the germinative layer and have undergone gradual change as they progressed towards the surface. Complete replacement of the epidermis takes about 40 days.

The maintenance of healthy epidermis depends upon three processes being synchronised:

Figure 14.1 The skin showing the main layers of the epidermis.

- desquamation (shedding) of the keratinised cells from the surface
- effective keratinisation of the cells approaching the surface
- continual cell division in the deeper layers with newly formed cells being pushed to the surface.

Hairs, secretions from sebaceous glands and ducts of sweat glands pass through the epidermis to reach the surface.

The surface of the epidermis is ridged by projections of cells in the dermis called the *papillae*. The pattern of ridges is different in every individual and the impression made by them is the 'fingerprint'. The downward projections of the germinative layer between the papillae are believed to aid nutrition of epidermal cells and stabilise the two layers, preventing damage due to shearing forces. *Blisters* develop when acute trauma causes separation of the dermis and epidermis and serous fluid collects between the two layers.

The colour of the skin is affected by three main factors.

- *Melanin*, a dark pigment derived from the amino acid tyrosine and secreted by *melanocytes* in the deep germinative layer, is absorbed by surrounding epithelial cells. The amount is genetically determined and varies between different parts of the body, between members of the same race and between races. The number of melanocytes is fairly constant so the differences in colour depend on the amount of melanin secreted. It protects the skin from the harmful effects of sunlight. Exposure to sunlight promotes synthesis of increased amounts of melanin.

- *The level of oxygenation of haemoglobin* and the amount of blood circulating in the dermis give the skin its pink colour.
- *Bile pigments* in blood and *carotenes* in subcutaneous fat give the skin a yellowish colour.

Dermis (Fig. 14.2)

The dermis is tough and elastic. It is formed from connective tissue and the matrix contains *collagen fibres* interlaced with *elastic fibres*. Rupture of elastic fibres occurs when the skin is overstretched, resulting in permanent *striae*, or stretch marks, that may be found in pregnancy and obesity. Collagen fibres bind water and give the skin its tensile strength, but as this ability declines with age, wrinkles develop. Fibroblasts, macrophages and mast cells are the main cells found in the dermis. Underlying its deepest layer there is areolar tissue and varying amounts of adipose tissue (fat). The structures in the dermis are:

- blood vessels
- lymph vessels
- sensory (somatic) nerve endings
- sweat glands and their ducts
- hairs, arrector pili muscles and sebaceous glands.

Blood vessels. Arterioles form a fine network with capillary branches supplying sweat glands, sebaceous glands, hair follicles and the dermis. The epidermis has no blood supply. It obtains nutrients and oxygen from interstitial fluid derived from blood vessels in the papillae of the dermis.

Lymph vessels. These form a network throughout the dermis.

Sensory nerve endings. Sensory receptors (specialised nerve endings) which are sensitive to *touch*, *change in temperature*, *pressure* and *pain* are widely distributed in the dermis. Incoming stimuli activate different types of sensory receptors shown in Figure 14.2 and Box 14.1. The skin is an important sensory organ through which individuals receive information about their environment. Nerve impulses, generated in the sensory receptors in the dermis, are conveyed to the spinal cord by sensory (*somatic cutaneous*) nerves, then to the sensory area of the cerebrum where the sensations are perceived.

Sweat glands

Sweat glands are found widely distributed throughout the skin and are most numerous in the palms of the hands, soles of the feet, axillae and groins. They are composed of epithelial cells. The bodies of the glands lie coiled in the subcutaneous tissue. Some ducts open onto the skin surface at tiny depressions, or pores, and others open into hair follicles. Glands opening into hair follicles

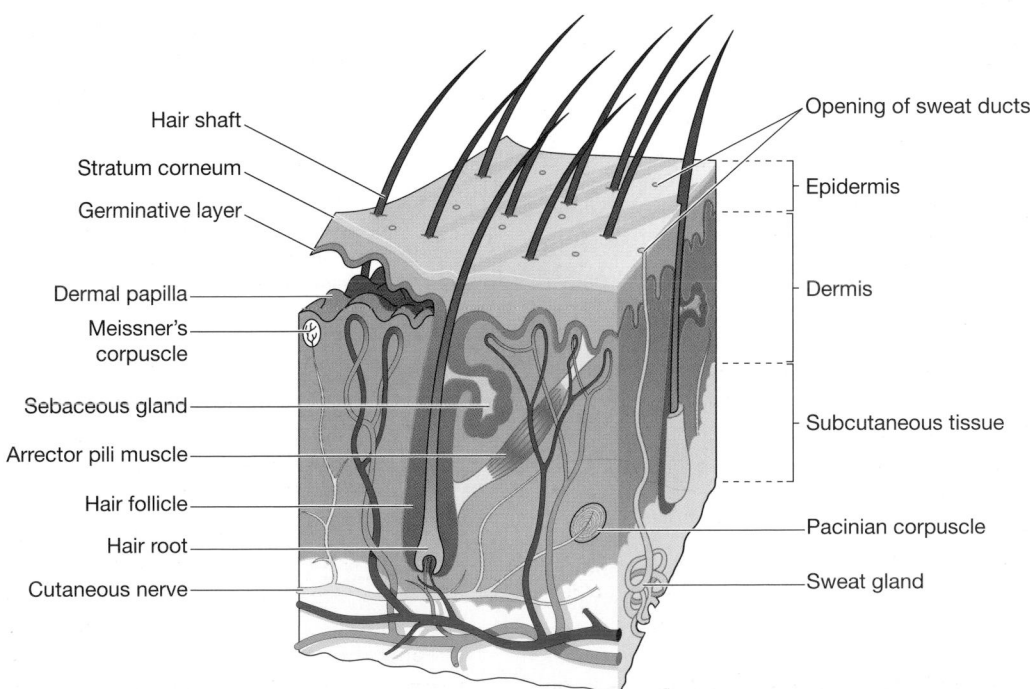

Figure 14.2 The skin showing the main structures in the dermis.

Box 14.1. Sensory receptors in the skin

Sensory receptor	Stimulus
Meissner's corpuscle	Light pressure
Pacinian corpuscle	Deep pressure
Free nerve ending	Pain

do not become active until puberty. In the axilla they secrete an odourless milky fluid which, if decomposed by surface microbes, causes an unpleasant odour. The functions of this secretion are not known. Sweat glands are stimulated by sympathetic nerves in response to raised body temperature and fear.

The most important function of sweat secreted by glands opening on to the skin surface is in the regulation of body temperature. Evaporation of sweat from body surfaces takes heat from the body and the amount of sweat produced is governed by the temperature-regulating centre in the hypothalamus. Excessive sweating may lead to dehydration and serious depletion of body sodium chloride unless intake of water and salt is appropriately increased. After 7 to 10 days' exposure to high environmental temperatures the amount of salt lost is substantially reduced but water loss remains high.

Hairs

These are formed by a down-growth of epidermal cells into the dermis or subcutaneous tissue, called *hair follicles*. At the base of the follicle is a cluster of cells called the *bulb*. The hair is formed by multiplication of cells of the bulb and as they are pushed upwards, away from their source of nutrition, the cells die and become keratinised. The part of the hair above the skin is the *shaft* and the remainder, the *root* (Fig. 14.2).

The colour of the hair is genetically determined and depends on the amount of melanin present. White hair is the result of the replacement of melanin by tiny air bubbles.

The arrector pili (Fig. 14.2). These are little bundles of smooth muscle fibres attached to the hair follicles. Contraction makes the hair stand erect and raises the skin around the hair, causing 'goose flesh'. The muscles are stimulated by sympathetic nerve fibres in response to fear and cold. Erect hairs trap air, which acts as an insulating layer. This is an efficient warming mechanism especially when accompanied by shivering, i.e. involuntary contraction of the skeletal muscles.

The sebaceous glands (Fig. 14.2). These consist of secretory epithelial cells derived from the same tissue as the

hair follicles. They secrete an oily substance, *sebum*, into the hair follicles and are therefore present in the skin of all parts of the body except the palms of the hands and the soles of the feet. They are most numerous in the skin of the scalp, face, axillae and groins. In regions of transition from one type of superficial epithelium to another, such as lips, eyelids, nipple, labia minora and glans penis, there are sebaceous glands that are independent of hair follicles, secreting sebum directly on to the surface.

Sebum keeps the hair soft and pliable and gives it a shiny appearance. On the skin it provides some waterproofing and acts as a bactericidal and fungicidal agent, preventing the successful invasion of microbes. It also prevents drying and cracking of skin, especially on exposure to heat and sunshine. The activity of these glands increases at puberty and is less at the extremes of age, rendering infants and the elderly prone to the effects of excessive moisture, e.g. nappy rash in infants.

Nails (Fig. 14.3)

The nails in human beings are equivalent to the claws, horns and hoofs of animals. They are derived from the same cells as epidermis and hair and consist of a hard, horny keratin plate. They protect the tips of the fingers and toes.

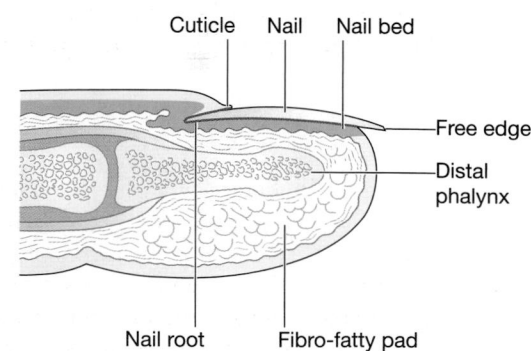

Figure 14.3 The nail and related skin.

The *root* of the nail is embedded in the skin, is covered by the *cuticle* and forms the hemispherical pale area called the *lunula*.

The *nail plate* of the nail is the exposed part that has grown out from the germinative zone of the epidermis called the *nail bed*.

Finger nails grow more quickly than toe nails and growth is quicker when the environmental temperature is high.

Functions of the skin

> **Learning outcome**
>
> After studying this section you should be able to:
>
> ■ explain the following functions of the skin: protection, regulation of body temperature, formation of vitamin D, sensation, absorption and excretion.

Protection

The skin forms a relatively waterproof layer that protects the deeper and more delicate structures. As an important non-specific defence mechanism it acts as a barrier against:

- invasion by microbes
- chemicals
- physical agents, e.g. mild trauma, ultraviolet light
- dehydration.

The dermis contains specialised immune cells called Langerhans cells. They phagocytose intruding antigens and travel to lymphoid tissue, where they present antigen to T-lymphocytes, thus stimulating an immune response (p. 379).

Due to the presence of the sensory nerve endings in the skin the body reacts by reflex action to unpleasant or painful stimuli, protecting it from further injury (p. 159).

Regulation of body temperature

The temperature of the body remains fairly constant at about 36.8°C (98.4°F) across a wide range of environmental temperatures. In health, variations are usually limited to between 0.5 and 0.75°C, although it is raised slightly in the evening, during exercise and in women just after ovulation. When metabolic rate increases body temperature rises and when it decreases body temperature falls.

To ensure this constant temperature a balance is maintained between heat produced in the body and heat lost to the environment.

Heat production

Some of the energy released in the cells during metabolic activity is in the form of heat and the most active organs, chemically and physically, produce the most heat. The principal organs involved are as follows.

- *The muscles*. Contraction of skeletal muscles produces a large amount of heat and the more strenuous the muscular exercise the greater the heat produced. Shivering involves muscle contraction and produces heat when there is the risk of the body temperature falling below normal.
- *The liver* is very chemically active, and heat is produced as a by-product. Metabolic rate and heat production are increased after eating.
- *The digestive organs* produce heat during peristalsis and by the chemical reactions involved in digestion.

Heat loss

Most of the heat loss from the body occurs through the skin. Small amounts are lost in expired air, urine and faeces.

Only the heat lost through the skin can be regulated to maintain a constant body temperature. There is no control over heat lost by the other routes.

Heat loss through the skin is affected by the difference between body and environmental temperatures, the amount of the body surface exposed to the air and the type of clothes worn. Air is a poor conductor of heat and when layers of air are trapped in clothing and between the skin and clothing they act as effective insulators against excessive heat loss. For this reason several layers of lightweight clothes provide more effective insulation against a low environmental temperature than one heavy garment. A balance is maintained between heat production and heat loss. Control is achieved mainly by thermoreceptors in the hypothalamus.

Mechanisms of heat loss. In *evaporation*, the body is cooled when heat is used to convert the water in sweat to water vapour.

In *radiation*, exposed parts of the body radiate heat away from the body.

In *conduction*, clothes and other objects in contact with the skin take up heat.

In *convection*, air passing over the exposed parts of the body is heated and rises, cool air replaces it and convection currents are set up. Heat is also lost from the clothes by convection.

365

Control of body temperature

Nervous control. The *temperature regulating centre* in the hypothalamus is responsive to the temperature of circulating blood. This centre controls body temperature through autonomic nerve stimulation of the sweat glands when body temperature rises.

The *vasomotor centre* in the medulla oblongata controls the diameter of the small arteries and arterioles, and therefore the amount of blood which circulates in the capillaries in the dermis. The vasomotor centre is influenced by the temperature of its blood supply and by nerve impulses from the hypothalamus. When body temperature rises the skin capillaries dilate and the extra blood near the surface increases heat loss by radiation, conduction and convection. The skin is warm and pink in colour. When body temperature falls arteriolar constriction conserves heat and the skin is whiter and feels cool.

Activity of the sweat glands. When the temperature of the body is increased by 0.25 to 0.5°C the sweat glands are stimulated to secrete sweat, which is conveyed to the surface of the body by ducts. When sweat droplets can be seen on the skin the rate of production is exceeding the rate of evaporation. This is most likely to happen when the environmental air is humid and the temperature high.

Loss of heat from the body by unnoticeable evaporation of water through the skin and expired air occurs even when the environmental temperature is low. This is called *insensible water loss* (around 500 ml per day) and is accompanied by insensible heat loss.

Effects of vasodilatation. The amount of heat lost from the skin depends to a great extent on the amount of blood in the vessels in the dermis. As heat production increases, the arterioles become dilated and more blood pours into the capillary network in the skin. In addition to increasing the amount of sweat produced the temperature of the skin is raised and there is an increase in the amount of heat lost by radiation, conduction and convection.

If the external environmental temperature is low or if heat production is decreased, vasoconstriction is stimulated by sympathetic nerves. This decreases the blood flow near the body surface, conserving heat.

Fever. This is often the result of infection and is caused by release of chemicals (*pyrogens*) from damaged tissue and the cells involved in inflammation. Pyrogens act on the hypothalamus, which releases prostaglandins that reset the hypothalamic thermostat to a higher temperature. The body responds by activating heat-promoting mechanisms, e.g. shivering and vasoconstriction until the new higher temperature is reached. When the thermostat is reset to the normal level, heat-loss mechanisms are activated. There is profuse sweating and vasodilatation accompanied by warm, pink (flushed) skin until body temperature falls to the normal range again.

Hypothermia. This is present when core temperature, e.g. the rectal temperature, is below 35°C (95°F). At a rectal temperature below 32°C (89.6°F), compensatory mechanisms to restore body temperature usually fail, e.g. shivering is replaced by muscle rigidity and cramps, vasoconstriction fails to occur and there is lowered blood pressure, pulse and respiration rates. Mental confusion and disorientation occur. Death usually occurs when the temperature falls below 25°C (77°F).

Individuals at the extremes of age are prone to hypothermia.

Formation of vitamin D

7-dehydrocholesterol is a lipid-based substance in the skin and ultraviolet light from the sun converts it to vitamin D. This circulates in the blood and is used, with calcium and phosphate, in the formation and maintenance of bone. Any vitamin D in excess of immediate requirements is stored in the liver.

Sensation

Sensory receptors consist of nerve endings in the dermis that are sensitive to touch, pressure, temperature or pain. Stimulation generates nerve impulses in sensory nerves that are transmitted to the cerebral cortex (see Fig. 7.20B, p. 153). Some areas have more sensory receptors than others causing them to be especially sensitive, e.g. the lips and fingertips.

Absorption

This property is limited but substances that can be absorbed include:

- some drugs, in transdermal patches, e.g. hormones used as replacement therapy in postmenopausal women, nicotine as an aid to stopping smoking
- some toxic chemicals, e.g. mercury.

Excretion

The skin is a minor excretory organ for some substances including:

- sodium chloride in sweat and excess sweating may lead to abnormally low blood sodium levels
- urea, especially when kidney function is impaired
- aromatic substances, e.g. garlic and other spices.

Wound healing

Conditions required for wound healing

Systemic factors. These include good nutritional status and general health. Infection, impaired immunity, poor blood supply and systemic conditions, e.g. diabetes mellitus and cancer, reduce the rate of wound healing.

Local factors. Local factors that facilitate wound healing include:

■ good blood supply providing oxygen and nutrients and removing waste products
■ freedom from contamination by, e.g., microbes, foreign bodies, toxic chemicals.

Primary healing (healing by first intention)

This method of healing follows minimal destruction of tissue when the damaged edges of a wound are in close apposition (Fig. 14.4). There are several overlapping stages in the repair process.

Inflammation. The cut surfaces become inflamed and blood clot and cell debris fill the gap between them in the first few hours. Phagocytes and fibroblasts migrate into the blood clot:

■ phagocytes begin to remove the clot and cell debris stimulating fibroblast activity
■ fibroblasts secrete collagen fibres which begin to bind the surfaces together.

Proliferation. There is proliferation of epithelial cells across the wound, through the clot. The epidermis meets and grows upwards until the full thickness is restored. The clot above the new tissue becomes the scab and separates after 3 to 10 days. *Granulation tissue*, consisting of new capillary buds, phagocytes and fibroblasts, develops, invading the clot and restoring the blood supply to the wound. Fibroblasts continue to secrete collagen fibres as the clot and any bacteria are removed by phagocytosis.

Maturation. The granulation tissue is replaced by fibrous scar tissue. Rearrangement of collagen fibres occurs and the strength of the wound increases. In time the scar becomes less vascular, appearing after a few months as a fine line.

The channels left when stitches are removed heal by the same process.

367

Inflammation   Proliferation   Maturation

Fibroblast
Phagocyte

Figure 14.4 Stages in primary wound healing.

Secondary healing (healing by second intention)

This method of healing follows destruction of a large amount of tissue or when the edges of a wound cannot be brought into apposition, e.g. varicose ulcers and pressure sores (decubitus ulcers). The stages of secondary healing are the same as in primary healing and the time taken for healing depends on the effective removal of the cause and on the size of the wound. There are several recognised stages in the repair process, e.g. of decubitus ulcers (Fig. 14.5):

Inflammation. This develops on the surface of the healthy tissue and separation of necrotic tissue (*slough*) begins, due mainly to the action of phagocytes in the inflammatory exudate.

Proliferation. This begins as granulation tissue, consisting of capillary buds, phagocytes and fibroblasts, develops at the base of the cavity. It grows towards the surface, probably stimulated by macrophages. Phagocytes in the plentiful blood supply tend to prevent infection of the wound by ingestion of bacteria after separation of the slough. Some fibroblasts in the wound develop a limited ability to contract, reducing the size of the wound and healing time. When granulation tissue reaches the level of the dermis, epithelial cells at the edges proliferate and grow towards the centre.

Maturation. This occurs as scar tissue replaces granulation tissue, usually over several months until the full thickness of the skin is restored. The fibrous scar tissue is shiny and does not contain sweat glands, hair follicles or sebaceous glands (p. 378).

Figure 14.5 Stages in secondary wound healing.

DISORDERS OF THE SKIN

Learning outcomes

After studying this section you should be able to:

- list the causes of diseases in this section

- explain the pathological features and effects of common conditions affecting the skin: infections, non-infective inflammatory conditions, pressure sores, burns and tumours.

Infections

Viral infections

Human papilloma virus (HPV)

This causes *warts* or *veruccas* that are spread by direct contact, e.g. from another lesion, or another infected individual. There is proliferation of the epidermis and development of a small firm growth. Common sites are the hands, the face and soles of the feet.

Herpes viruses

Chicken pox and shingles (p. 183) are caused by the herpes zoster virus. Other herpes viruses cause *cold sores* (HSV1) and *genital herpes* (HSV2). The latter cause genital warts affecting the genitalia and/or anus and are spread by direct contact during sexual intercourse.

Bacterial infections

Impetigo

This is a highly infectious condition commonly caused by *Staphylococcus aureus*. Superficial pustules develop, usually round the nose and mouth. It is spread by direct contact and affects mainly children and immunosuppressed individuals. When caused by *Streptococcus pyogenes* (group A β-haemolytic streptococcus) the infection may be complicated, a few weeks later, by an immune reaction causing glomerulonephritis (p. 351).

Cellulitis

This is a spreading infection caused by some anaerobic microbes or by *Streptococcus pyogenes* or *Clostridium perfringens*. The spread of infection is facilitated by the formation of enzymes that break down the connective tissue that normally isolates an area of inflammation. The microbes enter the body through a break in the skin. If untreated, the products of inflammation may enter the blood causing septicaemia. In severe cases *necrotising fasciitis* may occur, there is oedema and necrosis of subcutaneous tissue that usually includes the fascia in the affected area.

Fungal infections

Ringworm and tinea pedis

These are superficial infections of the skin. In ringworm there is an outward spreading ring of inflammation. It most commonly affects the scalp and is found in cattle from which infection is spread.

Tinea pedis (athlete's foot) affects the area between the toes. Both infections are spread by direct contact.

Non-infective inflammatory conditions

Eczema and dermatitis

These two terms are synonymous and describe inflammatory conditions which can be acute or chronic. In acute dermatitis there is redness, swelling and exudation of serous fluid usually accompanied by itching. This is often followed by crusting and scaling. If the condition becomes chronic, the skin thickens and may become leathery due to long-term scratching. Infection may complicate scratching.

Atopic dermatitis is caused by allergens and commonly affects atopic individuals. Children who may also suffer from hay fever or asthma (pp. 259 and 260) are often affected.

Contact dermatitis may be caused by:

- direct contact with irritants, e.g. cosmetics, soap, detergent, strong acids or alkalis, industrial chemicals
- a hypersensitivity reaction (see Fig. 15.9, p. 384) to, e.g., synthetic rubber, nickel, dyes and other chemicals.

Psoriasis

This condition is genetically determined and characterised by exacerbations and periods of remission of varying duration. It is a common condition, especially between the ages of 15 and 40 years. There is proliferation of the cells of the basal layers of the epidermis and the more rapid upward progress of these cells through the epidermis results in incomplete maturation of the upper layer. The skin is shiny, silver coloured and scaly. Bleeding may occur when scales are scratched or rubbed off. The elbows, knees and scalp are common sites but other parts can be affected. Triggering factors that lead to exacerbation of the condition include trauma, infection and sunburn. Sometimes psoriasis is associated with arthritis.

369

Acne vulgaris

This is a common condition in adolescents that is thought to be caused by increased levels of male sex hormones after puberty. It occurs when sebaceous glands in hair follicles become blocked and then infected leading to inflammation and pustule formation. In severe cases permanent scarring may result. The most common sites are the face, chest and upper back.

Pressure sores

Also known as *decubitus ulcers*, these occur over 'pressure points', areas where the skin is compressed for long periods between a bony prominence and a hard surface, e.g. a bed or chair. When this occurs, blood flow to the affected area is impaired and ischaemia develops. Initially the skin reddens, and later as ischaemia and necrosis occur the skin sloughs and an ulcer forms that may then enlarge into a cavity. If infection occurs, this can result in septicaemia. Healing takes place by second intention (p. 368).

Predisposing factors
These may be:

- extrinsic, e.g. pressure, shearing forces, trauma, immobility, moisture, infection
- intrinsic, e.g. poor nutritional status, emaciation, incontinence, infection, concurrent illness, sensory impairment, poor circulation, old age.

Burns

These may be caused by many types of trauma including: heat, cold, electricity, ionising radiation and chemicals, including strong acids or alkalis.

Local damage occurs disrupting the structure and functions of the skin. Infection is a common complication of any burn as the outer barrier formed by the epidermis is lost.

Burns are classified according to their depth:

- *partial thickness* (superficial) when only the epidermis is involved.
- *full thickness* (deep) when the epidermis and dermis are destroyed. These burns are usually relatively painless as the sensory nerve endings in the dermis are destroyed. After a few days the destroyed tissue coagulates and forms an *eschar*, or thick scab, which sloughs off after 2 to 3 weeks. In *circumferential burns* which encircle any area of the body complications may arise from constriction of the part by eschar,

e.g. respiratory impairment may follow circumferential burns of the chest, or the circulation to the distal part of an affected limb may be seriously impaired. Skin grafting is required except for small injuries. Otherwise, healing, which is prolonged, occurs by second intention (p. 368) and there is no regeneration of sweat glands, hair follicles or sebaceous glands. Resultant scar tissue often limits movement of affected joints.

The extent of burns in adults is roughly estimated using the 'rule of nines' (Fig. 14.6). In adults, hypovolaemic shock usually develops when 15% of the surface area is affected. Fatality is likely in adults with full thickness burns if the surface area affected is added to the patient's age and the total is greater than 80.

Complications of burns
Dehydration and hypovolaemia. These may occur in extensive burns due to excessive leakage of water and plasma proteins from the surface of the damaged skin.

Shock. This may accompany severe hypovolaemia.

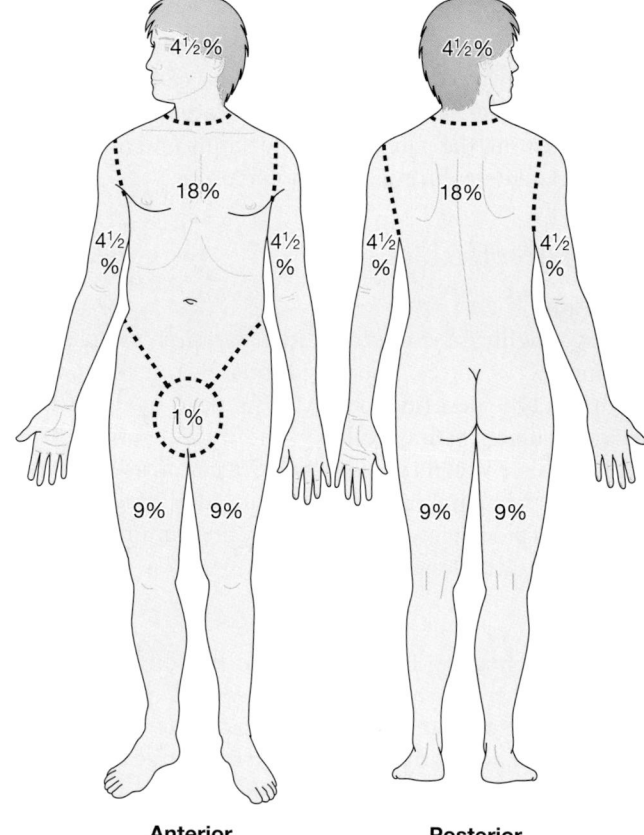

Anterior   **Posterior**

Figure 14.6 The 'rule of nines' for estimating the extent of burns.

370

Hypothermia. This develops when thermoregulation is impaired and excessive heat is lost.

Infection. Infection of the surface of a burn may result in septicaemia.

Renal failure. This occurs when the kidney tubules cannot deal with the amount of waste from haemolysed erythrocytes and damaged tissue.

Contractures. These may develop later as fibrous scar tissue contracts distorting the limbs, e.g. the hands, and impairing function.

Malignant tumours

Basal cell carcinoma

This is the least malignant and most common type of skin cancer. It is associated with long-term exposure to sunlight and is therefore most likely to occur on sun-exposed sites, usually the head or neck. It appears as a shiny nodule and later this breaks down, becoming an ulcer, commonly called a *rodent ulcer*. This is locally invasive but seldom metastasises.

Malignant melanoma

This is malignant proliferation of melanocytes, usually originating in a mole that may have an irregular outline. It may ulcerate and bleed and most commonly affects young and middle-aged adults. Predisposing factors are believed to be a fair skin and recurrent episodes of intensive exposure to sunlight including repeated episodes of sunburn in childhood. Likely sites for this tumour show a strong gender bias, with the lower leg being the commonest site in females and the torso being a common site in males. Metastases develop early and are frequently found in lymph nodes. The most common sites of blood-spread metastases are the liver, brain, lungs, bowel and bone marrow.

Kaposi's sarcoma

In this rare condition, a malignant tumour arises in the walls of lymphatic vessels. A small red-blue patch or nodule develops usually on the lower limbs.

It is also an AIDS-related disease and has thus become more common. In such cases, multiple lesions affect many sites of the body.

5

Resistance and immunity

An individual is under constant attack from an enormous range of potentially harmful invaders, from the months spent in the womb to the end of his life. These invaders include such diverse entities as bacteria, viruses, cancer cells, parasites and foreign (non-self) cells, e.g. in tissue transplant. The body therefore has developed a wide selection of protective measures, which can be divided into two categories.

Non-specific defence mechanisms. These protect against any of an enormous range of possible dangers.

Specific defence mechanisms. These are grouped together under the term *immunity*. Resistance is directed against only one particular invader. In addition, *immunological memory* develops, which confers long-term immunity to specific infections. An *antigen* is anything that stimulates an immune response.

NON-SPECIFIC DEFENCE MECHANISMS

Learning outcomes

After studying this section, you should be able to:

- describe the functions and features of the inflammatory response
- discuss the process of phagocytosis
- list the main antimicrobial substances of the body.

These are the first lines of general defence; they prevent entry and minimise further passage of microbes and other foreign material into the body.

There are four main non-specific defence mechanisms:

- defence at body surfaces
- phagocytosis
- natural antimicrobial substances
- the inflammatory response.

Defence at body surfaces

When skin and mucous membrane are intact and healthy they provide an efficient physical barrier to invading microbes. The outer layer of skin can be penetrated by only a few microbes and the mucus secreted by mucous membranes traps microbes and other foreign material on its sticky surface. Sebum and sweat secreted on to the skin surface contain antibacterial and antifungal substances.

Hairs in the nose act as a coarse filter and the sweeping action of cilia in the respiratory tract moves mucus and inhaled foreign materials towards the throat. Then it is expectorated or swallowed.

The one-way flow of urine from the bladder minimises the risk of microbes ascending through the urethra into the bladder.

Phagocytosis

The process of phagocytosis (cell eating) is shown in Figure 4.10, page 68. Phagocytic defence cells such as macrophages and neutrophils are attracted to sites of inflammation and infection by chemotaxis, when chemoattractants are released by injured cells and invading microbes. Phagocytes trap particles either by engulfing them with their body mass or by extending long pseudopodia towards them, which grasp them and reel them in (Fig. 15.1). These cells are non-selective in their targets; they will bind, engulf and digest foreign cells or particles.

Macrophages have an important role as a link between the non-specific and specific defence mechanisms. After ingestion and digestion of an antigen, they act as *antigen-presenting cells*, displaying their antigen on their own cell surface to stimulate T-lymphocytes and activate the immune response (p. 379).

Natural antimicrobial substances

Hydrochloric acid. This is present in high concentrations in gastric juice, and kills the majority of ingested microbes.

Lysozyme. This is a small molecule protein with antibacterial properties present in granulocytes, tears, and other body secretions. It is not present in sweat, urine and cerebrospinal fluid.

Antibodies. These are present in nasal secretions and saliva and are able to inactivate some microbes.

Saliva. This is secreted into the mouth and washes away food debris that may serve as culture medium for microbes. Its slightly acid reaction inhibits the growth of some microbes.

Interferons. These are substances produced by T-lymphocytes and by cells that have been invaded by viruses. They prevent viral replication within cells and spread of viruses to other cells.

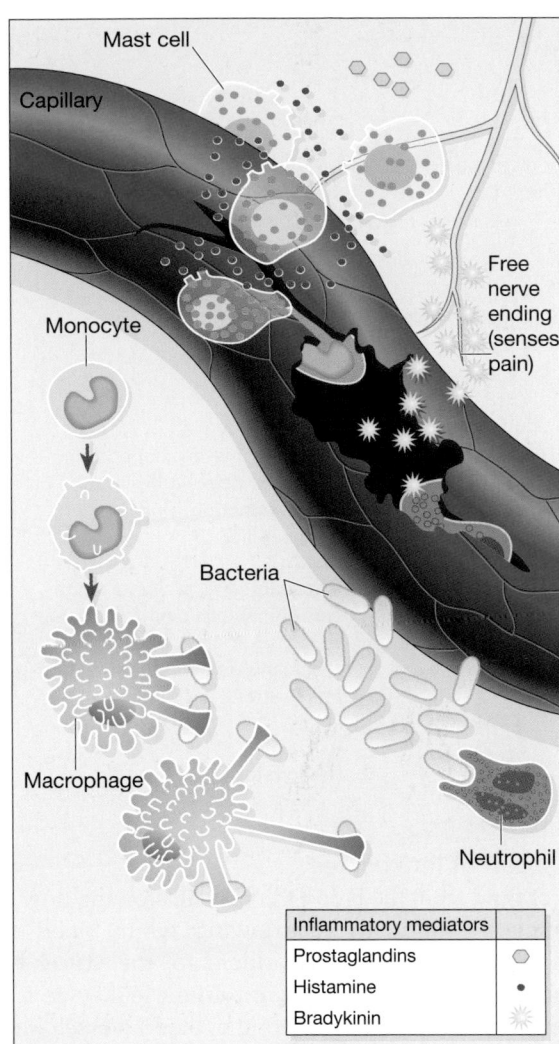

Mast cell

Capillary

Free nerve ending (senses pain)

Monocyte

Bacteria

Macrophage

Neutrophil

Inflammatory mediators	
Prostaglandins	⬡
Histamine	•
Bradykinin	✳

Figure 15.1 The inflammatory response.

Complement. Complement is a system of about 20 proteins found in the blood and tissues. It is activated by the presence of *immune complexes* (an antigen and antibody bound together) and by foreign sugars on bacterial cell walls. Complement:

- binds to, and makes holes in, bacterial cell walls, thus destroying the microbe
- binds to bacterial cell walls, stimulating phagocytosis by neutrophils and macrophages
- attracts phagocytic cells such as neutrophils into an area of infection.

The inflammatory response

This is the physiological response to tissue damage and is accompanied by a characteristic series of local changes (Fig. 15.1). It most commonly takes place when microbes have overcome the non-specific defence mechanisms. Its purpose is protective: to isolate, inactivate and remove both the causative agent and damaged tissue so that healing can take place.

Inflammatory conditions are recognised by their Latin suffix '-itis'; for example, appendicitis is inflammation of the appendix and laryngitis is inflammation of the larynx.

Causes of inflammation

The numerous causes of inflammation may be classified as follows:

- microbes, e.g. bacteria, viruses, protozoa, fungi
- physical agents, e.g. heat, cold, mechanical injury, ultraviolet and ionising radiation
- chemical agents
  - organic, e.g. microbial toxins and organic poisons, such as weedkillers
  - inorganic, e.g. acids, alkalis
- antigens that stimulate immunological responses.

Acute inflammation

Episodes of acute inflammation are usually of short duration, e.g. days to a few weeks, and may range from mild to very severe. The cardinal signs of inflammation are:

- redness
- heat
- pain
- swelling
- loss of function.

The acute inflammatory response is described in a series of overlapping stages: increased blood flow, increased formation of tissue fluid and migration of leukocytes. Some of the most important substances released in inflammation are summarised in Table 15.1.

Increased blood flow

Following injury, both the arterioles supplying the damaged area and the local capillaries dilate, increasing blood flow to the site.

This is caused mainly by the local release of a number of chemical mediators from damaged cells, e.g. histamine and serotonin. Increased blood flow to the area of tissue damage provides more oxygen and nutrients for the increased cellular activity that accompanies inflammation. Increased blood flow causes the increased temperature and reddening of an inflamed area.

Increased formation of tissue fluid

One of the cardinal signs of inflammation is swelling (oedema) of the tissues involved, which is caused by

Table 15.1 Summary of the principal substances released in inflammation

Substance	Made by	Trigger for release	Main pro-inflammatory actions
Histamine	Mast cells (in most tissues), basophils (blood); stored in cytoplasmic granules	Binding of antibody to mast cells and basophils	Vasodilatation, itching, ↑vascular permeability, degranulation, smooth muscle contraction (e.g. bronchoconstriction)
Serotonin (5-HT)	Platelets Mast cells and basophils (stored in granules) Also in CNS (acts as neurotransmitter)	When platelets are activated, and when mast cells/basophils degranulate	Vasoconstriction, ↑vascular permeability
Prostaglandins (PGs)	Nearly all cells; not stored, but made from cell membranes as required	Many different stimuli, e.g. drugs, toxins, other inflammatory mediators, hormones, trauma	Diverse, sometimes opposing, e.g. fever, pain, vasodilatation or vasoconstriction, ↑vascular permeability
Heparin	Liver, mast cells, basophils (stored in cytoplasmic granules)	Released when cells degranulate	Anticoagulant (prevents blood clotting), which maintains blood supply (nutrients, O_2) to injured tissue and washes away microbes and wastes
Bradykinin	Tissues and blood	When blood clots, in trauma and inflammation	Pain Vasodilatation

fluid leaving local blood vessels and entering the interstitial spaces. There are two main causes of oedema.

Increased permeability of small blood vessel walls. This is caused by inflammatory mediators, e.g. prostaglandins, histamine and serotonin, which are released by injured cells and cause the cells that form the single-layered venule wall to pull apart from one another. This opens channels that allow the movement of:

- excess fluid, which leaves the blood and enters the tissues, and
- plasma proteins, which are normally retained within the bloodstream and contribute to the osmotic pressure of the blood. When plasma proteins leave the blood, as in inflammation, the osmotic pressure of the blood falls and water moves from the bloodstream into the tissues.

Increased hydrostatic pressure. The increased blood flow into the capillary bed forces fluid out of the vessels and into the tissues.

Some interstitial fluid returns to the capillaries but most of the inflammatory exudate, phagocytes and cell debris are removed in lymph vessels because the pores of lymph vessels are larger, and the pressure inside is lower, than in blood capillaries.

Migration of leukocytes

Loss of fluid from the blood thickens it, slowing flow and allowing the normally fast-flowing white blood cells to make contact with, and adhere to, the vessel wall. In the acute stages, the most important leukocyte is the neutrophil, which adheres to the blood vessel lining, squeezes between the endothelial cells and enters the tissues, where its main function is in phagocytosis of antigens.

Later in the inflammatory response, after about 24 hours, macrophages become the predominant cell type at the inflamed site, and they persist in the tissues if the situation is not resolved, leading to chronic inflammation. Macrophages are larger and longer lived than the neutrophils. They phagocytose dead/dying tissue, microbes and other antigenic material, and dead/dying neutrophils.

Chemotaxis. This is the chemical attraction of leukocytes to an area of inflammation. The role of chemoattractants and the way in which they work is not fully understood.

It may be that chemoattractants act to retain passing leukocytes in the inflamed area, rather than actively attracting them from distant areas of the body. Known chemoattractants include microbial toxins, chemicals released from leukocytes, prostaglandins from damaged cells and complement proteins.

Benefits of acute inflammation

Most aspects of the inflammatory response are hugely beneficial, promoting removal of the harmful agent and setting the scene for healing to follow.

Promotion of phagocytosis (see Fig. 4.8). Neutrophils and macrophages in the tissues are actively recruited into inflamed areas. They engulf particles of biological and non-biological origin. Biological material includes dead and damaged cells, microbes, and damaged connective tissue fibres. Most biological material is digested by enzymes inside phagocytes. Phagocyte activity is promoted by the raised temperatures (local and systemic) associated with inflammation. Some microbes resist digestion and provide a possible source of future infection, e.g. *Mycobacterium tuberculosis*. Non-biological materials which cannot be digested include inhaled dust particles and chemical substances. Many phagocytes may die in an inflamed area if the material they ingest resists digestion, or if the number of particles is excessive. When this happens the phagocytes disintegrate and release material that may become fibrosed or cause further damage.

Promotion of the immune response. Formation of tissue exudate allows protective proteins such as antibodies to leave the bloodstream easily and collect at the site. The antibodies may promote phagocytosis of the microbes and neutralise their toxins.

Toxin dilution. Inflammatory exudate dilutes damaging and waste materials in the area, and assists their removal from the site. This is of particular importance when injurious chemicals and bacterial toxins are involved.

Increased core temperature. Body temperature rises when an endogenous pyrogen (interleukin 1) is released from macrophages and granulocytes in response to microbial toxins or immune complexes. Interleukin 1 is a chemical mediator that resets the temperature thermostat in the hypothalamus at a higher level, causing pyrexia and other symptoms that may also accompany inflammation, e.g. fatigue and loss of appetite. Pyrexia increases the metabolic rate of cells in the inflamed area and, consequently, there is an increased need for oxygen and nutrients. The increased temperature of inflamed tissues has the twin benefits of inhibiting the growth and division of microbes, whilst promoting the activity of phagocytes.

Fibrin formation. Fibrinogen, secreted by fibroblasts present in inflammatory exudate, is acted upon by thromboplastin released from damaged cells and forms an insoluble fibrin network. This may:

- wall off the inflamed area, preventing the spread of the cause
- bind together the cut edges of a wound during primary healing.

Some microbes such as *Streptococcus pyogenes*, which causes tonsillitis, pharyngitis and some skin infections, secrete toxins that break down fibrin, enabling infection to spread.

Harmful effects of acute inflammation

Tissue swelling. This is the result of the increased blood flow and exudation and is often accompanied by loss of function. The effects can be harmful, depending on the site:

- in a joint—limitation of movement
- in the larynx—interference with breathing
- in a confined space, such as inside the skull or under the periosteum of bone—severe pain due to pressure on nerves.

Pain. This occurs when local swelling compresses sensory nerve endings. It is exacerbated by chemical mediators of the inflammatory process, e.g. bradykinin, prostaglandins that potentiate the sensitivity of the sensory nerve endings to painful stimuli.

Suppuration (pus formation)

Pus consists of dead phagocytes, dead cells, cell debris, fibrin, inflammatory exudate and living and dead microbes. It is contained within a membrane of new blood capillaries, phagocytes and fibroblasts. The most common causative pyogenic microbes are *Staphylococcus aureus* and *Streptococcus pyogenes*. Small amounts of pus form *boils* and larger amounts form *abscesses*. *Staphylococcus aureus* produces the enzyme coagulase which converts fibrinogen to fibrin, localising the pus. *Streptococcus pyogenes* produces streptolysins that promote the breakdown of connective tissue, causing spreading infection. Healing, following pus formation, is by granulation and fibrosis (see Ch. 14).

Superficial abscesses tend to rupture through the skin and discharge pus. Healing is usually complete unless there is extensive tissue damage.

Deep-seated abscesses may have a variety of outcomes. There may be:

- early rupture with complete discharge of pus on to the surface, followed by healing
- rupture and limited discharge of pus on to the surface, followed by the development of a chronic abscess with an infected open channel or *sinus* (Fig. 15.2)

Figure 15.2 Sinus between an abscess and the surface of the body.

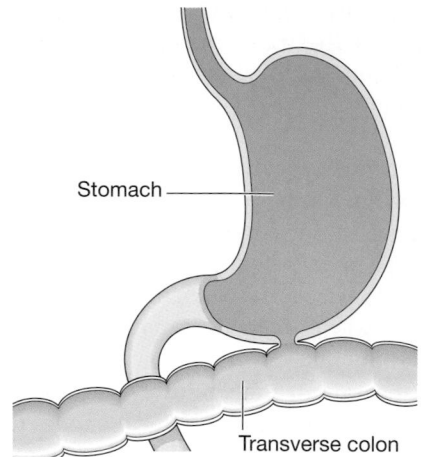

Figure 15.3 Fistula between the stomach and the colon.

- rupture and discharge of pus into an adjacent organ or cavity, forming an infected channel open at both ends or *fistula* (Fig. 15.3)
- eventual removal of pus by phagocytes, followed by healing
- enclosure of pus by fibrous tissue that may become calcified, harbouring live organisms which may become a source of future infection
- formation of fibrous adhesions between adjacent membranes, e.g. pleura, peritoneum
- shrinkage of fibrous tissue as it ages that may reduce the lumen or obstruct a tube, e.g. oesophagus, bowel, blood vessel.

Outcomes of acute inflammation

Resolution. This occurs when the cause has been successfully overcome. The inflammatory process is reversed and:

- damaged cells are phagocytosed
- fibrin strands are broken down by fibrinolytic enzymes
- waste material is removed in lymph and blood vessels
- repair is complete leaving only a small scar.

Development of chronic inflammation. (See below.) Any form of acute inflammation may develop into the chronic form if resolution is not complete, e.g. if live microbes remain at the site, as in some deep-seated abscesses, wound infections and bone infections.

Chronic inflammation

The processes involved are very similar to those of acute inflammation but, because the process is of longer duration, considerably more tissue is likely to be destroyed. The inflammatory cell types are mainly lymphocytes instead of neutrophils, and fibroblasts are activated, leading to the laying down of collagen, and *fibrosis*. If the body defences are unable to clear the infection, they may try to wall it off instead, forming nodules called *granulomas*, within which are collections of defensive cells. Tuberculosis is an example of an infection which frequently becomes chronic, leading to granuloma formation. The causative bacterium, *Mycobacterium tuberculosis*, is resistant to body defences and so pockets of organisms are sealed up in granulomas within the lungs.

Chronic inflammation may either be a complication of acute inflammation (see above) or a primary condition of slow onset.

Slow onset of inflammation

This may have several causes.

- There may be infection by low-virulence organisms in an area with a poor blood supply, e.g. endocarditis caused by non-haemolytic streptococci.
- Inorganic materials may be involved, for instance when:
  - an internal stitch has not dissolved
  - toxic silicic acid is formed when silicon, inhaled in dust, is dissolved.
- Hypersensitivity may develop following repeated exposure to some chemicals, e.g. in contact dermatitis skin proteins are altered when some chemicals are absorbed, the altered proteins act as antigens, stimulating the production of antibodies and initiating the inflammatory process.

Fibrosis (scar formation)

Fibrous tissue is formed during healing when there is loss of tissue or the cells destroyed do not regenerate, e.g. following chronic inflammation, persistent ischaemia, suppuration or large-scale trauma. The process begins with formation of granulation tissue, then, over time, the new capillaries and inflammatory material are removed leaving only the collagen fibres secreted by the fibroblasts. Fibrous tissue may have long-lasting damaging effects.

Adhesions consisting of fibrous tissue may limit movement, e.g. between the layers of pleura, preventing inflation of the lungs; between loops of bowel, interfering with peristalsis.

Fibrosis of infarcts. Blockage of an end-vessel by a thrombus or an embolus causes an infarct (area of dead tissue). Fibrosis of one large infarct or of numerous small infarcts may follow, leading to varying degrees of organ dysfunction, e.g. in heart, brain, kidneys, liver.

Tissue shrinkage occurs as fibrous tissue ages. The effects depend on the site and extent of the fibrosis, e.g.:

- Small tubes, such as blood vessels, air passages, ureters, the urethra and ducts of glands may become narrow or obstructed and lose their elasticity
- Contractures (bands of shrunken fibrous tissue) may extend across joints, e.g. in a limb or digit there may be limitation of movement or, following burns of the neck, the head may be pulled to one side.

IMMUNITY

Learning outcomes

After studying this section, you should be able to:

- discuss the roles of the different types of T-lymphocyte in providing cell-mediated immunity
- describe the process of antibody-mediated immunity
- distinguish between artificially and naturally acquired immunity, giving examples of each
- distinguish between active and passive immunity, giving examples of each.

The cell type involved in immunity is the lymphocyte (p. 67). This white blood cell is manufactured in the bone marrow, and has a characteristically large, single nucleus. Once released into the bloodstream from the bone marrow, lymphocytes are further processed to make two functionally distinct types: the T-lymphocyte and the B-lymphocyte.

T-lymphocytes. These are processed by the thymus gland, which lies between the heart and the sternum. The hormone thymosin, produced by the thymus, is responsible for promoting the processing, which leads to the formation of fully specialised (differentiated), mature, functional T-lymphocytes. It is important to recognise that a mature T-lymphocyte has been programmed to recognise only one type of antigen, and during its subsequent travels through the body will react to no other antigen, however dangerous it might be. Thus, a T-lymphocyte manufactured to recognise the chickenpox virus will not react to a measles virus, a cancer cell, or a tuberculosis bacterium.

T-lymphocytes provide *cell-mediated immunity*, discussed below.

B-lymphocytes. These are processed in the bone marrow. Their role is in production of *antibodies* (immunoglobulins), which are proteins designed to bind to, and cause the destruction of, an antigen. As with T-lymphocytes, each B-lymphocyte targets one specific antigen; the antibody released reacts with one type of antigen and no other. B-lymphocytes provide *antibody-mediated immunity*, discussed below.

From this description of T- and B-lymphocytes, it is clear that for every one of the millions of possible antigens that might be encountered in life there is one corresponding T- and B-lymphocyte. There is therefore a vast number of different T- and B-lymphocytes in the body, each capable of responding to only one antigen.

Cell-mediated immunity

T-lymphocytes that have been activated in the thymus gland are released into the circulation. When they encounter their antigen for the first time, they become sensitised to it. If the antigen has come from outside the body, it needs to be 'presented' to the T-lymphocyte on the surface of an antigen-presenting cell. There are different types of antigen-presenting cell, including macrophages. Macrophages are part of the non-specific defences, because they engulf and digest antigens indiscriminately, but they also participate in immune responses. To do this, after digesting the antigen they transport the most antigenic fragment to their own cell membrane and display it on their surface (Fig. 15.4). On their movement around the body, still displaying the antigen fragment, they eventually come into contact with

379

the T-lymphocyte that has been processed to target that particular antigen.

If the antigen is an abnormal body cell, such as a cancer cell, it too will be displaying foreign (non-self) material on its cell membrane that will stimulate the T-lymphocyte. Whichever way the antigen is presented to the T-lymphocyte, it stimulates the division and proliferation (*clonal expansion*) of the T-lymphocyte (Fig. 15.4). Three main types of specialised T-lymphocyte are produced, each of which is still directed against the original antigen, but which will tackle it in different ways.

Memory T-cells

These provide *cell-mediated immunity* by responding rapidly to another encounter with the same antigen.

Cytotoxic T-cells

These directly inactivate any cells carrying antigens. They attach themselves to the target cell and release powerful toxins, which are very effective because the two cells are so close together. The main role of cytotoxic T-lymphocytes is in destruction of abnormal body cells, e.g. infected cells and cancer cells.

Helper T-cells

These are essential for correct functioning of not only cell-mediated immunity, but also antibody-mediated immunity. Their central role in immunity is emphasised in situations where they are destroyed, as by the human immunodeficiency virus (HIV). When helper T-lymphocyte numbers fall significantly, the whole immune system is compromised. T-helpers are the commonest of the T-lymphocytes; their main functions include:

- production of special chemicals called *cytokines*, e.g. interleukins and interferons, which support and promote cytotoxic T-lymphocytes and macrophages
- cooperating with B-lymphocytes to produce antibodies; although B-lymphocytes are responsible for antibody manufacture, they require to be stimulated by a helper T-lymphocyte first.

Antibody-mediated (humoral) immunity

B-lymphocytes, unlike T-lymphocytes, which are free to circulate around the body, are fixed in lymphoid tissue (e.g. the spleen and lymph nodes). B-lymphocytes, unlike T-lymphocytes, recognise and bind antigen particles without having to be presented with them by an antigen-presenting cell. Once its antigen has been detected and bound, and with the help of a helper T-lymphocyte, the

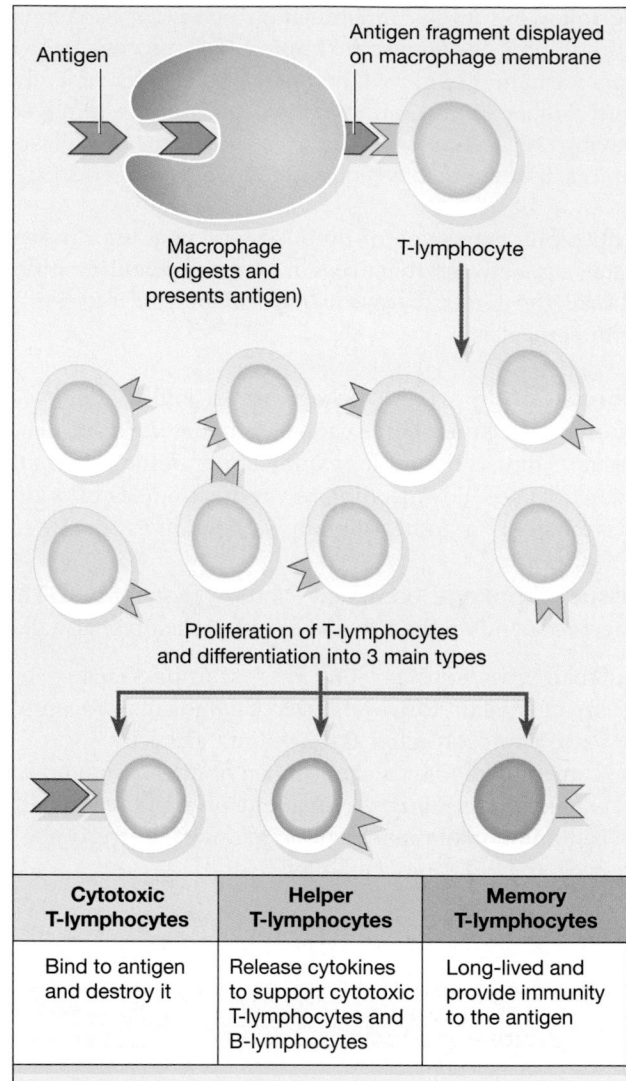

Cytotoxic T-lymphocytes	Helper T-lymphocytes	Memory T-lymphocytes
Bind to antigen and destroy it	Release cytokines to support cytotoxic T-lymphocytes and B-lymphocytes	Long-lived and provide immunity to the antigen

Figure 15.4 Clonal expansion of T-lymphocytes.

B-lymphocyte enlarges and begins to divide (clonal expansion, Fig. 15.5). It produces two functionally distinct types of cell, plasma cells and memory B-cells.

Plasma cells

These secrete antibodies into the blood. Antibodies are carried throughout the tissues, while the B-lymphocytes themselves remain fixed in lymphoid tissue. Plasma cells live no longer than a day, and produce only one type of antibody, which targets the specific antigen that originally bound to the B-lymphocyte. Antibodies:

- bind to antigens, labelling them as targets for other defence cells such as cytotoxic T-lymphocytes and macrophages
- bind to bacterial toxins, neutralising them
- activate complement (p. 375).

Figure 15.5 Clonal expansion of B-lymphocytes.

Plasma cells	Memory B-lymphocytes
Produce and release antibodies that bind to the antigen and cause its destruction	Long-lived and provide immunity to the antigen

Memory B-cells

These cells remain in the body long after the initial episode has been dealt with, and rapidly respond to another encounter with the same antigen by stimulating the production of antibody-secreting plasma cells.

The interdependence of the two parts of the immune system is summarised in Figure 15.6.

The fact that the body does not normally develop immunity to its own cells is due to the fine balance that exists between the immune reaction and its suppression. *Autoimmune diseases* are due to the disturbance of this balance.

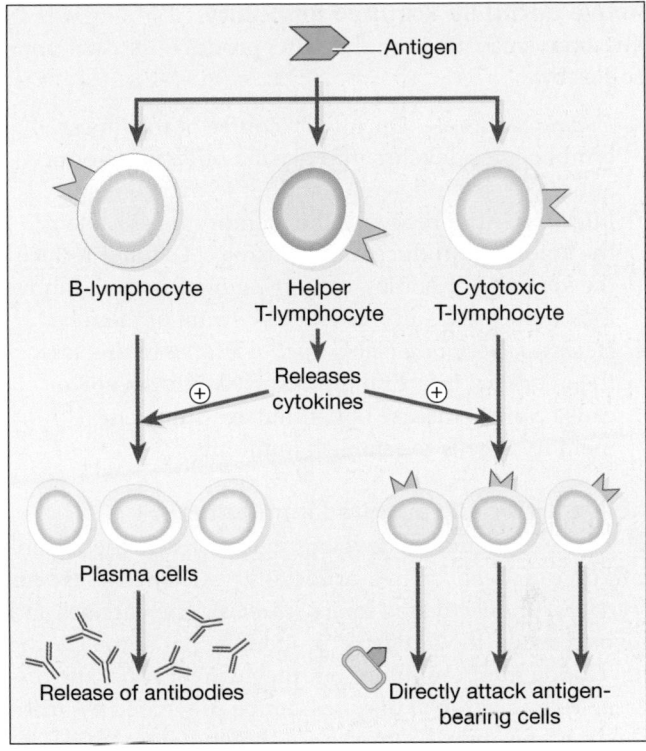

Figure 15.6 Interdependence of the T- and B-lymphocyte systems in the immune response.

Acquired immunity

When antigens, e.g. microbes, are encountered for the first time there is a *primary response* in which a low level of antibodies can be detected in the blood after about 2 weeks. Although the response may be sufficient to combat the antigen, the antibody levels then fall unless there is another encounter with the same antigen within a short period of time (2 to 4 weeks). The second encounter produces a *secondary response* in which there is a rapid response by memory B-cells resulting in a marked increase in antibody production (Fig. 15.7). Further increases can be achieved by later encounters but eventually a maximum is reached. This principle is used in active immunisation against infectious diseases.

Immunity may be acquired *naturally* or *artificially* and both forms may be *active* or *passive* (Fig. 15.8). Active immunity means that the individual has responded to an antigen and produced his own antibodies, lymphocytes are activated and the memory cells formed provide long-lasting resistance. In passive immunity the individual is given antibodies produced by someone else. The antibodies are then destroyed and unless lymphocytes are stimulated, passive immunity is short lasting.

Active naturally acquired immunity

The body may be stimulated to produce its own antibodies by:

- *Having the disease.* During the course of the illness, B-lymphocytes develop into plasma cells that produce antibodies in sufficient quantities to overcome the infection. After recovery, the memory B-cells retain the ability to produce more plasma cells that produce the specific antibodies, conferring immunity to future infection by the same microbe or strain of microbe.
- *Having a subclinical (subliminal) infection.* In this case the microbial infection is not sufficiently severe to cause clinical disease but stimulates sufficient memory B-cells to establish immunity.

Active artificially acquired immunity

This type of immunity develops in response to the administration of dead or live artificially weakened microbes (*vaccines*) or deactivated toxins (*toxoids*). The vaccines and toxoids retain the antigenic properties that stimulate the development of immunity but they cannot cause the disease. Many microbial diseases can be prevented by artificial immunisation. Examples are shown in Box 15.1.

Active immunisation against some infectious disorders confers lifelong immunity, e.g. diphtheria, whooping cough or mumps. In other infections the immunity may last for a number of years or for only a few weeks before revaccination is necessary. Apparent loss of immunity may be due to infection with a different strain of the same microbe, which has different antigenic properties but causes the same clinical illness, e.g. viruses that cause the common cold and influenza. In the elderly and when nutrition is poor the production of lymphocytes, especially B-lymphocytes, is reduced and the primary and secondary response may be inadequate.

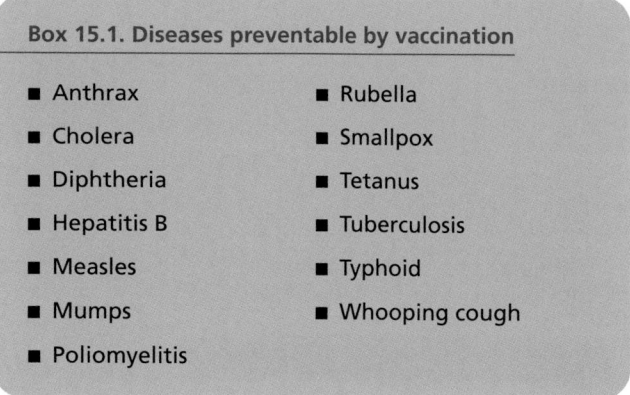

Box 15.1. Diseases preventable by vaccination

- Anthrax
- Cholera
- Diphtheria
- Hepatitis B
- Measles
- Mumps
- Poliomyelitis
- Rubella
- Smallpox
- Tetanus
- Tuberculosis
- Typhoid
- Whooping cough

Passive naturally acquired immunity

This type of immunity is acquired before birth by the passage of maternal antibodies across the placenta to the fetus and to the baby in breast milk. The variety of different antibodies provided depends on the mother's active immunity. The baby's lymphocytes are not stimulated and the immunity is short lived.

Passive artificially acquired immunity

In this type, ready-made antibodies, in human or animal serum, are injected into the recipient. The source of the antibodies may be an individual who has recovered from the infection, or animals, commonly horses, that have been artificially actively immunised. Specific immunoglobulins (antiserum) may be administered *prophylactically* to prevent the development of disease in people who have been exposed to the infection, or *therapeutically* after the disease has developed. Proteins in serum sometimes cause sensitisation of lymphocytes that may be damaging if encountered a second time, causing an abnormal immune reaction.

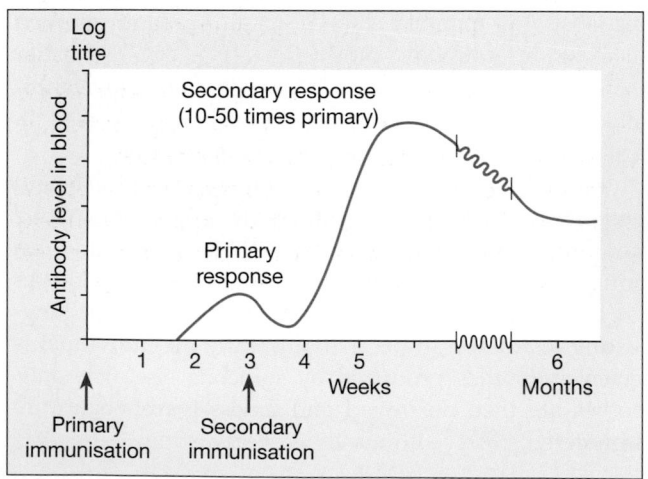

Figure 15.7 The antibody responses to immunisation.

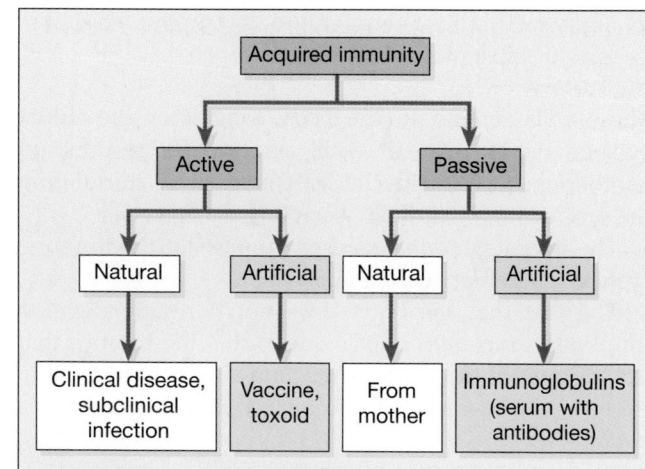

Figure 15.8 Summary of the types of acquired immunity.

HYPERSENSITIVITY (ALLERGY)

Learning outcome

After studying this section, you should be able to:

■ describe, with examples, the four types of allergic response.

Allergy is powerful immune response to an antigen (allergen). The allergen itself is usually harmless (e.g. house dust, animal dander, grass pollen). It is therefore usually the immune response that causes the damage to the body, not the allergen itself. Upon initial exposure to the allergen the individual becomes sensitised to it, and on second and subsequent exposures the immune system mounts a response entirely out of proportion to the perceived threat. It should be noted that these responses are exaggerated versions of normal immune function. Sometimes symptoms are mild, if annoying, e.g. the running nose and streaming eyes of hay fever. Occasionally the reaction can be extreme, overwhelming body systems and causing death (e.g. anaphylactic shock, p. 111).

There are four mechanisms of hypersensitivity, which are classified according to what parts of the immune system are involved. They are summarised in Figure 15.9.

Type I, anaphylactic hypersensitivity

This occurs in individuals who have inherited very high levels of a type of antibody called immunoglobulin E (IgE). When exposed to an allergen, e.g. house dust, these high levels of antibody activate mast cells and basophils (p. 66), which release their granular contents. The most important substance released is histamine, which constricts some smooth muscle (e.g. airway smooth muscle), causes vasodilatation and increases vascular permeability (leading to exudation of fluid and proteins into the tissues). Examples of type I reactions include the serious situation of anaphylaxis. There is profound bronchoconstriction and shock due to extensive vasodilatation. The condition can lead to death.

Type II, cytotoxic hypersensitivity

When an antibody reacts with an antigen on a cell surface, that cell is marked for destruction by a number of mechanisms, e.g. phagocytosis, or destruction by lytic enzymes. This is the usual procedure in the elimination of, for example, bacteria, but if the antibodies are directed against self-antigens the result is destruction of the body's own tissues (autoimmune disease). Type II mechanisms cause other conditions, e.g. haemolytic disease of the newborn (p. 71) and transfusion reactions (p. 72).

Type III, immune-complex-mediated hypersensitivity

Antibody–antigen complexes (immune complexes) are usually cleared efficiently from the blood by phagocytosis. If they are not, for example when there is phagocyte failure or an excessive production of immune complexes (e.g. in chronic infections), they can be deposited in tissues, e.g. kidneys, skin, joints and the eye, where they set up an inflammatory reaction. The kidney is a common site of deposition since it receives a large proportion of the cardiac output and filters the blood. Immune complexes collecting here lodge in and block the glomeruli (p. 351), impairing kidney function (glomerulonephritis). Sensitivity to penicillin is also a type III reaction; antibodies bind to penicillin (the antigen), and the symptoms are the result of deposition of immune complexes in tissues—rashes, joint pains and sometimes haematuria.

Type IV, delayed type hypersensitivity

Unlike types I–III, type IV hypersensitivity does not involve antibodies, but is an overreaction of T-lymphocytes to an antigen. When an antigen is detected by memory T-lymphocytes, it provokes clonal expansion of the T-lymphocyte (Fig. 15.4), and large numbers of cytotoxic T-lymphocytes are released to eliminate the antigen. Usually this system is controlled and the T-lymphocyte response is appropriate. If not, the actively aggressive cytotoxic T-lymphocytes damage normal tissues.

An example of this is contact dermatitis (p. 369). Graft rejection is also caused by T-lymphocytes; an incompatible skin graft, for instance, will become necrotic and slough off in the days following application of the graft.

384

Figure 15.9 The four types of hypersensitivity.

AUTOIMMUNE DISEASES

Learning outcomes

After studying this section, you should be able to:

■ describe the basis of autoimmune disease

■ discuss the specific examples of autoimmune disease.

Normally, an immune response is mounted only against foreign (non-self) antigens, but occasionally the body fails to recognise its own tissues and attacks itself. The resulting autoimmune disorders, examples of type II hypersensitivity, include a number of relatively common conditions.

Rheumatoid arthritis (p. 425)

The body produces antibodies to the membrane lining the joints, the synovial membrane. In most sufferers, the antibody can be detected in the blood; it is called *rheumatoid factor*. The antibodies bind to the synovial membrane, leading to chronically inflamed joints that are stiff, painful and swollen.

Hashimoto's disease (p. 230)

The body makes antibodies to thyroglobulin, leading to destruction of thyroid hormone, and hyposecretion of the thyroid.

Graves' disease

The body makes antibodies to the thyroid cells. Unlike Hashimoto's disease, however, the effect of the antibodies is to stimulate the gland, with a resultant hyperthyroidism (p.229).

Autoimmune haemolytic anaemia (p. 72)

In this, individuals make antibodies to their own red blood cells, leading to haemolytic anaemia.

Myasthenia gravis

This autoimmune condition of unknown origin affects more women than men, and usually those between 20 and 40 years. Antibodies are produced that bind to and block the acetylcholine receptors of neuromuscular junctions. The transmission of nerve impulses to muscle fibres is therefore blocked. This causes progressive and extensive muscle weakness, although the muscles are normal. Extraocular and eyelid muscles are affected first, causing *ptosis* (drooping of the eyelid) or *diplopia* (double vision), followed by those of the neck (possibly affecting chewing, swallowing and speech) and limbs. There are periods of remission, relapses being precipitated by, for example, strenuous exercise, infections or pregnancy.

IMMUNODEFICIENCY

Learning outcome

After studying this section, you should be able to:

■ discuss the causes and effects of acquired immune deficiency syndrome (AIDS).

When the immune system is compromised, there is a tendency to recurrent infections, often by microbes not normally pathogenic in humans (*opportunistic infections*). Immunodeficiency is classified as primary (usually occurring in infancy and genetically mediated) or secondary, that is, acquired in later life as the result of another disease, e.g. protein deficiency, acute infection, chronic renal failure, bone marrow diseases, following splenectomy or acquired immune deficiency syndrome (AIDS).

Acquired immune deficiency syndrome (AIDS)

This condition is caused by the human immunodeficiency virus (HIV), an RNA retrovirus which produces the enzyme *reverse transcriptase* inside the cells of the infected person (host cells). This enzyme transforms viral RNA to DNA and this new DNA, called the provirus, is incorporated into the host cell DNA. The host cell then produces new copies of the virus that pass out into tissue fluid and blood and infect other host cells. When infected host cells divide, copies of the provirus are integrated into the DNA of daughter cells, spreading the disease within the body.

HIV has an affinity for cells that have a protein receptor called CD_4 in their membrane, including T-lymphocytes, monocytes, macrophages, some B-lymphocytes and, possibly, cells in the gastrointestinal tract and neuroglial cells in the brain. Helper T-cells (Fig. 15.4) are the main cells involved. When infected their number is reduced, causing suppression of both antibody-mediated and cell-mediated immunity with the consequent development of widespread opportunistic infections, often by microbes of relatively low pathogenicity.

HIV has been isolated from semen, cervical secretions, lymphocytes, plasma, cerebrospinal fluid, tears, saliva, urine and breast milk. The secretions known to be especially infectious are semen, cervical secretions, blood and blood products.

Infection is spread by:

- sexual intercourse, vaginal and anal
- contaminated needles used:
  - during treatment of patients
  - when drug abusers share needles.
- an infected mother to her child:
  - across the placenta before birth
  - while the baby is passing through the birth canal
  - possibly by breast milk.

The presence of antibodies to HIV indicates that the individual has been exposed to the virus but *not* that a naturally acquired immunity has developed. Not all those who have antibodies in their blood develop AIDS although they may act as carriers and spread the infection to others.

A few weeks after infection there may be an acute influenza-like illness with no special features, followed by a period of two or more years without symptoms.

Chronic HIV infection may cause persistent generalised lymphadenopathy (PGL). Some patients may then develop AIDS-related complex (ARC) and experience chronic low-grade fever, diarrhoea, weight loss, anaemia and leukopenia.

When AIDS develops the main complications are widespread recurrent opportunistic infections and tumours. Outstanding features include the following.

- Pneumonia may be present, commonly caused by *Pneumocystis carinii*, but many other microbes may be involved.
- There may be persistent nausea, diarrhoea and loss of weight due to recurrent infections of the alimentary tract by a wide variety of microbes.
- Meningitis, encephalitis and brain abscesses may be recurrent, either caused by opportunistic microbes or possibly by HIV.
- There may be deterioration in neurological function characterised by forgetfulness, loss of concentration, confusion, apathy, dementia, limb weakness, ataxia and incontinence.
- Skin eruptions, often widespread, may be seen, e.g. eczema, psoriasis, cellulitis, impetigo, warts, shingles and 'cold sores'.
- Generalised lymphadenopathy may occur, i.e. non-infective enlargement of lymph nodes.
- There may be malignant tumours:
  - lymphomas, i.e. tumours of lymph nodes
  - Kaposi's sarcoma, consisting of tumours under the skin and in internal organs (p. 371).

6

The skeleton

BONE

Learning outcomes

After studying this section you should be able to:

- list five types of bones and give an example of each
- outline the general structure of a long bone
- describe the structure of compact and cancellous bone tissue
- describe the development of bone
- outline hormonal regulation of growth of bone
- state the functions of bones.

Bone is a strong and durable type of connective tissue. It consists of:

- water (25%)
- organic constituents including *osteoid* (the carbon-containing part of the matrix) and bone cells (25%)
- inorganic constituents, mainly calcium phosphate (50%).

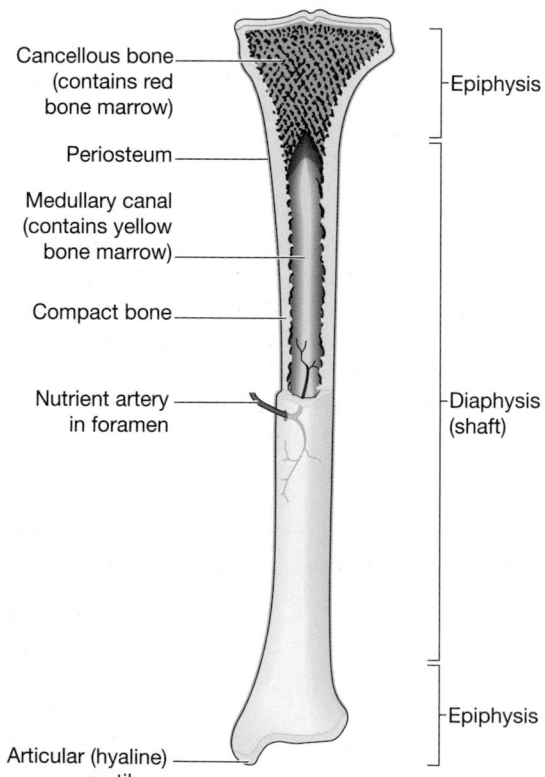

Figure labels:
Cancellous bone (contains red bone marrow) — Epiphysis
Periosteum
Medullary canal (contains yellow bone marrow)
Compact bone
Nutrient artery in foramen — Diaphysis (shaft)
— Epiphysis
Articular (hyaline) cartilage

Figure 16.1 A mature long bone – partially sectioned.

Although bones are often thought to be static or permanent they are highly vascular living structures that are continuously being remodelled.

Types of bones

Bones are classified as long, short, irregular, flat and sesamoid.

Long bones. These consist of a shaft and two extremities. As the name suggests the length is much greater than the width. Examples include the femur, tibia and fibula.

Short, irregular, flat and sesamoid bones. These have no shafts or extremities and are diverse in shape and size. Examples include:

- short bones—carpals (wrist)
- irregular bones—vertebrae and some skull bones
- flat bones—sternum, ribs and most skull bones
- sesamoid bones—patella (knee cap).

Bone structure

General structure of a long bone (Fig. 16.1)

These have a *diaphysis* or shaft and two *epiphyses* or extremities. The diaphysis is composed of *compact bone* with a central medullary canal, containing fatty *yellow bone marrow*. The epiphyses consist of an outer covering of compact bone with *cancellous bone* inside. The diaphysis and epiphyses are separated by *epiphyseal cartilages*, which ossify when growth is complete. Thickening of a bone occurs by the deposition of new bone tissue under the periosteum.

Long bones are almost completely covered by a vascular membrane, the *periosteum*. The outer layer is fibrous and the inner layer is osteogenic containing *osteoblasts* (bone-forming cells) and *osteoclasts* (bone-destroying cells), which are involved in maintenance and remodelling of bones; it gives attachment to muscles and tendons and protects bones from injury. *Hyaline cartilage* replaces periosteum on the articular surfaces of bones forming synovial joints.

Structure of short, irregular, flat and sesamoid bones

These have a relatively thin outer layer of compact bone with cancellous bone inside containing *red bone marrow* (Fig. 16.2). They are enclosed by periosteum except the inner layer of the cranial bones where it is replaced by dura mater.

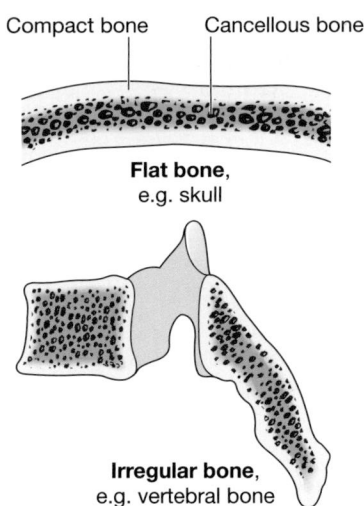

Figure 16.2 Sections of flat and irregular bones.

Figure 16.3 Microscopic structure of compact bone.

Microscopic structure of bone

Compact (cortical) bone

To the naked eye, compact bone appears solid but on microscopic examination large numbers of *Haversian systems* or *osteons* are seen (Fig. 16.3). These consist of a central Haversian canal, containing blood and lymph vessels and nerves, surrounded by concentric rings or plates of bone (*lamellae*). Between these are *lacunae*, tiny spaces, containing tissue fluid and spider-shaped *osteocytes* (mature bone cells). *Canaliculi* link the lacunae with each other and with the central Haversian canal. The tissue fluid nourishes the bone cells. The areas between Haversian systems contain *interstitial lamellae*, remains of older systems partially broken down during remodelling or growth of bone. The 'tubular' arrangement of lamellae gives bone greater strength than a solid structure of the same size.

Cancellous (trabecular, spongy) bone

To the naked eye, cancellous bone looks like a honeycomb. Microscopic examination reveals a framework formed from *trabeculae* (meaning 'little beams'), which consist of a few lamellae and osteocytes interconnected by canaliculi (Fig. 16.4). The spaces between the trabeculae contain *red bone marrow* that nourishes the osteocytes.

Bone cells

The cells responsible for bone formation are *osteoblasts* (these later mature into *osteocytes*). Osteoblasts and *chondrocytes* (cartilage-forming cells) develop from the same parent fibrous tissue cells. Differentiation into *osteogenic cells*, rather than *chondroblasts*, is believed to depend upon an adequate oxygen supply. This may be a factor affecting healing of fractures, i.e. if the oxygen supply is deficient there may be a preponderance of chondroblasts, resulting in a cartilaginous union of the fracture.

Osteoblasts

These are the bone-forming cells that secrete collagen and other constituents of bone tissue. They are present:

- in the deeper layers of periosteum
- in the centres of ossification of immature bone
- at the ends of the diaphysis adjacent to the epiphyseal cartilages of long bones
- at the site of a fracture.

Osteocytes

As bone develops, osteoblasts become trapped and remain isolated in lacunae. They stop forming new bone at this stage and are called *osteocytes*. Osteocytes are nourished by tissue fluid in the canaliculi that radiate from the Haversian canals. Their functions are not clear but they may be associated with the movement of calcium between the bones and the blood.

Osteoclasts

Their function is resorption of bone to maintain the optimum shape. This takes place at bone surfaces:

- under the periosteum, to maintain the shape of bones during growth and to remove excess callus formed during healing of fractures
- round the walls of the medullary canal during growth and to canalise callus during healing.

A fine balance of osteoblast and osteoclast activity maintains normal bone structure and functions.

389

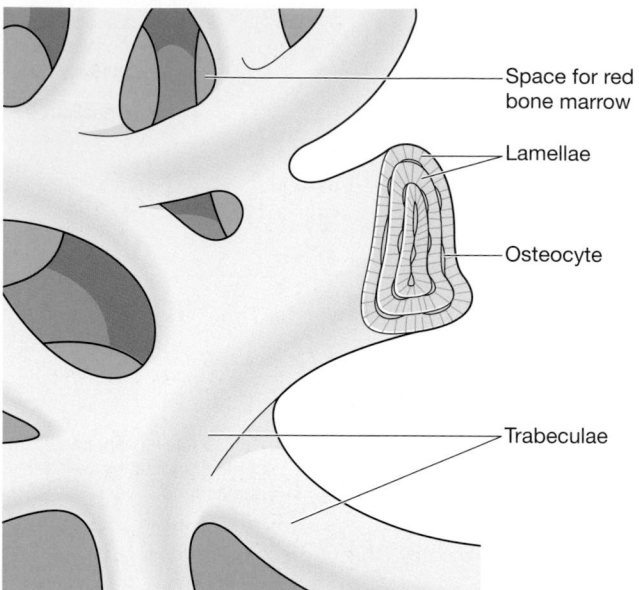

Figure 16.4 Microscopic structure of cancellous bone.

Development of bone tissue (osteogenesis or ossification)

This begins before birth and is not complete until about the 21st year of life (Fig. 16.5). Long, short and irregular bones develop from rods of cartilage, *cartilage models*. Flat bones develop from *membrane models* and sesamoid bones from *tendon models*. Bone development consists of two processes:

- secretion by osteoblasts of *osteoid*, i.e. collagen fibres in a mucopolysaccharide matrix which gradually replaces the original cartilage and membrane models
- calcification of osteoid immediately after its deposition.

There are two types of arrangement of collagen in osteoid.

Woven (non-lamellar) bone. Collagen fibres are deposited in irregular bundles, then ossified. This primitive bone structure is part of normal fetal development occurring during ossification of bones that originate as membrane models, e.g. skull bones. In adults it is also present in bone tumours and healing fractures (p. 407).

Lamellar bone. The collagen fibres are deposited as in woven bone, organised into characteristic lamellae found in compact and cancellous bone then ossified. This occurs when cartilage models are replaced by bone and in healing of fractures.

Figure 16.5 The stages of development of a long bone.

Development of long bones

In long bones the focal points from which ossification begins are small areas of osteogenic cells, or *centres of ossification* in the cartilage model. This is accompanied by development of a bone collar at about 8 weeks of gestation. Later the blood supply develops and bone tissue replaces cartilage as osteoblasts secrete osteoid components in the shaft. The bone lengthens as ossification continues and spreads to the epiphyses. Around birth, secondary centres of ossification develop in the epiphyses and the medullary canal forms when osteoclasts break down the central bone tissue in the middle of the shaft. After birth, the bone grows in length by ossification of the diaphyseal surface of the epiphyseal cartilages and growth is complete when the cartilages become completely ossified (Fig. 16.5).

Hormonal regulation of bone growth

Hormones that regulate the growth and consistency of size and shape of bones include the following.

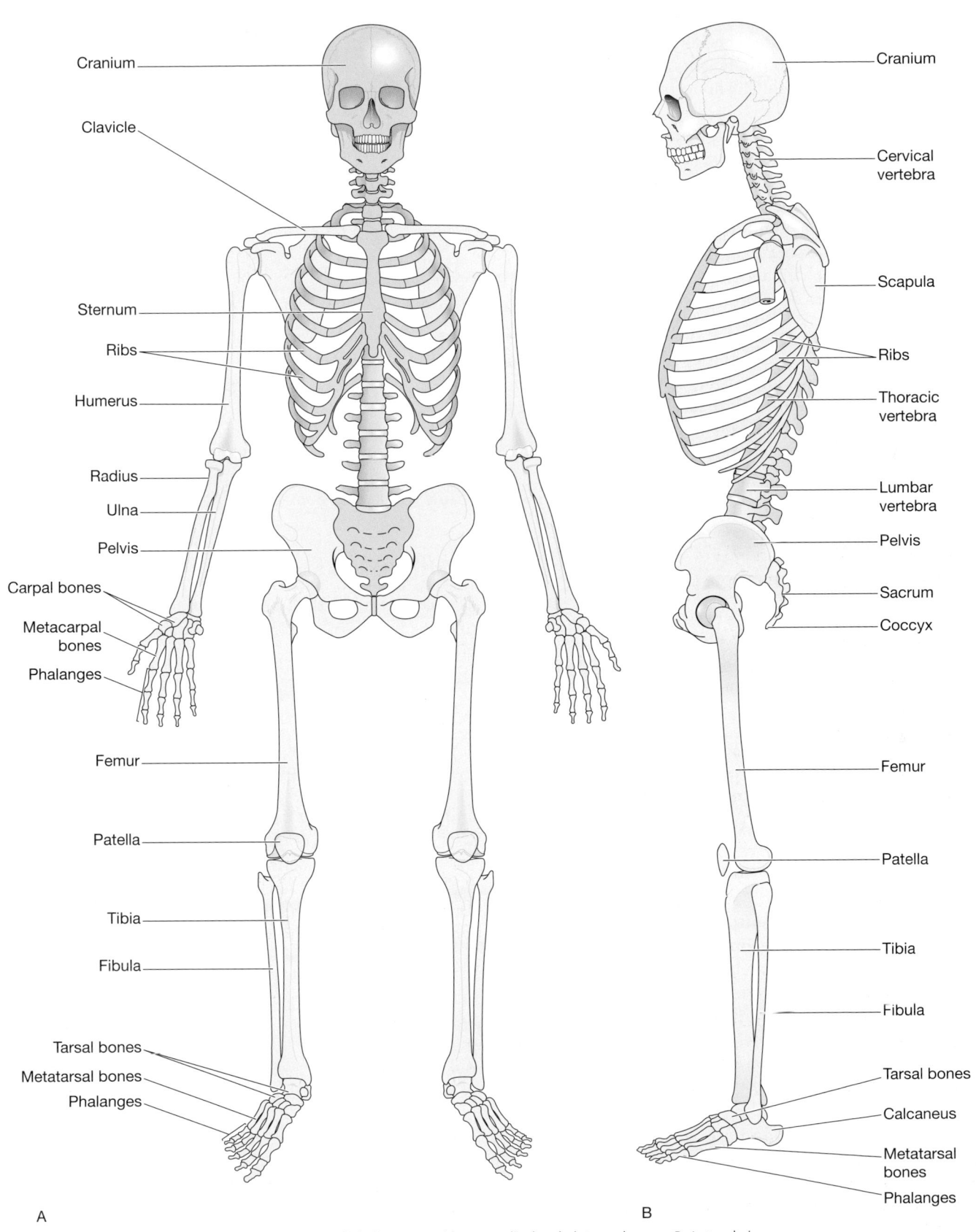

Cranium

Clavicle

Sternum

Ribs

Humerus

Radius

Ulna

Pelvis

Carpal bones

Metacarpal bones

Phalanges

Femur

Patella

Tibia

Fibula

Tarsal bones

Metatarsal bones

Phalanges

Cranium

Cervical vertebra

Scapula

Ribs

Thoracic vertebra

Lumbar vertebra

Pelvis

Sacrum

Coccyx

Femur

Patella

Tibia

Fibula

Tarsal bones

Calcaneus

Metatarsal bones

Phalanges

A

B

Figure 16.6 The skeleton. A. Anterior view: axial skeleton – gold; appendicular skeleton – brown. B. Lateral view.

- *Growth hormone* and the thyroid hormones, *thyroxine* and *triiodothyronine*, are especially important during infancy and childhood; deficient or excessive secretion of these results in abnormal development of the skeleton.
- *Testosterone* and *oestrogens* influence the physical changes that occur at puberty, i.e. the growth spurt and masculinising or feminising changes of specific parts of the skeleton, e.g. the pelvis.
- *Calcitonin* from the thyroid gland and *parathyroid hormone* from the parathyroid glands are involved in homeostasis of blood and bone calcium levels required for bone development.

Although the length and shape of bones does not normally change after ossification is complete, bone tissue is continually being remodelled and replaced when damaged. Osteoblasts continue to lay down osteoid and osteoclasts reabsorb it. The rate in different bones varies, e.g. the distal part of the femur is replaced gradually over a period of 5 to 6 months.

Functions of bones

Bones have a variety of functions. They:

- provide the framework of the body
- give attachment to muscles and tendons
- permit movement of the body as a whole and of parts of the body, by forming joints that are moved by muscles
- form the boundaries of the cranial, thoracic and pelvic cavities, protecting the organs they contain
- contain red bone marrow in which blood cells develop: haematopoiesis (see Fig. 4.2, p. 62)
- provide a reservoir of minerals, especially calcium phosphate.

Bone markings

Most bones have rough surfaces, raised protuberances and ridges which give attachment to muscle tendons and ligaments. These are not included in the following descriptions of individual bones unless they are of particular note, but many are marked on illustrations. Related terminology is defined on page 45.

The bones of the skeleton are divided into two groups: the *axial skeleton* and the *appendicular skeleton* (Fig. 16.6).

AXIAL SKELETON

Learning outcomes

After studying this section you should be able to:

- identify the bones of the skull (face and cranium)
- list the functions of the sinuses and fontanelles of the skull
- outline the characteristics of a typical vertebra
- describe the structure of the vertebral column
- explain the movements and functions of the vertebral column
- identify the bones that form the thoracic cage.

This part consists of the *skull, vertebral column, ribs* and *sternum*. Together the bones forming these structures constitute the central bony core of the body, the axis.

Skull (Figs 16.7 and 16.8)

The skull rests on the upper end of the vertebral column and its bony structure is divided into two parts: the cranium and the face.

Cranium

The cranium is formed by a number of flat and irregular bones that provide a bony protection for the brain. It has a *base* upon which the brain rests and a *vault* that surrounds and covers it. The periosteum inside the skull bones consists of the outer layer of dura mater. In the mature skull the joints (*sutures*) between the bones are immovable (fibrous). The bones have numerous perforations (e.g. foramina, fissures) through which nerves, blood and lymph vessels pass. The bones of the cranium are:

- 1 frontal bone
- 2 parietal bones
- 2 temporal bones
- 1 occipital bone
- 1 sphenoid bone
- 1 ethmoid bone.

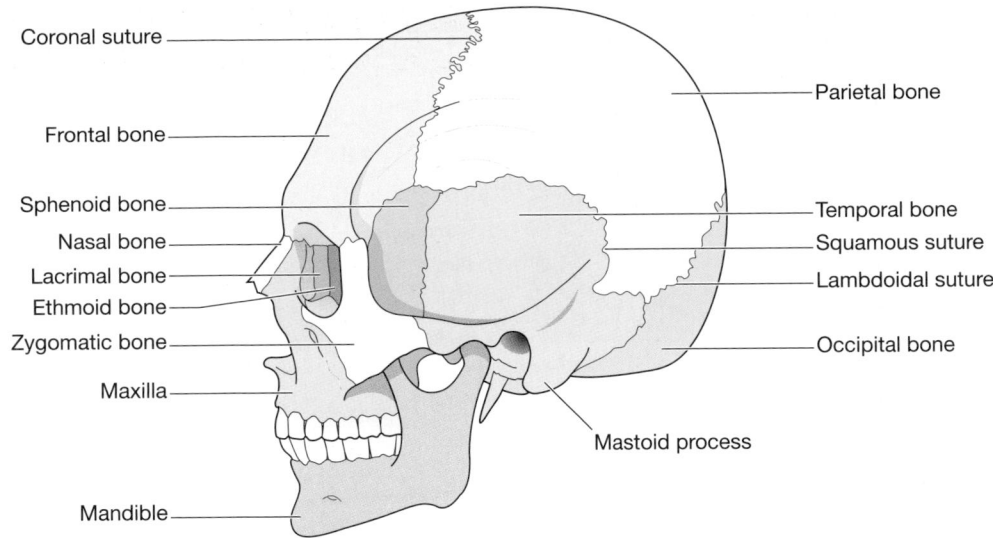

Figure 16.7 The bones of the skull and their sutures (joints).

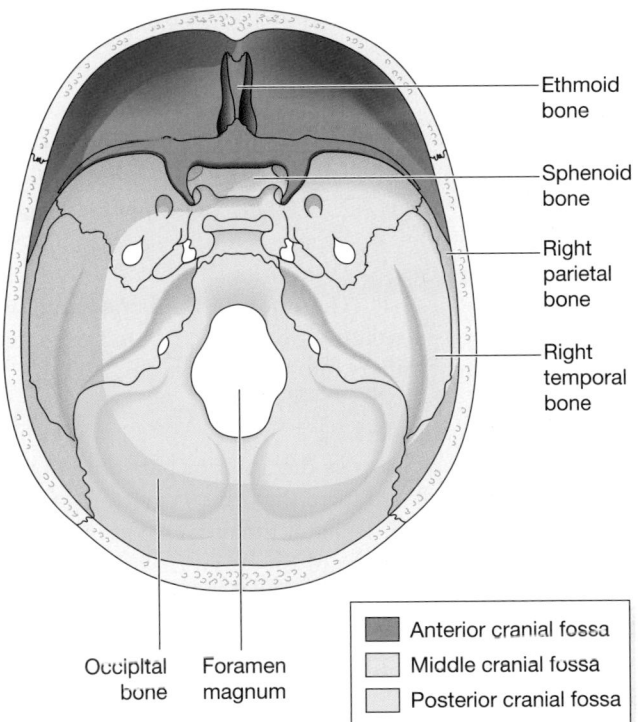

Figure 16.8 The bones forming the base of the skull and the cranial fossae. Viewed from above.

Frontal bone

This is the bone of the forehead. It forms part of the *orbital cavities* (eye sockets) and the prominent ridges above the eyes, the *supraorbital margins*. Just above the supraorbital margins, within the bone, there are two air-filled cavities or *sinuses* lined with ciliated mucous membrane which have openings into the nasal cavity.

The *coronal suture* joins the frontal and parietal bones and other fibrous joints are formed with the sphenoid, zygomatic, lacrimal, nasal and ethmoid bones. The bone originates in two parts joined in the midline by the *frontal suture* (Fig. 16.15).

Parietal bones

These bones form the sides and roof of the skull. They articulate with each other at the *sagittal suture*, with the frontal bone at the coronal suture, with the occipital bone at the *lambdoidal suture* and with the temporal bones at the *squamous sutures*. The inner surface is concave and is grooved by the brain and blood vessels.

Temporal bones (Fig. 16.9)

These bones lie one on each side of the head and form immovable joints with the parietal, occipital, sphenoid and zygomatic bones. Each temporal bone has several important features.

The *squamous part* is the thin fan-shaped part that articulates with the parietal bone. *The zygomatic process* articulates with the zygomatic bone to form the zygomatic arch (cheekbone).

The *mastoid part* contains the *mastoid process*, a thickened region behind the ear. It contains a large number of very small air sinuses which communicate with the middle ear and are lined with squamous epithelium.

The *petrous portion* forms part of the base of the skull and contains the organs of hearing (the spiral organ) and balance.

The temporal bone articulates with the mandible at the *temporomandibular joint*, the only movable joint of the skull. Immediately behind this articulating surface is the

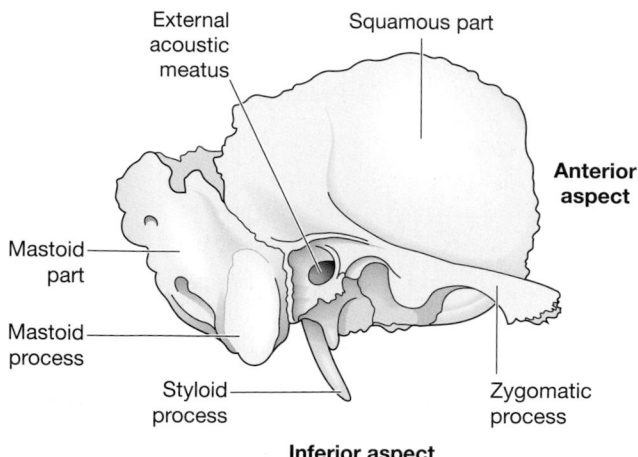

Figure 16.9 The right temporal bone. Lateral view.

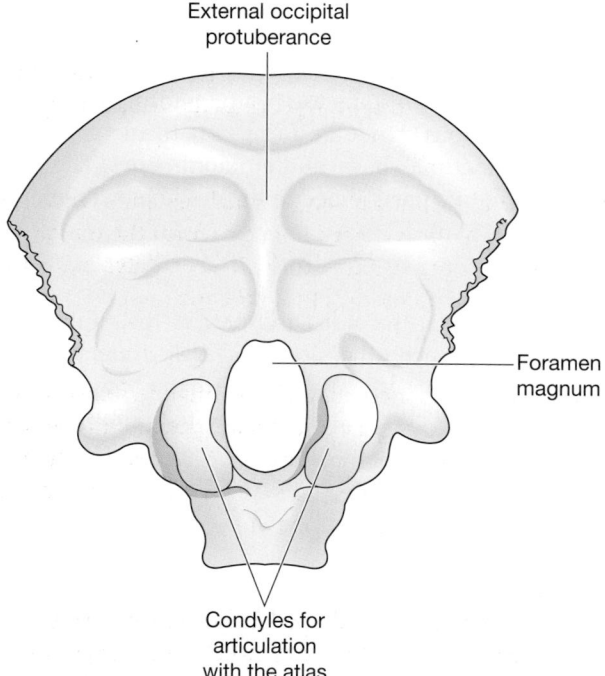

Figure 16.10 The occipital bone viewed from below.

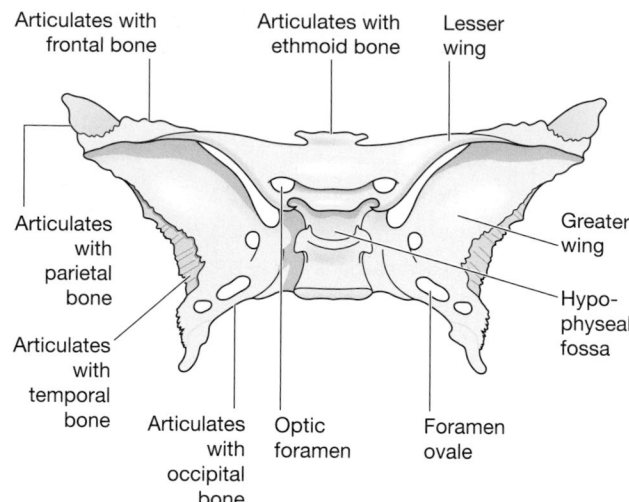

Figure 16.11 The sphenoid bone viewed from above.

condyles there is the *foramen magnum* (meaning 'large hole') through which the spinal cord passes into the cranial cavity.

Sphenoid bone (Fig. 16.11)

This bone occupies the middle portion of the base of the skull and it articulates with the occipital, temporal, parietal and frontal bones (Fig. 16.8). On the superior surface in the middle of the bone there is a little saddle-shaped depression, the *hypophyseal fossa* (*sella turcica*) in which the *pituitary gland* rests. The body of the bone contains some fairly large air sinuses lined by ciliated mucous membrane with openings into the nasal cavity.

Ethmoid bone (Fig. 16.12)

The ethmoid bone occupies the anterior part of the base of the skull and helps to form the orbital cavity, the nasal septum and the lateral walls of the nasal cavity. On each side are two projections into the nasal cavity, the *upper* and *middle conchae* or *turbinated processes*. It is a very delicate bone containing many air sinuses lined with ciliated epithelium and with openings into the nasal cavity. The horizontal flattened part, the *cribriform plate*, forms the roof of the nasal cavity and has numerous small foramina through which nerve fibres of the *olfactory nerve* (sense of smell) pass upwards from the nasal cavity to the brain. There is also a very fine *perpendicular plate* of bone that forms the upper part of the *nasal septum*.

Face

The skeleton of the face is formed by 13 bones in addition to the frontal bone, already described. Figure 16.13 shows the relationships between the bones:

external auditory meatus (auditory canal), which passes inwards towards the petrous portion of the bone.

Occipital bone (Fig. 16.10)

This bone forms the back of the head and part of the base of the skull. It has immovable joints with the parietal, temporal and sphenoid bones. Its inner surface is deeply concave and the concavity is occupied by the occipital lobes of the cerebrum and by the cerebellum. The occiput has two articular condyles that form hinge joints with the first bone of the vertebral column, the *atlas*. Between the

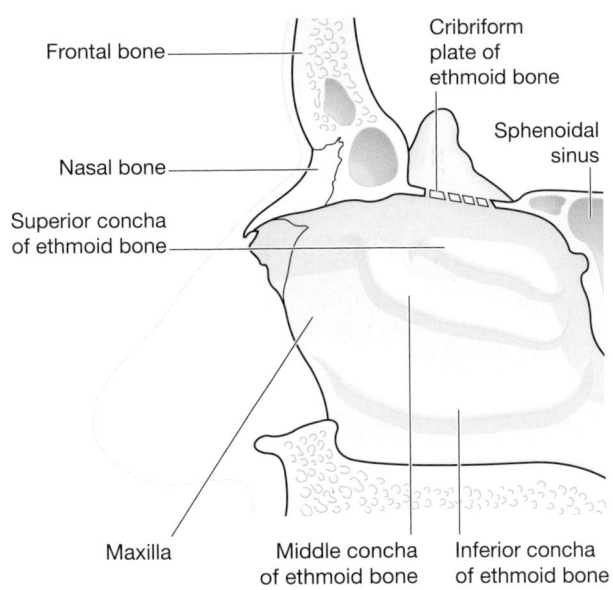

Figure 16.12 The right ethmoid bone and its related structures.

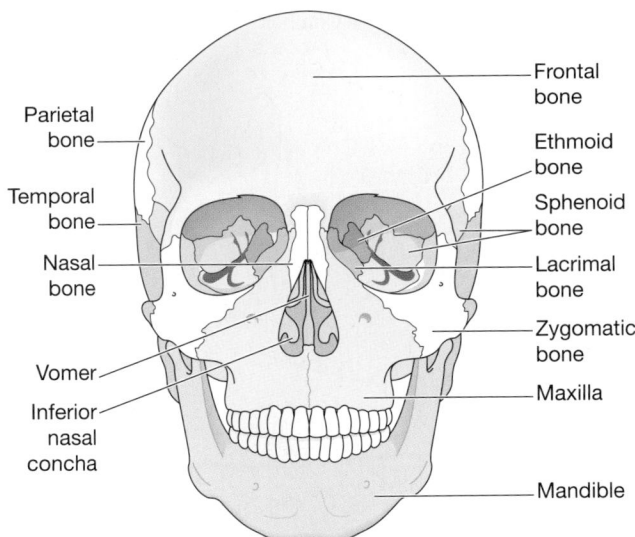

Figure 16.13 The bones of the face. Anterior view.

- 2 zygomatic or cheek bones
- 1 maxilla (originated as 2)
- 2 nasal bones
- 2 lacrimal bones
- 1 vomer
- 2 palatine bones
- 2 inferior conchae
- 1 mandible (originated as 2).

Zygomatic or cheek bones
The zygomatic bones form the prominences of the cheeks and part of the floor and lateral walls of the orbital cavities.

Maxilla or upper jaw bone
This originates as two bones but fusion takes place before birth. The maxilla forms the upper jaw, the anterior part of the roof of the mouth, the lateral walls of the nasal cavity and part of the floor of the orbital cavities. The *alveolar ridge*, or *process*, projects downwards and carries the upper teeth. On each side there is a large air sinus, the *maxillary sinus*, lined with ciliated mucous membrane and with openings into the nasal cavity.

Nasal bones
These are two small flat bones which form the greater part of the lateral and superior surfaces of the bridge of the nose.

Lacrimal bones
These two small bones are posterior and lateral to the nasal bones and form part of the medial walls of the orbital cavities. Each is pierced by a foramen for the

passage of the *nasolacrimal duct* which carries the tears from the medial canthus of the eye to the nasal cavity.

Vomer
The vomer is a thin flat bone which extends upwards from the middle of the hard palate to form the main part of the nasal septum. Superiorly it articulates with the perpendicular plate of the ethmoid bone.

Palatine bones
These are two L-shaped bones. The horizontal parts unite to form the posterior part of the hard palate and the perpendicular parts project upwards to form part of the lateral walls of the nasal cavity. At their upper extremities they form part of the orbital cavities.

Inferior conchae
Each concha is a scroll-shaped bone which forms part of the lateral wall of the nasal cavity and projects into it below the middle concha. The superior and middle conchae are parts of the ethmoid bone.

Mandible (Fig. 16.14)
This is the only movable bone of the skull. It originates as two parts which unite at the midline. Each half consists of two main parts: a *curved body* with the *alveolar ridge* containing the lower teeth and a *ramus* which projects upwards almost at right angles to the posterior end of the body.

At the upper end the ramus divides into the *condylar process* which articulates with the temporal bone to form the *temporomandibular* joint and the *coronoid process* that gives attachment to muscles and ligaments. The point where the ramus joins the body is the *angle* of the jaw.

395

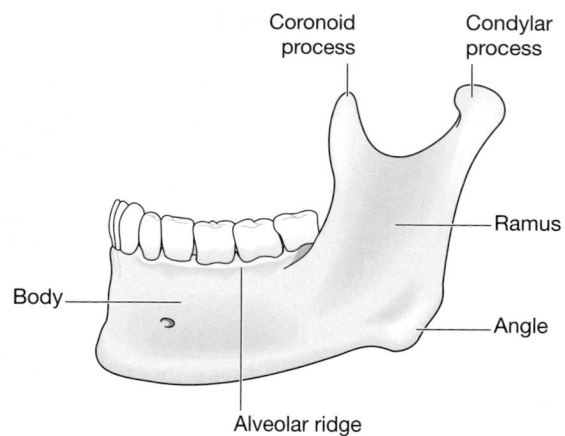

Figure 16.14 The left mandible. Lateral view.

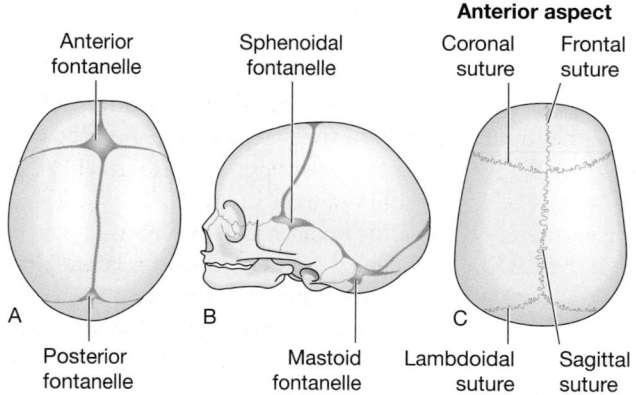

Figure 16.15 The skull showing the fontanelles and sutures. A. Fontanelles viewed from above. B. Fontanelles viewed from the side. C. Main sutures viewed from above when ossification is complete.

Hyoid bone

This is an isolated horse-shoe-shaped bone lying in the soft tissues of the neck just above the *larynx* and below the *mandible* (see Fig. 10.4, p. 242). It does not articulate with any other bone but is attached to the styloid process of the temporal bone by ligaments. It gives attachment to the base of the tongue.

Sinuses

Sinuses containing air are present in the sphenoid, ethmoid, maxillary and frontal bones. They all communicate with the nasal cavity and are lined with ciliated mucous membrane. Their functions are:

- to give resonance to the voice
- to lighten the bones of the face and cranium, making it easier for the head to balance on top of the vertebral column.

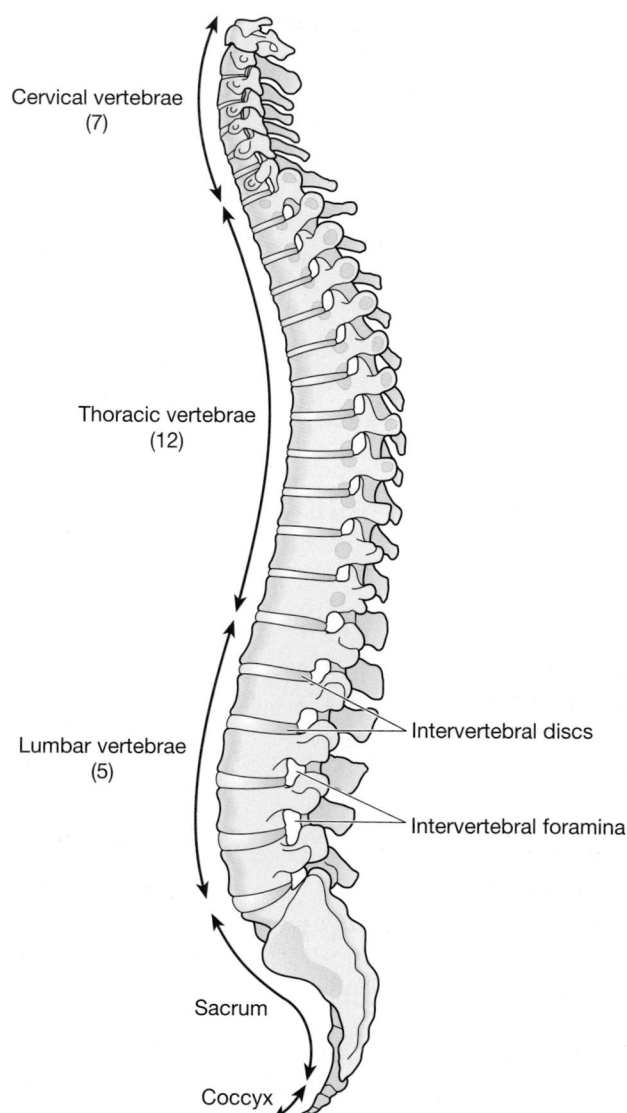

Figure 16.16 The vertebral column. Lateral view.

Fontanelles of the skull (Fig. 16.15)

At birth, ossification of the cranial sutures is incomplete. Where three or more bones meet there are distinct membranous areas, or *fontanelles*. The two largest are the *anterior fontanelle*, not fully ossified until the child is 12 to 18 months old, and the *posterior fontanelle*, usually ossified 2 to 3 months after birth. The skull bones do not fuse before birth to allow for moulding of the baby's head during its passage through the birth canal.

Vertebral column (Fig. 16.16)

The vertebral column consists of 24 separate movable, irregular bones, the *sacrum* (five fused bones) and the

Anterior aspect

Figure 16.17 A lumbar vertebra showing the features of a typical vertebra – viewed from above.

Anterior aspect

Figure 16.18 A cervical vertebra showing typical features viewed from above.

coccyx (four fused bones). The 24 separate bones are in three groups: 7 cervical, 12 thoracic and 5 lumbar.

The movable vertebrae have many characteristics in common but some groups have distinguishing features.

Characteristics of a typical vertebra (Fig. 16.17)

The body. The body of each vertebra is situated anteriorly. The size varies with the site. They are smallest in the cervical region and become larger towards the lumbar region.

The vertebral (neural) arch encloses a large *vertebral foramen*. The ring of bone consists of two *pedicles* that project backwards from the body and two *laminae*. Where the pedicles and laminae unite, *transverse processes* project laterally and where the two laminae meet in the midline posteriorly they form a *spinous process*. The neural arch has four articular surfaces: two articulate with the vertebra above and two with the one below. The vertebral foramina form the vertebral (neural) canal that contains the spinal cord.

Special features of vertebrae in different parts of the vertebral column

Cervical vertebrae (Fig. 16.18)
The transverse processes have a foramen through which a vertebral artery passes upwards to the brain. The first two cervical vertebrae are atypical.

The *atlas* (Fig. 16.19A) is the 1st cervical vertebra and it consists simply of a ring of bone with two short transverse processes. The anterior part of the large vertebral foramen is occupied by the *odontoid process* of the axis, which is held in position by a *transverse ligament* (Fig. 16.19C).

Thus the odontoid process forms the body of the atlas. The posterior part is the true vertebral foramen and is occupied by the spinal cord. On its superior surface the bone has two articular facets which form joints with the condyles of the occipital bone of the skull. The nodding movement of the head takes place at these joints.

The *axis* (Fig. 16.19B) is the 2nd cervical vertebra. The body is small and has the upward projecting *odontoid process* or *dens* that articulates with the first cervical vertebra, the atlas. The movement at this joint is turning the head from side to side.

Thoracic vertebrae (Fig. 16.20)
The bodies and transverse processes have facets for articulation with the ribs.

Lumbar vertebrae (Fig. 16.17)
These have no special features.

Sacrum (Fig. 16.21)
This consists of five rudimentary vertebrae fused to form a triangular or wedge-shaped bone with a concave anterior surface. The upper part, or base, articulates with the 5th lumbar vertebra. On each side it articulates with the ilium to form a *sacroiliac joint*, and at its inferior tip it articulates with the *coccyx*. The anterior edge of the base, the *promontory*, protrudes into the pelvic cavity. The vertebral foramina are present, and on each side of the bone there is a series of foramina for the passage of nerves.

Coccyx (Fig. 16.21)
This consists of the four terminal vertebrae fused to form a very small triangular bone, the broad base of which articulates with the tip of the sacrum.

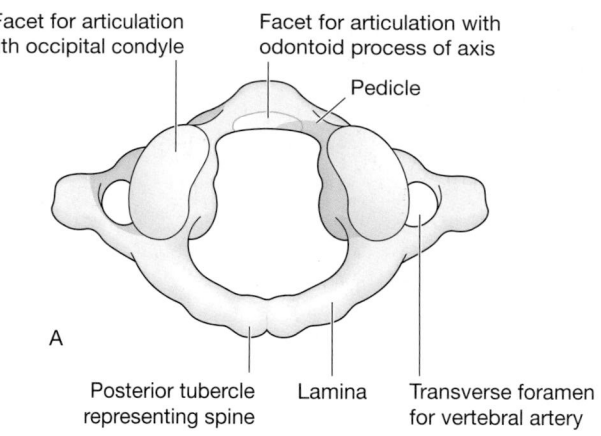

Anterior aspect

Facet for articulation with occipital condyle

Facet for articulation with odontoid process of axis

Pedicle

A

Posterior tubercle representing spine

Lamina

Transverse foramen for vertebral artery

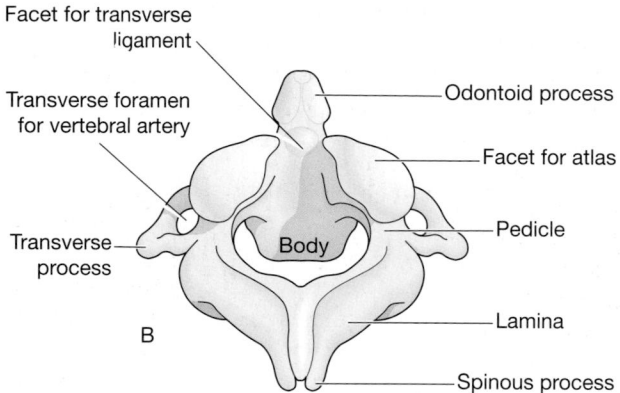

Anterior aspect

Facet for transverse ligament

Odontoid process

Transverse foramen for vertebral artery

Facet for atlas

Pedicle

Transverse process

Body

Lamina

B

Spinous process

Odontoid process of axis

Transverse ligament

Atlas

Axis

Vertebral foramen

Spine of axis

C

Figure 16.19 The upper cervical vertebrae viewed from above: A. The atlas. B. The axis. C. The atlas and axis in position showing the transverse ligament.

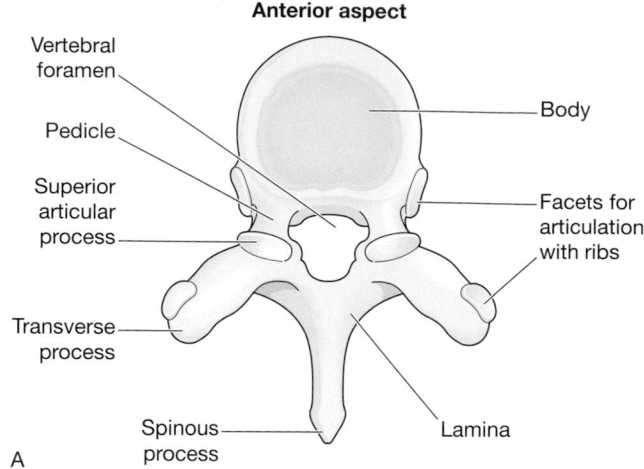

Anterior aspect

Vertebral foramen

Pedicle

Superior articular process

Transverse process

Body

Facets for articulation with ribs

Spinous process

Lamina

A

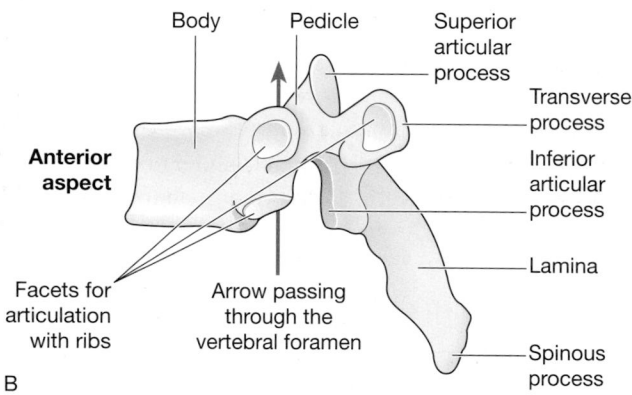

Body

Pedicle

Superior articular process

Transverse process

Inferior articular process

Anterior aspect

Facets for articulation with ribs

Arrow passing through the vertebral foramen

Lamina

Spinous process

B

Figure 16.20 A thoracic vertebra: A. Viewed from above. B. Viewed from the side.

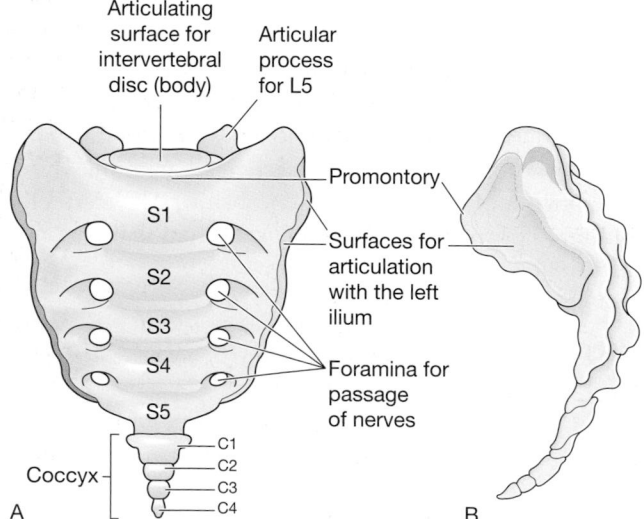

Articulating surface for intervertebral disc (body)

Articular process for L5

Promontory

S1

S2

S3

S4

S5

Surfaces for articulation with the left ilium

Foramina for passage of nerves

Coccyx

C1
C2
C3
C4

A

B

Figure 16.21 The sacrum and coccyx: A. Anterior view. B. Lateral view.

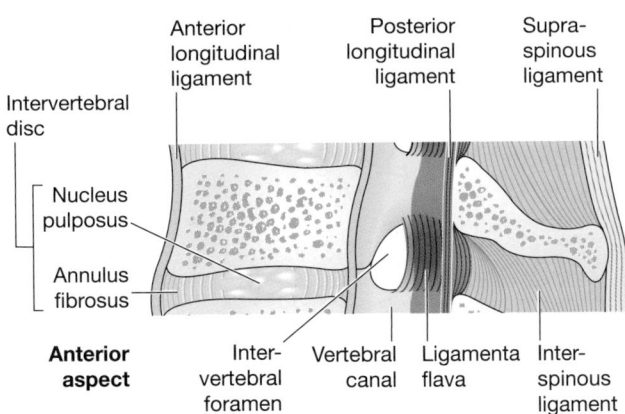

Figure 16.22 Section of the vertebral column showing the ligaments, intervertebral discs and intervertebral foramina.

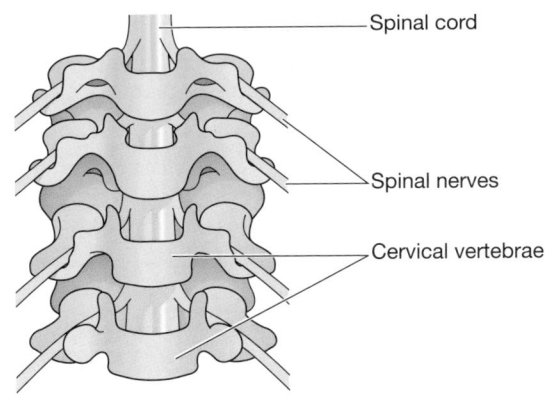

Figure 16.23 Lower cervical vertebrae separated to show the spinal cord and spinal nerves emerging through the intervertebral foramina. Anterior view.

Features of the vertebral column

Intervertebral discs

The bodies of adjacent vertebrae are separated by *intervertebral discs*, consisting of an outer rim of fibrocartilage (*annulus fibrosus*) and a central core of soft gelatinous material (*nucleus pulposus*) (Fig. 16.22). They are thinnest in the cervical region and become progressively thicker towards the lumbar region. The posterior longitudinal ligament in the vertebral canal helps to keep them in place. They have a shock-absorbing function and the cartilaginous joints they form contribute to the flexibility of the vertebral column as a whole.

Intervertebral foramina

When two adjacent vertebrae are viewed from the side, a foramen can be seen. Half of the wall is formed by the vertebra above and half by the one below (Fig. 16.23).

Throughout the length of the column there is an intervertebral foramen on each side between every pair of vertebrae, through which the spinal nerves, blood vessels and lymph vessels pass.

Ligaments of the vertebral column (Fig. 16.22)

These ligaments hold the vertebrae together and help to maintain the intervertebral discs in position.

The *transverse ligament* maintains the odontoid process of the axis in the correct position in relation to the atlas (Fig. 16.19C).

The *anterior longitudinal ligament* extends the whole length of the column and lies in front of the vertebral bodies.

The *posterior longitudinal ligament* lies inside the vertebral canal and extends the whole length of the vertebral column in close contact with the posterior surface of the bodies of the bones.

The *ligamenta flava* connect the laminae of adjacent vertebrae.

The *ligamentum nuchae* and the *supraspinous ligament* connect the spinous processes, extending from the occiput to the sacrum.

Curves of the vertebral column (Fig. 16.24)

When viewed from the side the vertebral column presents four curves, two *primary* and two *secondary*.

The fetus in the uterus lies curled up so that the head and the knees are more or less touching. This position shows the *primary curvature*. The secondary *cervical curve* develops when the child can hold up his head (after about 3 months) and the secondary *lumbar curve* develops when he stands upright (after 12 to 15 months). The thoracic and sacral primary curves are retained.

Movements of the vertebral column

The movements between the individual bones of the vertebral column are very limited. However, the movements of the column as a whole are quite extensive and include *flexion* (bending forward), *extension* (bending backward), *lateral flexion* (bending to the side) and *rotation*. There is more movement in the cervical and lumbar regions than elsewhere.

Functions of the vertebral column

These include the following.

- Collectively the vertebral foramina form the vertebral canal which provides a strong bony protection for the delicate spinal cord lying within it.
- The pedicles of adjacent vertebrae form intervertebral foramina, one on each side, providing access to the spinal cord for spinal nerves, blood vessels and lymph vessels.

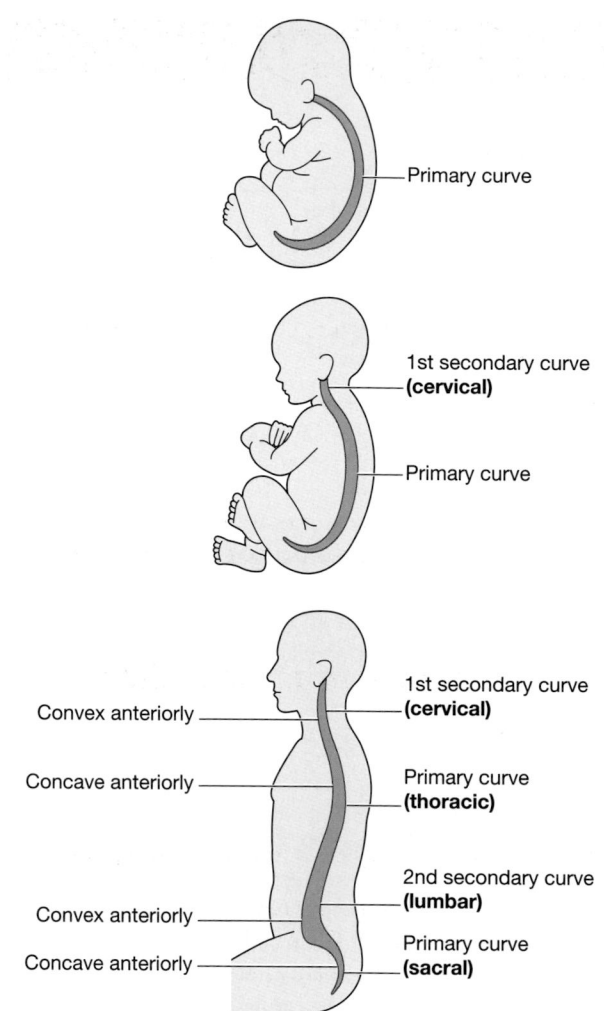

Figure 16.24 The order of development of the curves of the spine.

- The numerous individual bones enable a certain amount of movement.
- It supports the skull.
- The intervertebral discs act as shock absorbers, protecting the brain.
- It forms the axis of the trunk, giving attachment to the ribs, shoulder girdle and upper limbs, and the pelvic girdle and lower limbs.

Thoracic cage (Fig. 16.25)

The bones of the thorax or thoracic cage are:

- 1 sternum
- 12 pairs of ribs
- 12 thoracic vertebrae.

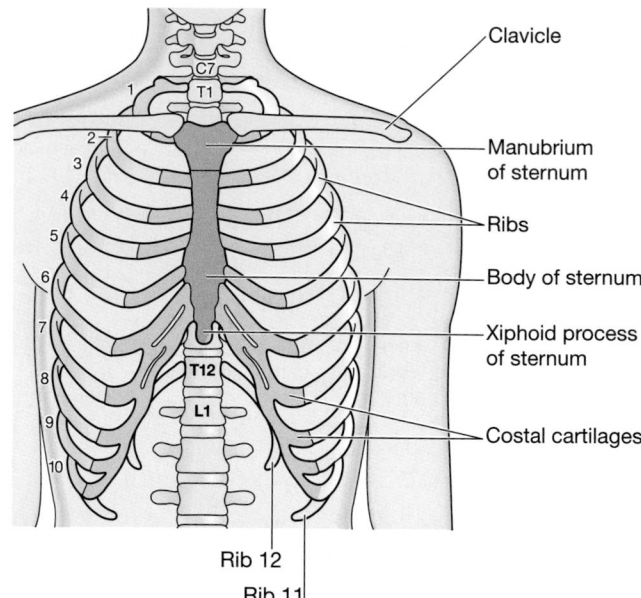

Figure 16.25 The thoracic cage. Anterior view.

Sternum or breast bone (Fig. 16.26)

This *flat bone* can be felt just under the skin in the middle of the front of the chest.

The *manubrium* is the uppermost section and articulates with the clavicles at the *sternoclavicular joints* and with the first two pairs of ribs.

The *body* or *middle portion* gives attachment to the ribs.

The *xiphoid process* is the tip of the bone. It gives attachment to the diaphragm, muscles of the anterior abdominal wall and the *linea alba*.

Ribs

There are 12 pairs of ribs which form the bony lateral walls of the thoracic cage and articulate posteriorly with the thoracic vertebrae. The first 10 pairs are attached anteriorly to the sternum by *costal cartilages*, some directly and some indirectly (Fig. 16.25).

The last two pairs (*floating ribs*) have no anterior attachment.

Characteristics of a rib (Fig. 16.27). The head articulates posteriorly with the bodies of two adjacent thoracic vertebrae and on the tubercle there is a facet that articulates with the transverse process of one. The sternal end is attached to the sternum by a costal cartilage, i.e. a band of hyaline cartilage. The superior border is rounded and smooth while the inferior border has a marked groove occupied by the intercostal blood vessels and nerves.

The first rib does not move during respiration. The spaces between the ribs are occupied by the intercostal muscles. During inspiration, when these muscles contract,

400

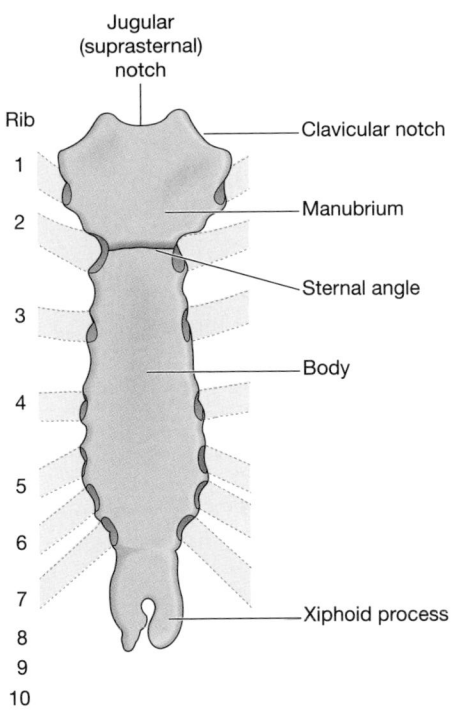

Figure 16.26 The sternum and its attachments.

Jugular (suprasternal) notch

Rib

1 — Clavicular notch

2 — Manubrium

— Sternal angle

3

— Body

4

5

6

7 — Xiphoid process

8

9

10

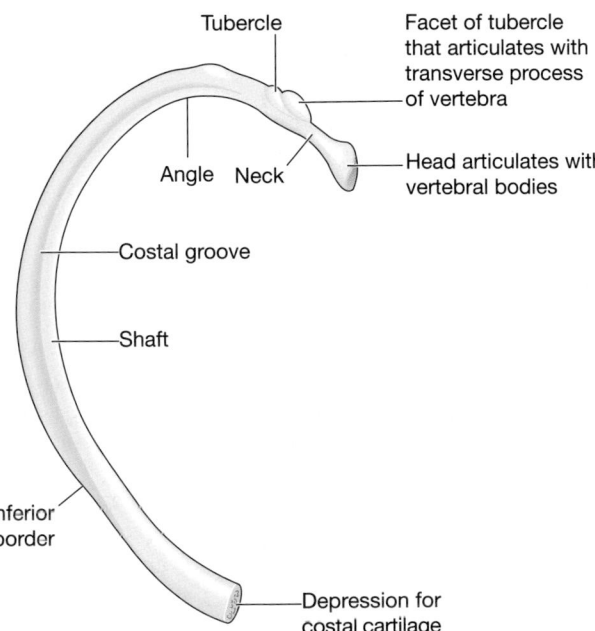

Figure 16.27 A typical rib viewed from below.

Tubercle

Facet of tubercle that articulates with transverse process of vertebra

Head articulates with vertebral bodies

Angle Neck

Costal groove

Shaft

Inferior border

Depression for costal cartilage

the ribs and sternum are lifted upwards and outwards, increasing the capacity of the thoracic cavity (see Fig. 10.21, p. 254).

Thoracic vertebrae

The 12 thoracic vertebrae are described on page 397.

APPENDICULAR SKELETON

Learning outcomes

After studying this section you should be able to:

- identify the bones that form the appendicular skeleton

- state the characteristics of the bones forming the appendicular skeleton

- outline the differences in structure between the male and female pelves.

The appendicular skeleton consists of the shoulder girdle with the upper limbs and the pelvic girdle with the lower limbs (Fig. 16.6).

Shoulder girdle and upper limb

Each shoulder girdle consists of:

- 1 clavicle
- 1 scapula.

Each upper limb consists of the following bones:

- 1 humerus
- 1 radius
- 1 ulna
- 8 carpal bones
- 5 metacarpal bones
- 14 phalanges.

Clavicle or collar bone (Fig. 16.28)
The clavicle is a long bone which has a double curve. It articulates with the manubrium of the sternum at the *sternoclavicular joint* and forms the *acromioclavicular joint* with the *acromion process* of the scapula. The clavicle provides the only bony link between the upper limb and the axial skeleton.

Scapula or shoulder blade (Fig. 16.29)
The scapula is a flat triangular-shaped bone, lying on the posterior chest wall superficial to the ribs and separated from them by muscles.

At the lateral angle there is a shallow articular surface, the *glenoid cavity* which, with the *head of the humerus*, forms the *shoulder joint*.

On the posterior surface there is a *spinous process* that projects beyond the lateral angle of the bone that overhangs the shoulder joint, called the *acromion process*. It articulates with the clavicle at the *acromioclavicular joint*. The *coracoid process*, a projection from the upper border of the bone, gives attachment to muscles that move the shoulder joint.

401

Acromial extremity (lateral)

Sternal extremity (medial)

Figure 16.28 The right clavicle.

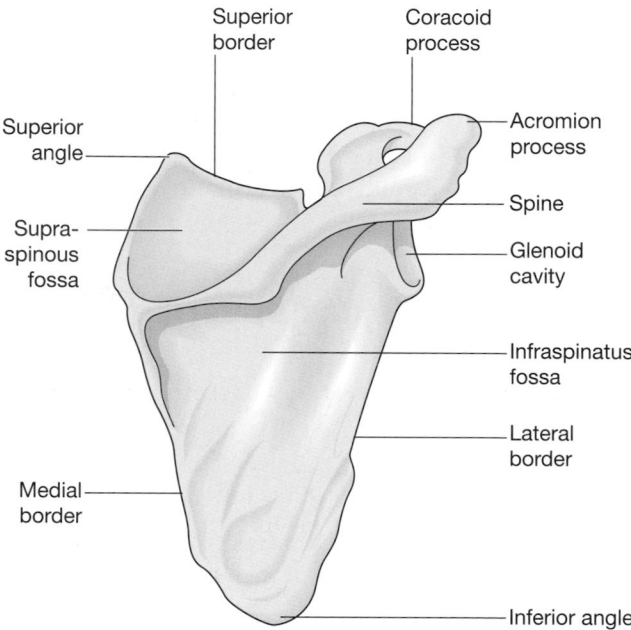

Superior border

Coracoid process

Superior angle

Acromion process

Supra-spinous fossa

Spine

Glenoid cavity

Infraspinatus fossa

Lateral border

Medial border

Inferior angle

Figure 16.29 The right scapula. Posterior view.

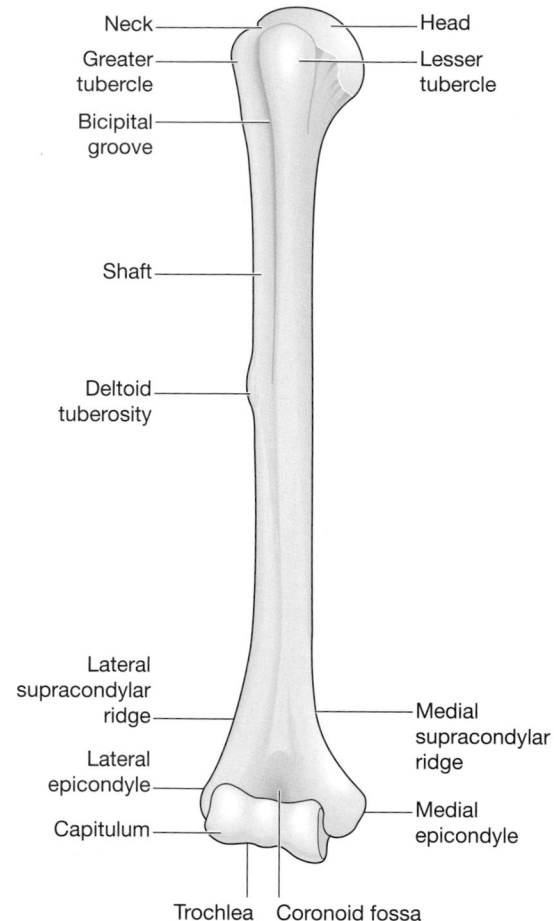

Neck

Head

Greater tubercle

Lesser tubercle

Bicipital groove

Shaft

Deltoid tuberosity

Lateral supracondylar ridge

Medial supracondylar ridge

Lateral epicondyle

Capitulum

Medial epicondyle

Trochlea   Coronoid fossa

Figure 16.30 The right humerus. Anterior view.

Humerus (Fig. 16.30)

This is the bone of the upper arm. The head articulates with the glenoid cavity of the scapula, forming the shoulder joint. Distal to the head there are two roughened projections of bone, the *greater* and *lesser tubercles,* and between them there is a deep groove, the *bicipital groove* or *intertubercular sulcus,* occupied by one of the tendons of the biceps muscle.

The distal end of the bone presents two surfaces that articulate with the radius and ulna to form the elbow joint.

Ulna and radius (Fig. 16.31)

These are the two bones of the forearm. The ulna is longer than and medial to the radius and when the arm is in the anatomical position, i.e. with the palm of the hand facing forward, the two bones are parallel. They articulate with the humerus at the *elbow joint,* the carpal bones at the *wrist joint* and with each other at the *proximal* and *distal radioulnar* joints.

Carpal or wrist bones (Fig. 16.32)

There are eight carpal bones arranged in two rows of four. From outside inwards they are:

- *proximal row*: scaphoid, lunate, triquetral, pisiform
- *distal row*: trapezium, trapezoid, capitate, hamate.

These bones are closely fitted together and held in position by ligaments which allow a certain amount of movement between them. The bones of the proximal row are associated with the wrist joint and those of the distal row form joints with the metacarpal bones. Tendons of muscles lying in the forearm cross the wrist and are held close to the bones by strong fibrous bands, called retinacula (see Fig. 17.8, p. 420).

Metacarpal bones or the bones of the hand

These five bones form the palm of the hand. They are numbered from the thumb side inwards. The proximal ends articulate with the carpal bones and the distal ends with the phalanges.

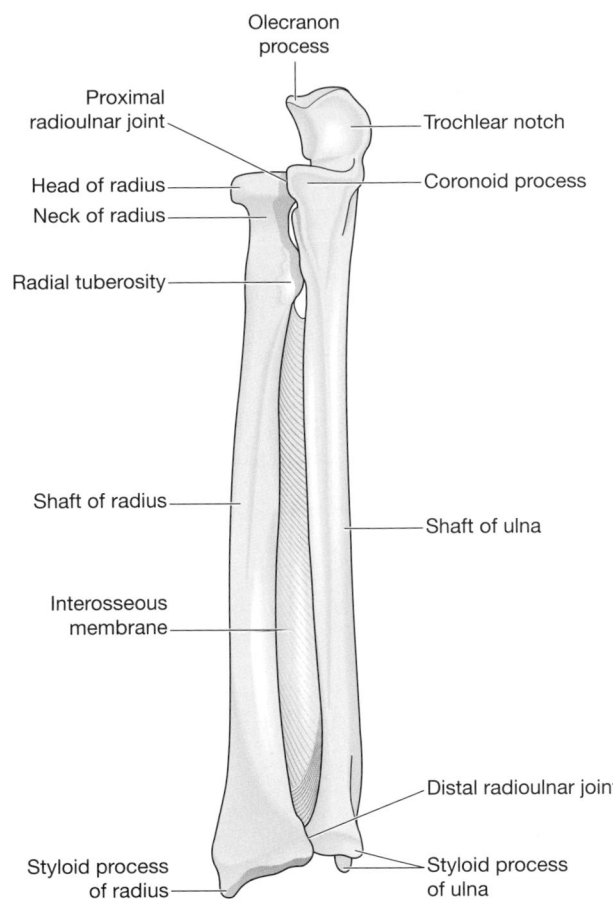

Figure 16.31 The right radius and ulna with the interosseous membrane. Anterior view.

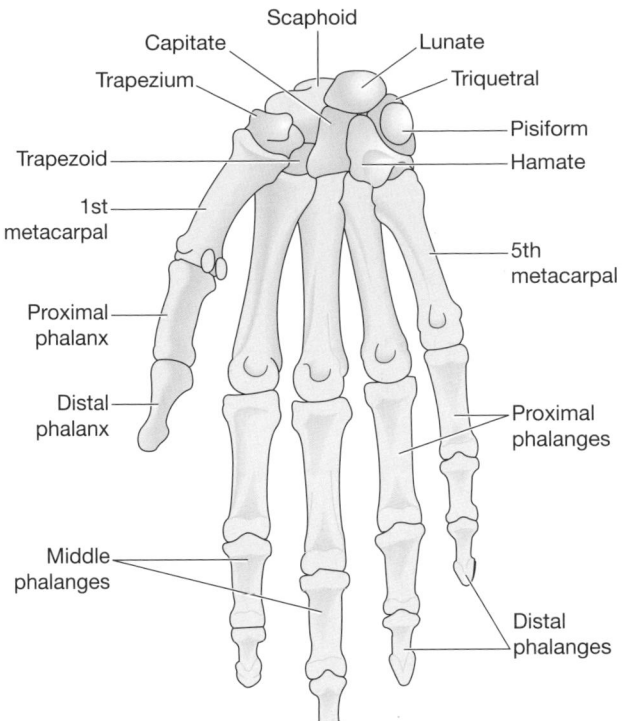

Figure 16.32 The bones of the wrist, hand and fingers. Anterior view.

403

Phalanges or finger bones

There are 14 phalanges, three in each finger and two in the thumb. They articulate with the metacarpal bones and with each other.

Pelvic girdle and lower limb

The bones of the pelvic girdle are:

- 2 innominate bones
- 1 sacrum.

The bones of the lower limb are:

- 1 femur
- 7 tarsal bones
- 1 tibia
- 5 metatarsal bones
- 1 fibula
- 14 phalanges.
- 1 patella

Innominate or hip bones (Fig. 16.33)

Each hip bone consists of three fused bones, the *ilium*, *ischium* and *pubis*. On its outer surface there is a deep

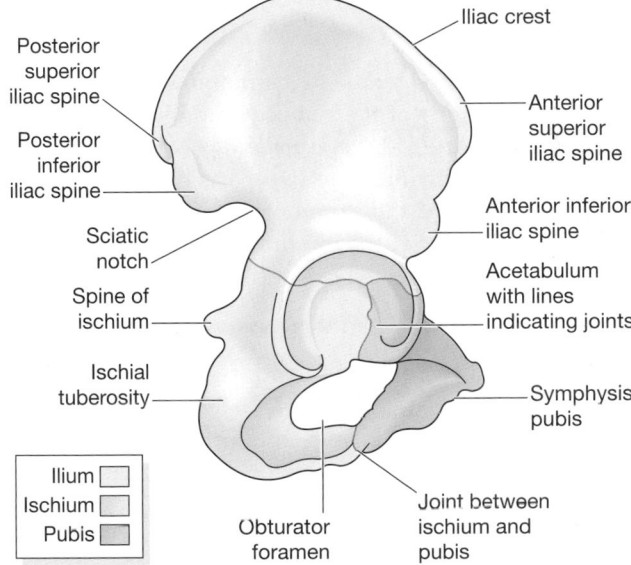

Figure 16.33 The right innominate bone. Lateral view.

depression, the *acetabulum*, which forms the hip joint with the almost-spherical head of femur.

The *ilium* is the upper flattened part of the bone and it presents the *iliac crest*, the anterior point of which is called the *anterior superior iliac spine*.

Figure 16.34 The bones of the pelvis and the upper part of the left femur.

The *pubis* is the anterior part of the bone and it articulates with the pubis of the other hip bone at a cartilaginous joint, the *symphysis pubis*.

The *ischium* is the inferior and posterior part.

The union of the three parts takes place in the *acetabulum*.

The pelvis (Fig. 16.34)

The pelvis is formed by the two innominate bones which articulate anteriorly at the symphysis pubis and posteriorly with the sacrum at the *sacroiliac joints* which are synovial joints. It is divided into two parts by the *brim of the pelvis*, consisting of the promontory of the sacrum and the *iliopectineal lines* of the innominate bones. The *greater* or *false pelvis* is above the brim and the *lesser* or *true pelvis* is below.

Differences between male and female pelves (Fig. 16.35).

The shape of the female pelvis allows for the passage of the baby during childbirth. In comparison with the male pelvis, the female pelvis has lighter bones, is more shallow and rounded and is generally more roomy.

Femur or thigh bone (Fig. 16.36)

The femur is the longest and strongest bone of the body. The head is almost spherical and fits into the *acetabulum* of the hip bone to form the *hip joint*. In the centre of the head there is a small depression for the attachment of the *ligament of the head of the femur*. This extends from the acetabulum to the femur and contains a blood vessel that

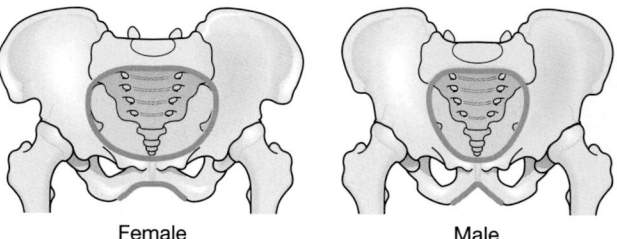

Figure 16.35 The difference in shape of the male and female pelves.

supplies blood to an area of the head of the bone. The neck extends outwards and slightly downwards from the head to the shaft and most of it is within the capsule of the hip joint.

The posterior surface of the lower third forms a flat triangular area called the *popliteal surface*. The distal extremity has two articular *condyles* which, with the tibia and patella, form the knee joint.

Tibia or shin bone (Fig. 16.37)

The tibia is the medial of the two bones of the lower leg. The proximal extremity is broad and flat and presents two *condyles* for articulation with the femur at the *knee joint*. The head of the fibula articulates with the inferior aspect of the lateral condyle, forming the *proximal tibiofibular joint*.

The distal extremity of the tibia forms the *ankle joint*. with the *talus* and the fibula. The *medial malleolus* is a downward projection of bone medial to the ankle joint.

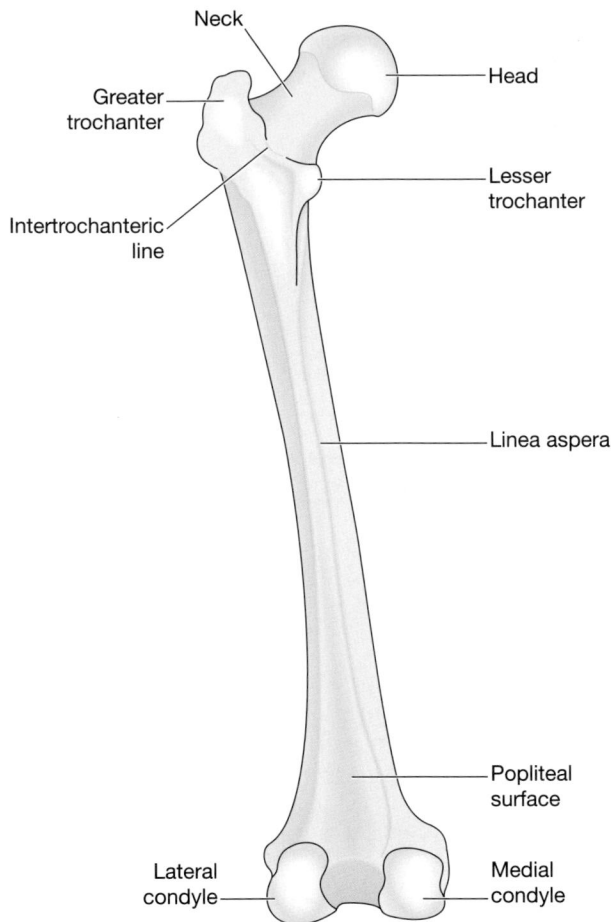

Figure 16.36 The left femur. Posterior view.

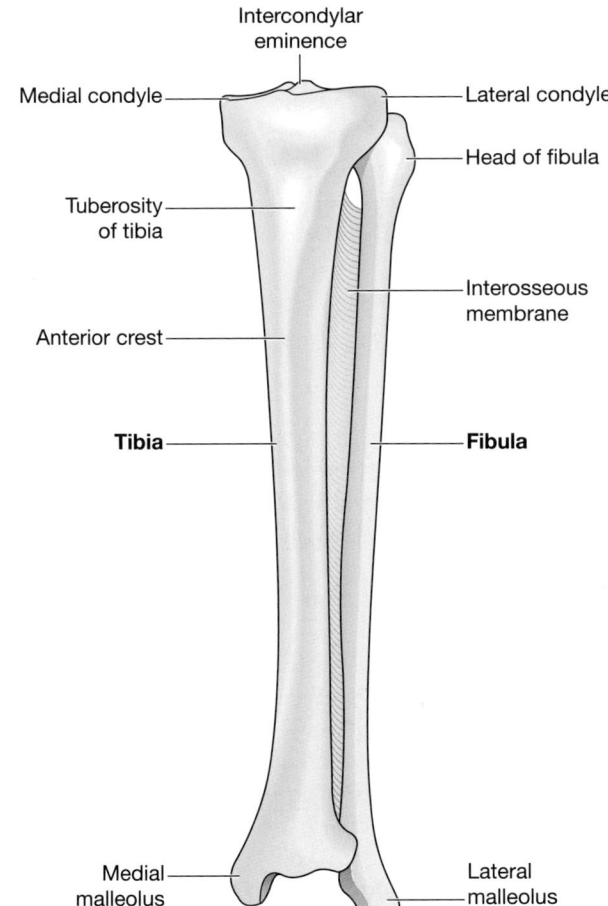

Figure 16.37 The left tibia and fibula with the interosseous membrane. Anterior view.

405

Fibula (Fig. 16.37)

The fibula is the long slender lateral bone in the leg. The head or upper extremity articulates with the lateral condyle of the tibia forming the proximal tibiofibular joint and the lower extremity articulates with the tibia then projects beyond it to form the *lateral malleolus*.

Patella or knee cap

This is a roughly triangular-shaped *sesamoid* bone associated with the knee joint. Its posterior surface articulates with the patellar surface of the femur in the knee joint and its anterior surface is in the *patellar tendon*, i.e. the tendon of the quadriceps femoris muscle.

Tarsal or ankle bones (Fig. 16.38)

There are seven tarsal bones which form the posterior part of the foot. They are:

- 1 talus
- 1 calcaneus
- 1 navicular
- 3 cuneiform
- 1 cuboid.

The *talus* articulates with the tibia and fibula at the ankle joint. The *calcaneus* forms the heel of the foot. The other bones articulate with each other and with the metatarsal bones.

Metatarsal bones of the foot (Fig. 16.38)

These are five bones, numbered from within outwards, which form the greater part of the dorsum of the foot. At their proximal ends they articulate with the tarsal bones and at their distal ends, with the phalanges. The enlarged distal head of the 1st metatarsal bone forms the 'ball' of the foot.

Phalanges of the toes (Fig. 16.38)

There are 14 phalanges arranged in a similar manner to those in the fingers, i.e. two in the great toe (the *halux*) and three in each of the other toes.

Arches of the foot. The arrangement of the bones of the foot is such that it is not a rigid structure. This point is

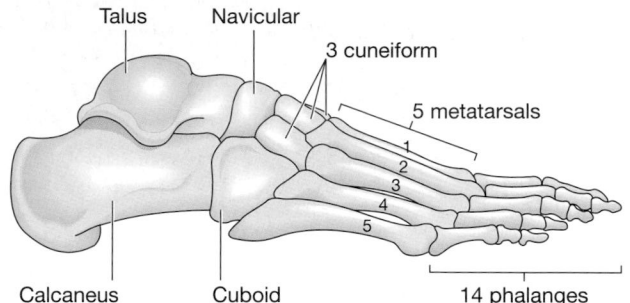

Figure 16.38 The bones of the foot. Lateral view.

Figure 16.39 The tendons and ligaments supporting the arches of the left foot. Medial view.

well illustrated by comparing a normal foot with a 'flat' foot. The bones have a bridge-like arrangement and are supported by muscles and ligaments so that four arches are formed, a *medial* and *lateral longitudinal arch* and two *transverse arches*.

Medial longitudinal arch. This is the highest of the arches and is formed by the calcaneus, talus, navicular, three cuneiform and first three metatarsal bones. Only the calcaneus and the distal end of the metatarsal bones should touch the ground.

Lateral longitudinal arch. The lateral arch is much less marked than its medial counterpart. The bony components are the calcaneus, cuboid and the two lateral metatarsal bones. Again only the calcaneus and metatarsal bones should touch the ground.

Transverse arches. These run across the foot and can be more easily seen by examining the skeleton than the live model. They are most marked at the level of the three cuneiform and cuboid bones.

Muscles and ligaments which support the arches of the foot (Fig. 16.39). As there are movable joints between all the bones of the foot, very strong muscles and ligaments are necessary to maintain the strength, resilience and stability of the foot during walking, running and jumping.

Posterior tibialis muscle. This is the most important muscular support of the medial longitudinal arch. It lies on the posterior aspect of the lower leg, originates from the middle third of the tibia and fibula and its tendon passes behind the medial malleolus to be inserted into the navicular, cuneiform, cuboid and metatarsal bones. It acts as a sling or 'suspension apparatus' for the arch.

Short muscles of the foot. This group of muscles is mainly concerned with the maintenance of the lateral longitudinal and transverse arches. They make up the fleshy part of the sole of the foot.

Plantar calcaneonavicular ligament or 'spring' ligament. This is a very strong thick ligament stretching from

the calcaneus to the navicular bone. It plays an important part in supporting the medial longitudinal arch.

Plantar ligaments and interosseous membranes. These structures support the lateral and transverse arches.

HEALING OF BONES

> **Learning outcomes**
>
> After studying this section you should be able to:
>
> - state three types of fractures
> - outline the process of bone healing
> - list the factors that delay healing of fractures
> - describe two complications of fractures.

Bone fractures are classified as:

- *simple*: the bone ends do not protrude through the skin
- *compound*: the bone ends protrude through the skin
- *pathological*: fracture of a bone weakened by disease.

Following a fracture, the broken ends of bone are joined by the deposition of new bone. This occurs in several stages (Fig. 16.40).

- A haematoma forms between the ends of bone and in surrounding soft tissues.
- There follows development of acute inflammation and accumulation of macrophages which phagocytose the haematoma, inflammatory exudate and small fragments of bone without blood supply (this takes about 5 days). Fibroblasts migrate to the site; granulation tissue and new capillaries develop.
- New bone forms as large numbers of osteoblasts secrete woven (non-lamellar) bone (p. 390), which is then quickly organised into lamellar bone and calcified, forming a *callus* (after about a week).
- Osteoblasts and osteoclasts remain active and the callus matures, reuniting the bone ends (after about 3 weeks).
- Reshaping of the bone continues and gradually the medullary canal is reopened through the callus (in weeks or months).
- In time the bone heals completely regaining its original features. Osteoblasts and osteoclasts are no longer present.

Factors that delay healing of fractures

Tissue fragments between the ends of bone. Splinters of dead bone (*sequestrae*) and soft tissue fragments not removed by phagocytosis delay healing.

Deficient blood supply. This delays growth of granulation tissue and new blood vessels. Hypoxia also reduces the number of osteoblasts and increases the number of chondrocytes that develop from their common parent cells. This may lead to cartilagenous union of the fracture, which results in a weaker repair. The most vulnerable sites, because of their normally poor blood supply, are the neck of femur, the scaphoid and the shaft of tibia.

Poor alignment of bone ends. This may result in the formation of a large and irregular callus which heals slowly and often results in permanent disability.

Continued mobility of bone ends. Continuous movement results in fibrosis of the granulation tissue followed by fibrous union of the fracture.

Inflamed area

Haematoma and bone fragments

1

Phagocytosis of clot and debris. Growth of granulation tissue begins

2

Osteoblasts begin to form new bone (callus)

3

Gradual spread and mineralisation of callus to bridge the gap

4

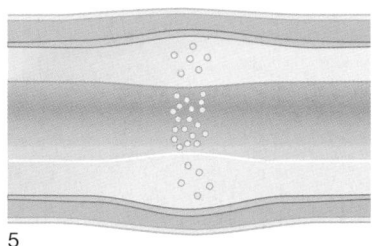

Bone almost healed. Osteoclasts reshape and canalise new bone

5

Figure 16.40 Stages in bone healing.

Miscellaneous. These include:

- infection (see below)
- systemic illness
- malnutrition
- drugs, e.g. corticosteroids
- ageing.

Complications of fractures

Infection (osteomyelitis). Microbes gain access through broken skin, although they may occasionally be blood-borne (p. 410). Healing will not occur until the infection resolves.

Fat embolism. Emboli consisting of fat from the marrow in the medullary canal may enter the circulation through torn veins. They are most likely to lodge in the lungs.

DISEASES OF BONES

Learning outcomes

After studying this section you should be able to:

- explain the pathological features of osteoporosis, Paget's disease, rickets and osteomalacia
- outline the causes and effects of osteomyelitis
- describe abnormalities of bone development
- explain the effects of bone tumours.

Box 16.1 Causes of decreased bone mass

Risk factors
Female gender
Increasing age
White ethnic origin
Family history
Lack of exercise/immobility
Diet (low calcium)
Smoking
Excess alcohol intake
Early menopause/oophorectomy
Thin build (small bones)

Drugs
Corticosteroids

Diseases
Cushing's syndrome
Hyperparathyroidism
Type I diabetes mellitus
Rheumatoid arthritis
Chronic renal failure
Chronic liver disease
Anorexia nervosa
Neoplasia

Osteoporosis

In this condition bone mass (the amount of bone tissue) is reduced because its deposition does not keep pace with resorption. Peak bone mass occurs around 35 years and then gradually declines in both sexes. Lowered oestrogen levels after the menopause are associated with a period of accelerated bone loss in women. Thereafter bone density in women is less than in men for any given age. Bone is progressively weakened with cancellous bone affected first by thinning and loss of trabeculae. In the postmenopausal period an imbalance of hormones probably causes bone weakening, i.e. between anabolic steroids (oestrogen and androgens) and antianabolic steroids (glucocorticoids). A range of environmental factors and diseases are associated with decreased bone mass and are implicated in development of osteoporosis (Box 16.1). Some can be influenced by changes in lifestyle. Exercise and calcium intake during childhood and adolescence are thought to be important in determining eventual bone mass of an individual. As bone mass decreases, susceptibility to fractures increases. Immobility causes reversible osteoporosis, the extent of which corresponds to the area of impaired movement, e.g.:

- localised – following immobilisation of a fractured limb or around a joint affected by rheumatoid arthritis
- generalised – in e.g. prolonged unconsciousness.

Common features of osteoporosis are:

- skeletal deformity – gradual loss of height with age, which is caused by compression of vertebrae
- bone pain
- fractures – especially of the hip (neck of femur), wrist (Colles fracture) and vertebrae.

Paget's disease

This disease can affect one bone, part of a bone or many bones. Osteocytes reabsorb excess bone, softening the tissue, and then overactive osteoblasts deposit abnormal new bone that is thickened or enlarged and structurally weak. This predisposes to deformities and fractures, commonly of the pelvis, femur, tibia and skull. Most cases occur after 40 years and the incidence increases with age. The cause is unknown and it often goes undetected until complications arise. These include:

- bone pain
- bony deformities, e.g. bowing of the tibia and femur
- fractures that are pathological (spontaneous) or follow minor trauma
- osteoarthritis due to bony deformities, especially in the hip joint
- osteosarcoma, which often occurs in the elderly and is associated with a poor prognosis (p. 411)
- compression of nerves in the diminished cranial foramina due to thickening of the bones, e.g. compression of the vestibulocochlear nerve causing deafness.

Rickets and osteomalacia

Rickets occurs in children and osteomalacia in adults after ossification is complete. They are caused by deficiency of vitamin D which promotes calcification of bone and absorption of calcium in the small intestine (see p. 274 and Table 11.1, p. 276). Deficiency may be due to:

- dietary deficiency of vitamin D
- malabsorption, e.g. coeliac disease or following gastrointestinal surgery

- lack of exposure to sunlight, e.g. pigmented skin, housebound people
- excessive loss of vitamin D or its precursors, e.g. in chronic renal failure, haemodialysis
- drugs that result in breakdown of vitamin D, e.g. anticonvulsants, including phenytoin.

In *rickets*, osteoid is deposited but calcification is incomplete. Although growth of the epiphyseal cartilage continues, growth is stunted. The bones remain soft and those of the lower limbs become bowed by the weight of the body.

In *osteomalacia* there is increased and abnormal turnover of bone. As in rickets, osteoid is not calcified and the bones become soft, bowed and prone to fractures.

Infection of bones

Osteomyelitis

Microbes gain access to bones:

- through the skin in compound fractures
- by spread from a local focus of infection, e.g. from an infected prosthesis or tooth abscess
- via the blood—commonly from a boil or paronychia (infection of the nail bed)
- during a surgical procedure.

The most common infecting organism is *Staphylococcus aureus*, which typically affects the growth regions of long bones in children. Infection of soft tissues of the feet, common in elderly diabetics, may spread to the bones. Infection of the bone causes inflammation that may completely resolve. In more severe cases healing may be delayed by the presence of *sequestra* (pieces of dead bone) in the wound. Complications include bone necrosis, suppuration (pus formation), local spread to the periosteum and then to surrounding soft tissues and joints. This may be followed by formation of a *subperiosteal abscess* that ruptures forming a sinus discharging pus to the skin, which in chronic cases can continue for several years.

Developmental abnormalities of bone

Achondroplasia

This is caused by a genetic abnormality. There is abnormal growth of cartilage, especially the epiphyseal cartilage of long bones, leading to characteristic dwarfism and under-development of the bones of the base of the skull (Fig. 16.41).

Figure 16.41 Achondroplasia.

Osteogenesis imperfecta ('brittle bone syndrome')

This is a group of conditions in which there is a congenital defect of osteoblasts, resulting in failure of ossification. The bones are brittle and fracture easily, either spontaneously or following very slight trauma.

Tumours of bone

Benign tumours

Single or multiple tumours may develop for unknown reasons in bone and cartilage. They may cause pathological fractures or pressure damage to soft tissues, e.g. a benign vertebral tumour may damage the spinal cord or a spinal nerve. Benign tumours of cartilage have a tendency to undergo malignant change.

Malignant tumours

Metastatic tumours

The most common malignancies of bone are metastases of primary carcinomas of the breast, lungs, thyroid, kidneys and prostate gland. The usual sites are those with the best blood supply, i.e. cancellous bone, especially the bodies of the lumbar vertebrae and the epiphyses of the humerus and femur. Tumour fragments are spread in blood, and possibly along the walls of the veins from pelvic tumours to vertebrae. The effects of the malignancy may be:

- destruction of bone, leading to pathological fractures
- collapse of vertebrae causing damage to the spinal cord and/or spinal nerves

- fibrosis of bone
- anaemia, leukopenia and thrombocytopenia but in most cases the link is not known.

Primary tumours

Osteosarcoma. This is a rapidly growing and often metastatic tumour believed to develop from the precursors of osteogenic cells. In young people between 10 and 25 years of age the tumour develops most commonly in the medullary canal of long bones, especially the femur.

It is usually well advanced before it becomes evident. In older people, usually over 60 years of age, it is often associated with Paget's disease and the bones most commonly affected are the vertebrae, skull and pelvis.

Chondrosarcoma. These relatively slow-growing tumours are usually the result of malignant change in benign tumours of cartilage cells. They occur mainly between the ages of 40 and 70 years.

17

The joints

A joint is the site at which any two or more bones articulate or come together. Some joints have no movement (*fibrous*), some only slight movement (*cartilaginous*) and some are freely movable (*synovial*).

TYPES OF JOINT

Learning outcomes

After studying this section you should be able to:

- state the characteristics of fixed and fibrous joints
- state the different types of synovial joints
- outline the movements possible at five types of synovial joints
- describe the structure and functions of a typical synovial joint.

Fibrous or fixed joints (Fig. 17.1)

These immovable joints have fibrous tissue between the bones, e.g. joints between the bones of the skull (sutures) and those between the teeth and the maxilla and mandible.

Cartilaginous or slightly movable joints (Fig. 17.2)

There is a pad of *fibrocartilage* between the ends of the bones that form the joint which allows for very slight movement where the pad of cartilage is compressed. Examples include the symphysis pubis and the joints between the vertebral bodies.

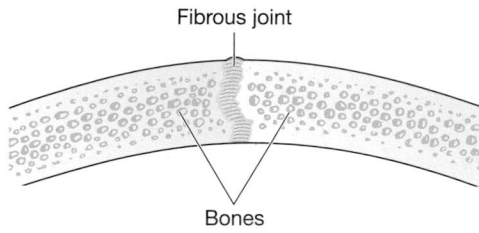

Figure 17.1 A fibrous or fixed joint, e.g. the sutures of the skull.

Figure 17.2 A cartilaginous or slightly movable joint, e.g. between the vertebral bodies.

Table 17.1 **Movements possible at synovial joints**	
Movement	**Definition**
Flexion	Bending, usually forward but occasionally backward, e.g. knee joint
Extension	Straightening or bending backward
Abduction	Movement away from the midline of the body
Adduction	Movement towards the midline of the body
Circumduction	Combination of flexion, extension, abduction and adduction
Rotation	Movement round the long axis of a bone
Pronation	Turning the palm of the hand down
Supination	Turning the palm of the hand up
Inversion	Turning the sole of the foot inwards
Eversion	Turning the sole of the foot outwards

Synovial or freely movable joints

Synovial joints have characteristic features that enable a wide range of movements (Table 17.1). They are classified according to the range of movement possible or to the shape of the articulating parts of the bones involved.

Ball and socket. The head or ball of one bone articulates with a socket of another and the shape of the bones allows for a wide range of movement. Those possible are flexion, extension, adduction, abduction, rotation and circumduction. Examples are the shoulder and hip.

Hinge joints. These allow the movements of flexion and extension only. They are the elbow, knee, ankle, the joints between the atlas and the occipital bone, and the interphalangeal joints of the fingers and toes.

Gliding joints. The articular surfaces glide over each other, e.g. sternoclavicular joints, acromioclavicular joints and joints between the carpal bones and those between the tarsal bones.

Pivot joints. Movement is round one axis (rotation), e.g. proximal and distal radioulnar joints and the joint between the atlas and the odontoid process of the axis.

Condyloid and saddle joints. Movements take place round two axes, permitting flexion, extension, abduction, adduction and circumduction, e.g. the wrist, temporomandibular, metacarpophalangeal and metatarsophalangeal joints.

Characteristics of a synovial joint (Fig. 17.3)

All synovial joints have certain characteristics in common.

Articular or hyaline cartilage

The parts of the bones which are in contact are always covered with hyaline cartilage. It provides a smooth articular surface and is strong enough to absorb compression forces and bear the weight of the body. The cartilage lining, which is up to 7 mm thick in young people, becomes thinner and less compressible with age. This leads to increasing stress on other structures in the joint. Cartilage has no blood supply and receives its nourishment from synovial fluid.

Capsule or capsular ligament

The joint is surrounded and enclosed by a sleeve of fibrous tissue which holds the bones together. It is sufficiently loose to allow freedom of movement but strong enough to protect it from injury.

Synovial membrane

This is composed of epithelial cells and is found:

- lining the capsule
- covering those parts of the bones within the joint not covered by articular cartilage
- covering all intracapsular structures that do not bear weight.

Synovial fluid. This is a thick sticky fluid, of egg-white consistency, secreted by synovial membranes into the *synovial cavity*, and it:

- provides nutrients for the structures within the joint cavity

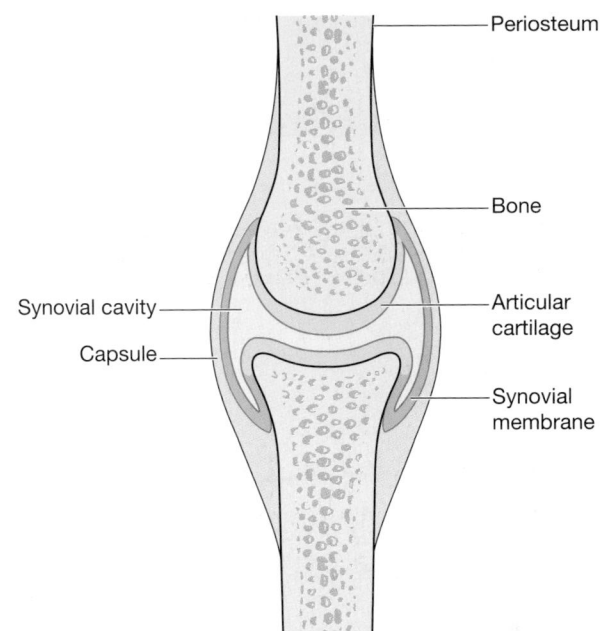

Figure 17.3 Diagram of the basic structure of a synovial joint.

- contains phagocytes, which remove microbes and cellular debris
- acts as a lubricant
- maintains joint stability
- prevents the ends of the bones from being separated, as does a little water between two glass surfaces.

Little sacs of synovial fluid or *bursae* are present in some joints, e.g. the knee. They act as cushions to prevent friction between a bone and a ligament or tendon, or skin where a bone in a joint is near the surface.

Other intracapsular structures

Some joints have structures within the capsule, but outside the synovial membrane, which assist in maintenance of stability, e.g. fat pads and menisci in the knee joint. When these structures do not bear weight they are covered by synovial membrane.

Extracapsular structures

- *Ligaments* that blend with the capsule provide additional stability at most joints.
- *Muscles* or their *tendons* also provide stability and stretch across the joints they move. When the muscle contracts it shortens, pulling one bone towards the other.

Nerve and blood supply

Nerves and blood vessels crossing a joint usually supply the capsule and the muscles that move it.

MAIN SYNOVIAL JOINTS OF THE LIMBS

Learning outcome

After studying this section you should be able to:

- describe the structure and movements of the following synovial joints: shoulder, elbow, wrist, hip, knee, ankle.

Individual synovial joints have the characteristics described above so only their distinctive features are included in this section.

Shoulder joint (Fig. 17.4)

This ball and socket joint is formed by the glenoid cavity of the scapula and the head of the humerus. The capsular ligament is very loose inferiorly to allow for the free movement normally possible at this joint. The glenoid cavity is deepened by a rim of fibrocartilage, the *glenoidal labrum*, which provides additional stability without limiting movement. The tendon of the long head of the *biceps muscle*, lying in the intertubercular (bicipital) groove of the humerus, extends through the joint cavity and is attached to the upper rim of the glenoid cavity. It has an important stabilising effect on the joint.

Synovial membrane forms a sleeve round the part of the tendon of the long head of the biceps muscles within the capsular ligament and covers the glenoidal labrum.

Extracapsular structures consist of:

- the *coracohumeral ligament*, extending from the coracoid process of the scapula to the humerus
- the *glenohumeral ligaments*, which blend with and strengthen the capsule
- the *transverse humeral ligament*, retaining the biceps tendon in the intertubercular groove.

The stability of the joint may be reduced if these structures, together with the tendon of the biceps muscle, are stretched by repeated dislocations of the joint.

Muscles and movements

Muscles (Fig. 17.5)

Coracobrachialis muscle. This lies on the upper medial aspect of the arm. It arises from the coracoid process of

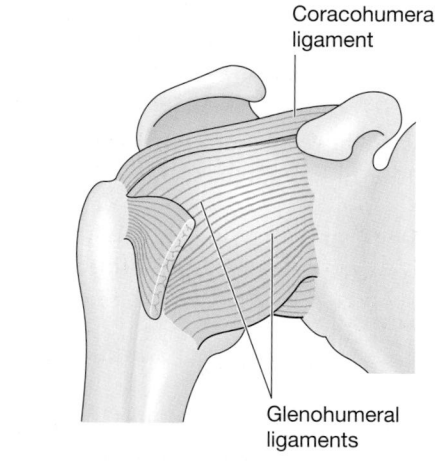

Figure 17.4 The right shoulder joint: A. Section viewed from the front. B. The position of glenoidal labrum with the humerus removed, viewed from the side. C. The supporting ligaments viewed from the front.

the scapula, stretches across in front of the shoulder joint and is inserted into the middle third of the humerus. It flexes the shoulder joint.

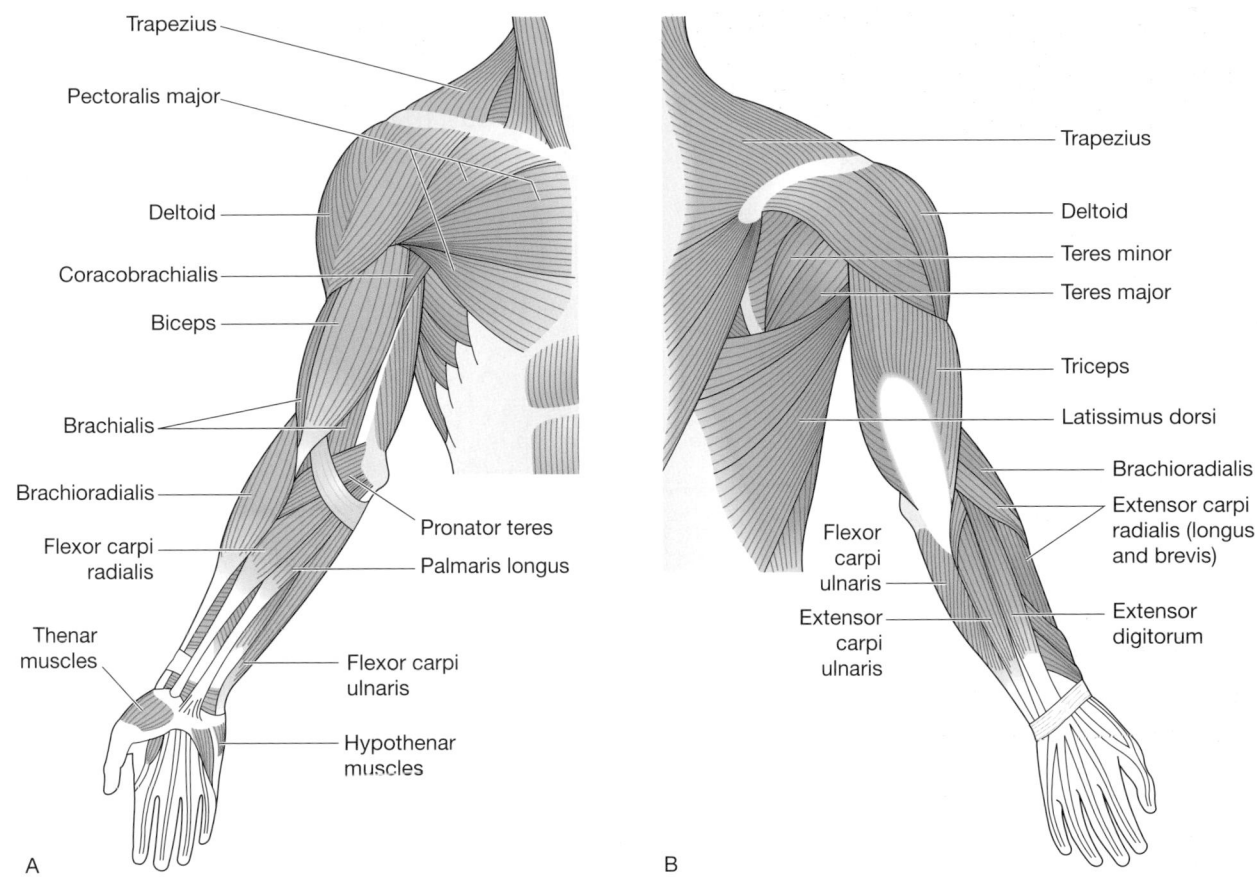

Figure 17.5 The main muscles that move the joints of the upper limb. A. Anterior view. B. Posterior view.

417

Deltoid muscle. These muscle fibres originate from the clavicle, acromion process and spine of scapula and radiate over the shoulder joint to be inserted into the deltoid tuberosity of the humerus. It forms the fleshy and rounded contour of the shoulder. The anterior fibres cause flexion, the middle or main part, abduction and the posterior fibres extend the shoulder joint.

Pectoralis major. This lies on the anterior thoracic wall. The fibres originate from the middle third of the clavicle and from the sternum and are inserted into the lip of the intertubercular groove of the humerus. It draws the arm forward and towards the body, i.e. flexes and adducts.

Latissimus dorsi. This arises from the posterior part of the iliac crest and the spinous processes of the lumbar and lower thoracic vertebrae. It passes upwards across the back then under the arm to be inserted into the bicipital groove of the humerus. It adducts, medially rotates and extends the arm.

Teres major. This originates from the inferior angle of the scapula and is inserted into the humerus just below the shoulder joint. It extends, adducts and medially rotates the arm.

Movements

Flexion: coracobrachialis, anterior fibres of deltoid and pectoralis major.
Extension: teres major, latissimus dorsi and posterior fibres of deltoid.
Abduction: deltoid.
Adduction: combined action of flexors and extensors.
Circumduction: flexors, extensors, abductors and adductors acting in series.
Medial rotation: pectoralis major, latissimus dorsi, teres major and anterior fibres of deltoid.
Lateral rotation: posterior fibres of deltoid.

Elbow joint (Fig. 17.6)

This *hinge* joint is formed by the trochlea and the capitulum of the humerus and the trochlear notch of the ulna and the head of the radius.

Extracapsular structures consist of anterior, posterior, medial and lateral strengthening ligaments.

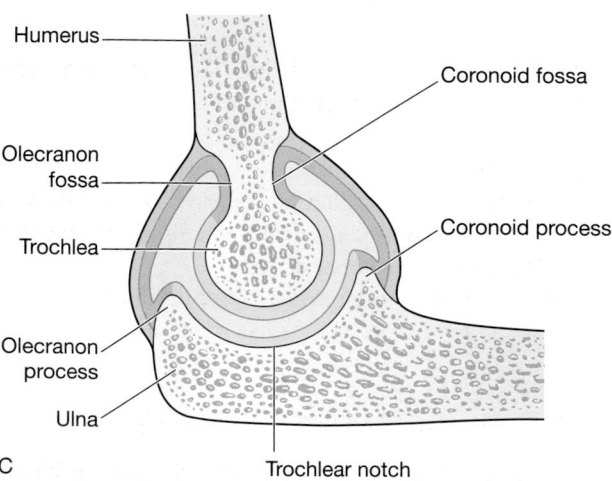

Figure 17.6 The elbow and proximal radioulnar joints. A. Section viewed from the front. B. The proximal radioulnar joint, viewed from above. C. Section of the elbow joint, partly flexed, viewed from the side.

Muscles and movements

Muscles (Fig. 17.5)

Biceps muscle. This lies on the anterior aspect of the upper arm. At its proximal end it is divided into two parts (heads) each of which has its own tendon. The short head rises from the coracoid process of the scapula and passes in front of the shoulder joint to the arm. The long head originates from the rim of the glenoid cavity and its tendon passes through the joint cavity and the bicipital groove of the humerus to the arm. It is retained in the bicipital groove by a transverse ligament which stretches across the groove. The distal tendon crosses the elbow joint and is inserted into the radial tuberosity. It helps to stabilise and flex the shoulder joint and at the elbow joint it assists with flexion and supination.

Brachialis muscle. This lies on the anterior aspect of the upper arm deep to the biceps. It originates from the shaft of the humerus, extends across the elbow joint and is inserted into the ulna just distal to the joint capsule. It is the main flexor of the elbow joint.

Triceps muscle. This lies on the posterior aspect of the humerus. It arises from three heads, one from the scapula and two from the posterior surface of the humerus. The insertion is by a common tendon to the olecranon process of the ulna. It helps to stabilise the shoulder joint, assists in adduction of the arm and extends the elbow joint.

Movements

Flexion: biceps and brachialis.
Extension: triceps.

Proximal and distal radioulnar joints

The *proximal radioulnar joint*, formed by the rim of the head of the radius rotating in the radial notch of the ulna, is in the same capsule as the elbow joint. The *annular ligament* is a strong extracapsular ligament which encircles the head of the radius and keeps it in contact with the radial notch of the ulna (Fig. 17.6B).

The distal *radioulnar joint* is a pivot joint between the distal end of the radius and the head of the ulna (Fig. 17.7).

Muscles and movements

Muscles (Fig. 17.5)

Pronator teres. This lies obliquely across the upper third of the front of the forearm. It arises from the medial epicondyle of the humerus and the coronoid process of the ulna and passes obliquely across the forearm to be inserted into the lateral surface of the shaft of the radius. It rotates the radioulnar joints, changing the hand from the anatomical to the writing position, i.e. pronation.

Supinator muscle. This lies obliquely across the posterior and lateral aspects of the forearm. Its fibres arise from the lateral epicondyle of the humerus and the upper part of the ulna and are inserted into the lateral surface of the upper third of the radius. It rotates the radioulnar joints, changing the hand from the writing to the anatomical position, i.e. supination. It lies deep to the muscles shown in Figure 17.5.

Movements

Pronation: pronator teres.
Supination: supinator and biceps.

Wrist joint (Fig. 17.7)

This is a *condyloid* joint between the distal end of the radius and the proximal ends of the scaphoid, lunate and triquetral. A disc of white fibrocartilage separates the ulna from the joint cavity and articulates with the carpal bones. It also separates the inferior radioulnar joint from the wrist joint.

Extracapsular structures consist of medial and lateral ligaments and anterior and posterior radiocarpal ligaments.

Muscles and movements

Muscles (Fig. 17.5)

Flexor carpi radialis. This lies on the anterior surface of the forearm. It originates from the medial epicondyle of the humerus and is inserted into the second and third metacarpal bones. It flexes the wrist joint, and when acting with the extensor carpi radialis, abducts the joint.

Flexor carpi ulnaris. This lies on the medial aspect of the forearm. It originates from the medial epicondyle of the humerus and the upper parts of the ulna and is inserted into the pisiform, the hamate and the fifth metacarpal bones. It flexes the wrist, and when acting with the extensor carpi ulnaris, adducts the joint.

Extensor carpi radialis longus and brevis. These lie on the posterior aspect of the forearm. The fibres originate from the lateral epicondyle of the humerus and are inserted by a long tendon into the second and third metacarpal bones. They extend and abduct the wrist.

Extensor carpi ulnaris. This lies on the posterior surface of the forearm. It originates from the lateral epicondyle of

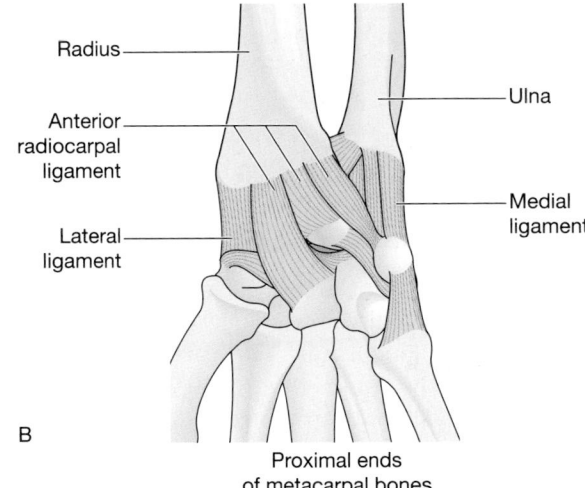

Figure 17.7 The wrist and distal radioulnar joints. Anterior view. A. Section. B. Supporting ligaments.

419

the humerus and is inserted into the fifth metacarpal bone. It extends and adducts the wrist.

Movements

Flexion: flexor carpi radialis and the flexor carpi ulnaris.
Extension: extensors carpi radialis (longus and brevis) and the extensor carpi ulnaris.
Abduction: flexor and extensors carpi radialis.
Adduction: flexor and extensor carpi ulnaris.

Joints of the hands and fingers

There are synovial joints between the carpal bones, between the carpal and metacarpal bones, between the metacarpal bones and proximal phalanges and between the phalanges. The powerful movements that occur at these joints are produced by muscles in the forearm which have tendons extending into the hand. Many of the finer movements of the fingers are produced by numerous small muscles in the hand.

The flexor retinaculum is a strong fibrous band that stretches across the front of the carpal bones, enclosing their concavity and forming the *carpal tunnel*. The tendons of flexor muscles of the wrist joint and the fingers and the median nerve pass through the carpal tunnel, the retinaculum holding them close to the bones. Synovial membrane forms sleeves around these tendons in the carpal tunnel and extends some way into the palm of the hand. Synovial sheaths also enclose the tendons on the flexor surfaces of the fingers. Synovial fluid prevents friction that might damage the tendons as they move over the bones (Fig. 17.8).

The extensor retinaculum is a strong fibrous band that extends across the back of the wrist. Tendons of muscles that extend the wrist and finger joints are encased in synovial membrane under the retinaculum. The synovial sheaths are less extensive than on the flexor aspect. The synovial fluid secreted prevents friction.

Hip joint (Fig. 17.9)

This ball and socket joint is formed by the cup-shaped acetabulum of the innominate bone and the almost spherical head of the femur. The capsular ligament includes most of the neck of the femur. The cavity is deepened by the *acetabular labrum,* a ring of fibrocartilage attached to the rim of the acetabulum. This adds stability to the joint without limiting its range of movement. The ligament of the head of the femur extends from the shallow depression in the middle of the head of the femur to the acetabulum. It conveys a blood vessel to the head of the femur. Synovial membrane covers both sides of the acetabular labrum and forms a sleeve around the ligament of the head of the femur. There are three important ligaments that surround and strengthen the capsule. They are the *iliofemoral, ischiofemoral* and *pubofemoral ligaments.*

Muscles and movements

Muscles (Figs 17.10 and 17.11)

Psoas muscle. This arises from the transverse processes and bodies of the lumbar vertebrae. It passes across the flat part of the ilium and behind the inguinal ligament to be inserted into the femur. Together with the iliacus it flexes the hip joint (Fig. 17.10).

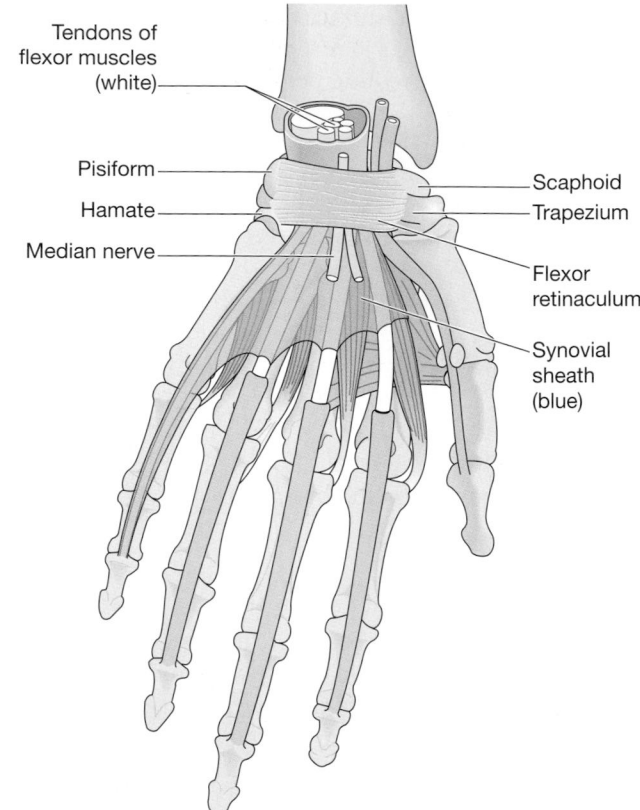

Figure 17.8 The carpal tunnel and synovial sheaths in the wrist and hand in green; tendons in white. Palmar view, left hand.

Iliacus muscle. This lies in the iliac fossa of the innominate bone. It originates from the iliac crest, passes over the iliac fossa and joins the tendon of the psoas muscle to be inserted into the lesser trochanter of the femur. The combined action of iliacus and psoas flexes the hip joint.

Quadriceps femoris. This is a group of four muscles lying on the front and sides of the thigh. They are the *rectus femoris* and three *vasti*. The rectus femoris originates from the ilium and the three vasti from the upper end of the femur. Together they pass over the front of the knee joint to be inserted into the tibia by the patellar tendon. Only the rectus femoris flexes the hip joint. Together the group acts as a very strong extensor of the knee joint.

Gluteal muscles. These consist of the *gluteus maximus, medius* and *minimus* which together form the fleshy part of the buttock. They originate from the ilium and sacrum and are inserted into the femur. They cause extension, abduction and medial rotation at the hip joint.

Sartorius. This is the longest muscle in the body and crosses both the hip and knee joints. It originates from the

A

B

C

Figure 17.9 The hip joint. Anterior view. A. Section. B. Supporting ligaments. C. Head of femur and acetabulum separated to show acetabular labrum and ligament of head of femur.

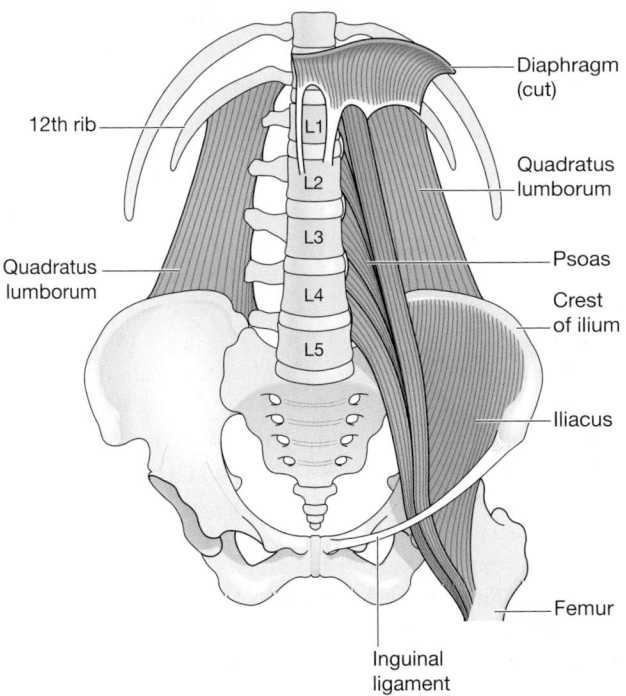

Figure 17.10 The muscles of the posterior abdominal wall and pelvis which flex the hip joint.

anterior superior iliac spine and passes obliquely across the hip joint, thigh and knee joint to be inserted into the medial surface of the upper part of the tibia. It is associated with flexion and abduction at the hip joint and flexion at the knee.

Adductor group. This lies on the medial aspect of the thigh. They originate from the pubic bone and are inserted into the linea aspera of the femur. They adduct and medially rotate the thigh.

Movements

Flexion: psoas, iliacus, rectus femoris and sartorius.
Extension: gluteus maximus and the hamstrings.
Abduction: gluteus medius and minimus, sartorius and others.
Adduction: adductor group.
Lateral rotation: mainly gluteal muscles and adductor group.
Medial rotation: gluteus medius and minimus and others.

Knee joint (Fig. 17.12)

This is the largest and most complex joint. It is a hinge joint formed by the condyles of the femur, the condyles of

421

Figure 17.11 The main muscles of the lower limb. A. Anterior view. B. Posterior view.

A

B

the tibia and the posterior surface of the patella. The anterior part of the capsule consists of the tendon of the quadriceps femoris muscle which also supports the patella. Intracapsular structures include two *cruciate ligaments* that cross each other, extending from the *intercondylar notch* of the femur to the *intercondylar eminence* of the tibia. They help to stabilise the joint.

Semilunar cartilages or *menisci* are incomplete discs of white fibrocartilage lying on top of the articular condyles of the tibia. They are wedge-shaped, being thicker at their outer edges. They help to stabilise the joint by preventing lateral displacement of the bones.

Bursae and pads of fat are numerous. They prevent friction between a bone and a ligament or tendon and between the skin and the patella. Synovial membrane covers the cruciate ligaments and the pads of fat. The menisci are not covered with synovial membrane because they are weight bearing. The most important strengthening ligaments are the *medial* and *lateral ligaments*.

Muscles and movements

Possible movements at this joint are flexion, extension and a rotatory movement which 'locks' the joint when it is fully extended. When the joint is locked, balance is maintained with less muscular effort than when it is flexed.

Muscles (Fig. 17.11)

Hamstring muscles. These lie on the posterior aspect of the thigh. They originate from the ischium and are inserted into the upper end of the tibia. They are *biceps femoris*, *semimembranosus* and *semitendinosus muscles*. They flex the knee joint.

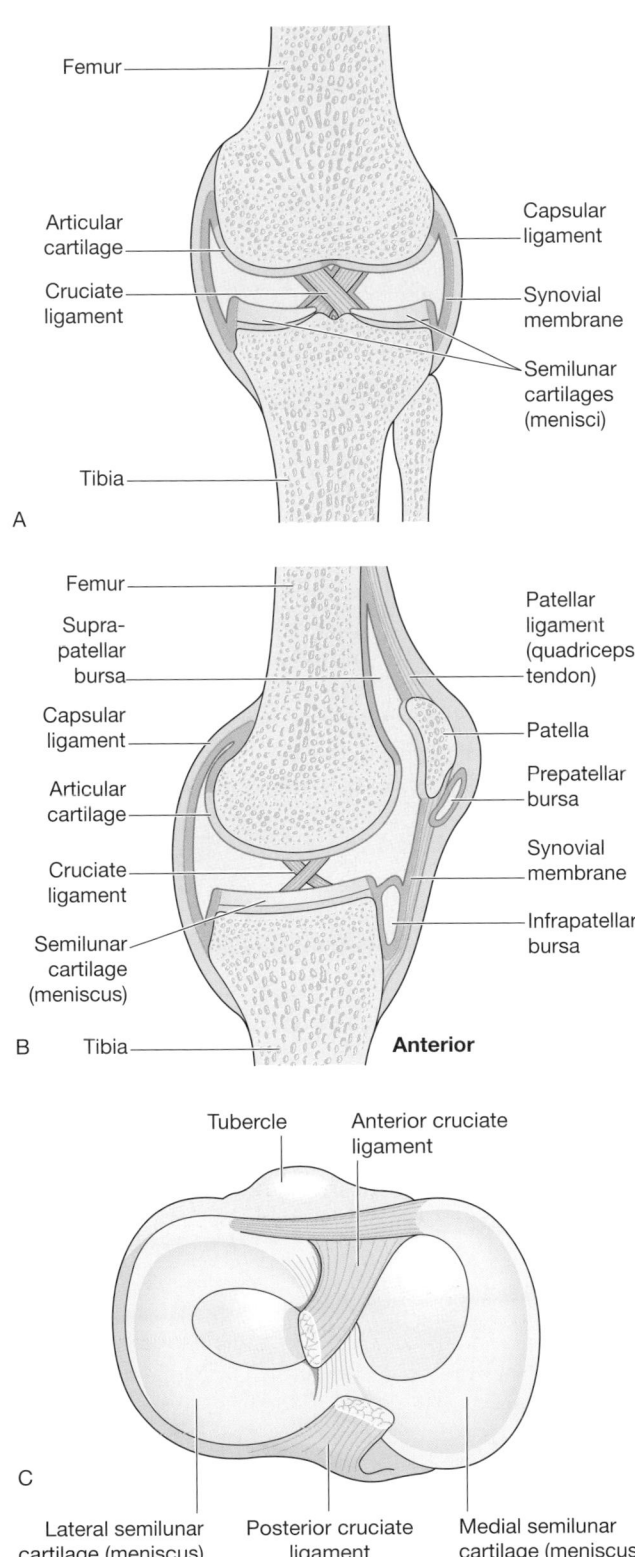

Figure 17.12 The knee joint. A. Section viewed from the front. B. Section viewed from the side. C. The superior surface of the tibia showing the semilunar cartilages and the cruciate ligaments.

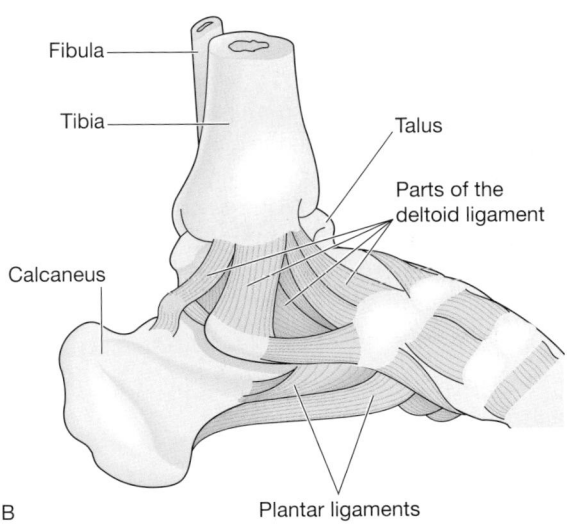

Figure 17.13 The left ankle joint. A. Section viewed from the front. B. Supporting ligaments. Medial view.

423

Gastrocnemius. This forms the bulk of the calf of the leg. It arises by two heads, one from each condyle of the femur, and passes down behind the tibia to be inserted into the calcaneus by the *calcanean tendon* (*Achilles tendon*). It crosses both knee and ankle joints, causing flexion at the knee and plantarflexion at the ankle.

Quadriceps femoris (described above). This extends the knee joint.

Movements

Flexion (bending backwards): gastrocnemius and hamstrings.
Extension (straightening): quadriceps femoris muscle.

Ankle joint (Fig. 17.13)

This *hinge* joint is formed by the distal end of the tibia and its malleolus (medial malleolus), the distal end of the fibula (lateral malleolus) and the talus. There are four important ligaments strengthening this joint. They are the deltoid and anterior, posterior, medial and lateral ligaments.

Muscles and movements

Muscles (Fig. 17.11)

Anterior tibialis muscle. This originates from the upper end of the tibia, lies on the anterior surface of the leg and is inserted into the middle cuneiform bone by a long tendon. It is associated with dorsiflexion of the foot.

Soleus. This is one of the main muscles of the calf of the leg, lying immediately deep to the gastrocnemius. It originates from the heads and upper parts of the fibula and the tibia. Its tendon joins that of the gastrocnemius so that they have a common insertion into the calcaneus by the calcanean (Achilles) tendon. It causes plantarflexion at the ankle and helps to stabilise the joint when standing.

Gastrocnemius. This (described above) is a powerful plantarflexor.

Movements

Flexion (dorsiflexion): anterior tibialis assisted by the muscles which extend the toes.
Extension (plantarflexion): gastrocnemius and soleus assisted by the muscles which flex the toes.

The movements of *inversion* and *eversion* occur between the tarsal bones and not at the ankle joint.

Joints of the foot and toes

There are a number of synovial joints between the tarsal bones, between the tarsal and metatarsal bones, between the metatarsals and proximal phalanges and between the phalanges. Movements are produced by muscles in the leg with long tendons which cross the ankle joint, and by muscles of the foot. The tendons crossing the ankle joint are encased in synovial sheaths and are held close to the bones by strong transverse ligaments. They move smoothly within their sheaths as the joints move. In addition to moving the joints of the foot these muscles support the arches of the foot and help to maintain body balance.

DISORDERS OF JOINTS

Learning outcomes

After studying this section you should be able to:

■ relate the features of the diseases in this section to abnormal anatomy and physiology

■ compare and contrast the features of rheumatoid arthritis and osteoarthritis.

The tissues involved in diseases of the synovial joints are synovial membrane, hyaline cartilage and bone.

Inflammatory diseases of joints (arthritis)

Rheumatoid arthritis (RA, rheumatoid disease)

This is a chronic progressive inflammatory autoimmune disease. It is a systemic disorder where inflammatory changes not only affect synovial joints but also many other sites including the heart, blood vessels and skin.

It is more common in females than males and can affect all ages, including children (Still's disease), although it usually develops between the ages of 35 and 55 years. The cause is not clearly understood but development of autoimmunity may be initiated by microbial infection, possibly by viruses, in genetically susceptible people. Antigen/antibody complexes (*rheumatoid factors*) are formed and are often found in the blood and synovial fluid (*seropositive RA*). Seropositive individuals tend to have a more aggressive form of RA than those without rheumatoid factors, i.e. seronegative RA. Rheumatoid factors appear early in severe cases of sudden onset, and later when the disease develops gradually. Acute exacerbations of rheumatoid arthritis are usually accompanied by fever, and are interspersed with periods of remission. The joints most commonly affected are those of the hands and feet, but in severe cases most of the synovial joints may be involved. With each febrile exacerbation there is additional and cumulative damage to the joints, leading to increasing deformity, pain and loss of function. The primary changes that may be reversible include hypertrophy and hyperplasia of synovial cells and fibrinous inflammatory effusion into the joint. If the disease progresses there are further secondary changes which may be irreversible, including:

■ erosion of articular cartilage and the growth of granulation tissue (*pannus*) that separates the bones and distorts the shape of the joint

■ fibrosis of pannus which causes adhesions between the bones, limiting movement

■ ossification of the fibrosed pannus, further restricting joint movement

■ spread of granulation tissue to tendons

■ weakening and atrophy of muscles possibly due to limited exercise

■ development of *rheumatoid nodules* (subcutaneous collagen nodules) outside the joints, e.g. in pressure areas such as the elbow, over the knuckles and in the lungs, pleura, heart and eyes

■ enlargement of lymph nodes and spleen (lymphadenopathy and splenomegaly).

In the later stages of the disease the inflammation and fever are less marked and movement is limited by deformity of the joint, muscle weakness and pain. The extent of disability varies between slight and severe. Table 17.2 highlights differences between osteoarthritis and rheumatoid arthritis.

425

Table 17.2 Features of the two main types of arthritis

	Osteoarthritis	Rheumatoid arthritis
Type of disease	Degenerative	Inflammatory and autoimmune
Tissue affected	Articular cartilage	Synovial membrane
Age of onset	Late middle age	Any age, mainly 30 to 55 years, occasionally children
Joints affected	Weight bearing, e.g. hip, knee; often only a single joint	Small, e.g. hands, feet; often many joints

Other types of polyarthritis

This group of autoimmune inflammatory arthritic diseases has many characteristics similar to rheumatoid arthritis but the rheumatoid factor is absent. The causes are not known but genetic features may be involved. The joints affected are mainly those of the axial skeleton.

Ankylosing spondylitis. In this the sacroiliac and vertebral joints become progressively ossified.

Psoriatic arthritis. This occurs in a proportion of people who suffer from psoriasis, especially if the nails are involved.

Reiter's syndrome (polyarthritis with urethritis and conjunctivitis). This syndrome, it is believed, may be precipitated by infection with *Chlamydia trachomatis*; the affected joints are usually those of the lower limb.

Rheumatic fever. Polyarthritis is a common presenting feature often involving the wrists, elbows, knees and ankles. Unlike cardiac effects, arthritis usually resolves spontaneously without complications (p. 122).

Infective arthritis

Microbes may be carried in the blood to the joints from foci of infection elsewhere in the body. In most cases of septic arthritis the joint has been damaged by previous injury or arthritic disease. The outcome may be:

- resolution without complications
- suppuration followed by healing with the formation of fibrous tissue that may become ossified
- development of chronic infection, especially in brucellosis, gonorrhoea and tuberculosis.

Traumatic injury to joints

Sprains, strains and dislocations

These damage the soft tissues, tendons and ligaments round the joint without penetrating the joint capsule. In dislocations there may be additional damage to intracapsular structures by stretching, e.g. long head of biceps muscle in the shoulder joint, cruciate ligaments in the knee joint, ligament of head of femur in the hip joint. If repair is incomplete there may be some loss of stability which increases the risk of repeated injury.

Penetrating injuries

These may be caused by a compound fracture of one of the articulating bones, or trauma caused by, e.g., gun shot. Healing may be uneventful or it may be delayed by:

- the presence in the joint of tissue fragments or sequestra (tiny pieces of bone) too large to be removed by phagocytes
- incomplete healing of torn ligaments inside the capsule
- infection that may be blood-borne or enter through broken skin.

When healing is incomplete there is a tendency for irreversible degenerative changes to occur.

Osteoarthritis (osteoarthrosis, OA)

This is a degenerative non-inflammatory disease that results in pain and restricted movement of affected joints. Osteoarthrosis is the more appropriate name but is less commonly used. Articular cartilage gradually becomes thinner because its renewal does not keep pace with its breakdown. Eventually the bony articular surfaces come in contact and the bones begin to degenerate. There is abnormal bone repair and the articular surfaces become misshapen. Chronic inflammation develops with effusion into the joint, possibly due to irritation caused by tissue debris not removed by phagocytes. Sometimes there is abnormal outgrowth of cartilage at the edges of bones which becomes ossified, forming *osteophytes*.

Primary osteoarthritis

This is the more common type and the cause is unknown. Changes may be due to acceleration of the normal ageing process in joints that have had excessive use. It usually develops in late middle age and affects large weight-bearing joints, i.e. the hips, knees and joints of the cervical and lower lumbar spine. In many cases only one joint is involved.

Osteoarthritis of spine
This condition is relatively common in the elderly. Degenerative changes cause narrowing of intervertebral discs and osteophytes may develop round the margins of joints of the vertebral column, commonly in the cervical region (*cervical spondylosis*). They may cause damage to the nervous system, varying from compression of individual spinal nerves to spinal cord injury.

Secondary osteoarthritis

This occurs in joints in which cartilage has already been damaged due to:

- congenital deformity of bones, e.g. in congenital dislocation of the hip
- trauma, e.g. intracapsular fracture of a bone, injury to intracapsular structures
- other conditions, e.g. inflammatory diseases, haemophilia following repeated haemorrhages into the joints, peripheral nerve lesions, gout, acromegaly, diabetic neuropathy.

Gout

This condition is more prevalent in males than females and there is a familial tendency. It is caused by the deposition of sodium urate crystals in joints and tendons that provokes an acute inflammatory response. It occurs in some people whose blood uric acid is abnormally high due to either overproduction or defective excretion by the kidneys. Uric acid is a waste product of the breakdown of nucleic acids, i.e. DNA and RNA, and is produced in excess when there is large-scale cell destruction, e.g. following trauma or treatment with cytotoxic drugs and in anaemia, starvation and malignancy. Defective excretion occurs in renal failure. In many cases only one joint is involved (monoarthritis) and it is typically red, hot and painful. The sites most commonly affected are the metatarsophalangeal joint of the big toe and the ankle, knee, wrist and elbow joints. Episodes of arthritis lasting days or weeks are interspersed with periods of remission. After repeated acute attacks permanent damage may occur with chronic deformity and loss of function of the affected joints. Gout is sometimes complicated by the development of renal calculi.

Connective tissue diseases

This group of disorders has common features. They:

- affect many systems of the body, especially the joints, skin and subcutaneous tissues

- tend to occur in early adult life
- usually affect more females than males
- are chronic conditions
- are autoimmune diseases in which abnormal autoantibodies are formed that attack the individual's tissues.

These disorders include the following.

- *Systemic lupus erythematosus* (SLE) — in this the affected joints are usually the hands, knees and ankles. A characteristic red 'butterfly' rash may occur on the face. Kidney involvement is common and can result in glomerulonephritis that may be complicated by chronic renal failure.
- *Systemic sclerosis* (*scleroderma*) — this is a group of disorders in which there is progressive thickening of connective tissue. There is increased production of collagen that affects many organs. In the skin there is dermal fibrosis and tightness that impairs the functioning of joints, especially of the hands. It also affects the walls of blood vessels, intestinal tract and other organs.
- *Polyarteritis nodosa* (p. 114).
- *Rheumatoid arthritis* (p. 425).
- *Ankylosing spondylitis* (p. 426).
- *Reiter's disease* (p. 426).

Carpal tunnel syndrome

This occurs when the median nerve is compressed in the wrist as it passes through the carpal tunnel (Fig. 17.8). It is a common condition, especially in women, between the ages of 30 and 50 years. There is pain and numbness in the hand and wrist affecting the thumb, index and middle fingers, and half of the ring finger. Many cases are idiopathic or secondary to other conditions, e.g. rheumatoid arthritis, diabetes mellitus, acromegaly and hypothyroidism. Repetitive flexion and extension of the wrist joint also cause the condition, e.g. following prolonged keyboard use.

427

18 The muscular system

The three types of muscle tissue, their features and the nomenclature of skeletal muscles are described on page 40.

This chapter considers the skeletal muscles not involved in the movements of the joints of the limbs:

- muscles of the face and neck
- muscles of the back
- muscles of the abdominal wall
- muscles of the pelvic floor.

Muscles of respiration are described on page 252. The muscles that move the joints are described in Chapter 17.

MUSCLES OF THE FACE AND NECK (Fig. 18.1)

Learning outcomes

After studying this section you should be able to:

- name the main muscles of the face and neck
- outline the functions of the main muscles of the face and neck.

430

Muscles of the face

There are many muscles involved in changing facial expression and with movement of the lower jaw during chewing and speaking. Only the main muscles are described here. Except where indicated the muscles are present in pairs, one on each side.

Occipitofrontalis (unpaired). This consists of a posterior muscular part over the occipital bone (*occipitalis*), an anterior part over the frontal bone (*frontalis*) and an extensive flat tendon or *aponeurosis* that stretches over the dome of the skull and joins the two muscular parts. It raises the eyebrows.

Levator palpebrae superioris. This muscle extends from the posterior part of the orbital cavity to the upper eyelid. It raises the eyelid.

Orbicularis oculi. This muscle surrounds the eye, eyelid and orbital cavity. It closes the eye and when strongly contracted 'screws up' the eyes.

Buccinator. This flat muscle of the cheek draws the cheeks in towards the teeth in chewing and in forcible expulsion of air from the mouth ('the trumpeter's muscle').

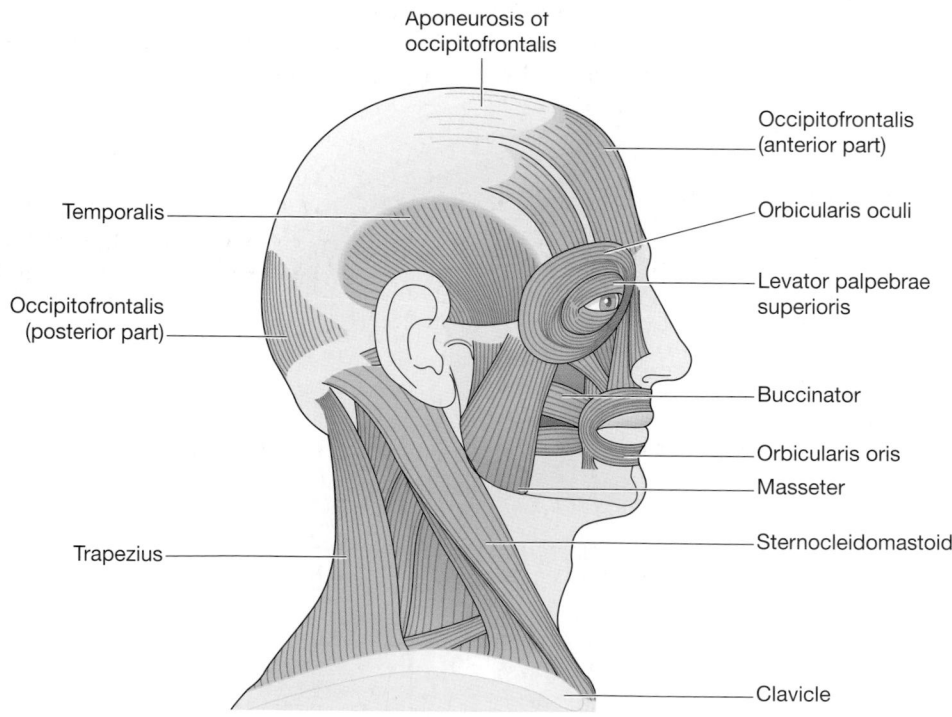

Figure 18.1 The main muscles on the right side of the face, head and neck.

Orbicularis oris (unpaired). This muscle surrounds the mouth and blends with the muscles of the cheeks. It closes the lips and, when strongly contracted, shapes the mouth for whistling.

Masseter. This is a broad muscle, extending from the zygomatic arch to the angle of the jaw. In chewing it draws the mandible up to the maxilla, closing the jaw, and exerts considerable pressure on the food.

Temporalis. This muscle covers the squamous part of the temporal bone. It passes behind the zygomatic arch to be inserted into the coronoid process of the mandible. It closes the mouth and assists with chewing.

Pterygoid. This muscle extends from the sphenoid bone to the mandible. It closes the mouth and pulls the lower jaw forward.

Muscles of the neck

There are many muscles situated in the neck but only the two largest are considered here.

Sternocleidomastoid. This muscle arises from the manubrium of the sternum and the clavicle and extends upwards to the mastoid process of the temporal bone. It assists in turning the head from side to side. When the muscle on one side contracts it draws the head towards the shoulder. When both contract at the same time they flex the cervical vertebrae or draw the sternum and clavicles upwards when the head is maintained in a fixed position, e.g. in forced respiration.

Trapezius. This muscle covers the shoulder and the back of the neck. The upper attachment is to the occipital protuberance, the medial attachment is to the transverse processes of the cervical and thoracic vertebrae and the lateral attachment is to the clavicle and to the spinous and acromion processes of the scapula. It pulls the head backwards, squares the shoulders and controls the movements of the scapula when the shoulder joint is in use.

MUSCLES OF THE BACK (Fig. 18.2)

Learning outcomes

After studying this section you should be able to:

- name the main muscles of the back

- outline the functions of the main muscles of the back.

There are six pairs of large muscles in the back in addition to those that form the posterior abdominal wall. The arrangement of these muscles is the same on each side of the vertebral column. They are:

- trapezius
- teres major   } described in Chapter 17
- psoas
- latissimus dorsi
- quadratus lumborum
- sacrospinalis.

Quadratus lumborum. This muscle originates from the iliac crest then it passes upwards, parallel and close to the vertebral column and it is inserted into the 12th rib (Fig. 18.5). Together the two muscles fix the lower rib during respiration and cause extension of the vertebral column (bending backwards). If one muscle contracts it causes lateral flexion of the lumbar region of the vertebral column.

Sacrospinalis (erector spinae). This is a group of muscles lying between the spinous and transverse processes of the vertebrae (Fig. 18.6). They originate from the sacrum and are finally inserted into the occipital bone. Their contraction causes extension of the vertebral column.

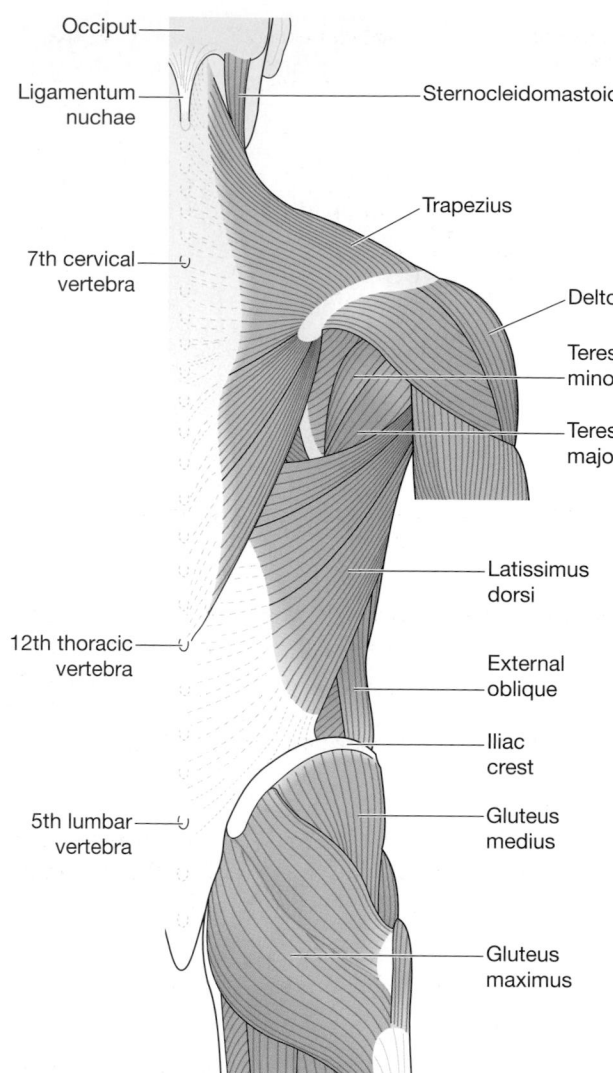

Figure 18.2 The main muscles of the back.

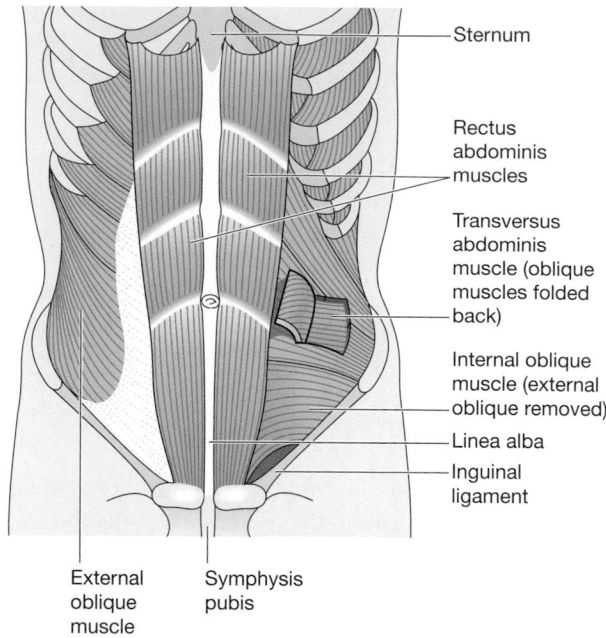

Figure 18.3 The muscles of the anterior abdominal wall.

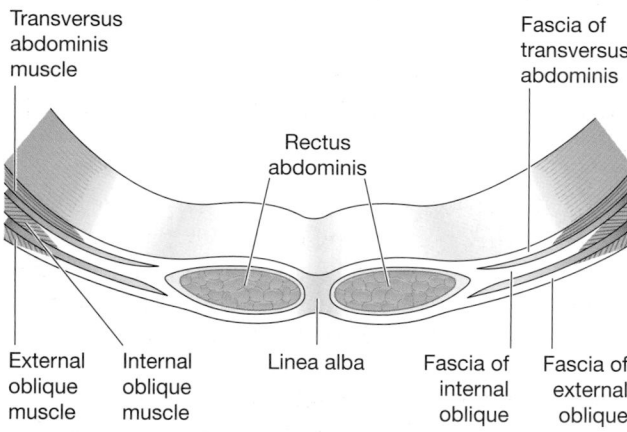

Figure 18.4 Transverse section of the muscles and fasciae of the anterior abdominal wall.

MUSCLES OF THE ABDOMINAL WALL (Figs 18.3, 18.4 and 18.5)

Learning outcomes

After studying this section you should be able to:

- name the main muscles of the abdominal wall

- outline the functions of the main muscles of the abdominal wall.

There are six pairs of muscles that form the abdominal wall. From the surface inwards they are:

- rectus abdominis
- external oblique
- internal oblique
- transversus abdominis
- quadratus lumborum
- psoas—described in Chapter 17.

The anterior abdominal wall is divided longitudinally by a very strong midline tendinous cord, the *linea alba* (meaning 'white cord') which extends from the xiphoid

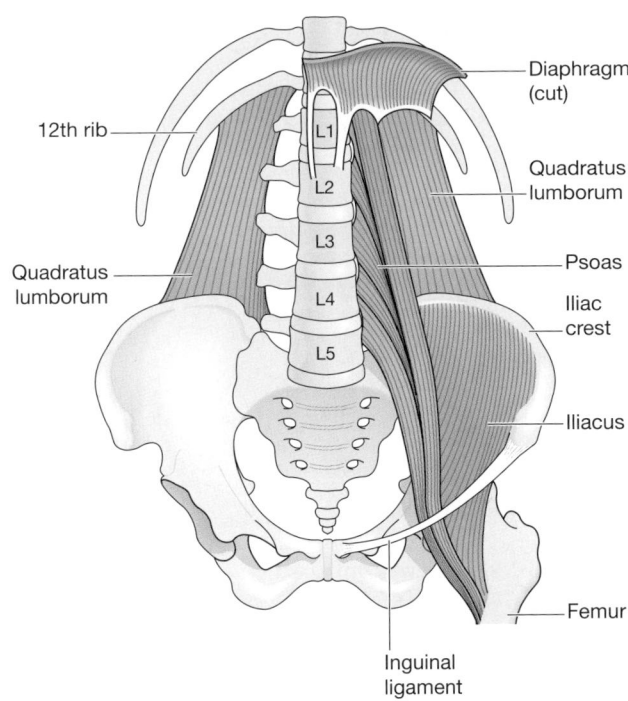

12th rib

Quadratus lumborum

Diaphragm (cut)

Quadratus lumborum

Psoas

Iliac crest

Iliacus

Femur

Inguinal ligament

Figure 18.5 The deep muscles of the posterior abdominal wall.

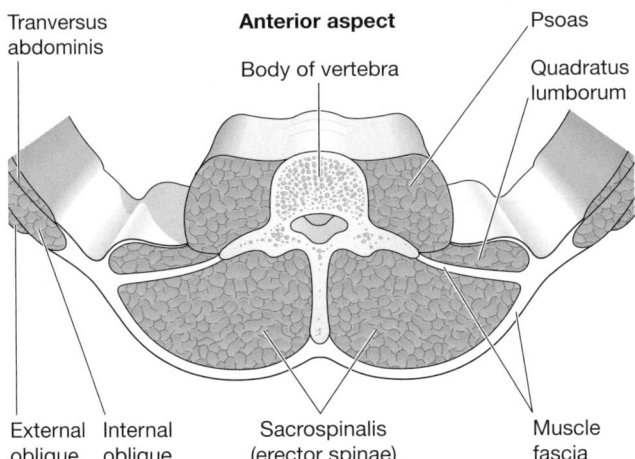

Tranversus abdominis

Anterior aspect

Psoas

Body of vertebra

Quadratus lumborum

External oblique

Internal oblique

Sacrospinalis (erector spinae)

Muscle fascia

Figure 18.6 Transverse section of the posterior abdominal wall: a lumbar vertebra and its associated muscles.

process of the sternum to the symphysis pubis. The structure of the abdominal wall on each side of the linea alba is identical.

Rectus abdominis. This is the most superficial muscle. It is broad and flat, originating from the transverse part of the pubic bone then passing upwards to be inserted into the lower ribs and the xiphoid process of the sternum. Medially the two muscles are attached to the linea alba.

External oblique. This muscle extends from the lower ribs downwards and forward to be inserted into the iliac crest and, by an aponeurosis, to the linea alba.

Internal oblique. This muscle lies deep to the external oblique. Its fibres arise from the iliac crest and by a broad band of fascia from the spinous processes of the lumbar vertebrae. The fibres pass upwards towards the midline to be inserted into the lower ribs and, by an aponeurosis, into the linea alba. The fibres are at right angles to those of the external oblique.

Transversus abdominis. This is the deepest muscle of the abdominal wall. The fibres arise from the iliac crest and the lumbar vertebrae and pass across the abdominal wall to be inserted into the linea alba by an aponeurosis. The fibres are at right angles to those of the rectus abdominis.

Functions

The main function of the four pairs of muscles is to form the strong muscular anterior wall of the abdominal cavity. When the muscles contract together they:

- compress the abdominal organs
- flex the vertebral column in the lumbar region (Fig. 18.6).

Contraction of the muscles on one side only bends the trunk towards that side. Contraction of the oblique muscles on one side rotates the trunk.

Inguinal canal

This canal is 2.5 to 4 cm long and passes obliquely through the abdominal wall. It runs parallel to and immediately in front of the transversalis fascia and part of the inguinal ligament (Fig. 18.5). In the male it contains the *spermatic cord* and in the female, the *round ligament*. It constitutes a weak point in the otherwise strong abdominal wall through which herniation may occur (see p. 330).

433

MUSCLES OF THE PELVIC FLOOR
(Fig. 18.7)

Learning outcomes

After studying this section you should be able to:

- name the main muscles of the pelvic floor
- outline the functions of the main muscles of the pelvic floor.

The pelvic floor is divided into two identical halves that unite along the midline. Each half consists of fascia and muscle. The muscles are:

- levator ani
- coccygeus.

Levator ani. This is a broad flat muscle, forming the anterior part of the pelvic floor. They originate from the inner surface of the true pelvis and unite in the midline. Together they form a sling which supports the pelvic organs.

Coccygeus. This is a triangular sheet of muscle and tendinous fibres situated behind the levator ani. They originate from the medial surface of the ischium and are inserted into the sacrum and coccyx. They complete the formation of the pelvic floor which is perforated in the male by the urethra and anus, and in the female by the urethra, vagina and anus.

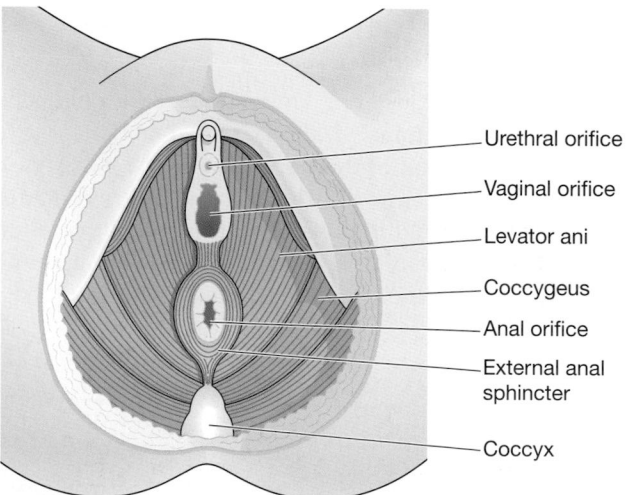

Figure 18.7 The muscles of the female pelvic floor.

- Urethral orifice
- Vaginal orifice
- Levator ani
- Coccygeus
- Anal orifice
- External anal sphincter
- Coccyx

Functions

The pelvic floor supports the organs of the pelvis and maintains continence, i.e. it resists raised intrapelvic pressure during micturition and defaecation.

HEALING OF MUSCLE

Learning outcome

After studying this section you should be able to:

- describe the healing of damaged muscle.

Muscle fibres may be damaged accidentally or be cut during surgery. The extent of the damage determines the mode and effectiveness of healing. In all cases, damaged tissue is removed by phagocytosis and replaced by granulation tissue.

- In *slight injury* the small gap in the muscle fibre is bridged by outgrowths from the surviving ends of the fibre, completely restoring its integrity.
- In *more extensive injury* the muscle fibre outgrowths may not be able to extend far enough into the granulation tissue to restore it completely. When this happens the remaining granulation tissue becomes fibrosed and scar tissue forms. In time this contracts and may restrict joint movement.
- In *very extensive injury* repair is by fibrosis. In *crush syndrome* (p. 436) there may also be serious systemic effects.

REPAIR OF NERVES SUPPLYING MUSCLES

Learning outcome

After studying this section you should be able to:

- describe how the nerve supply to muscles may be restored following injury.

A *motor unit* consists of a lower motor neurone (LMN) and the muscle fibres it supplies. When the nerve supply is cut the muscle cannot contract and gradually atrophies

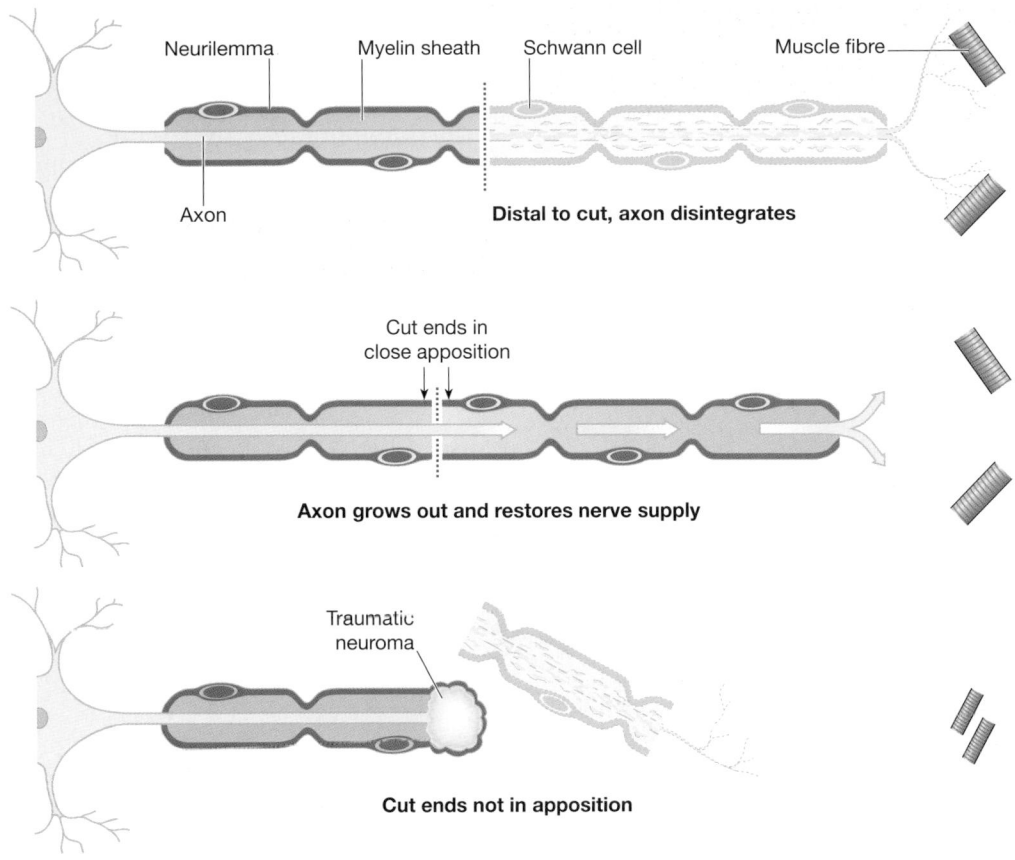

Figure 18.8 Regrowth of a peripheral nerve.

435

but, if the nerve regenerates, muscle fibre function is restored. The axon of the LMN in a peripheral nerve divides into numerous terminal branches, each of which supplies a muscle fibre. In a bundle of muscle fibres the nerve supply is derived from several LMNs (see Fig. 7.10, p. 147). Nerve supply to muscle fibres may be restored by:

- regeneration of the nerve if cut near the parent cell and if the cut ends are in close apposition (Fig. 18.8)
- the outgrowth of new terminal nerve fibres from the other axons supplying adjacent muscle fibres in the same bundle (Fig. 18.9).

When the neurilemma is out of position or destroyed a traumatic neuroma develops in which there is sprouting of axons and Schwann cells.

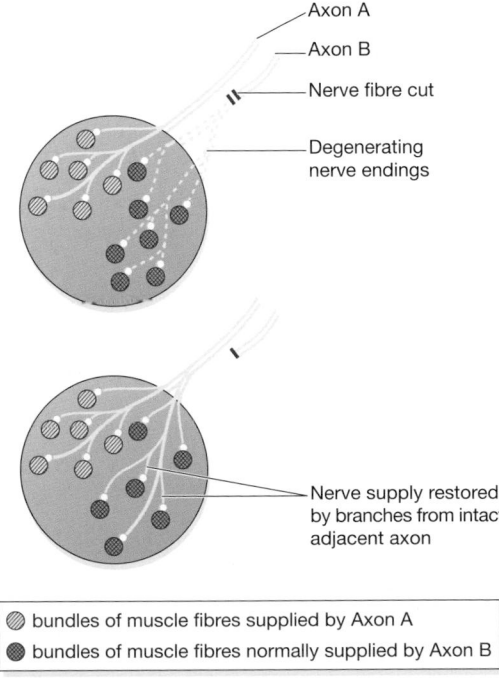

Figure 18.9 Restoration of nerve supply to muscle.

DISEASES OF MUSCLES

Learning outcomes

After studying this section you should be able to:

- list the causes of the diseases in this section
- compare and contrast the characteristics of different types of muscular dystrophy
- describe the effects of crush syndrome.

Myasthenia gravis

See page 385.

Myopathies

Muscular dystrophies

In this group of inherited diseases there is progressive degeneration of groups of muscles. The main differences in the types are:

- age of onset
- rate of progression
- groups of muscles involved.

Duchenne muscular dystrophy

Inheritance of this condition is sex linked, the affected gene being carried on the long X chromosome of female carriers. Their children may be affected by the condition if they are males (50% chance), or be carriers if they are females (50% chance) (see Fig. 4.12, p. 76).

The muscle abnormality is present before birth but may not be evident until the child is about 5 years of age. Wasting and weakness begin in muscles of the lower limbs then spread to the upper limbs, progressing rapidly without remission. Death usually occurs in adolescence, often from respiratory failure, cardiac arrhythmias or cardiomyopathy.

Facioscapulohumeral dystrophy

This disease affects both sexes. It usually begins in adolescence and the younger the age of onset the more rapidly it progresses. Muscles of the face and shoulders are affected first. This is a chronic condition that usually progresses slowly and may not cause complete disability. Life expectancy is normal.

Myotonic dystrophy

This disease usually begins in adult life and affects both sexes. Muscles contract and relax slowly, often seen as difficulty in releasing an object held in the hand. Muscles of the tongue and the face are first affected then muscles of the limbs. Systemic conditions associated with myotonic dystrophy include:

- cataracts
- atrophy of the gonads
- cardiomyopathy
- glucose intolerance.

The disease progresses without remission and with increasing disability. Death usually occurs in middle age from respiratory or cardiac failure.

Crush syndrome

Sustained pressure, on the trunk or a limb, causes ischaemia resulting in massive muscle necrosis. When pressure is relieved and the circulation is restored, myoglobin and other necrotic products are released from damaged muscle and enter the blood. This material is highly toxic to the kidneys and acute renal failure may develop. A common complication of this type of injury is infection, especially by anaerobic microbes, e.g. *Clostridium perfringens (Cl. welchii)* and other clostridia causing *gas gangrene*.

Healing of such extensive injury is by fibrosis.

19 The reproductive systems

The ability to reproduce is one of the properties which distinguishes living from non-living matter. The more primitive the animal, the simpler the process of reproduction. In human beings the process is one of sexual reproduction in which the male and female organs differ anatomically and physiologically.

Both males and females produce specialised reproductive germ cells, called *gametes*. The male gametes are called *spermatozoa* and the female gametes are called *ova*. They contain the genetic material, or *genes*, on *chromosomes*, which pass inherited characteristics on to the next generation. In other body cells there are 46 chromosomes arranged in 23 pairs but in the gametes there are only 23, one from each pair. Gametes are formed by *meiosis* (p. 33). When the ovum is fertilised by a spermatozoon the resultant *zygote* contains 23 *pairs* of chromosomes, one of each pair obtained from the father and one from the mother.

The zygote embeds itself in the wall of the uterus where it grows and develops during the 40-week *gestation period* before birth.

The functions of the female reproductive system are:

- formation of female gametes, ova
- reception of male gametes, spermatozoa
- provision of suitable environments for fertilisation of the ovum by spermatozoa and development of the resultant fetus
- parturition (childbirth)
- lactation, the production of breast milk, which provides complete nourishment for the baby in its early life.

The functions of the male reproductive system are:

- production of male gametes, spermatozoa
- transmission of spermatozoa to the female.

FEMALE REPRODUCTIVE SYSTEM

Learning outcomes

After studying this section, you should be able to:

- describe the main structures comprising the external genitalia
- explain the structure and function of the vagina
- describe the location, structure and function of the uterus and the uterine tubes
- discuss the process of ovulation and the hormones that control it
- outline the changes that occur in the female at puberty, including the physiology of menstruation
- describe the structure and function of the female breast.

The female reproductive organs, or genitalia, are divided into external and internal organs (Fig. 19.1).

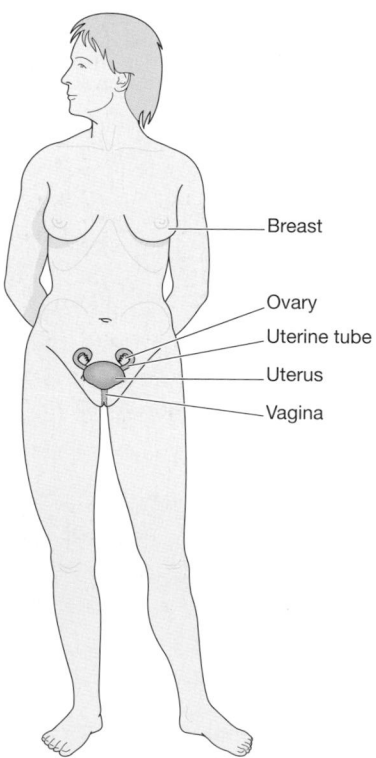

Breast

Ovary

Uterine tube

Uterus

Vagina

Figure 19.1 The female reproductive organs. Faint lines indicate the positions of the lower ribs and the pelvis.

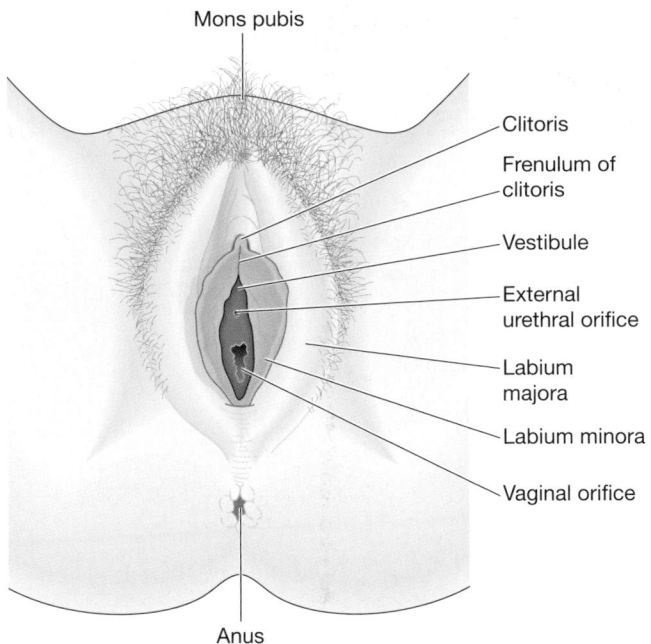

Labels: Mons pubis, Clitoris, Frenulum of clitoris, Vestibule, External urethral orifice, Labium majora, Labium minora, Vaginal orifice, Anus

Figure 19.2 The external genitalia of the female.

External genitalia (vulva)

The external genitalia (Fig. 19.2) are known collectively as the vulva, and consist of the labia majora and labia minora, the clitoris, the vaginal orifice, the vestibule, the hymen and the vestibular glands (Bartholin's glands).

Labia majora

These are the two large folds which form the boundary of the vulva. They are composed of skin, fibrous tissue and fat and contain large numbers of sebaceous glands. Anteriorly the folds join in front of the symphysis pubis, and posteriorly they merge with the skin of the perineum. At puberty hair grows on the mons pubis and on the lateral surfaces of the labia majora.

Labia minora

These are two smaller folds of skin between the labia majora, containing numerous sebaceous glands.

The cleft between the labia minora is the *vestibule*. The vagina, urethra and ducts of the greater vestibular glands open into the vestibule.

Clitoris

The clitoris corresponds to the penis in the male and contains sensory nerve endings and erectile tissue but it has no reproductive significance.

Hymen

The hymen is a thin layer of mucous membrane which partially occludes the opening of the vagina. It is normally incomplete to allow for passage of menstrual flow.

Vestibular glands

The vestibular glands (Bartholin's glands) are situated one on each side near the vaginal opening. They are about the size of a small pea and have ducts, opening into the vestibule immediately lateral to the attachment of the hymen. They secrete mucus that keeps the vulva moist.

Blood supply, lymph drainage and nerve supply

The arterial supply. This is by branches from the *internal pudendal arteries* that branch from the internal iliac arteries and by *external pudendal arteries* that branch from the femoral arteries.

The venous drainage. This forms a large plexus which eventually drains into the internal iliac veins.

Lymph drainage. This is through the superficial inguinal nodes.

Nerve supply. This is by branches from pudendal nerves.

Perineum

The perineum is the area extending from the base of the labia minora to the anal canal. It is roughly triangular and consists of connective tissue, muscle and fat. It gives attachment to the muscles of the pelvic floor (p. 434).

Internal genitalia

The internal organs of the female reproductive system (Figs 19.3 and 19.4) lie in the pelvic cavity and consist of the vagina, uterus, two uterine tubes and two ovaries.

Vagina

The vagina is a fibromuscular tube lined with stratified squamous epithelium, connecting the external and internal organs of reproduction. It runs obliquely upwards and backwards at an angle of about 45° between the bladder in front and rectum and anus behind. In the adult the anterior wall is about 7.5 cm (3 inches) long and the posterior wall about 9 cm long. The difference is due to the angle of insertion of the cervix through the anterior wall.

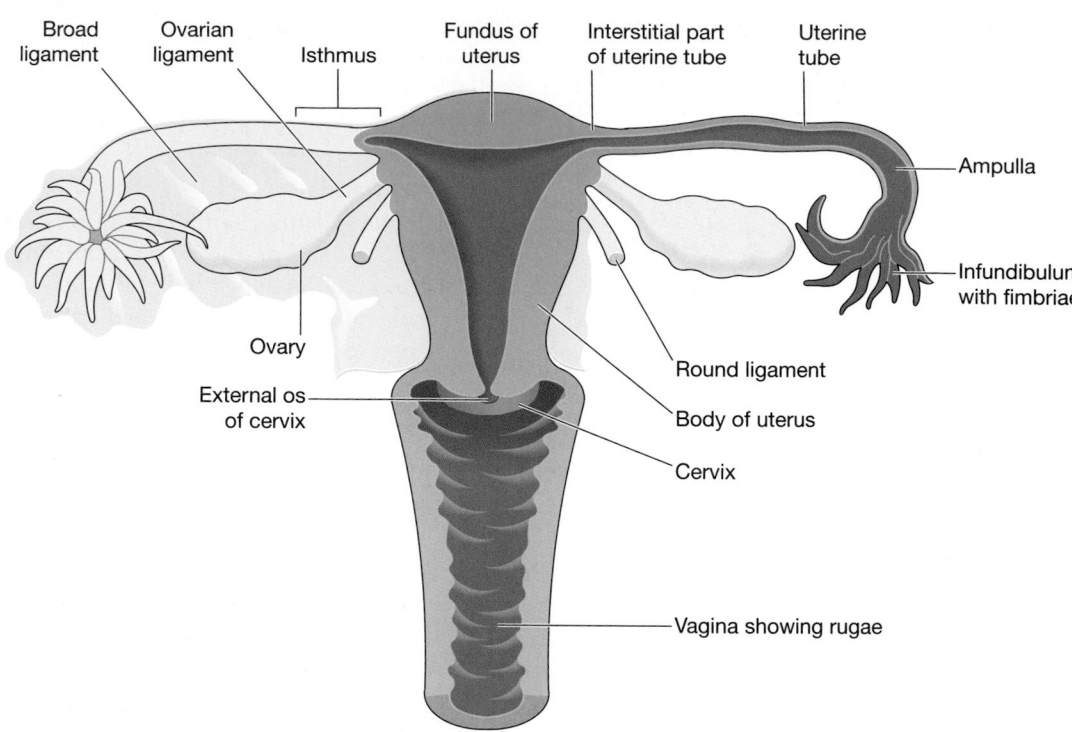

Figure 19.3 The female reproductive organs in the pelvis.

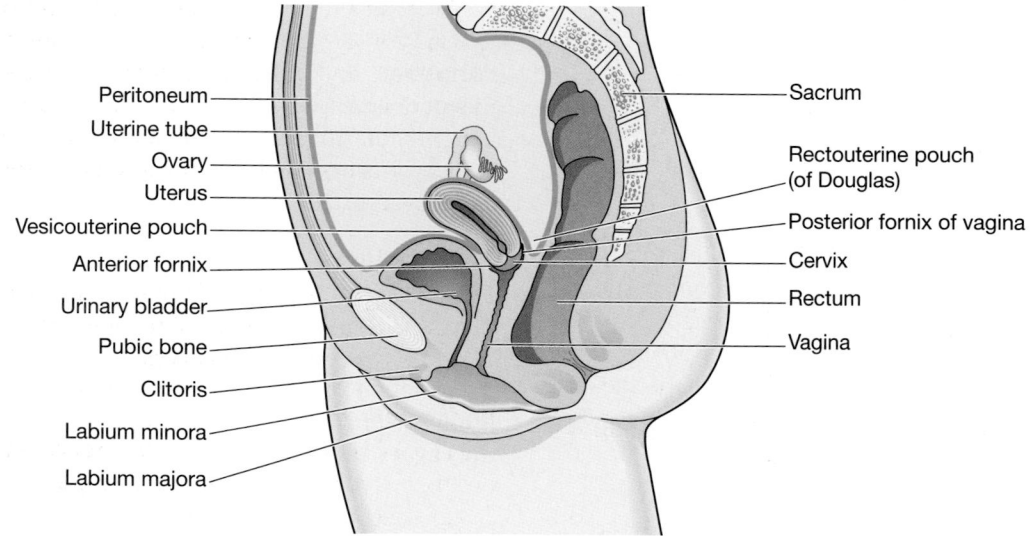

Figure 19.4 Lateral view of the female reproductive organs in the pelvis and their associated structures.

Structure of the vagina

The vagina has three layers: an outer covering of areolar tissue, a middle layer of smooth muscle and an inner lining of stratified squamous epithelium that forms ridges or *rugae*. It has no secretory glands but the surface is kept moist by cervical secretions. Between puberty and the menopause, *Lactobacillus acidophilus* bacteria are normally present, which secrete *lactic acid*, maintaining the pH between 4.9 and 3.5. The acidity inhibits the growth of most other microbes that may enter the vagina from the perineum.

Blood supply, lymph drainage and nerve supply

Arterial supply. An arterial plexus is formed round the vagina, derived from the uterine and vaginal arteries which are branches of the internal iliac arteries.

Venous drainage. A venous plexus, situated in the muscular wall, drains into the internal iliac veins.

Lymph drainage. This is through the deep and superficial iliac glands.

Nerve supply. This consists of parasympathetic fibres from the sacral outflow, sympathetic fibres from the lumbar outflow and somatic sensory fibres from the pudendal nerves.

Functions of the vagina

The vagina acts as the receptacle for the penis during coitus, and provides an elastic passageway through which the baby passes during childbirth.

Uterus

The uterus is a hollow muscular pear-shaped organ, flattened anteroposteriorly. It lies in the pelvic cavity between the urinary bladder and the rectum (Fig. 19.4).

In most women, it leans forward (*anteversion*), and is bent forward (*anteflexion*) almost at right angles to the vagina, so that its anterior wall rests partly against the bladder below, and forming the vesicouterine pouch between the two organs.

When the body is in the upright position the uterus lies in an almost horizontal position. It is about 7.5 cm long, 5 cm wide and its walls are about 2.5 cm thick. It weighs from 30 to 40 grams. The parts of the uterus are the fundus, body and cervix (Fig. 19.3).

The fundus. This is the dome-shaped part of the uterus above the openings of the uterine tubes.

The body. This is the main part. It is narrowest inferiorly at the *internal os* where it is continuous with the cervix.

The cervix ('neck' of the uterus). This protrudes through the anterior wall of the vagina, opening into it at the *external os.*

Structure of the uterus

The walls of the uterus are composed of three layers of tissue: perimetrium, myometrium and endometrium (Fig. 19.5).

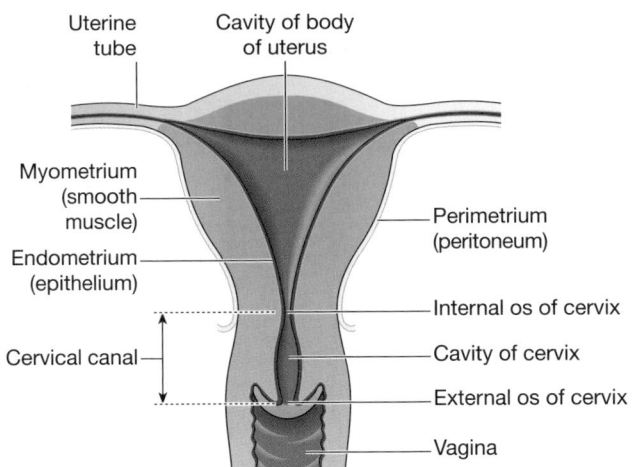

Figure 19.5 A section of the uterus.

Perimetrium
This is peritoneum, which is distributed differently on the various surfaces of the uterus (Fig. 19.4).

Anteriorly it extends over the fundus and the body where it is folded on to the upper surface of the urinary bladder. This fold of peritoneum forms the *vesicouterine pouch.*

Posteriorly the peritoneum extends over the fundus, the body and the cervix, then it continues on to the rectum to form the *rectouterine pouch* (of Douglas).

Laterally only the fundus is covered because the peritoneum forms a double fold with the uterine tubes in the upper free border. This double fold is the *broad ligament* which, at its lateral ends, attaches the uterus to the sides of the pelvis.

Myometrium
This is the thickest layer of tissue in the uterine wall. It is a mass of smooth muscle fibres interlaced with areolar tissue, blood vessels and nerves.

Endometrium
This consists of columnar epithelium containing a large number of mucus-secreting tubular glands. It is divided functionally into two layers.

- The functional layer is the upper layer and it thickens and becomes rich in blood vessels in the first half of the menstrual cycle. If the ovum is not fertilised and does not implant, this layer is shed during menstruation.
- The basal layer lies next to the myometrium, and is not lost during menstruation. It is the layer from which the fresh functional layer is regenerated during each cycle.

The upper two-thirds of the cervical canal is lined with this mucous membrane.

441

Further towards the vagina, however, the mucosa changes, becoming stratified squamous epithelium, which is continuous with the lining of the vagina itself.

Blood supply, lymph drainage and nerve supply

The arterial supply. This is by the *uterine arteries* which are branches of the internal iliac arteries. They pass up the lateral aspects of the uterus between the two layers of the broad ligaments. They supply the uterus and uterine tubes and join with the ovarian arteries to supply the ovaries. Branches pass downwards to anastomose with the vaginal arteries to supply the vagina.

Venous drainage. The veins follow the same route as the arteries and eventually drain into the internal iliac veins.

Lymph drainage. There are deep and superficial lymph vessels which drain lymph from the uterus and the uterine tubes to the aortic lymph nodes and groups of nodes associated with the iliac blood vessels.

Nerve supply. The nerves supplying the uterus and the uterine tubes consist of parasympathetic fibres from the sacral outflow and sympathetic fibres from the lumbar outflow.

Supports of the uterus

The uterus is supported in the pelvic cavity by surrounding organs, muscles of the pelvic floor and ligaments that suspend it from the walls of the pelvis.

Supporting structures (Fig. 19.6)

The broad ligaments. These are formed by a double fold of peritoneum, one on each side of the uterus. They hang down from the uterine tubes as though draped over them and at their lateral ends they are attached to the sides of the pelvis. The uterine tubes are enclosed in the upper free border and near the lateral ends they penetrate the posterior wall of the broad ligament and open into the peritoneal cavity. The ovaries are attached to the posterior wall, one on each side. Blood and lymph vessels and nerves pass to the uterus and uterine tubes between the layers of the broad ligaments.

The round ligaments. These are bands of fibrous tissue between the two layers of broad ligament, one on each side of the uterus. They pass to the sides of the pelvis then through the *inguinal canal* to end by fusing with the labia majora.

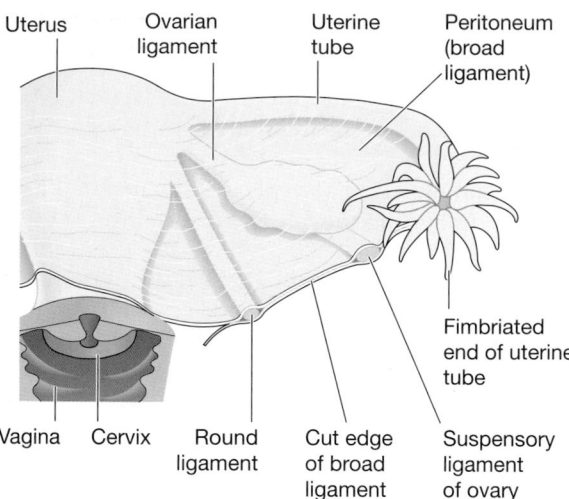

Figure 19.6 The main ligaments supporting the uterus. Only one side is shown.

The uterosacral ligaments. These originate from the posterior walls of the cervix and vagina and extend backwards, one on each side of the rectum, to the sacrum.

The transverse cervical ligaments (cardinal ligaments). These extend one from each side of the cervix and vagina to the side walls of the pelvis.

The pubocervical fascia. This extends forward from the transverse cervical ligaments on each side of the bladder and is attached to the posterior surface of the pubic bones.

Functions of the uterus

After puberty, the endometrium of the uterus goes through a regular monthly cycle of changes, the menstrual cycle, which is under the control of hypothalamic and anterior pituitary hormones (Ch. 9). The purpose of the cycle is to prepare the uterus to receive, nourish and protect a fertilised ovum. The cycle is usually regular, lasting between 26 and 30 days. If the ovum is not fertilised a new cycle begins with a short period of bleeding (menstruation).

If the ovum is fertilised the zygote embeds itself in the uterine wall. The uterine muscle grows to accommodate the developing baby, which is called an *embryo* during its first 8 weeks, and a *fetus* for the remainder of the pregnancy. Uterine secretions nourish the ovum before it implants in the endometrium, and after implantation the rapidly expanding ball of cells is nourished by the endometrial cells themselves. This is sufficient for only the first few weeks and the *placenta* is the organ that takes over thereafter. The placenta, which is attached to the fetus by the umbilical cord, is firmly attached to the wall of the uterus, and provides the means by which the growing baby receives oxygen and nutrients, and gets rid of its wastes. During pregnancy, which normally lasts about 40 weeks, the muscular walls of the uterus are prevented from contracting and expelling the baby early by high levels of the hormone progesterone secreted by the placenta. At the end of pregnancy (at term) the hormone oestrogen, which increases uterine contractility, becomes the predominant sex hormone in the blood. Additionally, oxytocin is released from the posterior pituitary, and also stimulates the uterine muscle. Control of oxytocin release is by positive feedback (see also Fig. 9.5, p. 219). During labour, the uterus forcefully expels the baby by means of powerful rhythmical contractions.

Uterine tubes (Fallopian tubes)

The uterine tubes (Fig. 19.3) are about 10 cm long and extend from the sides of the uterus between the body and the fundus. They lie in the upper free border of the broad ligament and their trumpet-shaped lateral ends penetrate the posterior wall, opening into the peritoneal cavity close to the ovaries. The end of each tube has fingerlike projections called *fimbriae*. The longest of these is the *ovarian fimbria* which is in close association with the ovary.

Structure of the uterine tubes

The uterine tubes have an outer covering of peritoneum (broad ligament), a middle layer of smooth muscle and are lined with ciliated epithelium.

Blood supply, lymph drainage and nerve supply
These are the same as for the uterus.

Function of the uterine tubes

The uterine tubes convey the ovum from the ovary to the uterus by peristalsis and ciliary movement. The mucus secreted by the lining membrane provides ideal conditions for movement of ova and spermatozoa. Fertilisation of the ovum usually takes place in the uterine tube, and the zygote is propelled into the uterus for implantation.

Ovaries

The ovaries (Fig. 19.4) are the female gonads, or glands, and they lie in a shallow fossa on the lateral walls of the pelvis. They are 2.5 to 3.5 cm long, 2 cm wide and 1 cm thick. Each is attached to the upper part of the uterus by the *ovarian ligament* and to the back of the broad ligament by a broad band of tissue, the *mesovarium*. Blood vessels and nerves pass to the ovary through the mesovarium (Fig. 19.7).

443

Figure 19.7 A section of an ovary showing the stages of development of one ovarian follicle.

Structure of the ovaries

The ovaries have two layers of tissue.

The medulla. This lies in the centre and consists of fibrous tissue, blood vessels and nerves.

The cortex. This surrounds the medulla. It has a framework of connective tissue, or *stroma*, covered by *germinal epithelium*. It contains *ovarian follicles* in various stages of maturity, each of which contains an ovum. Before puberty the ovaries are inactive but the stroma already contains immature (primordial) follicles, which the female has from birth. During the childbearing years, about every 28 days, one ovarian follicle (Graafian follicle) matures, ruptures and releases its ovum into the peritoneal cavity. This is called *ovulation* and it occurs during most menstrual cycles (Fig. 19.7).

Blood supply, lymph drainage and nerve supply

Arterial supply. This is by the *ovarian arteries*, which branch from the abdominal aorta just below the renal arteries.

Venous drainage. This is into a plexus of veins behind the uterus from which the ovarian veins arise. The right ovarian vein opens into the inferior vena cava and the left into the left renal vein.

Lymph drainage. This is to the lateral aortic and pre-aortic lymph nodes. The lymph vessels follow the same route as the arteries.

Nerve supply. The ovaries are supplied by parasympathetic nerves from the sacral outflow and sympathetic nerves from the lumbar outflow. Their precise functions are not yet fully understood.

Functions of the ovaries

Maturation of the follicle is stimulated by follicle stimulating hormone (FSH) from the anterior pituitary, and oestrogen secreted by the follicle lining cells. Ovulation is triggered by a surge of luteinising hormone (LH) from the anterior pituitary, which occurs a few hours before ovulation. After ovulation, the follicle lining cells develop into the *corpus luteum* (yellow body), under the influence of LH from the anterior pituitary. The corpus luteum produces the hormone progesterone and some oestrogen. If the ovum is fertilised it embeds itself in the wall of the uterus where it grows and develops and produces the hormone *human chorionic gonadotrophin* (hCG),

which stimulates the corpus luteum to continue secreting progesterone and oestrogen for the first 3 months of the pregnancy (Figs 19.8 and 19.9), after which time this function is continued by the placenta. If the ovum is not fertilised the corpus luteum degenerates and a new cycle begins with menstruation. At the site of the degenerate corpus luteum an inactive mass of fibrous tissue forms, called the *corpus albicans*. Sometimes more than one follicle matures at a time, releasing two or more ova in the same cycle. When this happens and the ova are fertilised the result is a multiple pregnancy.

Puberty in the female

Puberty is the age at which the internal reproductive organs reach maturity. This is called the *menarche*, and marks the beginning of the childbearing period. The ovaries are stimulated by the gonadotrophins from the anterior pituitary, follicle stimulating hormone and luteinising hormone.

The age of puberty varies between 10 and 14 years and a number of physical and psychological changes take place at this time:

- the uterus, the uterine tubes and the ovaries reach maturity
- the menstrual cycle and ovulation begin (menarche)
- the breasts develop and enlarge
- pubic and axillary hair begins to grow

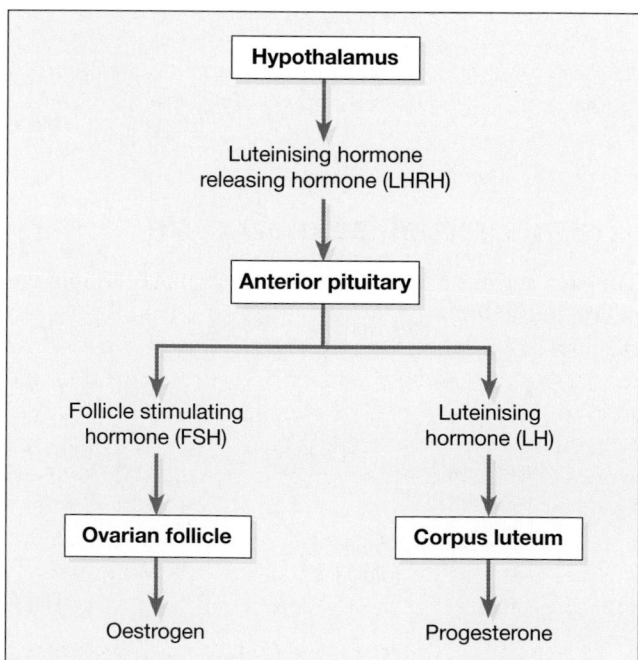

Figure 19.8 Female reproductive hormones and target tissues.

444

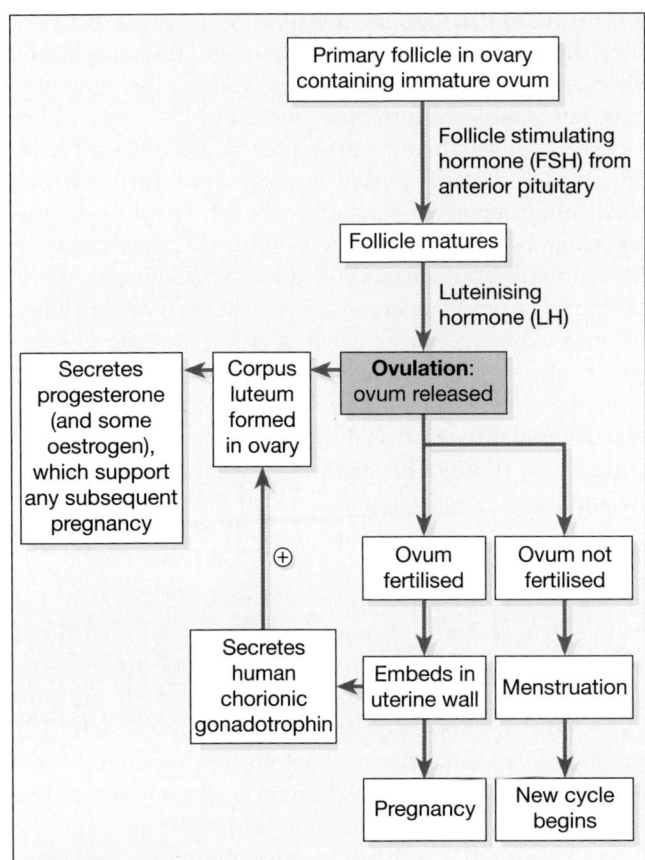

Figure 19.9 Summary of the stages of development of the ovum and the associated hormones.

- there is an increase in the rate of growth in height and widening of the pelvis
- there is an increase in the amount of fat deposited in the subcutaneous tissue, especially at the hips and breasts.

The menstrual (sexual) cycle

This is a series of events, occurring regularly in females every 26 to 30 days throughout the childbearing period of about 36 years (Fig. 19.10). The cycle consists of a series of changes that take place concurrently in the ovaries and uterine walls, stimulated by changes in the blood concentrations of hormones (Fig. 19.10B and D). Hormones secreted in the cycle are regulated by negative feedback mechanisms.

The hypothalamus secretes luteinising hormone releasing hormone (LHRH) which stimulates the anterior pituitary to secrete (see Table 9.1, p. 216):

- follicle stimulating hormone (FSH), which promotes the maturation of ovarian follicles and the secretion of oestrogen, leading to ovulation

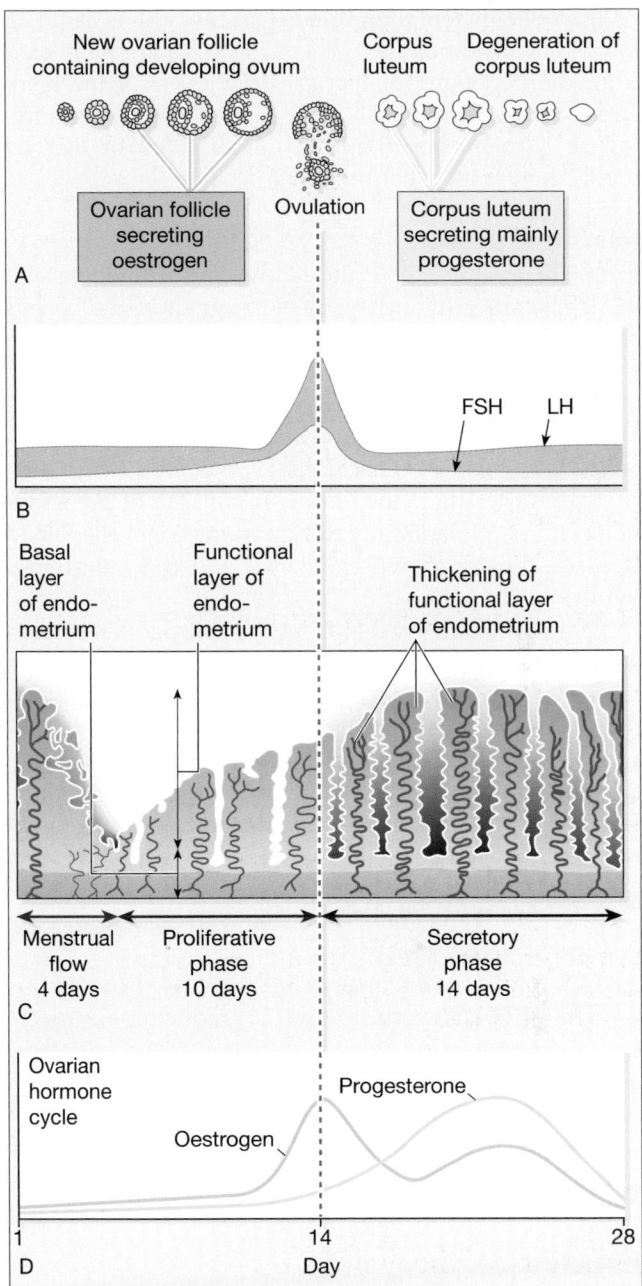

Figure 19.10 Summary of one female menstrual cycle: A. Ovarian cycle; maturation of follicle and development of corpus luteum. B. Anterior pituitary cycle; LH and FSH levels. C. Uterine cycle; menstrual, proliferative and secretory phases. D. Ovarian hormone cycle; oestrogen and progesterone levels.

- luteinising hormone (LH), which triggers ovulation, stimulates the development of the corpus luteum and the secretion of progesterone.

The hypothalamus responds to changes in the blood levels of oestrogen and progesterone. It is switched off by high levels and stimulated when they are low.

445

The average length of the menstrual cycle is about 28 days. By convention the days of the cycle are numbered from the beginning of the *menstrual phase* of the menstrual cycle which usually lasts about 4 days. This is followed by the *proliferative phase* (about 10 days), then by the *secretory phase* (about 14 days).

Menstrual phase

When the ovum is not fertilised, the corpus luteum starts to degenerate. (In the event of pregnancy, the corpus luteum is supported by human chorionic gonadotrophin (hCG) secreted by the developing embryo.) Progesterone and oestrogen levels therefore fall, and the functional layer of the endometrium, which is dependent on high levels of these ovarian hormones, is shed in menstruation (Fig. 19.10C). The menstrual flow consists of the secretions from endometrial glands, endometrial cells, blood from the broken down capillaries and the unfertilised ovum.

High circulating levels of ovarian progesterone and oestrogen inhibit the anterior pituitary, blocking the release of FSH and LH, and should pregnancy occur then rising oestrogen and progesterone levels therefore prevent the maturation and release of another ovum. After degeneration of the corpus luteum, however, falling levels of oestrogen and progesterone lead to resumed anterior pituitary activity, rising FSH levels and the initiation of the next cycle.

Proliferative phase

At this stage an ovarian follicle, stimulated by FSH, is growing towards maturity and is producing oestrogen. Oestrogen stimulates the proliferation of the functional layer of the endometrium in preparation for the reception of a fertilised ovum. The endometrium becomes thicker by rapid cell multiplication accompanied by an increase in the numbers of mucus-secreting glands and blood capillaries. This phase ends when ovulation occurs and oestrogen production declines.

Secretory phase

Immediately after ovulation, the lining cells of the ovarian follicle are stimulated by LH to develop the corpus luteum, which produces progesterone and some oestrogen. Under the influence of progesterone the endometrium becomes oedematous and the secretory glands produce increased amounts of watery mucus. This is believed to assist the passage of the spermatozoa through the uterus to the uterine tubes where the ovum is usually fertilised. There is a similar increase in the secretion of watery mucus by the glands of the uterine tubes and by cervical glands which lubricate the vagina.

The ovum may survive in a fertilisable form for a very short time after ovulation, probably as little as 8 hours. The spermatozoa, deposited in the vagina during coitus, may be capable of fertilising the ovum for only about 24 hours although they may survive for several days. This means that the period in each cycle during which fertilisation can occur is relatively short. The time of ovulation can be determined by observing certain changes in the woman's body around this period. Changes in cervical mucus, from thick and dry in consistency to thin, elastic and watery, are detected and, in addition, body temperature rises by a small but measurable amount immediately following ovulation. Some women experience some degree of abdominal discomfort in the middle of the cycle, thought to correspond to rupture of the follicle and release of its contents into the abdominal cavity.

If the ovum is not fertilised menstruation occurs and a new cycle begins.

If the ovum is fertilised there is no breakdown of the endometrium and no menstrual flow. The fertilised ovum (zygote) travels through the uterine tube to the uterus where it becomes embedded in the wall and produces human chorionic gonadotrophin (hCG), which is similar to anterior pituitary luteinising hormone. This hormone keeps the corpus luteum intact, enabling it to continue secreting progesterone and oestrogen for the first 3 to 4 months of the pregnancy, inhibiting the maturation of further ovarian follicles (Fig. 19.9). During that time the placenta develops and produces oestrogen, progesterone and gonadotrophins.

Menopause (climacteric)

The menopause usually occurs between the ages of 45 and 55 years, marking the end of the childbearing period. It may occur suddenly or over a period of years, sometimes as long as 10 years, and is caused by changes in sex hormone levels. The ovaries gradually become less responsive to FSH and LH, and ovulation and the menstrual cycle become irregular, eventually ceasing. Several other phenomena may occur at the same time including:

- short-term unpredictable vasodilatation with flushing, sweating and palpitations, causing discomfort and disturbance of the normal sleep pattern
- shrinkage of the breasts
- axillary and pubic hair become sparse
- atrophy of the sex organs
- episodes of uncharacteristic behaviour sometimes occur, e.g. irritability, mood changes
- gradual thinning of the skin

- loss of bone mass that predisposes to osteoporosis (p. 409)
- slow increase in blood cholesterol levels that predisposes postmenopausal women to cardiovascular disorders.

Similar changes occur after bilateral irradiation or surgical removal of the ovaries.

Breasts or mammary glands

The breasts or mammary glands are accessory glands of the female reproductive system. They exist also in the male but in only a rudimentary form.

In the female the breasts are small and immature until puberty. Thereafter they grow and develop to their mature size under the influence of oestrogen and progesterone. During pregnancy these hormones stimulate further growth. After the baby is born the hormone *prolactin* from the anterior pituitary stimulates the production of milk, and *oxytocin* from the posterior pituitary stimulates the release of milk in response to the stimulation of the nipple by the sucking baby, by a positive feedback mechanism.

Structure of the breast

The mammary glands (Fig. 19.11) consist of glandular tissue, fibrous tissue and fatty tissue.

Each breast consists of about 20 lobes of glandular tissue, each lobe being made up of a number of lobules that radiate around the nipple. The lobules consist of a cluster of alveoli which open into small ducts and these unite to form large excretory ducts, called *lactiferous ducts*. The lactiferous ducts converge towards the centre of the breast where they form dilatations or reservoirs for milk. Leading from each dilatation, or *lactiferous sinus*, is a narrow duct which opens on to the surface at the nipple. Fibrous tissue supports the glandular tissue and ducts, and fat covers the surface of the gland and is found between the lobes.

The nipple. This is a small conical eminence at the centre of the breast surrounded by a pigmented area, the *areola*. On the surface of the areola are numerous sebaceous glands (Montgomery's tubercles) which lubricate the nipple during lactation.

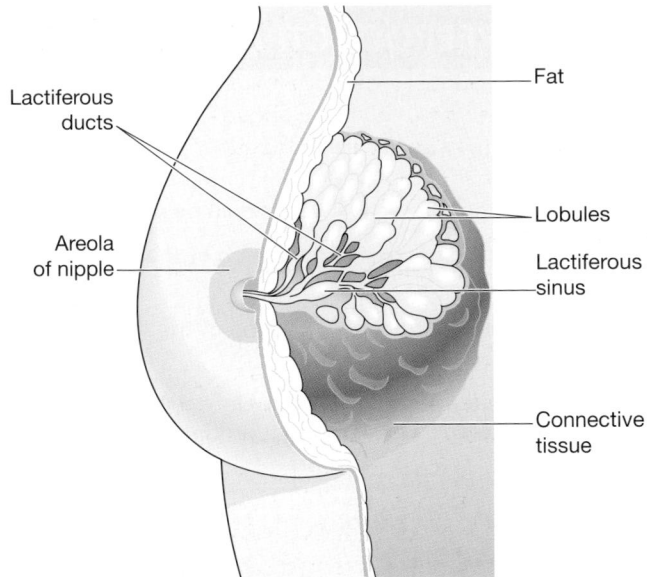

Figure 19.11 Structure of the breast.

Blood supply, lymph drainage and nerve supply

Arterial blood supply. The breasts are supplied with blood from the thoracic branches of the axillary arteries and from the internal mammary and intercostal arteries.

Venous drainage. This describes an anastomotic circle round the base of the nipple from which branches carry the venous blood to the circumference and end in the axillary and mammary veins.

Lymph drainage (see Fig. 6.1, p. 130). This is mainly into the axillary lymph vessels and nodes. Lymph may drain through the internal mammary nodes if the superficial route is obstructed.

Nerve supply. The breasts are supplied by branches from the 4th, 5th and 6th thoracic nerves which contain sympathetic fibres. There are numerous somatic *sensory nerve endings* in the breast especially around the nipple. When these *touch receptors* are stimulated by sucking, impulses pass to the hypothalamus and the flow of the hormone oxytocin is increased, promoting the release of milk.

Function of the breast

The mammary glands are only active during late pregnancy and after the birth of a baby when they produce milk (lactation). Lactation is stimulated by the hormone prolactin (p. 217).

447

MALE REPRODUCTIVE SYSTEM

Learning outcomes

After studying this section, you should be able to:

- describe the structure and function of the testes in the scrotum

- outline the structure and function of the spermatic cords

- describe the secretions that pass into the spermatic fluid, including the glands that produce them

- explain the process of ejaculation

- list the main changes occurring at puberty in the male.

The male reproductive system consists of the following organs (Fig. 19.12):

- 2 testes ⎫
- 2 epididymides ⎬ in the scrotum
- 2 deferent ducts (vas deferens)
- 2 spermatic cords
- 2 seminal vesicles
- 2 ejaculatory ducts
- 1 prostate gland
- 1 penis.

Scrotum

The scrotum is a pouch of deeply pigmented skin, fibrous and connective tissue and smooth muscle. It is divided into two compartments each of which contains one testis, one epididymis and the testicular end of a spermatic cord. It lies below the symphysis pubis, in front of the upper parts of the thighs and behind the penis.

Testes

The testes (Fig. 19.13A and B) are the reproductive glands of the male and are the equivalent of the ovaries in the female. They are about 4.5 cm long, 2.5 cm wide and 3 cm thick and are suspended in the scrotum by the spermatic cords. They are surrounded by three layers of tissue.

The tunica vaginalis. This is a double membrane, forming the outer covering of the testes, and is a downgrowth of the abdominal and pelvic peritoneum. During early fetal life the testes develop in the lumbar region of the abdominal cavity just below the kidneys. They then descend into the scrotum taking with them coverings of peritoneum, blood and lymph vessels, nerves and the deferent duct. The peritoneum eventually surrounds the testes in the scrotum, and becomes detached from the abdominal peritoneum. Descent of the testes into the scrotum should be complete by the 8th month of fetal life.

The tunica albuginea. This is a fibrous covering beneath the tunica vaginalis that surrounds the testes. Ingrowths form septa dividing the glandular structure of the testes into *lobules*.

Figure 19.12 The male reproductive organs and their associated structures.

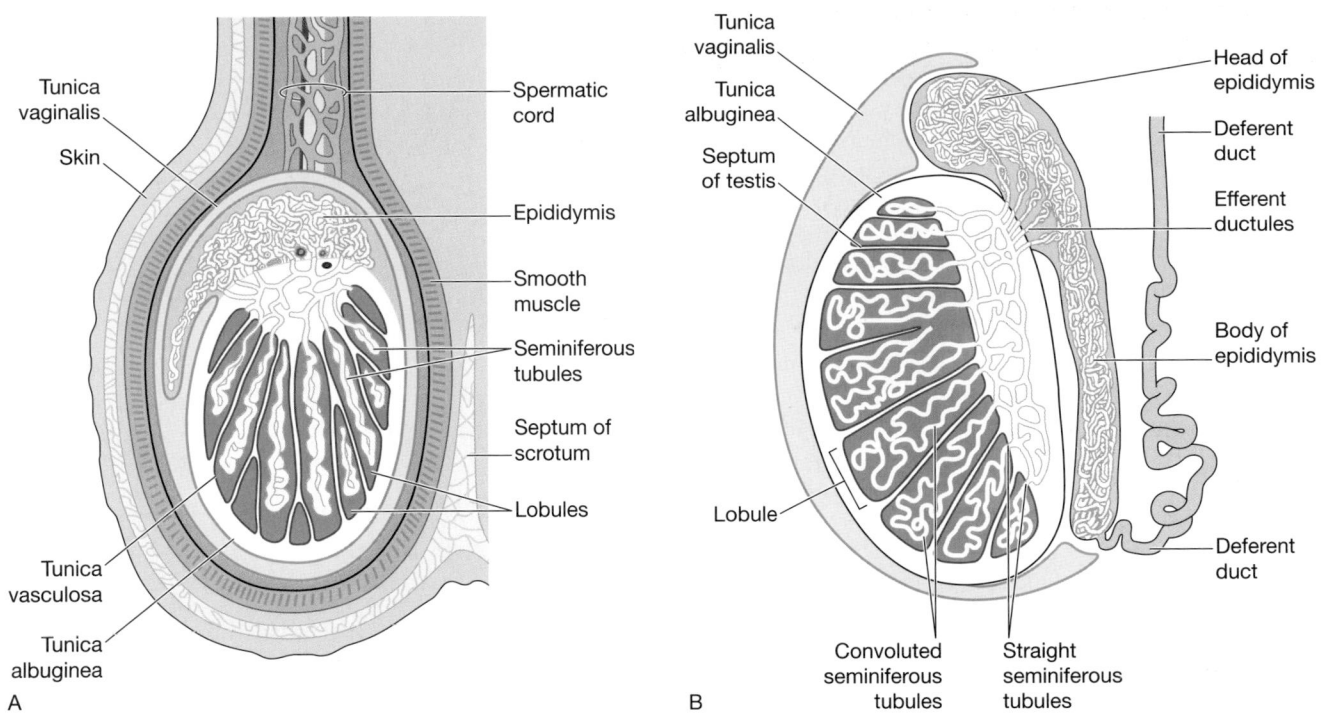

Figure 19.13 The testis: A. A section of the testis and its coverings. B. A longitudinal section of a testis and deferent duct.

The tunica vasculosa. This consists of a network of capillaries supported by delicate connective tissue.

Structure of the testes

In each testis are 200 to 300 lobules and within each lobule are 1 to 4 convoluted loops composed of *germinal epithelial cells*, called *seminiferous tubules*. Between the tubules there are groups of *interstitial cells (of Leydig)* that secrete the hormone testosterone after puberty. At the upper pole of the testis the tubules combine to form a single tubule. This tubule, about 6 m in its full length, is repeatedly folded and tightly packed into a mass called the epididymis. It leaves the scrotum as the *deferent duct* (vas deferens) in the *spermatic cord*. Blood and lymph vessels pass to the testes in the spermatic cords.

Functions of the testes

Spermatozoa (sperm) are produced in the seminiferous tubules of the testes, and mature as they pass through the long and convoluted epididymis, where they are stored. The hormone controlling sperm production is FSH from the anterior pituitary (p. 218). A mature sperm (Fig. 19.14) has a head, a body, and a long whip-like tail that is used for motility. The head is almost completely filled by

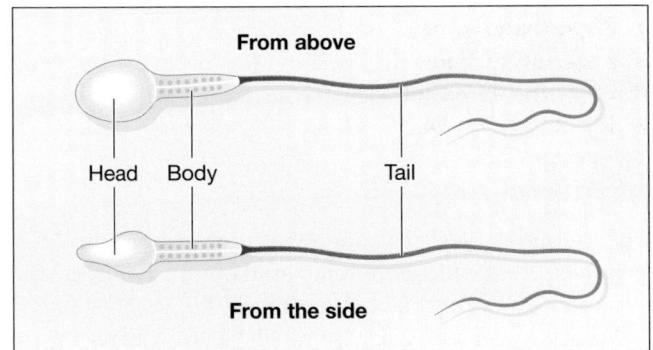

Figure 19.14 A spermatozoon.

the nucleus, containing its DNA. It also contains the enzymes required to penetrate the outer layers of the ovum to reach, and fuse with, its nucleus. The body of the sperm is packed with mitochondria, which fuel the propelling action of the tail that powers the sperm on its journey into the female reproductive tract.

Successful spermatogenesis takes place at a temperature about 3°C below normal body temperature. The testes are cooled by their position outside the abdominal cavity, and the thin outer covering of the scrotum has very little insulating fat.

The spermatic cords

The spermatic cords suspend the testes in the scrotum. Each cord contains a testicular artery, testicular veins, lymphatics, a deferent duct and testicular nerves, which come together to form the cord from their various origins in the abdomen. The cord, which is covered in a sheath of smooth muscle and connective and fibrous tissues, extends through the inguinal canal (p. 433) and is attached to the testis on the posterior wall.

The testicular artery. This branches from the abdominal aorta, just below the renal arteries.

The testicular vein. This passes into the abdominal cavity. The left vein opens into the left renal vein and the right into the inferior vena cava.

Lymph drainage. This is through lymph nodes around the aorta.

The deferent duct. This is some 45 cm long. It passes upwards from the testis through the inguinal canal and ascends medially towards the posterior wall of the bladder where it is joined by the duct from the *seminal vesicle* to form the *ejaculatory duct* (Fig. 19.15).

The nerve supply. This is provided by branches from the 10th and 11th thoracic nerves.

Seminal vesicles

The seminal vesicles are two small fibromuscular pouches lined with columnar epithelium, lying on the posterior aspect of the bladder (Fig. 19.15).

At its lower end each seminal vesicle opens into a short duct which joins with the corresponding deferent duct to form an ejaculatory duct.

Functions of the seminal vesicles

The seminal vesicles contract and expel their stored contents, seminal fluid, during ejaculation. Seminal fluid, which forms 60% of the bulk of the fluid ejaculated at male orgasm, contains nutrients to support the sperm during their journey through the female reproductive tract.

Ejaculatory ducts

The ejaculatory ducts are two tubes about 2 cm long, each formed by the union of the duct from a seminal vesicle

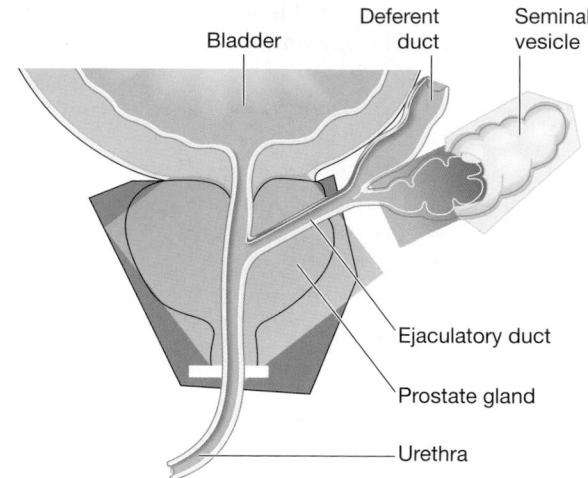

Figure 19.15 Section of the prostate gland and associated reproductive structures on one side.

and a deferent duct. They pass through the prostate gland and join the prostatic urethra, carrying seminal fluid and spermatozoa to the urethra (Fig. 19.15).

The ejaculatory ducts are composed of the same layers of tissue as the seminal vesicles.

Prostate gland

The prostate gland (Fig. 19.15) lies in the pelvic cavity in front of the rectum and behind the symphysis pubis, surrounding the first part of the urethra. It consists of an outer fibrous covering, a layer of smooth muscle and glandular substance composed of columnar epithelial cells.

Functions of the prostate gland

The prostate gland secretes a thin, milky fluid that makes up about 30% of *semen*, and gives it its milky appearance. It is slightly acidic, which provides a protective local environment for sperm arriving in the acidic vagina. It also contains a clotting enzyme, which thickens the semen in the vagina, increasing the likelihood of semen being retained in the vicinity of the cervix.

Urethra and penis

Urethra

The male urethra provides a common pathway for the flow of urine and semen, the combined secretions of the male reproductive organs. It is about 19 to 20 cm long and consists of three parts. The *prostatic urethra* originates at the urethral orifice of the bladder and passes through the prostate gland. The *membranous urethra* is the shortest and narrowest part and extends from the prostate gland to the bulb of the penis, after passing through the perineal membrane. The *spongiose* or *penile urethra* lies within the corpus spongiosum of the penis and terminates at the external urethral orifice in the *glans penis*.

There are two urethral sphincters (Fig. 19.16). The *internal sphincter* consists of smooth muscle fibres at the neck of the bladder above the prostate gland. The *external sphincter* consists of skeletal muscle fibres surrounding the membranous part.

Penis

The penis (Fig. 19.16) has a *root* and a *body*. The root lies in the perineum and the body surrounds the urethra. It is formed by three cylindrical masses of *erectile tissue* and involuntary muscle. The erectile tissue is supported by fibrous tissue and covered with skin and has a rich blood supply.

The two lateral columns are called the *corpora cavernosa* and the column between them, containing the urethra, is the *corpus spongiosum*. At its tip it is expanded into a triangular structure known as the *glans penis*. Just above the glans the skin is folded upon itself and forms a movable double layer, the *foreskin* or *prepuce*. Arterial blood is supplied by deep, dorsal and bulbar arteries of the penis which are branches from the internal pudendal arteries. A series of veins drain blood to the internal pudendal and internal iliac veins. The penis is supplied by autonomic and somatic nerves. Parasympathetic stimulation leads to filling of the spongy erectile tissue with blood, caused by arteriolar dilatation and venoconstriction, which increases blood flow into the penis and obstructs outflow. The penis therefore becomes engorged and erect, an essential prerequisite for coitus to occur.

Ejaculation

During ejaculation, which occurs at the point of male orgasm, spermatozoa are expelled from the epididymis and pass through the deferent duct, the ejaculatory duct and the urethra. The semen is propelled by powerful rhythmical contraction of the smooth muscle in the walls of the deferent duct; the muscular contractions are sympathetically mediated. Muscle in the walls of the seminal vesicles and prostate gland also contracts, adding their contents to the fluid passing through the genital ducts. The force generated by these combined processes leads to emission of the semen through the external urethral sphincter (Fig. 19.17).

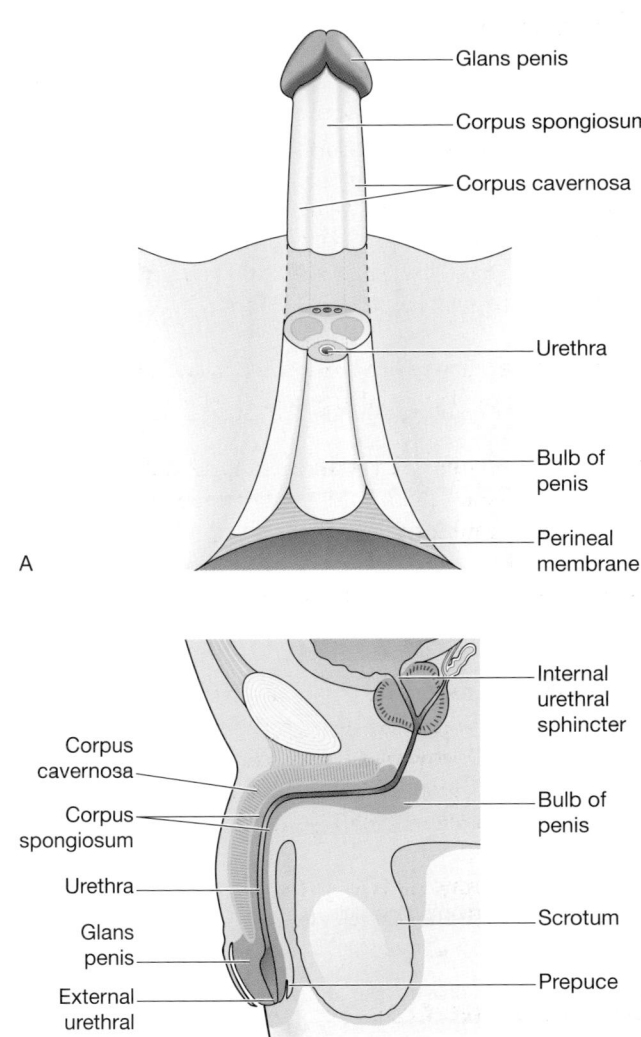

Figure 19.16 The penis: A. Viewed from below. B. Viewed from the side.

451

Sperm comprise only 10% of the final ejaculate, the remainder being made up of seminal and prostatic fluids, which are added to the sperm during male orgasm, as well as mucus produced in the urethra. Between 2 and 5 ml of semen are produced in a normal ejaculate, and contain between 40 and 100 million spermatozoa per ml. If not ejaculated, sperm gradually lose their fertility after several months and are reabsorbed by the epididymis.

Puberty in the male

This occurs between the ages of 10 and 14. Luteinising hormone from the anterior lobe of the pituitary gland stimulates the interstitial cells of the testes to increase the

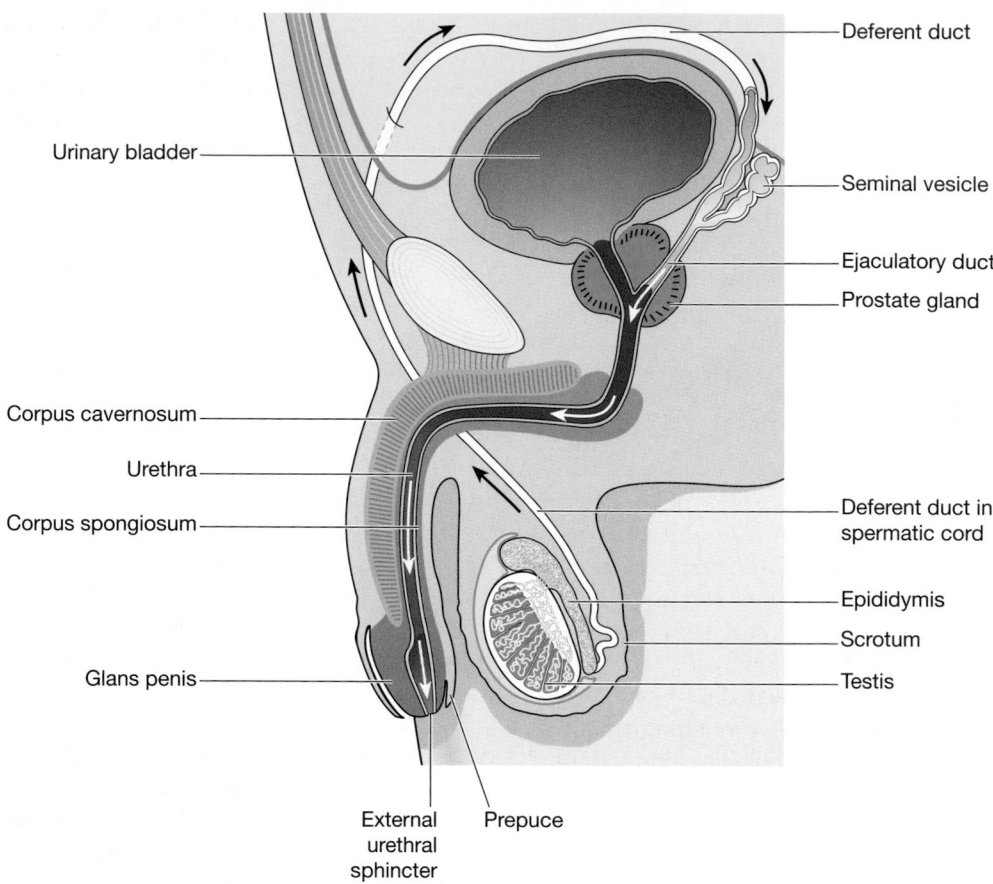

Urinary bladder

Corpus cavernosum

Urethra

Corpus spongiosum

Glans penis

External urethral sphincter

Prepuce

Deferent duct

Seminal vesicle

Ejaculatory duct

Prostate gland

Deferent duct in spermatic cord

Epididymis

Scrotum

Testis

Figure 19.17 Section of the male reproductive organs. Arrows show the route taken by spermatozoa during ejaculation.

production of testosterone. This hormone influences the development of the body to sexual maturity. The changes which occur at puberty are:

- growth of muscle and bone and a marked increase in height and weight
- enlargement of the larynx and deepening of the voice—it 'breaks'
- growth of hair on the face, axillae, chest, abdomen and pubis

- enlargement of the penis, scrotum and prostate gland
- maturation of the seminiferous tubules and production of spermatozoa
- the skin thickens and becomes more oily.

In the male, fertility and sexual ability tend to decline gradually with ageing. The secretion of testosterone gradually declines, usually beginning at about 50 years of age. There is no period comparable to the female menopause.

SEXUALLY TRANSMITTED DISEASE (VENEREAL DISEASE)

Learning outcomes

After studying this section, you should be able to:

- list the principal causes of sexually transmitted diseases
- explain the effects of sexually transmitted diseases.

Infection of the reproductive system may be classified as:

- *non-specific*, usually caused by a mixture of microbes, e.g. staphylococci, streptococci, coliform bacteria, *Clostridium perfringens (Cl. welchii)*
- *specific*, caused by sexually transmitted microbes, the most common of which being *Neisseria gonorrhoeae, Trichomonas vaginalis*, chlamydia, herpes viruses, human immunodeficiency virus (HIV) and hepatitis B.

In general, the microbes that cause sexually transmitted diseases:

- are unable to survive outside the body for long periods
- have no intermediate host
- produce lesions in the genital area which discharge the infecting microbes.

Chlamydia

The microbe *Chlamydia trachomatis* causes inflammation of the female cervix, which may ascend through the reproductive tract and cause pelvic inflammatory disease, and urethritis in the male, which may also ascend and lead to epididymitis. *Chlamydia* infection is often present in conjunction with other sexually transmitted diseases. The same organism causes trachoma, an infection of the eye that is the primary cause of blindness world-wide (p. 210).

Gonorrhoea

This is the most commonly occurring venereal disease and affects men and women. It is caused by *Neisseria gonorrhoeae* which affects the mucosa of the reproductive and urinary tracts. In the male, suppurative urethritis occurs and the infection may spread to the prostate gland, epididymis and testes. In the female the infection may spread from vulvar glands, vagina and cervix to the body of the uterus, uterine tubes, ovaries and peritoneum. Healing by fibrosis in the female may cause obstruction of the uterine tubes, leading to infertility. In the male it may cause urethral stricture.

Non-venereal transmission of gonorrhoea may cause *neonatal ophthalmia* in babies born to infected mothers. The eyes are infected as the baby passes through the vagina.

Syphilis

This disease is caused by *Treponema pallidum*. There are three clearly marked stages although the third is now rarely seen in Britain. After an incubation period of several weeks, the *primary sore* (chancre) appears at the site of infection, e.g. the vulva, vagina, perineum, penis or round the mouth. In the female the primary sore may be undetected if it is internal. After several weeks the chancre subsides spontaneously. *Secondary lesions* appear 3 to 4 months after infection. They consist of skin rashes and raised papules (condylomata lata) on the external genitalia and vaginal walls. These subside after several months and are followed by a latent period of a variable number of years. *Tertiary lesions* (gummas) develop in many organs and in a few cases the nervous system is involved, leading to general paralysis.

Sexual transmission occurs during the primary and secondary stages when discharge from lesions contains microbes. Congenital transmission occurs when microbes from an infected mother cross the placenta to the fetus, often with fatal consequences. Accidental spread of infection may occur by blood transfusion if a donor's blood is taken during the incubation period after microbes have spread to the blood from the site of infection.

Trichomonas vaginalis

These *protozoa* cause acute vulvovaginitis. It is usually sexually transmitted and is commonly present in women with gonorrhoea.

Candidiasis

The yeast *Candida albicans* (see also p. 319) is frequently a commensal in the normal vagina and causes no problems. It is normally prevented from flourishing by, e.g., vaginal acidity, but in certain circumstances it proliferates, causing candidiasis (thrush). Common precipitating factors include:

- antibiotic therapy, which kills the bacteria that keep vaginal pH low
- pregnancy
- reduced immune function.

Acquired immune deficiency syndrome (AIDS) and hepatitis B infection

These viral conditions may be sexually transmitted but there are no local signs of infection. For a description of AIDS and HIV see page 385 and hepatitis B page 334.

453

DISEASES OF THE FEMALE REPRODUCTIVE SYSTEM

Learning outcomes

After studying this section, you should be able to:

- describe the causes and consequences of pelvic inflammatory disease

- discuss the disorders of the vulva

- define the term imperforate hymen

- outline the causes and effects of cervical carcinoma

- discuss the main pathologies of the uterus and uterine tubes

- describe the causes and effects of ovarian disease

- describe the causes of female infertility

- discuss the principal disorders of the female breast.

Pelvic inflammatory disease (PID)

This infection may be specific or non-specific. It usually begins as vulvovaginitis, including the vulvar glands, then it may spread to the cervix, uterus, uterine tubes and ovaries. Upward spread is most common when microbes are present in the vagina before a surgical procedure, childbirth or abortion, especially if some of the products of conception are retained.

Complications of PID include:

- infertility due to obstruction of uterine tubes
- peritonitis
- intestinal obstruction due to adhesions between the bowel and the uterus and/or uterine tubes
- bacteraemia which may lead to meningitis, endocarditis or suppurative arthritis
- Bartholin's gland abscess or cyst formation if the duct is blocked.

Vulvar dystrophies

Atrophic dystrophy

This is thinning of vulvar epithelium and the formation of fibrous tissue, occurring after the menopause due to oestrogen withdrawal. It predisposes to infection, especially in debilitated women, and to malignant epithelial neoplasia.

Vulvar intraepithelial neoplasia (VIN)

The extent of development of hyperplasia and dysplasia of cells of the skin of the vulva varies considerably. It is often associated with human papilloma virus infection. In the majority of cases the neoplasia are benign. Some VIN cases progress to invasive carcinoma while others regress spontaneously. In elderly women and immuno-suppressed young women malignant tumours may develop which spread locally with early involvement of inguinal lymph nodes. Because of the anastomoses between lymph vessels on the two sides of the vulva, bilateral lymph node involvement is common.

Imperforate hymen

This is a congenital abnormality which may not be noticed until the onset of menstruation. When complete (imperforate), the hymen forms a barrier in the vagina. Blood accumulates in the vagina, uterus and uterine tubes with each menstrual cycle, and it may enter the peritoneal cavity and cause peritonitis. The uterine tubes may become obstructed by coagulated blood, leading to infertility.

Disorders of the cervix

Cervical carcinoma

Dysplastic changes referred to as cervical intraepithelial neoplasia (CIN) begin in the deepest layer of cervical epithelium, usually at the junction of the stratified squamous epithelium of the lower third of the cervical canal with the secretory epithelium of the upper two-thirds. Dysplasia may progress to involve the full thickness of epithelium, called *carcinoma-in-situ*. The cancer may develop further and spread locally to the vagina, uterine body and other pelvic structures. More widespread metastases occur late in the disease. Not all cases in which dysplastic changes are observed develop to the cancerous stage but it is not possible to predict how far development will go, and whether it will remain static or regress. Three degrees of dysplasia have been described, although clear distinction between them is not always possible:

- CIN 1 = mild dysplasia
- CIN 2 = moderate dysplasia
- CIN 3 = carcinoma-in-situ.

CIN 3 may progress to invasive carcinoma. Early spread is via lymph nodes and local spread is commonly to the uterus, vagina, bladder and rectum. In the late stages spread via the blood to the liver, lungs and bones may occur.

The disease takes 15 to 20 years to develop and it occurs mostly between 35 and 50 years of age. It is likely that a significant proportion of cases are due to the transmission of some carcinogenic factor to the female during sexual intercourse. This is supported by the observations that the disease occurs more frequently in women who commence sexual activity at an early age, who have many partners, who have many pregnancies or have frequent sexual intercourse. Additionally, barrier contraceptives protect against the disease. The human papillomavirus (HPV), which causes genital warts, is strongly associated with this cancer (see also p. 369).

Disorders of the uterine body

Acute endometritis

This is usually caused by non-specific infection, following parturition or abortion, especially if fragments of membranes or placenta have been retained in the uterus. A variety of microbes may be involved, e.g. staphylococci, streptococci, *Escherichia coli* or *Pseudomonas*. The inflammation may subside after removal of retained products. The infection may spread to:

- myometrium, perimetrium and surrounding pelvic tissues which may lead to thrombosis of iliac veins
- uterine tubes, causing salpingitis, fibrosis, obstruction and infertility
- any of the above-mentioned areas, causing peritonitis and possibly adhesions.

Chronic endometritis

This may follow an acute attack or be due to spread of pelvic inflammatory disease. It may follow abortion or parturition and may be associated with chronic salpingitis, endometrial carcinoma or the use of intrauterine contraceptive devices.

Endometriosis

This is the growth of endometrial tissue outside the uterus, most commonly in the ovaries, uterine tubes and other pelvic structures. The ectopic tissue, like the uterine endometrium, is responsive to the fluctuations in sex hormone levels of the menstrual cycle, causing menstrual-type bleeding into the lower abdomen and, in the ovaries, the formation of coloured cysts, 'chocolate cysts'. There is intermittent pain due to swelling, and recurrent

haemorrhage causes fibrous tissue formation. Ovarian endometriosis may lead to pelvic inflammation, infertility and extensive pelvic adhesions, involving the ovaries, uterus, uterine ligaments and the bowel. The cause is not clear but it has been suggested that there may have been:

- abnormal cell differentiation in the fetus
- regurgitation of menstrual material through the uterine tubes
- spread of endometrial cells in lymph and blood during menstruation.

Adenomyosis

This is the growth of endometrium within the myometrium. The ectopic tissue may cause general or localised uterine enlargement. The lesions may cause dysmenorrhoea and irregular excessive bleeding (menorrhagia), usually beginning between 40 and 50 years of age.

Endometrial hyperplasia

The hyperplasia may affect endometrial glands, causing cyst formation and/or focal hyperplasia of atypical cells. The focal type frequently undergoes malignant change. Both types are associated with a sustained high blood oestrogen level, which may be due to:

- failure of ovarian follicles to mature and release their ova
- oestrogen-secreting ovarian tumours
- prolonged oestrogen therapy.

Leiomyoma (fibroid, myoma)

These are very common, often multiple, benign tumours of myometrium. They are firm masses of smooth muscle encapsulated in compressed muscle fibres and they vary greatly in size. Large tumours may undergo degenerative changes if they outgrow their blood supply, leading to necrosis, fibrosis and calcification. They develop during the reproductive period and may be hormone dependent, enlarging during pregnancy and when oral contraceptives are used. They tend to regress after the menopause. Large tumours may cause pelvic discomfort, frequency of micturition, menorrhagia, irregular bleeding, dysmenorrhoea and reduced fertility. Malignant change is rare.

Endometrial carcinoma

This occurs mainly in nulliparous women (i.e. women who have never been pregnant) between 50 and 60 years of age. The cause is not known but there is some evidence that oestrogen may be involved. The incidence of carcinoma is increased when an oestrogen-secreting tumour is present and in women who are obese, hypertensive or diabetic, because they tend to have a high level of blood oestrogen. The tumour may develop as a diffuse mass, a localised plaque or a polyp and there is often ulceration and bleeding. Endometrium has no lymphatics, so lymph spread is delayed until there is extensive local spread that involves other pelvic structures. Distant metastases, spread in blood or lymph, develop later, most commonly in the liver, lungs and bones. Invasion of the ureters leads to hydronephrosis and uraemia which is commonly the cause of death.

Disorders of the uterine tubes and ovaries

Acute salpingitis

Salpingitis is inflammation of the uterine tubes, and is usually due to infection spreading from the uterus, and only occasionally from the peritoneal cavity. The outcome may be:

- uneventful recovery
- chronic inflammation, leading to fibrous tubal obstruction and infertility
- pus formation (*pyosalpinx*) and further spread to the ovaries and peritoneal cavity, leading to fibrous tubal obstruction, infertility and/or pelvic adhesions.

Ectopic pregnancy

This is the implantation of a fertilised ovum outside the uterus, most commonly in a uterine tube. As the fetus grows the tube ruptures and its contents enter the peritoneal cavity, causing acute inflammation (peritonitis) and possibly severe intraperitoneal haemorrhage.

Ovarian tumours

The majority of ovarian tumours are benign, usually occurring between 20 and 45 years of age. The remainder occur mostly between 45 and 65 years and are divided between borderline malignancy (low-grade cancer) and frank malignancy. There are three main types of cells involved: epithelial cells, germ cells and hormone-secreting cells (sex-cord stroma cells).

Epithelial cell tumours
Most of these are borderline or malignant tumours. They vary greatly in size from very large to quite small and some are partly cystic. Large tumours may

cause pressure, leading to gastrointestinal disturbances, frequency of micturition, dysuria and ascites. Those suspended by a pedicle may twist, causing ischaemia, necrosis, haemorrhage or rupture of a cyst. The principal methods of spread are invasion of local and peritoneal structures. Later lymph- and blood-spread metastases may develop.

The prevalence is higher in developed societies and in the higher socio-economic groups. Pregnancy and suppression of ovulation by medicinal contraceptives, e.g. the oral contraceptive pill, may have a protective effect due to a reduction in the number of ovulatory menstrual cycles.

Germ cell ovarian tumours
These occur mainly in children and young adults and only a few are malignant. Benign *dermoid cysts* are the most common type. These are thick-walled cysts containing a variety of uncharacteristic tissues, e.g. hair, skin, epithelium or teeth. They are usually small and have a tendency to twist on a pedicle, causing ischaemia and necrosis.

Sex-cord stroma cell tumours
These cells are the precursors of the ovarian follicle lining cells, luteal cells and fibrous supporting cells. Mixed tumours develop, some of which secrete hormones. Oestrogen-secreting tumours cause precocious sexual development in children. In adults the excess oestrogen may cause endometrial hyperplasia, endometrial carcinoma, cystic disease of the breast or breast cancer. Androgen-secreting tumours occasionally develop, causing atrophy of the breast and genitalia and the development of male sex characteristics.

Metastatic ovarian tumours
The ovaries are a common site of metastatic spread from primary malignant tumours in other pelvic organs, the breast, stomach, pancreas and biliary tract.

Female infertility

This may be due to:

- blockage of uterine tubes, often the consequence of pelvic inflammatory disease
- anatomical problems, e.g. retroversion (tilting backwards) of the uterus
- endocrine factors; any abnormalities of the glands and hormones governing the menstrual cycle can interfere with, for example, ovulation or the uterine cycle
- low body weight or severe malnourishment
- endometriosis.

Disorders of the breast

Mastitis (inflammation of the breast)

Acute non-suppurative mastitis

This occurs during lactation and is associated with painful congestion and oedema of the breast. It is of hormonal origin.

Acute suppurative (pyogenic) mastitis

The microbes enter through a nipple abrasion caused by the infant sucking. The most common causative microbes are *Staphylococcus aureus* and *Streptococcus pyogenes* usually acquired by the infant while in hospital. The infection spreads along the mammary ducts of a lobe causing localised swelling and redness. If it does not resolve it can become chronic and an abscess may form.

Tumours of the breast

Benign tumours

Most breast tumours (90%) are benign. Fibroadenomas are the commonest type and occur any time after puberty; incidence peaks in the third decade. Some are cystic and some solid and they usually occur in women nearing the menopause. They may originate from secretory cells, fibrous tissue or from ducts.

Malignant tumours

The most common types of tumour are usually painless lumps found in the upper outer quadrant of the breast. There is considerable fibrosis around the tumour that may cause retraction of the nipple and necrosis and ulceration of the overlying skin. It is increasingly common between 35 and 70 years.

Early spread beyond the breast is via lymph to the axillary and internal mammary nodes. Local invasion involves the pectoral muscles and the pleura. Blood-spread metastases may occur later in many organs and bones, especially lumbar and thoracic vertebrae. The causes of breast cancer are not known, but an important predisposing factor appears to be high oestrogen exposure. Women with an early menarche, a late menopause, and no pregnancies have a higher than normal risk because they experience more menstrual cycles in their lifetimes, and each monthly cycle brings with it the oestrogen surge seen in the proliferative phase of the cycle. A genetic component is also likely, with close relatives of cancer sufferers having a significantly elevated risk of developing the disease. One per cent of all breast cancer occurs in men.

DISEASES OF THE MALE REPRODUCTIVE SYSTEM

Learning outcomes

After studying this section, you should be able to:

- outline the causes and effects of penile and urethral infections
- describe the main pathologies of the testis
- discuss the principal disorders of the prostate gland
- list the main causes of male infertility.

Infections of the penis

Inflammation of the glans and prepuce may be caused by a specific or non-specific infection. In non-specific infections, or *balanitis*, lack of personal hygiene is an important predisposing factor, especially if *phimosis* is present, i.e. the orifice in the foreskin (prepuce) is too small to allow for its normal retraction. If the infection becomes chronic there may be fibrosis of the foreskin, which increases the phimosis.

Infections of the urethra

Gonococcal urethritis is the most common specific infection. Non-specific infection may be spread from the bladder (cystitis) or be introduced during catheterisation, cystoscopy or surgery. Both types may spread throughout the system to the prostate, seminal vesicles, epididymis and testes. If infection becomes chronic, fibrosis may cause urethral stricture or obstruction, leading to retention of urine.

Epididymis and testes

Infections

Non-specific epididymitis and orchitis are usually due to spread of infection from the urethra, commonly following prostatectomy. The microbes may spread either through the deferent duct (vas deferens) or via lymph.

Specific epididymitis. This is usually caused by gonorrhoea spread from the urethra.

Orchitis (inflammation of the testis). This is more commonly caused by mumps viruses, bloodborne from the

457

parotid glands. Acute inflammation with oedema occurs about 1 week after the appearance of parotid swelling. The infection is usually unilateral but, if bilateral, severe damage to germinal epithelium of the seminiferous tubules may result in sterility.

Undescended testis (cryptorchidism)

During embryonic life the testes develop within the abdominal cavity, but descend into the scrotum prior to birth. If they fail to do this and the condition is not corrected, infertility is likely to follow and the risk of testicular cancer is increased.

Hydrocele

This is the most common form of scrotal swelling and is accumulation of serous fluid in the tunica vaginalis. The onset may be acute and painful or chronic. It may be congenital or be secondary to another disorder of the testis or epididymis.

Testicular tumours

Most testicular tumours are malignant and are the commonest malignancies in young men. They occur in children and young adults in whom the affected testis has not descended or has been late in descending into the scrotum. The tumour tends to remain localised for a considerable time but eventually spreads in lymph to pelvic and abdominal lymph nodes, and more widely in blood. Occasionally hormone-secreting tumours develop and may cause precocious development in children.

Prostate gland

Infections

Acute prostatitis is usually caused by non-specific infection, spread from the urethra or bladder, often following catheterisation, cystoscopy, urethral dilatation or surgery in which part of the gland is removed. Chronic infection may follow an acute attack, but it may develop insidiously and is not associated with known microbes. Fibrosis of the gland may occur during healing, causing urethral stricture or obstruction.

Benign prostatic enlargement

Hyperplastic nodules form around the urethra and may cause constriction or obstruction to the flow of urine, causing retention of urine. Urethral stricture may prevent the bladder emptying completely during micturition, predisposing to infection which may spread upwards and cause pyelonephritis and other complications.

Prostatic enlargement is common in men over 50, affecting up to 70% of men aged over 70. The cause is not clear, but it may be an acceleration of the ageing process associated with the decline in androgen secretion which changes the androgen/oestrogen balance.

Malignant prostatic tumours

These are a relatively common cause of death in men over 50. The carcinogen is not known but changes in the androgen/oestrogen balance may be significant or viruses may be involved. Invasion of local tissues is widespread before lymph-spread metastases develop in pelvic and abdominal lymph nodes. Blood-spread metastases in bone are common and bone formation rather than bone destruction is a common feature. Lumbar vertebrae are a common site, possibly due to retrograde spread along the walls of veins. In many cases bone metastases are the first indication of malignant prostatic tumours.

Breast

Breast tissue in men consists of ducts and stroma only.

Gynaecomastia

This is proliferation of breast tissue in men. It usually affects only one breast and is benign. It is common in adolescents and older men, and is often associated with:

- endocrine disorders, especially those associated with high oestrogen levels
- cirrhosis of the liver (p. 335)
- malnutrition
- some drugs, e.g. chlorpromazine, spironolactone, digoxin
- Klinefelter's syndrome, a genetic disorder in which there is testicular atrophy and absence of spermatogenesis.

Malignant tumours

These develop in a small number of men, usually in the older age groups.

Male infertility

This may be due to:

- endocrine disorders
- obstruction of the deferent duct
- failure of erection or ejaculation during intercourse
- surgical vasectomy
- suppression of spermatogenesis by, e.g., ionising radiation, chemotherapy and other drugs.

Normal values

Note. *Some biological measures have been extracted from the text and listed here for easy reference. In some cases slightly different 'normals' may be found in other texts and used by different medical practitioners.*

Metric measures, units and SI symbols

Name	SI unit	Symbol
Length	metre	m
Mass	kilogram	kg
Amount of substance	mole	mol
Pressure	pascal	Pa
Energy	joule	J

Decimal multiples and submultiples of the units are formed by the used of standard prefixes.

Multiple	Prefix	Symbol	Submultiple	Prefix	Symbol
10^6	mega	M	10^{-1}	deci	d
10^3	kilo	k	10^{-2}	centi	c
10^2	hecto	h	10^{-3}	milli	m
10^1	deca	da	10^{-6}	micro	μ
			10^{-9}	nano	n
			10^{-12}	pico	p
			10^{-15}	femto	f

Conversion table for kPa/mmHg (for e.g. capillary pressures)

1 mmHg	=	0.13 kPa
1 kPa	=	7.5 mmHg
35 mmHg	=	4.7 kPa
25 mmHg	=	3.3 kPa
15 mmHg	=	2.0 kPa
10 mmHg	=	1.3 kPa

Hydrogen ion concentration (pH)

Neutral = 7   Acid = 0 to 7   Alkaline = 7 to 14

Normal pH of some body fluids	
Blood	7.35 to 7.45
Saliva	5.4 to 7.5
Gastric juice	1.5 to 3.5
Bile	6.0 to 8.5
Urine	4.5 to 8.0

Some normal plasma levels in adults

Calcium	2.12 to 2.62 mmol/l	(8.5 to 10.5 mg/100 ml)
Chloride	97 to 106 mmol/l	(97 to 106 mEq/l)
Cholesterol	3.6 to 6.7 mmol/l	(140 to 260 mg/100 ml)
Glucose	3.5 to 8 mmol/l	(63 to 144 mg/100 ml)
Fasting glucose	3.6 to 5.8 mmol/l	(65 to 105 mg/100 ml)
Potassium	3.3 to 4.7 mmol/l	(3.3 to 4.7 mEq/l)
Sodium	135 to 143 mmol/l	(135 to 143 mEq/l)
Urea	2.5 to 6.6 mmol/l	(15 to 44 mg/100 ml)

Arterial blood gases

PO_2	12 to 15 kPa	(90 to 110 mmHg)
PCO_2	4.5 to 6 kPa	(34 to 46 mmHg)
Bicarbonate	21 to 27.5 mmol/l	
H^+ ions	36 to 44 nmol/l	(7.35 to 7.45 pH units)

Blood pressure

Normal adult 120/80 mmHg

Hypertension, i.e. above 'normal' maximum for age	
20 years	140/90 mmHg
50 years	160/95 mmHg
75 years	170/105 mmHg

Heart rate

At rest 60 to 80/min
Sinus bradycardia   < 60/min
Sinus tachycardia   > 100/min

Respiration rate

At rest 15 to 18/min
Tidal volume   500 ml
Dead space   150 ml
Alveolar ventilation   15 (500 – 150) = 5.25 l/min

Blood count

Leukocytes	$4 \times 10^9/l$	to	$11 \times 10^9/l$
Neutrophils	$2.1 \times 10^9/l$	to	$7.2 \times 10^9/l$
Eosinophils	$0.04 \times 10^9/l$	to	$0.44 \times 10^9/l$
Basophils	$0.015 \times 10^9/l$	to	$0.2 \times 10^9/l$
Monocytes	$0.2 \times 10^9/l$	to	$0.8 \times 10^9/l$
Lymphocytes	$1.5 \times 10^9/l$	to	$4.0 \times 10^9/l$
Erythrocytes			
female	$3.8 \times 10^{12}/l$	to	$5 \times 10^{12}/l$
male	$4.5 \times 10^{12}/l$	to	$6.5 \times 10^{12}/l$
Thrombocytes	$150 \times 10^9/l$	to	$440 \times 10^9/l$

Diet

Vitamins. Daily requirements see pages 276 and 277
1 kilocalorie (kcal)   =   4.182 kilojoules (kJ)
1 kilojoule   =   0.24 kilocalories

Engergy source	Energy released	Recommended proportion in diet
Carbohydrate	1 g = 17 kJ = 4 kcal	55–75%
Protein	1 g = 17 kJ = 4 kcal	10–15%
Fat	1 g = 38 kJ = 9 kcal	15–30%

Urine

Specific gravity   1.020 to 1.030
Volume excreted   1000 to 1500 ml/day
Glucose is normally absent, but appears in urine when blood glucose levels exceed 9 mmol/l

Body temperatures

Normal   36.8°C (98.4°F): axillary
Hypothermia   32°C (89.6°F): axillary
                        35°C (95°F): core temperature
Death when below   25°C (77°F)

Cerebrospinal fluid pressure

Lying on the side 50 to 180 mm

Intraocular pressure

1.3 to 2.6 kPa (10 to 20 mmHg)

Bibliography

Bourke S J, Brewis R A L 1998 Respiratory medicine, 5th edn. Blackwell Science, Oxford

Bull P D 1996 Diseases of the ear, nose and throat, 8th edn. Blackwell Science, Oxford

Burkitt H G, Young B, Health J W 1993 Wheater's functional histology, 3rd edn. Churchill Livingstone, New York

Burns M V 1998 Pathophysiology. A self-instructional program. Appleton and Lange, Connecticut

Department of Health 1991 Dietary reference values of food energy and nutrients for the UK: COMA report. HMSO, London

Drake-Lee A 1996 Clinical otorhinolaryngology. Churchill Livingstone, New York

Forrest A P M, Carter D C, Macleod I B 1995 Principles and practice of surgery, 3rd edn. Churchill Livingstone, New York

Ganong W D 1999 Review of medical physiology, 19th edn. Appleton and Lange, Connecticut

Govan A D T, Macfarlane P S, Callander R 1995 Pathology illustrated, 4th edn. Churchill Livingstone, New York

Guyton A C, Hall J E 1996 Textbook of medical physiology, 9th edn. W B Saunders, New York

Haslett C, Chilvers R C, Hunter J A A, Boon N A (eds) 1999 Davidson's principles and practice of medicine, 3rd edn. Churchill Livingstone, New York

Hinchliff S M, Montague S E, Watson R 1996 Physiology for nursing practice, 2nd edn. Baillière Tindall, New York

James B, Chew C, Bron A 1997 Ophthalmology, 8th edn. Blackwell Science, Oxford

Kumar P, Clark M (eds) 1998 Clinical medicine. A textbook for medical students and doctors, 4th edn. W B Saunders, New York

Macsween R N M, Whaley K (eds) 1992 Muir's textbook of pathology, 13th edn. Edward Arnold, London

Marieb E N 1998 Human anatomy and physiology, 4th edn. Addison Wesley Longman, New York

Mathews C K, van Holde K E, Ahern K G 2000 Biochemistry, 3rd edn. Benjamin Cummings, San Francisco

Merck manual of diagnosis and therapy 1999 17th edn. Merck Research Laboratories, New Jersey

Mirpuri N, Patel P 1998 Crash course: renal and urinary systems. Mosby, New York

Pocock G, Richards C D 1999 Human physiology — the basis of medicine. Oxford University Press, Oxford

Rogers A W 1992 Textbook of anatomy. Churchill Livingstone, New York

Roitt I, Brostoff J, Male D 1998 Immunology, 5th edn. Mosby, New York

Schaechter M, Engleberg N C, Eisenstein B I, Medoff G 1998 Mechanisms of microbial disease, 3rd edn. Williams and Wilkins, Baltimore

Smith A F, Beckett G J, Walker S W, Rae P W H 1998 Lecture notes on clinical biochemistry, 6th edn. Blackwell Science, Oxford

Spector W G 1989 An introduction to general pathology, 3rd edn. Churchill Livingstone, Edinburgh

Sutton J 1998 Biology. Macmillan, London

Thibodeau G A, Patton K T 1999 Anatomy and physiology, 4th edn. Mosby, New York

Tortora G J 1999 Principles of human anatomy, 8th edn. Addison Wesley Longman, New York

Tortora G J, Grabowski S R 1996 Principles of anatomy and physiology, 8th edn. Addison Wesley Longman, New York

Underwood J C E (ed) 1996 General and systematic pathology, 2nd edn. Churchill Livingstone, New York

Vander A J, Sherman J H, Luciano D 1998 Human physiology — the mechanisms of body function, 7th edn. McGraw-Hill, Boston

Weir D M, Stewart J 1997 Immunology, 8th edn. Churchill Livingstone, New York

Whitney E N, Rolfe S R 1999 Understanding nutrition, 8th edn. Wadsworth, Belmont, CA

Williams P L, Bannister L H, Berry M M et al (eds) 1995 Gray's anatomy — the anatomical basis of medicine and surgery, 38th edn. Churchill Livingstone, New York

Index

Page numbers in **bold** refer to main discussions of anatomy and physiology. Those in ***bold italics*** refer to main discussions of diseases. Page numbers referring to anatomy and physiology are in ordinary type. Those referring to diseases are in *italics*.

A

Abdominal cavity, **50–51**
  arterial supply, 104–105
  contents, 50–51
  lymph nodes, 133
  regions, 51
  venous return, 105
Abdominal wall
  muscles, **432–433**
  nerves, 166, 167
Abducent nerve (cranial nerve VI), **168**, 169
Abduction, 414
ABO blood group system, 64, 65
Abscess, *377–378*
  brain, *183*
  liver, *335*
  lung, *263–264*
  pelvic, *325*
  subperiosteal, *410*
  subphrenic, *324, 325*
Absorption, 283, **311–312**
  in large intestine, 305
  by skin, 366
  in small intestine, 131, **302–303**
  in stomach, 299
Accessory nerve (cranial nerve XI), **168**, 169
Accommodation, of eyes to light, **202**
Acetabular labrum, 420
Acetabulum, 403, 404, 420
Acetylcholine, 144
  in autonomic nervous system, 146, 170, 171
  in neuromuscular transmission, 145, 146, 159
Acetyl co-enzyme A, 317
Achalasia, *322*
Achilles (calcanean) tendon, 422, 423
Achondroplasia, *410*
Acid–base balance, 23, 346
Acidosis, 22–23, *354*
Acid reserve, 22
Acids, **21–23**
Acne vulgaris, *370*
Acquired disease, *15*
Acquired immune deficiency syndrome, *see* AIDS
Acromegaly, *227, 228*
Acromioclavicular joint, 401
Acromion process, 401, 402
ACTH, *see* Adrenocorticotrophic hormone
Actin, 40
Action potential, 141, **142–143**
Acute disease, *15*
Acute disseminating encephalomyelitis, *185*
Acute idiopathic inflammatory polyneuropathy, *188*
Acute renal failure, ***353–354***
Acute tubular necrosis (ATN), *353–354*
Adam's apple, 244
Addisonian crisis, *233*

Addison's disease, *233*
Adduction, 414
Adductor muscles of hip, 421, 422
Adenohypophysis, see Pituitary gland, anterior
Adenoids (pharyngeal tonsils), 243
  enlarged, *258*
Adenomyosis, uterine, *455*
Adenosine diphosphate (ADP), 25, 67
Adenosine triphosphate (ATP), 25, 32, 315
ADH, *see* Antidiuretic hormone
Adhesions, *325, 379*
Adipocytes, 37
Adipose tissue, 37–38
ADP (adenosine diphosphate), 25, 67
Adrenal (suprarenal) arteries, 104, 222
Adrenal cortex, **222–223**
  acute insufficiency, *233*
  chronic insufficiency, *233*
  disorders, *126, 232–233*
Adrenal glands, **222–224**
  autonomic stimulation, 173
  response to stress, 224
Adrenaline, 173, 223, **224**, 315
  excess secretion, *126*
  heart rate and, 87
Adrenal medulla, 222, **223–224**
  disorders, *126, 234*
  tumours, *234*
Adrenal (suprarenal) vein, 105, 222
Adrenocorticoids, 222–223
Adrenocorticotrophic hormone (ACTH), 216, **217**, 218, 222
  deficiency, *233*
  hypersecretion, *126, 232*
Adult respiratory distress syndrome (ARDS), *268*
Aerobic metabolism, 23, 315
Aetiology, 14, 15
Afferent nerves, *see* Sensory nerves
Afterload, 90
Age
  heart rate and, 87
  varicose veins and, *116*
Agranulocytes, 64, 65, **66–67**
Agranulocytosis, *73*
AIDS (acquired immune deficiency syndrome), *184, 371, **385–386**, 453*
Air, 240
  alveolar, 255
  composition, **255**
  entry into bronchi/bronchioles, 248–249
  expired, 255
  filtering/cleaning, 242, 246, 247
  humidification, 242, 243, 246, 247, 249
  passages, 36, 241–242, 243, **246–249**
  warming, 242, 243, 246, 247, 249
Airflow resistance, 254
Air (paranasal) sinuses, 45, 241, 393, 396
  fractures involving, *179*
  infection/inflammation (sinusitis), *258*
  tumours, *259*

Airway obstruction, *267–268*
Albinos, 198
Albumin, 61
Alcohol (ethanol) metabolism, 309
Aldosterone, 223
  function, 223, 344, 346
  regulation of secretion, 223, 345
Aldosteronism
  primary (Conn's syndrome), *126, 233*
  secondary, *233*
Alimentary canal, 11, 282, **283–288**
  adventitia, 284–285
  blood supply, 286–288
  mucosa, 285–286
  muscle layer, 285
  nerve supply, 286
  submucosa, 285
  venous drainage, 288
  see also specific organs
Alkali reserve, 22
Alkalis, **21–23**
Alkalosis, 22–23
Allergen, 66, *383*
Allergic reactions, 13, *111*, **383**, *384*
α_1-antitrypsin deficiency, *261*
α_2-macroglobulin, 61
Altitude, high, 73
Alveolar ducts, 248, 249
Alveolar hypoventilation, *268*
Alveolar ridges, 289, 395
Alveolar ventilation, 254–255, 460
Alveoli, 11, 248, **249**
  air in, 255
  blood supply, 251–252
Alveolitis, extrinsic allergic, *266*
Alzheimer's disease, *181*
Amino acids, 23–24, 272, **316–317**
  absorption, 303
  deamination, 273, 309, 316
  energy release, 316–317
  essential/non-essential, 272, 316
  pool, 316
  utilisation, 273
Ammonia, 316, 346
Amoebic dysentery, *327*
Ampulla, hepatopancreatic, 299–300, 306, 310, 311
Amylase
  pancreatic, 302, 312
  salivary, 293, 312
Anabolism, 12, 313
Anaemia, 64, ***69–72***
  aplastic, *70–71*
  in chronic renal failure, *354*
  folic acid deficiency, *70*
  haemolytic, *69, 71–72*
  hypochromic, *69*
  hypoplastic, *70–71*
  iron deficiency, *69–70, 278*
  in liver failure, *336*
  macrocytic, *69*
  megaloblastic, *70*

Main anatomy and physiology: **bold.** Main diseases: ***bold italics.*** Anatomy & physiology: ordinary type. Diseases: *italics.*

465

Main anatomy and physiology: **bold**. Main diseases: ***bold italics***. Anatomy & physiology: ordinary type. Diseases: *italics*.

Bronchial veins, 103–104, 248
Bronchiectasis, **260–261**, *263*
Bronchioles, **248–249**
  respiratory, 248, 249
  terminal, 248
Bronchitis
  acute, *259*
  chronic, *259–260*
Bronchopneumonia, *262*, **263**
Bronchospasm, *260*
Buccinator muscle, 430
Buerger's disease, *114*
Buffers, 22, 23
Bundle branches, 87
Bundle of His (atrioventricular bundle), 87
Burkitt's lymphoma, *137*
Burns, **370–371**
  complications, *370–371*
  hypovolaemic shock, *111*
  'rule of nines', *370*
Bursae, 415, 422
Busulphan, *266*
Byssinosis, *266*

C

Cachexia, tumour, *55*
Caecum, 300, 304
Calcanean tendon, 422, 423
Calcaneus, 405, 406
Calciferol, *see* Vitamin D
Calcitonin, 220, **221**, 222, 344, 392
Calcium, 276–278
  homeostasis, 221–222
  low blood, *231–232*
  plasma, 27–28, 459
  renal excretion, 344
Calculi
  renal, **354–355**, *356*, *357*
  salivary gland, *320*
  see also Gallstones
Callus, fracture, 407
Calories, 313
Calyces, renal, 341
Campylobacter food poisoning, *327*
Canal of Schlemm, 199
Cancer, *see* Malignant tumours
Candidiasis (thrush)
  oesophageal, *322*
  oral, *319*
  vaginal, *453*
Canine teeth, 290, 291
Capillaries, 8–9, **79**
  cell nutrition, 81–82
  fluid dynamics, 81–82
  gas exchange, 80–81
  glomerular, 342, 343
  increased permeability, *118*, 376
  lymph, 82, 131
  pulmonary, 251–252
Capitate, 402, 403
Capsular ligament, 415
Capsule, joint, 415
Carbaminohaemoglobin, 256
Carbohydrates, 23, **271–272**, 313, 460
  absorption, 303, 312
  digestion, 302, 312
  functions of digestible, 272
  metabolism, 309, **314–316**

Carbon dioxide (CO$_2$), 12, 240
  in acid–base balance, 23, 346
  in air, 255
  exchange, 255–256
  formation, 314, 316
  partial pressure (PCO$_2$), 255, 459
  transport in blood, 61, 81, **256**
Carbonic acid, 20, 22, 23, 346
Carcinogenesis, *53*
Carcinogens, *53*
Carcinoid syndrome, *329*
Carcinoid tumours, *329*
Carcinoma-in-situ, cervical, *454*
Carcinomatosis, *55*
Cardiac arrest, *123*
Cardiac arrhythmias, **123–124**
Cardiac cycle, **88–89**
Cardiac failure, **119–120**, *121*
  acute, *120*
  chronic, *120*
  left-sided (left ventricular), *120*
  right-sided (congestive), *120*
Cardiac muscle, **41**, 83–84
Cardiac output, **89–90**, 91
Cardiac reserve, 89
Cardiac sphincter, 294, 296
Cardinal ligaments, 442
Cardiogenic shock, *111*
Cardiovascular centre (CVC), 87, 91–92, 154
Cardiovascular system, **77–127**
  autonomic stimulation, 173
  in diabetes mellitus, *236*
Carina, 246, 247
Carotene, 274, 276, 309, 363
Carotid arteries, 96–97
Carotid bodies, 96, 257
Carotid sheath, 96
Carotid sinuses, 92, 96
Carpal bones, 402, 403
Carpal tunnel, 420
Carpal tunnel syndrome, *427*
Cartilage, **38–39**
  elastic, 39
  epiphyseal, 388
  hyaline (articular), 39, 388, 415
Caruncle, 205, 206
Catabolism, 12, 313, 315
Cataract, *211*
Catecholamines, see also Adrenaline;
    Noradrenaline
Cation, 20
Cauda equina, 161
Caustic materials, swallowed, *321*
Cavities, body, **49–51**
Cell(s), 4
  differentiation, 54
  disorders, **53–55**
  division, 32–33
  labile, 42
  membrane, *see* Plasma membrane
  nutrition, **81–82**
  organelles, 30, 31–32
  permanent, 42
  specialisation, 4
  stable, 42
Cellulitis, *369*
Cement, dental, 291
Central nervous system (CNS), 9, 140,
    145–149
  effect of poisons, *176*

infections, *181*, **182–184**
  see also Brain; Spinal cord
Central retinal artery, 166, 199
Central retinal vein, 166, 199
Central sulcus, 150, 151
Cephalic vein, 102–103
Cereals, 270, 271
Cerebellum, 148, **155**, 196, 200
Cerebral aqueduct, 148, 149
Cerebral cortex, 150
Cerebral hemispheres, 151
  motor areas, 151, 152
  sensory areas, 152
Cerebral hypoxia, 177, **180**
Cerebral infarction, *113*, *178*, *180*
Cerebral oedema, **178**, *179*
Cerebrospinal fluid (CSF), 147, **148–149**
  functions, 149
  increased volume, *178*
  obstructed flow, *178*
  pressure, 149, 460
  sampling, 155
Cerebrovascular disease (stroke), *127*, **180–181**
Cerebrum, **150–153**
  functional areas, 151–153
  functions, 151
  interior of, 150–151
  motor areas, 151–152
  sensory areas, 152
Cerumen, 193
Cervical lymph nodes, 132, 133
Cervical mucus, 446
Cervical plexus, 161, **162**
Cervical spondylosis, *426*
Cervix, uterine, 440, 441
  carcinoma, *454–455*
  disorders, **454–455**
  intra-epithelial neoplasia (CIN), *454–455*
Chalazion, *209*
Cheek (zygomatic) bone, 47, 395
Cheilitis, angular, *319*
Chemicals
  carcinogens, *53*
  haemolytic anaemia due to, *71–72*
  leukaemia due to, *74*
  lung diseases induced by, *266–267*
  see also Toxins
Chemoreceptors, 92, 94, 96, **256–257**
  central, 257
  olfactory, 206
  peripheral, 257
  taste, 207
Chemotaxins, 65
Chemotaxis, leukocyte, 376
Chenodeoxycholic acid, 310
Chewing, 294, 295
Chicken pox, *183*, *369*
Chlamydia trachomatis, *210*, *426*, *453*
Chloride, plasma, 21, 459
Cholangitis, *337*
  ascending, *335*
Cholecystitis, *71*, *337*
  acute, *337*
  chronic, *337*
Cholecystokinin (CCK), 298, 301, 302, 311
Cholelithiasis (gallstones), *71*, *336–337*
Cholera, *327*
Cholesteatoma, *208*
Cholesterol, 273, 459
Cholic acid, 310

Main anatomy and physiology: **bold**. Main diseases: ***bold italics***. Anatomy & physiology: ordinary type. Diseases: *italics*.

Main anatomy and physiology: **bold**. Main diseases: ***bold italics***. Anatomy & physiology: ordinary type. Diseases: *italics*.

D

Dacryoadenitis, acute, *212*
Dacryocystitis, *212*
Dairy products, 270, 271
Dark adaptation, 203
Dead space, anatomical, 254, 460
Deafness, *209*
  conductive, *209*
  sensorineural, *209*
Deamination, 273, 309, 316
Decubitus ulcers (pressure sores), *370*
Deep palmar arch, 102
Deep peroneal nerve, 164, 165
Deep vein thrombosis (DVT), *115–116*
Defecation, 12, 173, **306**
Defence mechanisms, 374
  at body surfaces, 374
  digestive system, 299, 301
  hepatic, 309
  non-specific, 13, **374–379**
  respiratory, 249
  salivary, 293, 374
  skin, 365, 374
  specific, 13, 374
Deferent duct (vas deferens), 14, 449, 450
Degeneration, *15*
Deglutition (swallowing), 294–295
Dehydration, *355, 370*
7-Dehydrocholesterol, 366
Deltoid ligament, 423
Deltoid muscle, 417
Dementia, *181–182*
  multi-infarct, *180, 181*
  secondary, *181–182*
Demyelinating diseases, *184–185*
Dendrites, **141–142**
Dens, 397
Dentine, 291
Dentition, 290
Deoxyribonucleic acid (DNA), 24, 25, 31
Depolarisation, 142
Dermal papillae, 362
Dermatitis, *369*
  atopic, *369*
  contact, *369, 378*
Dermatomes, 161, 163, 165
Dermis, 13, **363–365**
Dermoid cysts, *456*
Detoxification, 309
Detrusor muscle, 348, 350
Diabetes insipidus, *228*
Diabetes mellitus, ***234–236****, 317*
  complications, *235–236*
  effects, *235*, 346
  gestational, *235*
  kidney disease, *236, 352*
  macroangiopathy, *236*
  microangiopathy, *236*
  retinopathy, *211, 236*
  secondary, *235*
  type I, insulin-dependent (IDDM), *234*
  type II, non-insulin-dependent (NIDDM), *235*
Diabetic ketoacidosis, *235–236*
Diaphragm, 47, 252, **253**, 254
Diaphragmatic hernia, *330*
Diaphysis, 388
Diarrhoea, severe, *111*

Diastole, 88
  complete cardiac, 88, 91
Diet, 270, 460
  balanced, **270–271**
  see also Food; Nutrition
Dietary intake, 11–12
Differentiation, cell, 54
Diffusion, 26–27, 33–34
  facilitated, 33–34
  from capillaries, 81
  of gases, 255
  nutrient absorption by, 303
Digestion, 11, 282, **311–312**
  defective, *332*
  in small intestine, 301–302
  in stomach, 298, 299
Digestive juices, 285–286
Digestive system, 11, 12, **281–338**
  accessory organs, 282, 283
  autonomic control, 173
  functions, 282–283
  organs, 282, **283**
  see also Alimentary canal; *specific organs*
Digital arteries, 102
1,1-Dimethyl-4,4 bipyridylium chloride (paraquat), 266
2,3-Diphosphoglycerate (2,3-DPG), 81, 256
Diphtheria, *259*
Diploid number (of chromosomes), 33
Diplopia, *202, 385*
Disaccharides, 23, 272
Disease
  study of, **14–15**
  terminology, *15*
Dislocations, *426*
Disseminated intravascular coagulation (DIC), *75*
Disseminated (multiple) sclerosis, *176,* ***184–185***
Distal, 44
Diuresis, 218, *354*
Diverticular disease, *328*
Diverticulitis, *328*
Diverticulosis, *328*
DNA (deoxyribonucleic acid), 24, 25, 31
Dopamine (prolactin inhibiting hormone), 216, 217, 218
Dorsal, 44
Dorsalis pedis artery, 107, 108
Dorsal venous arch, 108
Drugs
  detoxification, 309
  haemolysis caused by, *71*
  hypertension due to, *126*
  leukopenia due to, *73*
  thrombocytopenia due to, *75*
Duchenne muscular dystrophy, *436*
Duct, 43
Ductus arteriosus, 124
  patent, *124*
Duodenum, 299–300
Dural venous sinuses, 100, 101
Dura mater, **147–148**, 155, 161
Dwarfism
  achondroplasia, *410*
  pituitary, *227, 228*
Dysentery, *327*
  amoebic, *327*
  bacillary, *327*
Dysplasia, *54*

Dyspnoea (breathlessness), *118, 260*
  in anaemia, *69*
  paroxysmal nocturnal, *120*
Dysuria, *357*

E

Ear, **192–196**
  diseases, ***208–209***
  drum (tympanic membrane), 192, 193
  inner, 192, 194–195
  middle, 192, 193–194
  outer, 192–193
  structure, 192–195
  wax, 193
Ectopic pregnancy, *456*
Eczema, *369*
Efferent nerves, *see* Motor nerves
Effusions, *118–119*
Ejaculation, **451**, 452
Ejaculatory duct, 450
Elastic fibres, 37, 38, 39, 363
Elastic tissue, 38
Elbow joint, 402, **417–418**
  muscles and movements, 418
Electrocardiogram (ECG), 89, 123
Electrolytes, 20–21
  balance, **346**
  movement within body, 26–27
  in renal failure, *354*
Electromagnetic spectrum, 200, 201
Electron, 18
  configuration, 19
Elements, 18
  inert, 19
Elimination of waste, 7, **12**, 283
Emboli (embolus), 117
  atheromatous, *113*
  tumour, 54
Embolism, *15,* ***117–118***
  aneurysms causing, *115*
  fat, *408*
  pulmonary, *116*
  septic, *264*
Embryo, 442
Emetropic eye, *212*
Emotional states, 87, 92
Emphysema, *260,* ***261–262***
  centrilobular, *261*
  interstitial, *262*
  panacinar, *261*
  pulmonary, *261*
Empyema, *263*
Enamel, tooth, 291
Encephalitis, *182*
  herpes simplex, *183*
  pyogenic, *183*
  viral, *183*
Encephalomyelitis, acute disseminating, *185*
Encephalopathy
  hepatic, *335*
  hypertensive, *127*
End-arteries, 79
Endocarditis, infective, *122–123*
  acute, *123*
  subacute, *123*
Endocardium, 83, 84
Endocrine glands, 10, 43, 214
  disorders, *126,* ***227–236***

Main anatomy and physiology: **bold.** Main diseases: ***bold italics.*** Anatomy & physiology: ordinary type. Diseases: *italics.*

469

Main anatomy and physiology: **bold**. Main diseases: ***bold italics***. Anatomy & physiology: ordinary type. Diseases: *italics*.

Main anatomy and physiology: **bold**. Main diseases: ***bold italics***. Anatomy & physiology: ordinary type. Diseases: *italics*.

471

Main anatomy and physiology: **bold**. Main diseases: ***bold italics***. Anatomy & physiology: ordinary type. Diseases: *italics*.

472

Main anatomy and physiology: **bold**. Main diseases: ***bold italics***. Anatomy & physiology: ordinary type. Diseases: *italics*.

Main anatomy and physiology: **bold**. Main diseases: ***bold italics***. Anatomy & physiology: ordinary type. Diseases: *italics*.

Main anatomy and physiology: **bold**. Main diseases: ***bold italics***. Anatomy & physiology: ordinary type. Diseases: *italics*.

Main anatomy and physiology: **bold**. Main diseases: ***bold italics***. Anatomy & physiology: ordinary type. Diseases: *italics*.

477

Main anatomy and physiology: **bold**. Main diseases: ***bold italics***. Anatomy & physiology: ordinary type. Diseases: *italics*.

Main anatomy and physiology: **bold**. Main diseases: ***bold italics***. Anatomy & physiology: ordinary type. Diseases: *italics*.

Main anatomy and physiology: **bold**. Main diseases: ***bold italics***. Anatomy & physiology: ordinary type. Diseases: *italics*.

Main anatomy and physiology: bold. Main diseases: ***bold italics***. Anatomy & physiology: ordinary type. Diseases: *italics*.

Main anatomy and physiology: **bold**. Main diseases: ***bold italics***. Anatomy & physiology: ordinary type. Diseases: *italics*.

Main anatomy and physiology: **bold**. Main diseases: ***bold italics***. Anatomy & physiology: ordinary type. Diseases: *italics*.

483

Main anatomy and physiology: **bold**. Main diseases: ***bold italics***. Anatomy & physiology: ordinary type. Diseases: *italics*.

Main anatomy and physiology: **bold.** Main diseases: ***bold italics.*** Anatomy & physiology: ordinary type. Diseases: *italics.*